ADVANCED TECHNIQUES IN MUSCULOSKELETAL MEDICINE AND PHYSIOTHERAPY

USING MINIMALLY INVASIVE THERAPIES IN PRACTICE

Fermín Valera Garrido PT MSc PhD

Co-director MVClinic; FREMAP Hospital, Department of Physical Therapy, Madrid, Spain
Programme Director and Professor Master's degree in Invasive Physiotherapy Techniques, Department of Physiotherapy, Faculty of Medicine, San Pablo CEU University, Madrid, Spain
Editor, *Journal of Invasive Techniques in Physical Therapy*

Francisco Minaya Muñoz PT MSc PhD

Co-director MVClinic; FREMAP Hospital, Department of Physical Therapy, Madrid, Spain
Programme Coordinator and Professor Master's degree in Invasive Physiotherapy Techniques, Department of Physiotherapy, Faculty of Medicine, San Pablo CEU University, Madrid, Spain
Associate Editor, *Journal of Invasive Techniques in Physical Therapy*

TRANSLATED BY
Isabel Quintero

ELSEVIER

Edinburgh   London   New York   Oxford   Philadelphia   St Louis
Sydney   Toronto   2016

ELSEVIER

Notices

Knowledge and best practice in this field are constantly changing. As new research and experience broaden our understanding, changes in research methods, professional practices, or medical treatment may become necessary.

Practitioners and researchers must always rely on their own experience and knowledge in evaluating and using any information, methods, compounds, or experiments described herein. In using such information or methods they should be mindful of their own safety and the safety of others, including parties for whom they have a professional responsibility.

With respect to any drug or pharmaceutical products identified, readers are advised to check the most current information provided (i) on procedures featured or (ii) by the manufacturer of each product to be administered, to verify the recommended dose or formula, the method and duration of administration, and contraindications. It is the responsibility of practitioners, relying on their own experience and knowledge of their patients, to make diagnoses, to determine dosages and the best treatment for each individual patient, and to take all appropriate safety precautions.

To the fullest extent of the law, neither the Publisher nor the authors, contributors, or editors, assume any liability for any injury and/or damage to persons or property as a matter of products liability, negligence or otherwise, or from any use or operation of any methods, products, instructions, or ideas contained in the material herein.

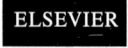

ELSEVIER your source for books, journals and multimedia in the health sciences

www.elsevierhealth.com

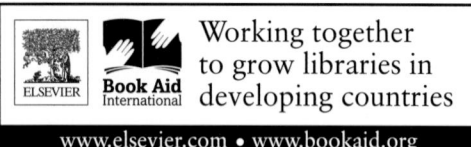

Working together to grow libraries in developing countries

www.elsevier.com • www.bookaid.org

The publisher's policy is to use paper manufactured from sustainable forests

Printed in China

Advanced Techniques in
MUSCULOSKELETAL MEDICINE & PHYSIOTHERAPY

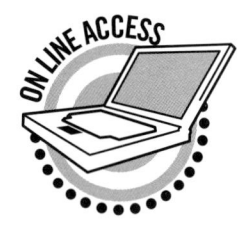

Fermín Valera Garrido
Francisco Minaya Muñoz

Your purchase entitles you to access the following online resources which are designed to enhance the material in your book:

- bank of 22 procedural videos
- bank of over 300 colour images
- 84 MCQs for self-testing

Your online resources are available at

www.advancedtechniquesonline.com

Please register and follow the log in instructions.

CONTENTS

PART I
INVASIVE TECHNIQUES IN PHYSIOTHERAPY AND MUSCULOSKELETAL MEDICINE

PART II
CADAVER-BASED APPROACHES IN PHYSIOTHERAPY

PART III
MUSCULOSKELETAL ULTRASOUND

PART IV
DRY NEEDLING

COMPANION WEBSITE:
www.advancedtechniquesonline.com

- video bank
- colour image bank
- MCQs.

VIDEO LIST

Access to the videos can be found online at: www.advancedtechniquesonline.com.

Videos are referred to throughout the text using the following icon: 📹

ACKNOWLEDGEMENTS

Our special thanks go out to all the chapter authors who have made possible the publication of this work, together with the rest of the collaborators: Isabel Vinuesa Lara (design of the original figures), Carolina Redondo González (design of the original electronic content), Alberto Sánchez González (illustration), Jesús Redondo Linares (original review), M. Ángeles Valera Garrido (pedagogic review) and V. Rey V. (bibliographic review).

We would also like to thank Isabel Quintero for her dedication and commitment to the translation of this work, as well as Rita Demetriou-Swanwick of Elsevier UK for her helpful encouragement and guidance in the preparation of this edition. Special thanks are also extended to Manuel Júlbez Campos, Ana Martin Rubio and David Hough of Elsevier Spain, whose support has enabled *Fisioterapia Invasiva* to become the first original Spanish title on physiotherapy to be translated into English.

FOREWORD TO THE SPANISH EDITION, *FISIOTERAPIA INVASIVA*

Writing the foreword to a work is always hard, as an excess of compliments directed towards the authors or editors is inappropriate and a cold factual presentation can detract from the reader's curiosity.

In the case of *Invasive Techniques in Physiotherapy (Fisioterapia Invasiva)*, this role becomes a moral obligation, due to the level of commitment shown by Professors Valera and Minaya who, at the forefront of a new physiotherapy, offer a compendium of the array of techniques that, grouped under the heading of 'invasive', present a new frontier of knowledge in the science of physiotherapy.

They face a challenge, together with the rest of their coauthors and collaborators, among who it is necessary to highlight the figure of José Manuel Sánchez-Ibáñez, creator of the EPI® technique who, without a doubt, has made the most important Spanish contribution to worldwide physiotherapy this century, representing a historical landmark that deserves recognition and support. The challenge is to advance towards a new scientific paradigm, modernizing a profession that has evolved into a science, while contributing the values of effectiveness, evidence and low cost. These attributes place this group of techniques into a high rank with regard to the optimization of therapeutic resources.

Throughout this book, the reader advances progressively from the necessary anatomical stage that frames the work of the physiotherapist to the quantitative verification of therapeutic results through ultrasound. This reaches its theoretical high point with the chapters dedicated to EPI® and dry needling, not forgetting associated complementary techniques, such as acupuncture and mesotherapy.

Without doubt, we are producing a singular piece of work bringing order to the intervention area of invasive physiotherapy and, above all, which constitutes a brave effort that can only receive critiques from those who wish to place our science in the straitjacket of outdated parameters of competency.

All that remains is to thank the authors for their great efforts. This book is the product of a decade of dedicated and meticulous work, verified by a long list of previous scientific publications that entirely support the publication of this book, which is fresh, technical and easy to read and understand. I am delighted to have been a part of the creation, development and future growth of this novel therapeutic concept, with its indisputable Spanish stamp.

Prof. Dr José A. Martín Urrialde
President of the General Council of
Physiotherapy Boards of Spain

FOREWORD

All methods are sacred if they are internally necessary. All methods are sins if they are not justified by internal necessity.

WASSILY KANDINSKY

This foreword is written for the prospective reader of this book.

Not surprisingly, in the history of scientific and medical progress, the quality of the questions posed has very often been the determining factor for the quality of the answers found. Many scientific breakthroughs have only been made possible after open-minded and careful observers have effectively challenged the 'conventional' ideas of their time, be it Aristotle, the medieval church, gold standards of academies and colleges, or even today's peer-reviewed and respectable publications.

In the broad field of musculoskeletal medicine, the last 50 years have seen significant progress in our understanding of clinical conditions manifesting in the complex musculoskeletal system.

Mechanistic models – inherited from the origins of Western medicine – are now slowly being replaced by neurological models that better reflect the realities of human physiology, particularly with regard to the miscellaneous conditions we term 'functional disorders' that, arguably, constitute most of the challenging clinical problems that most 'manual medicine practitioners' face every day.

Not only are techniques evolving, but also professions, and this book is a welcome platform for a conjoined effort to disseminate new vital knowledge for the practitioners of manual medicine worldwide. Manual medicine is quickly becoming an international umbrella term to describe the daily practice of professionals with diverse denominations and licences, who use their hands and some, or all, of the tools and techniques presented in this book, to assess and treat musculoskeletal disorders. Practitioners of manual medicine form an ever-growing multidisciplinary collective that includes physiotherapists, chiropractors, osteopaths, naprapaths, sports medicine physicians, physical medicine and rehabilitation physicians, nurses, integrative acupuncture practitioners, and a broad array of miscellaneous licensed massage therapists and body workers.

Despite the still predominant structural approach to the diagnosis and treatment of musculoskeletal problems (so well covered by many of the chapters presented in this book), ongoing new insights from neurology are paving the way for an additional array of new approaches to the evaluation and categorization of functional musculoskeletal disorders, many of which will continue to evolve from the key diagnostic and treatment techniques presented by the authors of this book, namely ultrasound-guided interventions, miscellaneous electrical tissue stimulations with and without needles, and injections of physiological substances to improve the biochemical environment when and where needed.

Meanwhile, the development of these new 'technology-based' diagnostic and treatment techniques that allow new access to the effectors of the musculoskeletal system (specifically muscles, tendons, bones, joints and peripheral nerves) is also contributing to clarify some of the fundamental structural dimensions associated with these complex – and still incompletely understood – functional musculoskeletal disorders.

In this manner, with the contributions of many researchers and practitioners, 'the heart' of the musculoskeletal system is gradually opening itself to those who approach it properly, like the authors of this book. Simplicity, clarity and a scientifically inquisitive mind are the main tools in this quest.

Like many other fields of medicine and science, the main reward for the researcher and practitioner is the excitement of finding the connections between the visible and invisible worlds. For the manual medicine practitioner it is the art of discovering the pathways left on the soft tissues of the body by gravitational and reaction forces, the art of finding the dysfunctional spinal segments inhibiting proper motor function and metabolic activities of the peripheral tissues (and even the viscera), and the art of restoring normal metabolic capabilities to specific peripheral tissues that have lost their vitality and optimal structural arrangement.

This spirit is clearly behind the many interesting and exciting chapters presented in this book. Many authors have generously contributed their time and expertise to the production of this unique professional text for manual medicine practitioners, the core being a group of Spanish physiotherapists at the forefront of their profession.

Spain has never been a scientific power, but historically it has been the land of some of the most original and creative thinkers in the history of medicine and science: Nobel prize physician Santiago Ramon y Cajal represents them all. Still young in years but rich in clinical experience, the editors of this exciting book (as well as the main contributors), Fermín Valera-Garrido and Francisco Minaya-Muñoz have proven to be worthy heirs to this tradition. Thanks to their efforts you now have the unique opportunity of being exposed to the latest approaches and techniques in the understanding and treatment of musculoskeletal disorders, all in one book, which is both comprehensive and richly illustrated.

It was another Spaniard, philosopher Jose Ortega y Gasset, who said: 'to be surprised, to wonder, is to begin to understand'. And this is how a book like this should be approached, by an intelligent reader like yourself. Not as an authoritative source of consolidated knowledge, but as a rich tapestry of science-based wonders in the field of musculoskeletal medicine, a major work still in progress.

Just a final comment for the overly enthusiastic reader, as perhaps 'Advanced Techniques' in the title may be slightly misleading. Techniques are means to an end, and as such they are at the service of a definite purpose. All techniques should be precise, safe and effective. It is the advanced understanding of the problems being tackled, in this case musculoskeletal pain and dysfunction, that gives the techniques their ultimate meaning, not the other way around.

The power of excellent manual medicine practitioners, like the chess master, the artful writer, the accomplished musician, or the genius sculptor and painter – the secret that makes their 'technique' advanced or superior – is simply their ability to master the elemental components of their craft, specifically the ability to combine these elements in a timely fashion for the service of a higher purpose. This is the only secret of all mastery.

As it is often the case, to master such a simple recipe requires a lifetime of intelligent observation of our own modus operandi and purposeful determination to apply this controlled experience to refine our next output. This is, and has always been, the essence of science. Patience, passion, vision, determination and purposefulness can infuse quality and even immortal life to a chess piece, a collection of words or musical notes, a piece of marble, a canvas, or in our case, in your case (as a manual medicine practitioner), a minimally invasive technique performed with clarity and accuracy.

If you are reading this now, while holding with anticipation this valuable addition to your medical library, the choice is literally in your hands.

Dr. Alejandro Elorriaga Claraco, Sports Medicine Specialist (Spain)
Founding Director McMaster University Contemporary Medical Acupuncture Program, Hamilton, Ontario, Canada
www.mcmasteracupuncture.com

PREFACE

The basis of all art consists of bringing reality closer to one's dreams.

ANDRÉ MAUROIS

Rotterdam (2007), Marbella and Elche (2008) mark the beginning of what is, today, a reality captured by this book. These were the 'seeds' of a line of training in invasive physiotherapy which changed our way of perceiving the professional and the patients' results, and these seeds are what produced the Spanish version of the book *Fisioterapia Invasiva* (Elsevier, 2013).

Our presence and scientific contribution to a range of international events, in London and Vancouver (2012) and Toronto (2014), together with other international engagements marked the 'ripening' of a new 'fruit', this book, *Advanced Techniques in Musculoskeletal Medicine and Physiotherapy: using minimally invasive therapies in practice.*

Similar to the pieces of a puzzle, each and every one of the minimally invasive therapies fits together to form an area of knowledge in musculoskeletal medicine and physiotherapy that integrates dry needling, percutaneous needle tenotomy (PNT), acupuncture, percutaneous needle electrolysis, mesotherapy, injection therapy and high-volume image-guided injections (HVIGIs), among others. This book is the first worldwide reference to integrate minimally invasive therapies within musculoskeletal medicine and physiotherapy from a clinical, evidence-based perspective.

Around the world, minimally invasive therapies have the support of a range of institutions such as the Chartered Society of Physiotherapy, the Australian Physiotherapy Association, the Canadian Physical Therapy Association, the Federation of State Boards of Physical Therapy, the Irish Association of Physical Therapists, the General Council of Physiotherapy Boards in Spain, the Spanish Association of Physiotherapists and the American Physical Therapy Association, which consider the application of manual therapy interventions with a needle as an advanced-extended scope of practice.

The incorporation of invasive techniques within the scope of physiotherapy is supported by the curricula of current entry-level and postgraduate educational programmes, scientific evidence and established practice. These techniques are a reflection of the experiences and realities of specialized care in many countries, such as Spain, Portugal, Greece, Sweden, Norway, Ireland, the Netherlands, Belgium, Switzerland, the UK, Argentina, Chile, Brazil, South Africa, Zimbabwe, Canada, Australia, New Zealand, the USA, India, the United Arab Emirates-Dubai and Hong Kong.

In Spain, the University San Pablo CEU and MVClinic are the worldwide pioneers organizing, since 2012, the Master's degree in Invasive Physiotherapy Techniques, in which many of the procedures that today make up the physiotherapy scope of practice are integrated.

On the other hand, within the physiotherapy collective there is a growing interest in invasive techniques, due to their effectiveness and efficiency in the treatment of many dysfunctions of the neuromusculoskeletal system that are difficult to resolve using conventional techniques.

This work begins with an introduction of the different invasive physiotherapy techniques, incorporating important aspects regarding history, education, training and regulation of invasive techniques within the physiotherapy profession, and with a description of the theoretical and practical considerations that must be considered for a correct praxis (Part I: Chapter 1 and 2). In Part II, the areas of vasculonervous conflict are described, together with the most important anatomical landmarks in the application of puncture techniques (Chapter 3).

Part III covers the applicability of musculoskeletal ultrasound in physiotherapy (Chapter 4), anatomical–ultrasound integration (sonoanatomy) (Chapter 5), the use of new imaging methods such as elastography (Chapter 6) and the practice of ultrasound-guided procedures with the goal of improving the effectiveness and safety of interventions (Chapter 7).

In Parts IV to X, the mechanisms of action, application methodology and effects of invasive techniques are described, such as dry needling (Chapter 8), Dry Needling for Hypertonia and Spasticity (DNHS®) (Chapter 9), needling techniques for segmental dysfunction (Chapter 10), PNT (Chapter 11), Intratissue Percutaneous Electrolysis (EPI®) (Chapters 12–14), clinical acupuncture (Chapters 15 and 16), mesotherapy (Chapter 17), injection therapy (Chapter 18) and HVIGI (Chapter 19).

Finally, part XI is designed to teach the professional to assess the results obtained objectively from the perspective of functionality (Chapter 20) and the changes achieved in the treated tissue (Chapter 21).

This book is designed as a teaching tool and includes a glossary, explaining the most important terms. Each chapter also contains real clinical cases. Additional online material is available, including videos of the interventions and the figures (in colour) from the book.

Lastly, we would like to express our gratitude to our close associate Françesc Medina i Mirapeix, who, for many years, has shown us the scientific value of physiotherapy, and to all the authors who have contributed towards this editorial project. This work paves the way for new research and discoveries.

Without a present there is no future.

Fermín Valera Garrido
Francisco Minaya Muñoz

CONTRIBUTORS

Ferrán Abat González MD
Orthopedic Sports Specialist
CEREDE Center
Orthopedic Surgeon, ACTUA Medical
    Services
Barcelona, Spain

Diana Marcela Aguirre Rueda Ms
Physiology
Laboratory research
Department of Physiology
University of Valencia
Valencia, Spain

María Elena del Baño Aledo PT PhD
Department of Physiotherapy, Central Unit of
    Anatomy
San Antonio Catholic University (UCAM)
Murcia, Spain
Research Assistant
Preventive Ultrasonography, Morpho-
    densitometry and Research in Physiotherapy
    and Manual Therapy (ECOFISTEM)
    Research Group
Murcia, Spain

Adrián Benito Domingo PT
Department of Physiotherapy
FREMAP Clinic
Villalba, Madrid, Spain
Assistant Coordinator, Master's degree in
    Invasive Physiotherapy Techniques
University San Pablo CEU
Boadilla del Monte, Madrid, Spain

Anders Boesen MD PhD
Institute of Sports Medicine – Copenhagen
Bispebjerg Hospital
Denmark

Morten Boesen MD PhD
Teres Parkens Private Hospital
Copenhagen
Denmark

Sandra Calvo Carrión PT
Professor, Physiotherapy Degree
Clinical Researcher, Invasive Physiotherapy
    Research Group
San Jorge University
Zaragoza, Spain

Otto Chan MD
The London Independent Hospital and The
    Royal Free Hospital
London, UK

Andrew Chang MD
Resident, Department of Obstetrics and
    Gynecology
St Barnabas Medical Center
New Jersey, USA

Pilar Escolar Reina PhD PT
Department of Physiotherapy
University of Murcia
Murcia, Spain
Research Assistant
Physiotherapy and Disability Research Group
Murcia, Spain

José María Estrela Arigüel PhD
Professor, Department of Physiology
University of Valencia
Valencia, Spain

Antonio García Godino PT
Acupuncturist; Associate Professor, Department
    of Physiotherapy
Faculty of Physiotherapy and Nursery 'Salus
    Infirmorum'
Pontifical University of Salamanca
Madrid, Spain
Department of Physiotherapy
FREMAP Hospital
Majadahonda, Madrid, Spain
Vocal of Commission on Acupuncture
Council of Physiotherapy Boards of Madrid
Madrid, Spain

Sergio García Herreros PT
Research Assistant
Department of Physiology
University of Valencia
Valencia, Spain

Pilar García Palencia PhD
Anatomopathologist; Research Assistant
Department of Medicine and Animal Surgery
Faculty of Veterinary Medicine
Complutense University of Madrid
Madrid, Spain

John Georgy MD MBA
Resident Physician, Physical Medicine and
    Rehabilitation
Department of Physical Medicine and
    Rehabilitation
Albert Einstein College of Medicine/
    Montefiore Medical Center
Bronx, NY, USA

Ana de Groot Ferrando PT
Director Khronos Physiotherapy
Department of Physiotherapy
Elche, Alicante, Spain
Research Assistant
Preventive Ultrasonography, Morpho-
    densitometry and Research in Physiotherapy
    and Manual Therapy (ECOFISTEM)
    Research Group
Murcia, Spain

Juliana Heimur BA
Research Assistant
Rehabilitation Medicine Department
Clinical Center
National Institutes of Health
Bethesda, Maryland, USA

Pablo Herrero Gallego PT PhD
Vice-Dean and Professor, Physiotherapy
    Degree
Director, Invasive Physiotherapy Research
    Group
San Jorge University
Zaragoza, Spain

Henning Langberg PT DMSc PhD MSc
Professor, CopenRehab, Department of Public
    Health
Faculty of Heath Sciences
University of Copenhagen
Denmark

Peter Malliaras PT PhD
Centre for Sports and Exercise Medicine,
    William Harvey Research Institute, Bart's
    and the London School of Medicine and
    Dentistry
Queen Mary University of London
Mile End Hospital
London, UK

Jacinto J. Martínez Payá PT PhD
Department of Physiotherapy, Central Unit of
    Anatomy
San Antonio Catholic University (UCAM)
Murcia, Spain
Research Assistant
Preventive Ultrasonography, Morpho-
    densitometry and Research in Physiotherapy
    and Manual Therapy (ECOFISTEM)
    Research Group
Murcia, Spain

Orlando Mayoral del Moral PT
Department of Physiotherapy
Provincial Hospital
Toledo, Spain
Board Chair
International Myopain Society
Florida, USA
Honorary Chairman
Spanish Association of Myofascial Pain and
    Dry Needling
Toledo, Spain
Director Travell & Simons Seminars®
Toledo, Spain

Francesc Medina Mirapeix PT PhD
Professor, Department of Physiotherapy
University of Murcia
Murcia, Spain
Research Director
Physiotherapy and Disability Research Group
Murcia, Spain

Francisco Minaya Muñoz PT MSc PhD
Co-Director, MVClinic
Madrid, Spain
Department of Physiotherapy
FREMAP Hospital,
Majadahonda, Madrid, Spain
Academic Coordinator and Professor, Master's
    degree in Invasive Physiotherapy Techniques
Department of Physiotherapy
Faculty of Medicine
San Pablo CEU University
Madrid, Spain
Research Assistant
Physiotherapy and Disability Research Group
Murcia, Spain

Dylan Morrissey PT PhD MSc MMACP MCSP BSc(Hons)
NIHR/HEE Consultant physiotherapist and senior clinical lecturer
Physiotherapy, Bart's Health NHS Trust
Centre for Sports and Exercise Medicine, Bart's and the London School of Medicine and Dentistry, QMUL
London
UK

María Ortiz Lucas PT PhD
Professor, Physiotherapy Degree
Co-director, Invasive Physiotherapy Research Group
San Jorge University
Zaragoza, Spain

Patricio Paredes Bruneta
Research Assistant
Department of Physiology
University of Valencia
Valencia, Spain

Shounuck I. Patel DO
Sports Medicine and Interventional Spine Fellow
OSS Health
York, PA, USA

Fernando Polidori PT
Associate Professor
Department of Physiotherapy
University of Mendoza
Mendoza, Argentina

José Ríos Díaz PT MSc PhD BSc
Department of Physiotherapy
San Antonio Catholic University (UCAM)
Research Director, Preventive Ultrasonography, Morpho-densitometry and Research in Physiotherapy and Manual Therapy (ECOFISTEM) Research Group
Murcia, Spain

Juan Ruiz Alconero MD
Associate Professor
Department of Medical Pathology
Faculty of Health Sciences
University of Alfonso X 'El Sabio'
Madrid, Spain
Medical Director, Capilae Clinic
Madrid, Spain

Isabel Salvat Salvat PT PhD
Associate Professor
Faculty of Medicine and Health Sciences
University of Rovira i Virgili
Reus, Tarragona, Spain
Associate Professor
Travell & Simons Seminars®
Toledo, Spain

José Manuel Sánchez Ibáñez PT PhD
Chief Physiotherapy Officer , CEREDE Center
Chief Executive Officer, EPI Advanced Medicine®
Associate Professor
Master's degree in High Performance FC Barcelona
University of Barcelona
Barcelona, Spain

Stephanie Saunders FCSP FSOM
Private practitioner
Course Director, Orthopaedic Medicine Seminars
Fellow of Chartered Society of Physiotherapist, London, UK

Roberto Sebastián Ojero PT
Acupuncturist; Honorary Professor
Department of Cell Biology, Histology and Pharmacology
Faculty of Medicine
University of Valladolid
Valladolid, Spain
Department of Physiotherapy
FREMAP Clinic
Valladolid, Spain

Jay P. Shah MD PhD FAAPMR
Senior Staff Physiatrist and Clinical Investigator
Rehabilitation Medicine Department
Clinical Center
National Institutes of Health
Bethesda, Maryland
USA

Todd P. Stitik MD
Professor, Physical Medicine and Rehabilitation
Co-director, Musculoskeletal/Pain
  Management Fellowship
Director, Occupational/Musculoskeletal
  Medicine
Co-director, Interventional Spine Injection
  Clinic
Department of Physical Medicine and
  Rehabilitation
University of Medicine and Dentistry of New
  Jersey
New Jersey Medical School
Newark, New Jersey, USA

Nikki Thaker BS
Rehabilitation Medicine Department
Clinical Center
National Institutes of Health
Bethesda, Maryland, USA

Francisco J. Valderrama Canales PhD
Anatomist; Associate Professor
Department of Human Anatomy and
  Embryology
Faculty of Medicine
Complutense University of Madrid
Madrid, Spain
Member of Spanish Society of Anatomy, Spain

Fermín Valera Garrido PT MSc PhD
Co-director, MVClinic
Madrid, Spain
Department of Physiotherapy
FREMAP Hospital,
Majadahonda, Madrid, Spain
Director and Professor, Master's degree in
  Invasive Physiotherapy Techniques
Department of Physiotherapy
Faculty of Medicine
San Pablo CEU University
Madrid, Spain
Research Assistant
Physiotherapy and Disability Research Group
Murcia, Spain

Soraya Vallés Martí PhD
Assistant Professor
Department of Physiology
University of Valencia
Valencia, Spain

Milin Vora MD
Sports Medicine and Interventional Spine
  Research and Clinical Fellow
Center for Advance Pain Management and
  Rehabilitation
Graduate of the Medical University of Lublin,
  Poland

PART I

INVASIVE TECHNIQUES IN PHYSIOTHERAPY AND MUSCULOSKELETAL MEDICINE

CHAPTER 1

INVASIVE TECHNIQUES IN PHYSIOTHERAPY: GENERAL CONCEPTS

Fermín Valera Garrido • Francisco Minaya Muñoz

Evidence is the most decisive proof.
CICERO

CHAPTER OUTLINE

KEYWORDS

acupuncture; informed consent; adverse events; percutaneous needle electrolysis; invasive physiotherapy; minimally invasive physiotherapy; injection therapy; high-volume injection; mesotherapy; dry needling; biomedical waste; needlestick; safety.

1.1 INTRODUCTION

1.1.1 Concept of invasive techniques in physiotherapy

The use of physical agents and modalities such as heat and manual therapy is as ancient as humanity itself. Today, physiotherapy is a well-recognized profession, which has evolved and developed successfully since its remote beginnings.[1–3] Indeed, the role of the physiotherapists has expanded in recent years, becoming increasingly diverse,[4,5] particularly in response to reforms in health and education[6] and based on the changing needs of patients and the population at large.[7,8]

The complex and broad nature of the physiotherapy profession has outgrown the reach of general practice. Continuous professional development is now essential in order to guarantee quality of care, and this has become a professional responsibility. Physiotherapists must seek to create new and innovative ways of working that are efficient and effective, while guaranteeing patient safety. At the same time, it is important for professionals not to forget the historic roots of physiotherapy and to understand how these support the development of the profession.

The broad nature of physiotherapy is apparent in the definition of physiotherapy provided by the World Confederation for Physical Therapy (WCPT) as:

services to individuals and populations to develop, maintain and restore maximum movement and functional ability throughout the lifespan. This includes providing services in circumstances where movement and function are threatened by ageing, injury, disease or environmental factors. Functional movement is central to what it means to be healthy.[9]

The concept of needling techniques or invasive techniques (both terms are used interchangeably) is defined by Valera & Minaya as:

manual therapy interventions in which a filiform/hollow needle is used to diagnose and treat neuromuscular pain and functional movement deficits.

Within the scope of physiotherapy practice, these techniques can be referred to as (minimally) invasive physiotherapy. Examples of these are dry needling, percutaneous needle electrolysis (PNE), injection therapy or acupuncture in physiotherapy practice. The Spanish term *fisioterapia invasiva* (invasive physiotherapy) was first used in 2001 by Mayoral,[10] and it is indeed the original title of this book, published in Spain in 2013 by Valera and Minaya.[11]

During invasive techniques, the needle becomes the active element of movement, a sort of extension of the professional's hands used to apply mobilization, vibration or pressure on to the soft tissue. A mechanical effect is sought, which may be: (1) isolated: for example in the case of acupuncture, dry needling or percutaneous needle tenotomy (PNT) techniques; (2) combined with physical agents such as heat (moxibustion), electricity (e.g. PNE, electrolipolysis); or (3) combined with medication that is injected into the subcutaneous tissue (mesotherapy) at a greater depth (injection techniques). In each country, the development of professional competencies and the official training programmes define the scope of practice for physiotherapists and other professionals who perform needling techniques.

Physiotherapists who perform invasive techniques base their intervention on sound clinical reasoning processes and these techniques are supported by an evidence-based and best-practice approach within the scope of physiotherapy. There is growing research to suggest that invasive techniques are effective in the management of neuromusculoskeletal conditions[12–15]; however ongoing research is needed in order to expand the knowledge base regarding the effectiveness of these interventions.

1.1.2 Physiotherapy scope of practice changes

Scope of practice, as described by the Pew Health Professions Commission,[16] is the:

> *definition of the rules, the regulations, and the boundaries within which a fully qualified practitioner with substantial and appropriate training, knowledge, and experience may practice in a field of medicine or surgery, or other specifically defined field. Such practice is also governed by requirements for continuing education and professional accountability.*

The WCPT indicates that the physiotherapy profession itself is responsible for defining the profession's scope of practice and the roles of physiotherapists. National physiotherapy associations are a key figure for seeking legislative and public support for their members, which in itself contributes to the autonomous figure of physiotherapists and the establishment of a defined scope of practice.

There are many factors which may limit scope of practice, such as training, experience and competency, but also local customs and practice. Interestingly, in Australia the legislation does not provide a definition of physiotherapy scope of practice and it is therefore the responsibility of the profession to define the practice. The Australian Physiotherapy Association (APA) supports a broad definition of physiotherapy which recognizes the presence of a diversity of clinical specialities in order to meet the needs of a variety of client groups:

> *Physiotherapy involves a holistic approach to the prevention, diagnosis, and therapeutic management of disorders of movement or optimisation of function to enhance the health and welfare of the community from an individual or population perspective. The practice of physiotherapy encompasses a diversity of clinical specialties to meet the unique needs of different client groups.[17]*
>
> *The APA believes it is inappropriate to list the activities which are considered either within or outside the current scope of practice. The scope of physiotherapy in Australia may include both existing and emerging practices. Physiotherapists may practice any activity that falls within the broad scope of physiotherapy providing that they are appropriately educated, trained, credentialed and competent to practice. Physiotherapists working in new and innovative roles must at all times be able to demonstrate how their activities align with the professional practice of physiotherapy. Education providers should be encouraged to develop courses for physiotherapists that equip them with the appropriate skills and competencies to expand their scope of practice.[17]*

The scope of physiotherapy practice should be dynamic and responsive to the patient's/client's and societal health needs.[18–20] For instance, when scope of practice is defined too rigidly or concisely, problems may arise later on, as there will be little room for innovation. This becomes increasingly difficult for the profession to evolve together with contextual changes in society and healthcare policies. It is equally important for scope of practice to undergo periodic review and, in doing so, the latest evidence base should be considered as well as the health needs of the population.

There is a lack of consensus in the literature surrounding the definition of advanced and extended scope of practice,[21–27] although there was general agreement that it involved an expansion of traditional roles in physiotherapy, in terms of diagnostics, management and interventions (first-line physiotherapy). The APA[28] supports the following definitions:

Advanced Scope of Practice – A role that is within the currently recognised scope of practice for that profession, but that through custom and practice has been performed by other professions. The advanced role may require additional training as well as significant professional experience and competency development.

Extended Scope of Practice – A role that is outside the currently recognised scope of practice and one that requires some method of credentialing following additional training, competency development and significant professional experience, as well as legislative change.

The WCPT offers further details regarding the use of the term extended scope of practice[29]:

physical therapists may develop a scope of practice beyond the usual and customary physical therapist's practice as a result of attaining significant additional education, professional experience, and/or enhanced competencies. It may also be referred to as extended scope of practice. Specialisation is an example of advanced scope of practice.

Indeed, clinical specialization[30–32] 'recognizes physical therapists with advanced clinical knowledge, experience, and skills in a special area of practice, assists consumers and the health care community in identifying physical therapists who are specialists, and meet a specific area of patient need.'[33]

A useful definition of extended scope of practice could also include the term role enhancement 'as increasing the depth of a job by extending the role or skills of a particular group of workers'.[34] In the UK, especially in the case of physiotherapists, new roles in advanced and extended scope of practice have been rapidly adopted.[22] The use of injection therapy[35] for physiotherapists since 1995 is an example of role enhancement. In July 2012 UK physiotherapists were the first in the world to be granted the right to prescribe medication in the management of their patient's care without needing a doctor to sign off on their decision.

An extended scope practice physiotherapist is a clinical specialist, who has the opportunity to develop and demonstrate expertise beyond the currently recognized scope of practice, including some aspect of job enhancement or expansion, involving the areas of extended therapeutics, diagnostics and practice consultation.[23,26]

In Canada, the physiotherapy scope of practice is under review. Some recent interventions included within the scope of practice, such as spinal manipulation, dry needling or acupuncture, are not considered entry-level and require additional postgraduate training following graduation to add them to physiotherapy practice.[36] Regarding invasive techniques, a survey of Canadian physiotherapists in 2008 found that these techniques (dry needling, acupuncture) are considered to be an advanced practical skill.[37]

KEY POINTS

Invasive techniques in physiotherapy practice should be considered an advanced-extended scope of practice.

In the UK, the Chartered Society of Physiotherapy (CSP)[38] defined scope of practice based on the four pillars of practice contained within the Royal Charter[39]: massage, exercise, electrotherapy and kindred forms of treatment.

any activity undertaken by an individual physiotherapist that may be situated within the four pillars of physiotherapy practice where the individual is educated, trained and competent to perform that activity. Such activities should be linked to existing or emerging occupational and/ or practice frameworks acknowledged by the profession, and be supported by a body of evidence.

Although the first three pillars are quite well defined and specific, the fourth pillar offers the possibility for physiotherapists to expand their knowledge base according to the needs of their patients.

By keeping a broad perspective, ultimately patient care benefits, as physiotherapists can extend the treatment options available to their patients.

In 2006, in the USA, the Federation of State Medical Boards published a joint report[40] together with the Association of Social Work Boards, the Federation of State Boards of Physical Therapy (FSBPT), the National Board for Certification in Occupational Therapy, the National Council of State Boards of Nursing and the National Association of Boards of Pharmacy on changes in healthcare professions scope of practice. Within this document[40] they issued the following statement:

if a profession can provide supportive evidence in the four foundational areas: historical basis, education and training, evidence, and regulatory environment, then the proposed changes are likely to be in the public's best interest.

One activity does not define a profession, but it is the entire scope of activities within the practice that makes any particular profession unique. Simply because a skill or activity is within one profession's skill set does not mean another profession cannot and should not include it in its own scope of practice.[40]

Furthermore, the CSP[38] establishes the scope of practice of the individual physiotherapist; in other words, they give their members the choice to work as either generalists or as specialist practitioners. Therefore it is up to physiotherapists whether or not they decide to extend their practice into the so-called fourth pillar, developing further clinical skills.

The CSP states that the fourth pillar includes an advanced and extended scope of practice, which requires further training and development beyond undergraduate or immediate postgraduate training. According to the CSP, doctors typically provide extended-scope physiotherapists with the necessary mentorship, training and supervision.

KEY POINTS

Advanced and extended scope of practice requires additional postgraduate training in order to include these within physiotherapy practice.

These models of advanced practice or extended scope of practice have existed for nurses[41-44] since World War I and for physiotherapists in the USA since the Vietnam War. There are many other professions looking to increase their current scope of practice. In recent years radiologist assistants,[45] optometrists[46] and podiatrists[47] have successfully expanded into new areas. Physiotherapists can draw on the experiences of these professions when undertaking strategic advocacy.

A recent systematic review published in 2012 focused on advanced-practice roles in physiotherapy in the management of patients with musculoskeletal disorders.[48] The authors found that physiotherapists in advanced-practice roles tend to provide equal or improved care in comparison to physicians in terms of diagnostic accuracy, effectiveness of treatment, use of healthcare resources, economic costs and patient satisfaction.

Around the world, the changes to the physiotherapy scope of practice are supported by the curricula of current entry-level and postgraduate educational programmes, scientific evidence and established practice. The incorporation of the invasive techniques within the scope of physiotherapy is also a reflection of the experiences and realities of specialized care in many countries, such as Spain, Portugal, Greece, Sweden, Norway, Ireland, the Netherlands, Belgium, Switzerland, the UK, Argentina, Chile, Brazil, South Africa, Zimbabwe, Canada, Australia, New Zealand, the USA, India, the United Arab Emirates-Dubai and Hong Kong.

The USA is not foreign to this new reality of physiotherapy. In updating their guidelines, the American Physical Therapy Association (APTA) Board of Directors (March 2014) formally listed dry needling within the scope of practice.[49] More specifically, they added under section two:

Physical therapy, which is limited to the care and services provided by or under the direction and supervision of a physical therapist, includes: Alleviating impairment and functional limitation by designing, implementing, and modifying therapeutic interventions that include, but are not limited to: dry needling.

Currently, there is enough evidence to include dry needling in the next edition of the *Guide to Physical Therapist Practice*,[50] developed by the APTA.

Since 2007 and up until 2014, KinetaCore® (a postgraduate education company) alone has certified almost 4000 North American providers in functional dry needling techniques across the USA, which is indicative of the growing interest raised within the physiotherapy collective.

According to the APA,[51] over 25% of registered physiotherapists currently employ needling techniques as part of the repertoire of treatment modalities used to manage conditions within their scope of practice. Aware of the surge in popularity of this treatment modality, the APA has recognized the need to establish a framework to ensure proper training for those who practise needling techniques, performed in line with the core competencies taught within physiotherapy entry-level education.

In South Africa, of the approximately 9000 registered physical therapists, over 75% are estimated to employ the technique at least once daily.[52] Furthermore, South African physiotherapists and those from the UK are allowed to perform botulinum toxin injections[53] in the management of individuals with focal spasticity and dystonia.

In 1984, the UK Acupuncture Association of Chartered Physiotherapists (AACP) was formed, becoming the largest professional network of the CSP. This association was formed for the practice of Western research-based acupuncture in physiotherapy; around 6000 members were registered in 2014.

In Europe, the Bologna process[54] is the process of creating the European Higher Education Area by making academic degree standards and quality assurance standards more comparable and compatible throughout Europe, in particular under the Lisbon Recognition Convention.[55] In countries such as Spain, Portugal, Greece, the UK, Ireland, Switzerland, the Netherlands, Belgium, Norway and Sweden, physiotherapists have been applying invasive techniques within the scope of physiotherapy practice for many years and are indeed a reference for the future.

1.2 HISTORY, EDUCATION, TRAINING AND REGULATION OF INVASIVE TECHNIQUES WITHIN THE PHYSIOTHERAPY PROFESSION

1.2.1 History

Acupuncture in physiotherapy practice

Acupuncture (including conventional acupuncture, electroacupuncture [EA] and moxibustion) has been used as a physiotherapy intervention modality in Canada, the UK, Australia, New Zealand, South Africa and Sweden since the early 1980s.[56] More recently, in other countries such as Spain, Portugal and Brazil,[57] physiotherapists have begun to use acupuncture as part of an integrated approach with conventional physiotherapy treatments.

KEY POINTS

Acupuncture is considered within the scope of practice for physiotherapists.

In 1999, the World Health Organization (WHO) published *Guidelines on Basic Training and Safety in Acupuncture*.[58] These guidelines assist national health authorities to establish the basic requirements for training physicians, non-physician acupuncturists and other health professionals. These also promote the practice of acupuncture in their profession as a part of modern Western medicine.

The International Acupuncture Association of Physical Therapists (IAAPT), founded in 1991, has been a subgroup of the WCPT since 1999. The IAAPT aims to develop standards of safe acupuncture practice and educational and training programmes, and promote sharing of information and research between individual and group members. Currently, 11 core member countries (Australia, South Africa, New Zealand, Sweden, the UK, Argentina, Hong Kong,

Canada, Zimbabwe, Ireland and Greece) form a part of the association.

Since 1986, the Acupuncture Association of the South African Society of Physiotherapy has been hosting training courses, organized with the assistance of the IAAPT. As the practice of acupuncture was regulated by act of Parliament in November 2000 (Act 50 of 2000, published on 1 December 2000 in Gazette 21825), physiotherapists who have completed the course are now applying for registration as acupuncturists with the Chiropractors, Homeopaths and Allied Health Service Professions Council of South Africa.

In 1997, the first book was published specifically for physiotherapists, entitled *Acupuncture and Related Techniques in Physical Therapy*.[59] This was a collaboration between clinicians, researchers and teachers who were members of the IAAPT.

In 2003, the IAAPT published *Standards of Safe Acupuncture Practice by Physiotherapists*[60] for the application of acupuncture, EA, moxa, cupping and auricular needles, press needles and beads.

In Canada, the Acupuncture Division of the Canadian Physiotherapy Association supports physiotherapists in advancing the use of acupuncture as an established core competency in physiotherapy clinical practice.

In the UK, all physiotherapists practising acupuncture should be eligible to join and maintain membership of the AACP.

In 2007 (reviewed in 2013), the Australian Society of Acupuncture Physiotherapists developed *Guidelines for Safe Acupuncture and Dry Needling Practice* as a guide to safe practice for physiotherapists and other allied health practitioners practising acupuncture in Australia.[61] The guideline was developed based on Australian and international acupuncture guidelines, including the minimum standards set by the IAAPT. In these guidelines, acupuncture practitioners include professionally trained and qualified Chinese medicine and acupuncture practitioners, and other qualified professionals who have received acupuncture training, including physiotherapists. The physiotherapist cannot use the title of acupuncturist.

According to the APTA, acupuncture is not within the scope of practice for physiotherapists and is not in the *Guide to Physical Therapist Practice*.[50] To practise acupuncture, physiotherapists would need to contact each state agency responsible for acupuncture licensing to establish the training requirements. Most states that license acupuncture or traditional Chinese medicine practitioners use standards set by the Accreditation Commission of Acupuncture and Oriental

Medicine (ACAOM). The USA is far behind in allowing physiotherapists to use invasive techniques in their scope of practice compared to countries such as Canada, the UK, Ireland and Australia. The present situation has similarities to the use of manual therapy techniques in the USA.[61] Initially, many US state boards of physiotherapy opposed the use of manual therapy. Although for several decades, manual physiotherapy had already been an essential part of the scope of physiotherapy practice in Europe, Australia and New Zealand, manual therapy did not make its debut in the USA until the 1960s. During the past few years, physical therapists, the APTA and the American Academy of Orthopaedic Manual Physical Therapists (AAOMPT) have had to defend the right to practise manual therapy, especially when challenged by the chiropractic community. A similar situation may be evolving with the relatively new invasive techniques.

Electroacupuncture. EA[60] (see chapter 16) was first used in China in the 1950s as an extension of hand manipulation of acupuncture needles. The term EA refers to the application of a pulsating electrical current through acupuncture needles to provide continued stimulation of the acupoints (acupuncture points).[62,63] The Chinese developed this method to be used for acupuncture-induced surgical anaesthesia. In the 1960s EA was introduced into clinical practice, especially for the treatment of chronic pain and neurological diseases. Today EA is used mostly in the treatment of nociceptive musculoskeletal pain, in both acute and chronic cases. It is based on the use of low-frequency electric currents such as transcutaneous electrical nerve stimulation (TENS) or microcurrents administered through the needle.

Dry needling in physiotherapy practice

Dry needling has been practised by physiotherapists for over 20 years in countries such as Canada, the UK, Ireland, Spain, Norway, Switzerland and South Africa, among others, with minimal numbers of adverse effects reported.[64] In 1984, the Maryland Board of Physical Therapy Examiners was the first physiotherapy board in the USA to approve dry needling by physiotherapists. Currently, dry needling is probably the invasive technique most used by physiotherapists around the world.

The AAOMPT[65] defines dry needling as:

a neurophysiological evidence-based treatment technique that requires effective manual assessment of the neuromuscular system. Physical

therapists are well trained to utilize dry needling in conjunction with manual physiotherapy interventions. Research supports that dry needling improves pain control, reduces muscle tension, normalizes biochemical and electrical dysfunction of motor endplates, and facilitates an accelerated return to active rehabilitation.

Since the 1970s several dry needling approaches have been developed for the treatment of myofascial trigger points (see chapters 8 and 10) within the scope of physiotherapy practice. Currently, dry needling is also used with intramuscular needle stimulation[65] ('electroneedling') in order to evoke further muscular relaxation. The use of the needles as electrodes offers many advantages over traditional stimulation[62] (the resistance of the skin to electrical currents is eliminated, with results in some cases that are more rapid and longer lasting). Several studies[66–68] have demonstrated that percutaneous stimulations is more effective for pain relief and improving functionality over traditional TENS. Moreover, relevant clinical studies[69–74] have combined dry needling with autologous blood injection therapy as a method of tendinopathy treatment, with excellent results. In these cases, dry needling consists of repeatedly passing a needle through the tendon to disrupt the fibres, induce bleeding and activate healing and regeneration. If local anesthesia is injected and a hollow needle is used, this technique is referred to as PNT[75,76] (see chapter 11).

In the USA, dry needling, within the scope of physiotherapy, is also defined as intramuscular manual therapy, intramuscular stimulation or functional dry needling, such as manual therapy techniques performed on the inside of the muscle.

In January 2012, the APTA published an educational resource paper entitled *Physical Therapists and the Performance of Dry Needling*[77] to assist practitioners on this issue. This document was meant to provide background information for state chapters, regulatory entities and providers dealing with the issue of dry needling. In February 2013, the APTA published a second paper regarding dry needling, entitled *Description of Dry Needling in Clinical Practice: An Educational Resource Paper.*[78]

KEY POINTS

Dry needling is considered an invasive physiotherapy technique and is consistent with the practice of physiotherapy.

At this point in time (July 2014), dry needling in the USA[79] is formally within the scope of physiotherapy practice in the District of Columbia and in 34 states (Alabama, Alaska, Arizona, Colorado, Connecticut, Georgia, Illinois, Indiana, Iowa, Kentucky, Louisiana, Maryland, Michigan, Minnesota, Mississippi, Montana, Nebraska, Nevada, New Hampshire, New Jersey, New Mexico, North Carolina, North Dakota, Ohio, Oklahoma, Oregon, Rhode Island, South Carolina, Texas, Utah, Virginia, West Virginia, Wisconsin and Wyoming). Currently the only states that have made a ruling against dry needling for physiotherapists are California, Florida, Hawaii, Idaho and New York, mainly due to verbiage in the practice act against puncturing the skin.

The FSBPT's Examination, Licensure and Disciplinary Database has no entries in any jurisdiction of discipline for harm caused by dry needling performed by physiotherapists.[78]

In the USA, controversy exists between physiotherapists and acupuncturists regarding dry needling techniques.[80–82] The ACAOM affirms that, historically, dry needling derives from acupuncture techniques; however, the practices of acupuncture and dry needling differ in terms of their historical, philosophical, indicative and practical contexts. Modern dry needling, performed by physiotherapists, is based on Western neuroanatomy and modern scientific study of the musculoskeletal and nervous systems. Physiotherapists who perform dry needling do not use traditional acupuncture theories or acupuncture terminology.

In another example, chiropractors sometimes argue that spinal manipulations are within their exclusive scope of practice; however, osteopathic physicians and physiotherapists use these techniques daily all over the world.[82] These days, it is quite common for many professions to share some skills or procedures with other professions. Therefore, the federations of state boards now recognize that it is no longer reasonable to expect each profession to have a completely unique scope of practice that is exclusive of all others. However, commonly:

> *one profession may perceive another profession as 'encroaching' into their area of practice. The profession may be economically or otherwise threatened and therefore oppose the other profession's legislative effort to change scope of practice.*

Specifically, in the case of dry needling, some acupuncture societies and associations in the USA may feel threatened by the growing numbers of physical therapists using this technique within their scope of practice.

Ultrasound-guided percutaneous needle electrolysis in physiotherapy practice

In recent years, physiotherapists have also incorporated additional needling techniques, such as PNE techniques (EPI®, EPTE®, MEP®) within their practice. These techniques are based on the combination of mechanical and electrical stimulation using a galvanic current through an acupuncture needle. Percutaneous needle electrolysis provides a controlled microtrauma to the affected soft-tissue structures under direct visualization via the ultrasound machine. These techniques stimulate a local inflammatory response, with increased cellular activity and repair of the affected area.[83] Since 2008, more than 2000 physiotherapists have received training in this technique in Spain, together with other therapists based in Europe and South America.

Injection therapy in physiotherapy practice

Injection therapy involves regular injections of beneficial substances which are administered by injection to intra- and extra-articular tissues and joint spaces, also including aspiration of joint spaces.

Injection therapy has been formally accepted within the scope of physiotherapy practice since 1995 in the UK for registered physiotherapists who firstly, have received and successfully completed specific, appropriate supervised training and secondly, have been assessed and proved their competency in the administration of injections in accordance with a Patient Group Direction and recommendations issued by the CSP.[84,85] Physiotherapists must prove their competency to practise by obtaining a qualification in injection therapy from a recognized postgraduate institution.

The Association of Chartered Physiotherapists in Orthopaedic Medicine and Injection Therapy (ACPOMIT), a professional network recognized by the CSP, supports postgraduate education courses for physiotherapists and promotes high standards of practice. The Orthopaedic Medicine Seminars® (Stephanie Saunders; since 1995), the Society of Musculoskeletal Medicine (SOMM) and different universities in the UK (Cardiff, Coventry, Essex, Hertfordshire, Keele, Nottingham, Plymouth, Queen Mary, Southampton and ULCAN) provide credited courses and diplomas for injection therapy approved by the CSP (e.g. the Advanced Professional Practice in Physiotherapy postgraduate programme of Plymouth University includes a module on injection therapy). Entry qualifications include completion of specialist musculoskeletal training or postgraduate clinical experience in a musculoskeletal setting, prior to injection training.

The SOMM has been training UK physiotherapists and doctors in injection therapy skills since 2000 through an advanced programme, validated as part of the Master's degree in Musculoskeletal Medicine at Middlesex University in London. In 2013, the SOMM trained physiotherapists from outside the UK in injection therapy for the first time in Norway. Other European countries are now expanding the scope of physiotherapy, creating a demand for established injection training courses.

Injection therapy is an example of activities that have transferred from one professional group to another with the change of professional roles. Initially, it was doctors who trained physiotherapists in injection therapy. In the UK, an audit of injections performed by physiotherapists between 1999 and 2008 showed that it was a safe, cost-effective intervention for pain relief, especially for musculoskeletal conditions.[86,87]

Injection therapy, when performed within the context of physiotherapy practice,[84–91] has several therapeutic purposes: (1) inflammatory pain from a range of orthopaedic and rheumatological conditions; (2) spasticity and dystonia due to a range of neurological conditions; (3) chronic headache with a musculoskeletal or neurological origin; and (4) bladder disorders in women's health physiotherapy.

There are several different types of therapeutic injections that are used by physiotherapists in the UK.[83–89] These are: corticosteroid injections, viscosupplementation with hyaluronic acid or Botulinum toxin A (Botox®), among others. Furthermore, the use of adjunctive guidance such as ultrasound or electromyography studies is recommended. The ACPOMIT included musculoskeletal ultrasound and ultrasound-guided injections.

In 1999, the CSP published its first clinical guideline[84] for the use of injection therapy by physiotherapists. In 2008, the CSP, in collaboration with the Medicines and Healthcare products Regulatory Agency and the Department of Health, produced a comprehensive review of the use of medicines in physiotherapy injection therapy in National Health Service settings.[85]

Since 1993, in the USA, the Maryland Board of Physical Therapy Examiners has approved trigger point injections by physiotherapists and, during the past 20 years, Maryland has been the only jurisdiction in the USA allowing physiotherapists to use trigger point injections, with no reports of adverse effects during this time. Ultrasound-guided trigger point injections for myofascial trigger points have good clinical results[92–94] based on the available evidence. In South Africa and Australia,[91] physiotherapists also perform injections with botulinum toxin for the management of focal spasticity and dystonia. In Spain and Portugal, physiotherapists have been using mesotherapy since 2011. In other parts of the world, although the model practice act does not specifically mention injection therapy, there is nothing specifically to exclude these techniques. Indeed, physiotherapists are starting to use them as a type of advanced/extended scope of practice.[91]

1.2.2 Education and training

Over time, the entry-level credential for physiotherapy around the world has evolved to the current entry-level, master's degree and doctorate study programmes. The credential progression has been a response to advances within the profession and the increasing responsibilities undertaken by physiotherapists.

The WCPT *Guideline for Qualifications of Faculty for Physical Therapist Professional Entry Level Programmes*[5] provides a professional foundation whereby the use of needles can be legitimately incorporated into physiotherapy practice. The interventions that may be used in curriculum development may include, but are not limited to, acupuncture and dry needling.[5]

Needle techniques are safe procedures when conducted by trained and skilled practitioners and when appropriate precautions are taken to identify and manage adverse reactions or side effects occurring to patients. Needle techniques, as advanced skills performed by the physiotherapist, require postgraduate education and training programmes. Currently, in Australia, Canada, the UK and the USA, needle techniques are not specifically included within entry-level education, requiring additional education and training after graduation.[95–100] However other possibilities for approaching this subject are available; for example, several universities in Spain include initial training in dry needling within their entry-level education programmes, as part of physiotherapy training in subjects within their curriculum.[101,102] According to the federations of state boards[40] in the USA, 'it is not realistic to require a skill or activity to be taught in an entry-level program before it becomes part of a profession's scope of practice. If this were the standard, there would be few, if any, increases in scope of practice'.

The standards for postgraduate educational programmes are developed in close coordination with many universities and other postgraduate education companies in Europe, the USA, Australia, Canada and South Africa, among others. For example, in Spain, many universities (e.g. Alcalá de Henares, Rovira i Virgili, Castilla-La Mancha) offer specialist certification programmes in myofascial trigger point therapy, which include dry needling, and the University of San Jorge offers a Clinical Acupuncture programme for physiotherapists. Since 2012, a Master's degree in Invasive Physiotherapy Techniques is taught by CEU San Pablo University in Spain. This is the premier postgraduate education course around the world, with an intensive and practitioner-oriented programme designed to acquire knowledge and develop skills and abilities to perform invasive techniques (acupuncture, dry needling, PNE, mesotherapy, percutaneous electrical stimulation, percutaneous electrical nerve stimulation, musculoskeletal ultrasound) within the physiotherapist's scope of practice. In the UK, Coventry University, Hertfordshire University, Nottingham University, Queen Mary University of London and the University of Essex, among others, and the Orthopaedic Medicine Seminars® include injection therapy for physiotherapists as part of their continuing education programmes. In the USA, KinetaCore® and Myopain Seminars® and GEMt® in Australia are postgraduate continuing education companies with a focus on myofascial pain syndrome, manual trigger point therapy and dry needling. In Portugal, the Master Physical Therapy® company offers courses on acupuncture, dry needling, PNE and mesotherapy. In Canada, for example, McMaster University has been offering the Contemporary Medical Acupuncture Programme for physiotherapists and other healthcare professionals since 1998.

Recommendations for education and training in invasive (needle) techniques

In preparation for this chapter, a thorough review of the physiotherapy curricula from relevant countries around the world was conducted to provide comparisons of educational programmes, scope of practice, accreditation and practice environments. Specifically, the situation in Canada,[95] the UK,[96] the USA,[97] Australia,[98] New Zealand[99] and the European Union[100] was analysed, generating the following recommendations in matters of education and training in invasive techniques:

- Postgraduate education and training programmes should include a theoretical and a practical component, as well as an assessment of theoretical knowledge and practical skills.
- Local regulatory agencies should provide credits for postgraduate training programmes, and establish a minimum number of face-to-face training hours (online study is not considered appropriate training), as a prerequisite for practice. In this sense, the physiotherapy entry-level education programme includes biological science, physical science, behavioural science and clinical science. Currently, there is no apparent difference in the curricular content[95-100] between academic programmes in Europe, including the UK, Canada, Australia, New Zealand and the USA and there is minimal variance in practice standards.[103-108] The length of the minimal training required bears in mind the fact that the clinical reasoning basis for invasive techniques (such as dry needling or contemporary acupuncture) does not differ from the knowledge in anatomy and neurophysiology that physiotherapists already possess. Rather, the specific needle technique skills are supplemental to that knowledge. For example, the AACP requires its members to undergo a minimum of 80 hours of acupuncture training and has an additional strict code of practice, whereas advanced members have a minimum of 200 hours of acupuncture training. Furthermore, in 2003, a minimum of 80 hours of acupuncture training for physiotherapists was decided by consensus at a meeting of the IAAPT at the World Congress of Physical Therapy in Spain. In another example, the CSP in the UK has set formal expectations since 2011 as to training standards for the use of injection therapy in general. In Spain, the General Council for Physiotherapy Boards has established a minimal training duration of 60–75 hours in courses on dry needling.[109] In this sense, a recent study[64] was conducted to investigate the adverse events associated with dry needling when performed by physiotherapists. This study revealed that the risk of a significant adverse event occurring due to dry needling carried out by a physiotherapist was 0.04% in 7629 dry needling treatments with 64 hours' training.
- Training in invasive techniques should be an integrated educational continuum. This continuum should start at the entry-level programme and continue throughout postgraduate education and professional practice. The evidence

currently available[12–15,35,48,63,83,86,89,90] in relation to the safety and effectiveness of invasive techniques in physiotherapy practice should be included within entry-level physiotherapy curricula worldwide. Historically, a similar situation has occurred with manual therapy techniques, including thrust and non-thrust mobilizations/manipulations.[82,110]

- Advanced courses must only be open to physiotherapists who are already using invasive techniques.
- The course attendees should participate as both clinicians and patients because it is vital to have experienced these techniques before practising them on patients.
- Local regulatory agencies should establish a register for physiotherapists formed in invasive techniques, as a prerequisite for practice. For example, the College of Physiotherapists of Ontario (Canada) has a roster (list) for each of the authorized activities that may be performed by physiotherapists (e.g. acupuncture). This information is available on the public register and online, allowing patients to see which authorized activities a physiotherapist is qualified to perform (therefore promoting public confidence) and also supporting the College's assessment of competencies and practices. In the UK, all physiotherapists practising acupuncture should be eligible to join and maintain membership of the AACP.

KEY POINTS

Needling techniques must follow the practice guidelines taught on a recognized accredited training course.

- Ongoing continuing professional development must be kept up to date in line with local regulatory requirements. Maintenance of competency should be assessed annually by peer-assessed competency review. All trained physiotherapists should continue their education in invasive techniques via course work, conference attendance and by staying up to date with the literature. For example, members of the AACP are required to complete a stated minimum number of hours (10) of continuing professional development each year in order to remain on the register. The Australian Society of Acupuncture Physiotherapists[111] recommends completion of 30 hours of continuing professional development in acupuncture or dry needling every 3 years to remain competent in this field of practice.
- 'Life-long learning and professional development is the hallmark of a competent physical therapist, participation in continuing education contributing to the development and maintenance of quality practice.'[112]

KEY POINTS

Physiotherapists must have the knowledge, skill, ability and documented competency to perform needling techniques that are within the physiotherapy scope of practice.

The Constitutional Court of Spain has highlighted the link between the professional competencies and the training of graduates. Considering that health professions are by nature in constant evolution, there is no closed competency profile, but rather:

> the determination of the competency fields is closely linked to the content of the different training programmes, in the measure that it is via these programmes that the knowledge, attitudes, abilities and techniques that form the essential content of each speciality are determined and, thereby also their respective fields of action.

In this regard, statutes STC 187/1991[113] and 155/1997[114] declare that the directive regulating study plans to obtain official titles must correspond with 'the essential knowledge that must be learnt in order to obtain an official title that is valid in the entire national territory'.

1.2.3 Physiotherapy practice and regulation

Many practising physiotherapists around the world possess skills in the area of invasive techniques. These physiotherapists work in diverse fields, such as musculoskeletal, sports, respiratory therapy, neurology, women's health and animal physiotherapy.

Physiotherapists employ a wide range of intervention strategies to reduce patients' pain and improve function. Invasive techniques performed by physiotherapists are a manual therapy intervention that involves the use of needles. In our opinion, needles are a valuable tool to add to the physiotherapist's toolbox, which includes, for example, the thumbs. According to our clinical experience, it is one of the most powerful techniques at hand, therefore safe and precise use is necessary. For the same reason, these techniques must be considered as advanced scope and therefore must be performed by clinical specialists or advanced practitioners.

Within the scope of physiotherapy practice, invasive techniques are limited to areas of practice for which the individual has received education and training and gained experience, and in which competency has been demonstrated.

KEY POINTS

Physiotherapists around the world use invasive (needle) techniques as part of their clinical practice in combination with other physiotherapy interventions.

Recommendations for physiotherapy practice and practice regulation

- The physiotherapist performing needle techniques should have significant professional experience and competency development. We recommend 1 year of practice as a licensed physiotherapist prior to using needling techniques.
- Physiotherapists should perform invasive techniques in a manner that is consistent with generally accepted standards of practice[103–108] (patient informed consent, clean needle technique and universal precautions) (see section 1.3) and guidelines developed by associations and entities responsible for the clinical practice of each country and at an international level. Such guidelines are intended to encourage high standards of practice and to reduce variation in practice. For example, the CSP, the Australian Society of Acupuncture Physiotherapists and the Swiss Association of Dry Needling have developed guidelines for the application of acupuncture,[111] dry needling[115] and injection therapy[84,85,116,117] by physiotherapists.
- A Master's level qualification and/or advanced training in the relevant speciality area (e.g. musculoskeletal) are desirable.
- Physiotherapists should only apply invasive techniques if they are completely sure that they can apply them to the best of their knowledge and ability.
- Physiotherapists should only apply invasive techniques in areas of the body for which they have been trained. This is important, as in most countries there are short courses

(2–3 days) taught at basic or introductory levels (e.g. dry needling). Our opinion is that it is necessary to establish a minimum standard for safe practice.
- Physiotherapists must be vaccinated against hepatitis B (see section 1.6.15 on needle-stick injury).
- Our recommendation is that recently trained physiotherapists in invasive techniques or professionals who have not practised within the last 12 months must liaise with their local regulatory agencies in order to identify a mentor for the first 6 months of their practice. The professionals and the mentor should meet at least once a month to review practice and discuss clinical cases.
- The physiotherapy practice should be covered by professional liability insurance cover, subject to the terms of the policy. The terms of most professional and public liability insurance covers (subject to the terms of the national policy of each country) provide coverage for members working within the scope of practice of physiotherapy. For example, dry needling or acupuncture falls within the overall scope of the physiotherapy profession in the UK, Canada, Australia, New Zealand, South Africa, Brazil, Switzerland, Sweden, Spain and Portugal, among others. The CSP in the UK makes no further distinction as to what types of injections may be performed, beyond saying that only therapeutic purposes are considered to be within scope. For example, in rule 1 of the Professional Conduct Code, the CSP[118] establishes:

Chartered Physiotherapists shall only practise to the extent that they have established and maintained their ability to work safely and competently and shall ensure that they have appropriate professional liability cover for that practice.

- In some countries invasive techniques are not allowed within physiotherapy practice (for example, in France). It is the responsibility of the physiotherapists themselves to check the legal situation of the country in which they are practising.
- Physiotherapists should limit the use of these modalities to the treatment of generally accepted physical disorders within the scope of practice for physiotherapists (musculoskeletal, neuromuscular and cardiorespiratory systems).

KEY POINTS

Physiotherapists are required to adhere to the regulatory requirements for the education and use of these interventions in the local/national jurisdiction in which they practise.

In the absence of specific statutory or regulatory prohibitions, it is within the scope of practice for physiotherapists to perform generally accepted professional activities for which they have been prepared by entry-level education, appropriate continuing education, training/experience, and for which they have demonstrated competency to perform safely and effectively. Physiotherapists must be prepared to accept responsibility and accountability.

1.3 SAFETY MEASURES

Needle techniques are usually a safe procedure,[119–121] with few contraindications and complications (see sections 1.5 and 1.6) in the hands of physiotherapists who have completed professional training. However, they do carry a potential risk for the patient, the professional and third persons (related to waste handling) (see section 1.7). Many of the potential risks in relation to needle techniques are not associated with conventional physiotherapy treatments, such as the risk of infection or pneumothorax. For this reason, it is necessary to establish safety standards in relation to these techniques.

KEY POINTS

Safety is the most important aspect of the care provided. Invasive techniques are a safe technique for patients in the hands of physiotherapists who have completed professional training.

The correct and safe application of the puncture technique depends on the following conditions (similar to the practice of subcutaneous or intramuscular injections)[111,122–125]:
- a clean work environment
- hand hygiene on the part of the professional
- correct preparation of the needle application sites
- sterile needles and equipment and appropriate storage
- aseptic technique
- careful manipulation and disposal of used needles.

1.3.1 Clean and safe work space

Treatment room

The treatment room must meet the following standards:
- It must have sufficient space to allow for safe practice.
- It must be free from dirt and dust, have sufficient light and ventilation and have a special work area, for example, a table or tray, upon which the sterile equipment must be placed.
- It must be constructed with materials that are washable and can be easily cleaned and disinfected, as required.
- The room must have a facility located close by where needles can be disposed of safely.

Protective clothing

- Protective clothing must be worn, whether this be a lab coat or scrubs.
- Professionals should wear protective work clothes while at the workplace, and remove them before leaving.
- These work clothes must be cleaned separately from other domestic clothing, with hot water at 70°C for at least 25 minutes. Diluted bleach can be used for increased sanitizing.
- Protective clothing contaminated with blood should be treated with hypochlorite solution (bleach) before laundering.

Material

- The disposable plinth covers must be changed with each new patient, even though they may appear clean. Another option is to cover the treatment bed with single-use paper towels.

Climatization system

- The climatization system must guarantee the patient's comfort and achieve a quality of air that is free from contaminating particles and microorganisms as a result of appropriate filtration. Health work locations must have highly efficient filter systems (not inferior to 85%) that filter all recirculated and fresh air. It is recommended that the filters are changed at least every 2 years.
- A temperature of 21–24°C and a relative humidity of 30% in winter and 50% in summer is recommended.

1.3.2 Hand hygiene

Hand hygiene is considered the most important intervention to prevent transmission of infectious agents (bacteria, viruses, fungi, protozoa, prions) and professionals should receive education regarding the same. Several factors could contribute to the transmission of pathogens by healthcare workers (HCWs). The most obvious factor is failure of HCWs to clean their hands,[126–131] and another is the improper use of gloves.[131,132]

The *World Health Organization (WHO) Guidelines on Hand Hygiene in Health Care*[134] provide a thorough review of evidence on hand hygiene in healthcare and specific recommendations to improve practice and reduce the transmission of pathogenic microorganisms to patients and HCWs. Healthcare practitioners must adhere to the national safety guidelines and local legal requirements.

The most important recommendations regarding needle techniques are as follows:

Prior

- Nails must be short (with nail tips less than 0.5 cm long or approximately $\frac{1}{4}$ inch) and clean.
- Do not wear coloured nail polish or artificial nails.
- Do not wear rings, bracelets or watches.
- Shirt sleeves must be short or rolled up.

Specifications for hand hygiene[134–137]

- Wash hands with soap and water when visibly dirty or visibly soiled with blood and after using the toilet.
  - Preferably an antimicrobial soap must be used, as regular soap eliminates visible dirt but is not effective in preventing antimicrobial activity.
  - Different forms of soap are acceptable (liquid, bar, leaf or powdered forms). When bar soap is used, small bars of soap in racks that facilitate drainage should be used to allow the bars to dry.
  - Hot water should not be used. Repeated exposure to hot water may increase the risk of dermatitis, resulting in more frequent colonization by pathogenic microorganisms in the skin on the hands.
- If hands are not visibly soiled, use an alcohol-based handrub as the preferred means of routine hand antisepsis: before and after touching the patient, immediately prior to performing any needle technique, regardless of whether gloves are used, and after removing gloves. If alcohol-based handrub is not obtainable, wash hands with soap and water.
  - Alcohol-based handrubs should contain 60–95% alcohol alone, or 50–95% when combined with small amounts of a quaternary ammonium compound, and hexachlorophene or chlorhexidine gluconate. This reduces bacterial counts on the skin immediately postscrub more effectively than other agents.
- Soap and alcohol-based handrubs should not be used concomitantly.
- Hands should be dried using individual paper towels, rather than the roll type or hanging paper towels. Multiple-use cloth towels are not appropriate. Reusing or sharing towels should be avoided because of the risk of cross-infection.
- Carefully dry the hands. Wet hands are a critical factor contributing to acquiring and spreading microorganisms associated with contact via touch after hand cleansing.
- Use hand lotions or creams to minimize the occurrence of irritant contact dermatitis associated with hand antisepsis or handwashing.
- The workplace should have sufficient hand hygiene facilities.

Hand hygiene technique[134–138]

Handwashing with soap (figure 1.1)
1. Wet hands with water and apply enough soap to cover all hand surfaces.
2. Rub hands for at least 15 seconds, covering all surfaces of the hands, fingers and fingernails (the subungual region, in particular, harbours a greater number of microorganisms than other areas of the hands. This area is often neglected during routine hand cleansing).
3. Rinse hands with water.
4. Dry hands thoroughly with a single-use towel.
5. Use towel to turn off the faucet and then dispose of it in a bin.

Handrubbing (figure 1.2)
1. Apply a palm full of alcohol-based handrub in a cupped hand, covering all surfaces.
2. Rub hands – palms, fingers and fingernails – for at least 15 seconds.
3. Leave to dry.

KEY POINTS

Hand hygiene still remains the basic and most effective measure to prevent pathogen transmission and infection.

HAND HYGIENE TECHNIQUE WITH SOAP AND WATER

🕐 Duration of the entire procedure: 40-60 seconds.

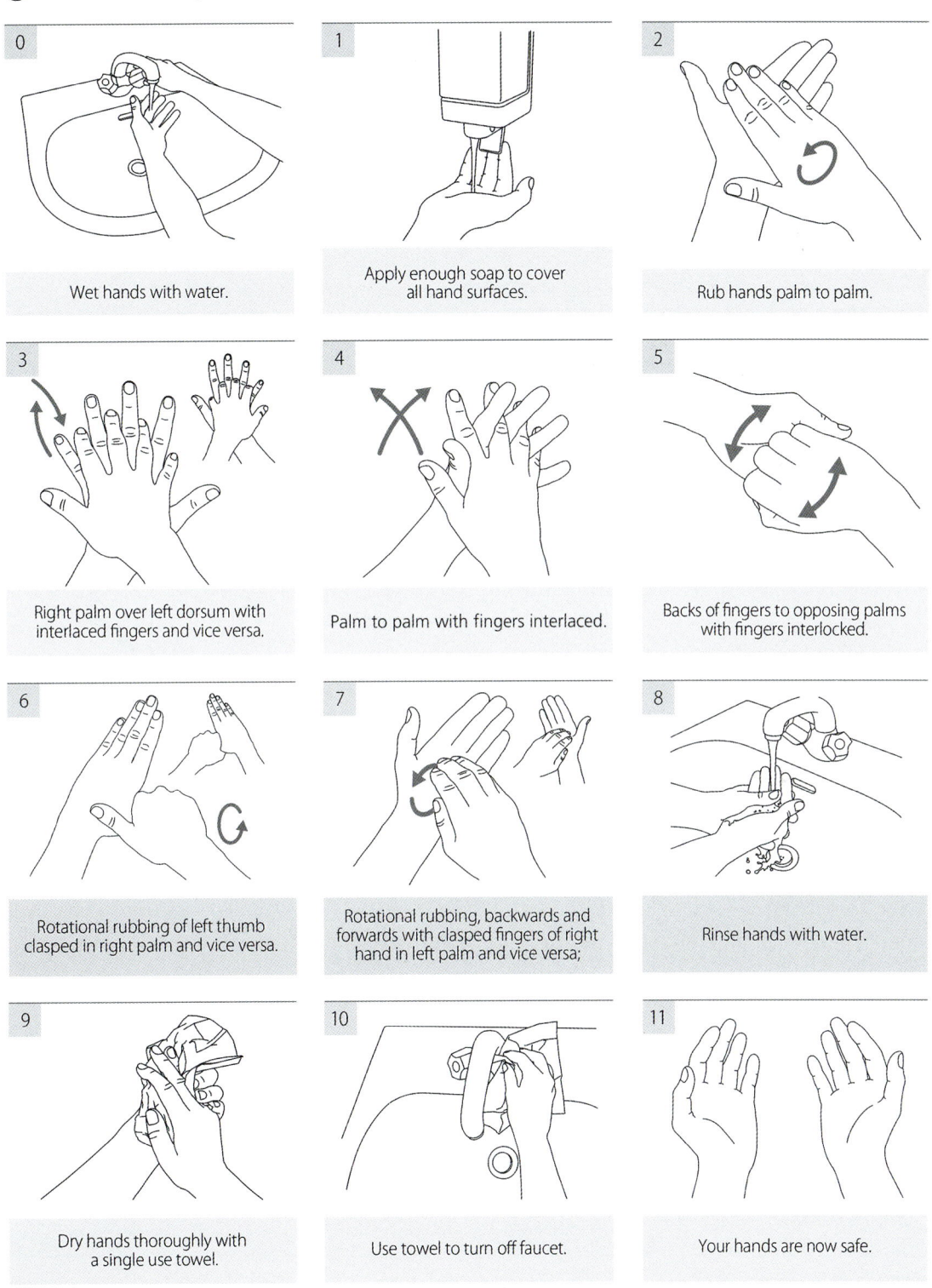

0 Wet hands with water.	**1** Apply enough soap to cover all hand surfaces.	**2** Rub hands palm to palm.
3 Right palm over left dorsum with interlaced fingers and vice versa.	**4** Palm to palm with fingers interlaced.	**5** Backs of fingers to opposing palms with fingers interlocked.
6 Rotational rubbing of left thumb clasped in right palm and vice versa.	**7** Rotational rubbing, backwards and forwards with clasped fingers of right hand in left palm and vice versa;	**8** Rinse hands with water.
9 Dry hands thoroughly with a single use towel.	**10** Use towel to turn off faucet.	**11** Your hands are now safe.

FIGURE 1.1 ■ **Handwashing with soap.** (Reproduced, with the permission of the publisher, from the *WHO Guidelines on Hand Hygiene in Health Care*. Geneva, World Health Organization, 2009 (Fig. II.2, page 156 http://whqlibdoc.who.int/publications/2009/9789241597906_eng.pdf, accessed 20 April 2013).)

HAND HYGIENE TECHNIQUE WITH ALCOHOL-BASED FORMULATION.

🕐 Duration of the entire procedure: 20-30 seconds.

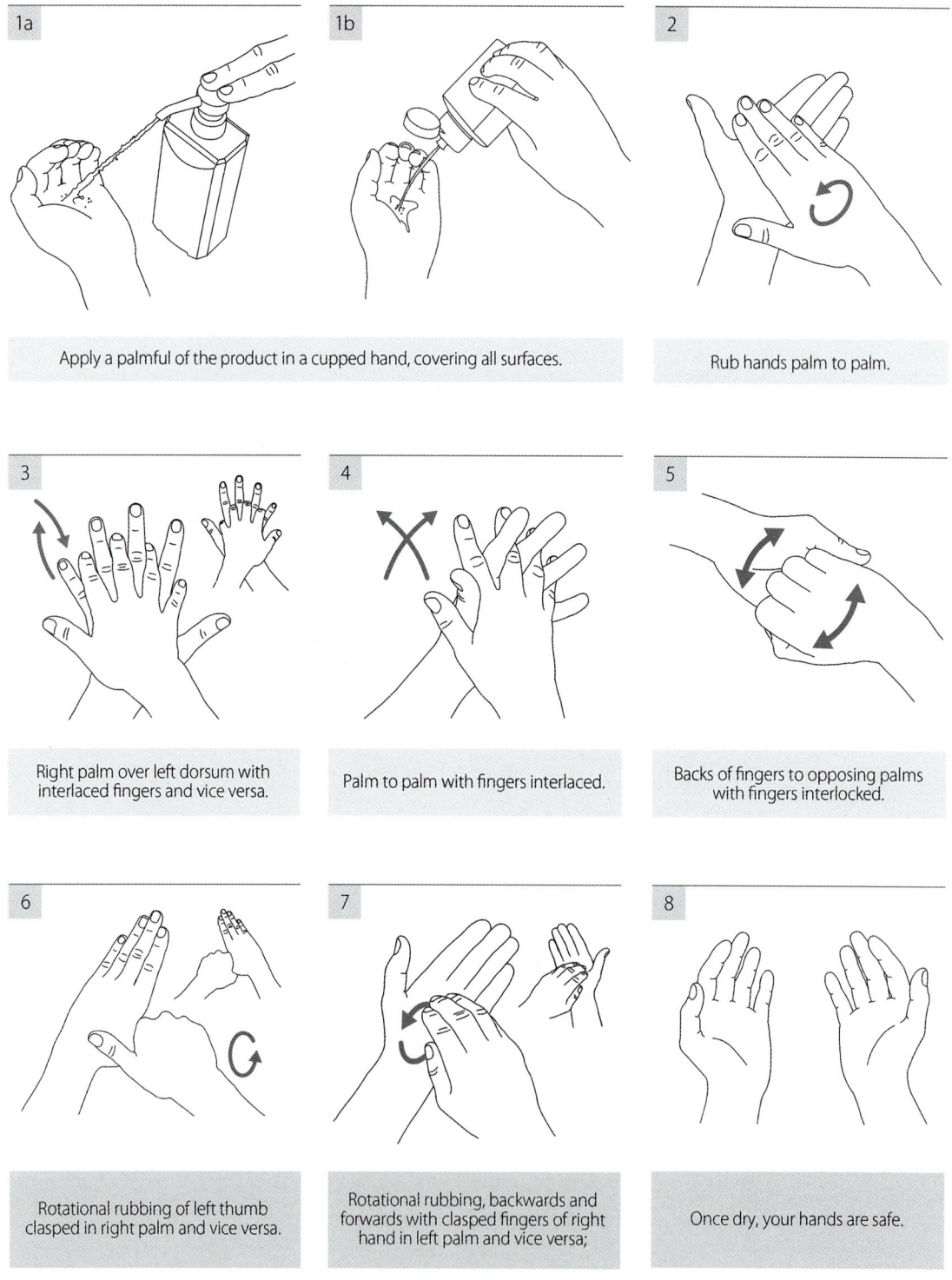

1a / **1b** Apply a palmful of the product in a cupped hand, covering all surfaces.		**2** Rub hands palm to palm.
3 Right palm over left dorsum with interlaced fingers and vice versa.	**4** Palm to palm with fingers interlaced.	**5** Backs of fingers to opposing palms with fingers interlocked.
6 Rotational rubbing of left thumb clasped in right palm and vice versa.	**7** Rotational rubbing, backwards and forwards with clasped fingers of right hand in left palm and vice versa;	**8** Once dry, your hands are safe.

FIGURE 1.2 ■ **Handrubbing.** (Reproduced, with the permission of the publisher, from the *WHO Guidelines on Hand Hygiene in Health Care*. Geneva, World Health Organization, 2009 (Fig. II.1, page 155 http://whqlibdoc.who.int/publications/2009/9789241597906_eng.pdf, accessed 20 April 2013).) (Colour version of figure is available online).

1.3.3 Gloves

Medical gloves used by professionals during invasive techniques are recommended for two main reasons:

1. To reduce the risk of contaminating professionals' hands with blood. In this regard, the US National Institute for Occupational Safety and Health Administration mandates that gloves be worn during all patient-care activities involving exposure to blood and body fluids.[139] The risk of transmission is related to the degree of blood exposure or frequency of needle exposure, and not to patient contact per se. If it is reasonably expected that the professional may have hand contact with blood when the needles are inserted or removed (e.g. dry needling, PNE, PNT, injection techniques), wear gloves.

2. To reduce the risk of germ dissemination to the environment and of transmission from the professionals to the patient and vice versa, as well as from one patient to another. In no way does glove use modify hand hygiene indications or substitute for hand hygiene, washing with soap and water or handrubbing with an alcohol-based handrub. In this sense, the risk of pathogen transmission via unused non-sterile gloves has been demonstrated in a recent study[140]; the unused gloves were contaminated prior to use due to contact with an unclean HCW's hands.

KEY POINTS

Examination gloves are recommended in clinical situations where there is a possibility of touching blood.

KEY POINTS

Gloves represent a risk for pathogen transmission and infection if used inappropriately.

Amongst professionals (especially acupuncture practitioners) there is a debate regarding 'to glove or not to glove' for several reasons:

- Standard puncture needles (acupuncture needles or similar; a solid, filiform needle) are very fine and need fingertip control. Wearing gloves when handling needles could prove to be hazardous because the needles cannot be properly controlled with a gloved hand.

- The use of gloves during the insertion of needles increases the risk of a needlestick injury due to clumsiness caused by the gloves.
- Gloves may hamper the ability to place needles safely into a container, as many needle handles stick to latex.
- Gloves provide protection from blood and body fluids but do not protect against a needle penetrating the latex or vinyl barrier.
- The risk of infection and transmission is considered to be minimal.

KEY POINTS

The use of gloves does not prevent accidental injuries by direct puncture.

The AACP recommends that disposable gloves need only be worn if one of the following applies:

- The patient is bleeding profusely.
- Vomit/urine is present.
- The patient has a known contagious disease.
- The therapist has lesions on the hand which cannot be covered with a waterproof dressing.
- The therapist is handling blood-soiled items, body fluids, excretions or secretions.

In any case, three factors must be considered:

1. Hypodermic and acupuncture needles are completely different with regard to their uses and handling techniques. In many cases, infection control officers have developed standardized nursing and medical procedures and rules (such as with intramuscular or intravenous injections). It is therefore important to understand the differences between these. For instance, the risk of bleeding is greater with hypodermic needles, as these always have a greater diameter together with a bevelled tip that causes a greater skin lesion. For this reason, gloves must be used during any injection therapy technique.

2. The risk of exposure to blood will depend on the type of local stimulation; in other words, the needle insertion and manipulation technique. For instance, if deep dry needling is performed, the risk of bleeding is greater in comparison to superficial dry needling.

3. In techniques with less risk of bleeding, such as acupuncture techniques, the greatest risk exists when removing needles; therefore gloves should be used at least during this part of the treatment.

Indications for the use of gloves

- Gloves should be single-use. It is not advisable to reuse gloves.
- Non-sterile gloves are recommended.
- Use natural rubber latex or synthetic non-latex materials such as vinyl, nitrile and neoprene. Latex-free gloves should be used for HCWs and with patients with a known latex sensitivity or allergy. Vinyl gloves are an alternative because they have less sticking power.
- The use of gloves does not replace handwashing.
- Gloves must be disposed of after use and discarded in the container for sanitary waste.
- Hands must be washed after removing the gloves.
- If a glove breaks, remove it and, after washing and drying the hands again, put on a new pair.
- Shear forces associated with wearing or removing gloves and allergy to latex proteins may also contribute to dermatitis of the hands.
- Use a glove box that has a flap covering the opening in order to reduce contamination via unused non-sterile gloves.

Procedure

How to put on and take off non-sterile gloves (figure 1.3). Our recommendation is that the use of gloves be consistent with universal precautions recommended by disease control experts in order to provide the best protection for both the professional and the patient.

1.3.4 Preparation of the application sites for needling

- The application sites must be clean and without cuts, wounds or infections.
- If skin is swabbed, use an individually packaged swab of isopropyl alcohol or ethanol or an antiseptic spray, from the centre towards the surrounding area, scrubbing using a rotating movement and leaving the alcohol to dry.
- Clean visibly dirty skin with clean water and dry the skin carefully with individual paper towels or clean cotton cloths.
- Ensure skin is free of oils, creams and lotions.

1.3.5 Puncture technique

Aseptic technique

- The use of disposable gloves is recommended to facilitate the manipulation of needles without contamination.
- The needles must be manipulated in a manner that avoids the professional's fingers touching the shaft. With longer needles, the shaft must be maintained steady on the insertion point using cotton or manipulation techniques with a guide (see chapter 2, figures 2.13 and 2.14).
- The use of containers with multiple needles is not recommended, as this increases the risk of touching the needle shafts (see chapter 2, figures 2.5d and 2.5e).
- Apply pressure on to the insertion point using cotton wool or sterile gauze when withdrawing the needle from the skin, thus protecting the patient's open skin surface from contact with possible pathogens, and protecting the professional from exposure to the used needle shaft and the patient's bodily fluids. All the compresses or cotton wool balls that are contaminated by blood or bodily fluids must be removed in a special container for infected waste.
- If a needle comes into contact with bone or perforates the joint capsule, withdraw it and replace it with another to avoid possible infection. When applying PNE, give a minimal dosage due to the antibacterial and germicidal properties of the technique itself.
- Use bleach to disinfect immediately any blood stains affecting the clinical material or other material in the treatment room, such as the plinth. The beginning of an infection can be due to an accidental stick or contact with the patient's blood via the professional's skin erosions. The skin has small invisible wounds and microlesions which make the epithelial layer lose its continuity.
- Use a high-level disinfectant to immediately clean any surface that has been contaminated with blood or body fluids. Practitioners are reminded that viruses such as hepatitis B can survive on surfaces at room temperature for 1 week or more.

KEY POINTS

The needle shaft must be kept in sterile conditions.

I. HOW TO DON GLOVES

1

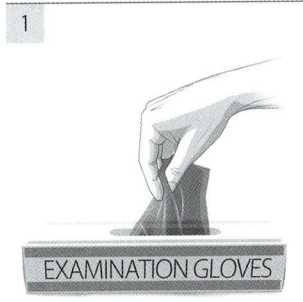

Take out glove from its original box.

2

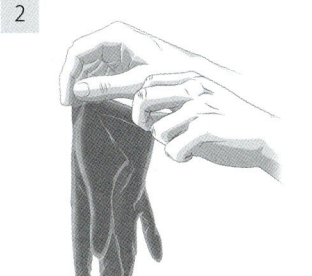

Touch only a restricted surface of the glove corresponding to the wrist (at the top edge of the cuff).

3

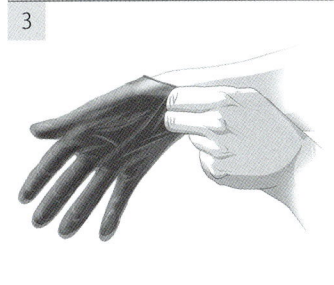

Don the first glove.

4

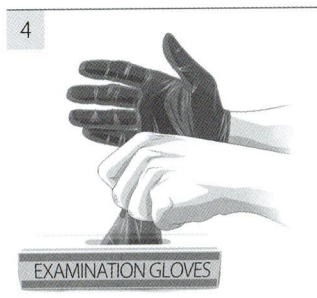
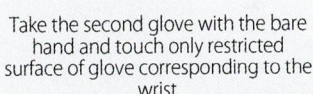

Take the second glove with the bare hand and touch only restricted surface of glove corresponding to the wrist.

5

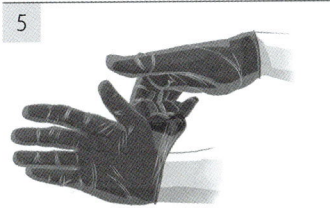

To avoid touching the skin of the foream with the gloved hand, turn the external surface of the glove to be donned on the folded fingers of the gloved hand, thus permitting to glove the second hand.

6

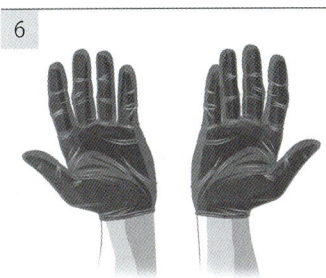

Once gloved, hands should not touch anything else that is not defined by indications and conditions for glove use.

II. HOW TO REMOVE GLOVES

1

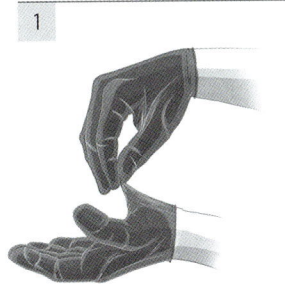

Pinch one glove at the wrist level to remove it, wothut touching the skin of the forearm, and peel away from the hand, thus allowing the glove to turn inside out.

2

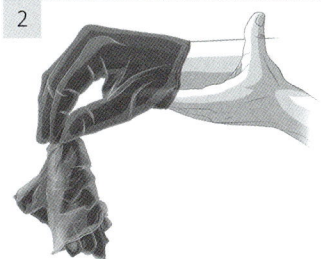

Hold the removed glove in the gloved hand and slide the fingers of the ungloved hand inside betwen the glove and the wrist. Remove the second glove by rolling it down the hand and fold into the first glove.

3

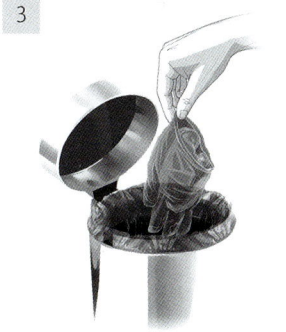

Discard the removed gloves.

4

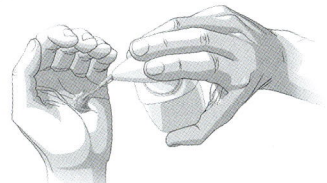

Then perform hand hygiene by rubbing with an alcohol-based handrub or by washing with soap and water.

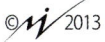

FIGURE 1.3 ■ **How to put on and take off non-sterile gloves.** (Adapted, with the permission of the publisher, from the *WHO Guidelines on Hand Hygiene in Health Care*. Geneva, World Health Organization, 2009 (Fig. I.23.2, page 141 http://whqlibdoc.who.int/publications/2009/9789241597906_eng.pdf, accessed 20 April 2013).) (Colour version of figure is available online).

Asepsis of the probe or ultrasound transducer

- In ultrasound-guided processes (see chapter 7, section 7.4.2), the contact surface of the transducer with the patient's skin must be covered with a protective sleeve (probe covers) to avoid the contamination of the same with bleeding.

1.3.6 Sterilization and storage of needles

- In all cases, the use of disposable needles and guide tubes is recommended (see chapter 2). However, the use of these kinds of needles does not mean that the adoption of aseptic techniques in other aspects of clinical practice can be overlooked.
- Check the expiry dates of sterile needles before use and make sure the packages are intact.
- The package should be opened just before use to prevent contamination.
- All disposable needles must be discarded immediately after use and disposed of in a special container (see section 1.7).
- Perform a single puncture with a needle, rather than several punctures in different points.
- In acupuncture, it is common to place the needles in metallic trays, or trays made of cardboard and plastic. These must be sterilized at the end of the day or disposed of, as they can become contaminated if used during treatment.
- In acupuncture, plum blossom needles, or seven-star needles can be used repeatedly on the same patient, but must be sterilized before use on another patient, or disposable plum blossom heads must be used.
- If any blister pack (see chapter 2) remains open, the needle must be disposed of.

KEY POINTS

Check each package for tears or damage.

1.3.7 Transducer cleaning and disinfection

- Cleaning and disinfection of probes should be performed before use and between patient exams.
- Cleaning is the removal of all visible soil or contaminants from the ultrasound transducer. After every exam, ensure the acoustic coupling gel is completely wiped off the probe. Transducers should not be left soaking in gel. Use a lint-free soft and clean dry cloth or wipe to dry the probe thoroughly.
- After cleaning the transducer, wipe or spray the transducer with a low- and intermediate-level disinfectant. Disinfectant products may damage or discolour the transducer. Disinfectant products should be as close to neutral pH as possible. Transducers must not be soaked in isopropyl alcohol (rubbing alcohol). This will cause damage to the transducer. An acceptable cleaning process would be to wipe only the distal tip of the transducer (housing) with a cloth dampened with isopropyl alcohol solution (only 70% alcohol or less). The use of any type of brush is not recommended as bristles may damage lens materials.
- Do not use any alcohol or alcohol-based products on the cable. Use a soft cloth lightly dampened in a mild soap or a detergent solution to clean the cable and the connector.

1.3.8 Training in resuscitation measures

It is important for the professional to have the knowledge and skills necessary to perform an emergency cardiopulmonary resuscitation and be able to employ instrumental measures such as the Guedel airway tube or the Ambu bag. The professional should also be able to administer an adrenaline injection (e.g. EpiPen®) in the case of an anaphylactic reaction, as the result of a complication.

1.4 APPLICATION CRITERIA

1.4.1 Training

Needle techniques are within the profession's authorized scope of practice but are not considered entry-level. They require additional education and appropriate training. See section 1.2.2.

1.4.2 Professional and public liability insurance

In order to practise invasive techniques, physiotherapists need to be able to demonstrate adequate training and competency in the technique (e.g. dry needling, acupuncture) and that they have appropriate professional liability cover for that practice in a local/national jurisdiction where needling techniques are considered within the scope of physiotherapy practice. See section 1.2.3.

1.4.3 Informed consent

It is necessary to inform patients of the procedure and request their informed consent (see section 1.8) before applying the technique. The authors' recommendation is that this should be in writing.

1.4.4 The workplace

The application of invasive physiotherapy techniques should be performed in a place designed for this purpose, and which allows the treatment to be personalized in ideal conditions of visual and auditory intimacy.

1.4.5 Patient positioning

- The patient must be in a comfortable position and lying down (side lying, prone or supine). The sitting or standing positions are forbidden in order to guarantee the patient's safety in the event of an unexpected movement or fainting.
- The use of pillows and roll cushions is advised in order to ensure a relaxed patient position.
- Whenever possible, the patient's position should allow the professional to see the patient's face for feedback. In any case, verbal communication with the patient should be sought in order to assess the patient's response to the invasive procedure.

KEY POINTS

The application of invasive physiotherapy techniques is contraindicated in sitting and standing.

1.4.6 Information regarding the procedure

Prior to the application of the technique it is necessary to inform the patient that single-use, sterile, disposable needles will be used, as well as to explain the procedure of needle insertion, the application of needle stimulation (for example, via manual stimulation or electrical stimulation), and forewarn of the possibility of transient symptoms appearing during and/or after treatment. Patients should be advised to stay still and avoid abruptly changing their position during the invasive procedure, as this could cause the

professional to lose control over the needle. This is especially important in any procedures taking place in the trunk structures (for example, the inferior trapezius) in order to reduce the risk of pneumothorax or rupture of the needle. Along these lines, it is important to assess the patient's mental condition.

KEY POINTS

During the procedure, warn patients against performing sudden movements that may cause needlestick injuries.

1.4.7 Application

- The application of the invasive technique must be performed following the safety rules established for this purpose (i.e. clean needle technique; see section 1.3).
- Allow enough time to carry out procedures safely.
- Have a clear treatment plan.
- Have appropriate knowledge of the relevant anatomical structures, such as the areas of vasculonervous conflict, the organs (liver, kidneys, lung) and pleura in order to be aware of any associated precautions required when needling and ensure that the techniques of invasive physiotherapy are provided with safety (see chapter 2).
- Insert the needle using the proper angle and depth and adjust the needle in response to the patient's reaction.
- The treatment intensity must adapt to the patient's tolerance (especially if this is the patient's first experience) and also consider the clinical picture and the individual characteristics of each person (e.g. age, body shape, associated illnesses such as diabetes[14]). The parameters that can be used as criteria for controlling the application are: the total number of needle insertions per structure, the number of structures (e.g. muscle, tendon) treated in a single session, the intensity of the techniques, the stimulation and the amount of local twitch responses, the application time. In any case, after the first session it is necessary to assess the patient's response to invasive treatment in order to plan the following sessions. It is also helpful to gather feedback from patients regarding any previous invasive physiotherapy treatments they may have received (see chapter 2, table 2.7).
- The physiotherapist must maintain active communication with the patient during

treatment. Patients must be monitored during the treatment session and must not be left alone in the treatment area.

- Have adequate support or know how to respond in the event of an adverse reaction.

KEY POINTS

The patient's response to invasive treatment must be analyzed after the first session in order to plan the following sessions.

1.4.8 Postapplication

- After the application of techniques that involve needle manipulation, perform haemostasis on the area for 30–60 seconds.
- If a small amount of bleeding appears after this application, apply pressure and clean the area with alcohol.
- Patients should be allowed sufficient time to rest and recover safely after treatment, especially if they feel drowsy and are driving.
- Massage or heat should not be applied to a site immediately after a puncture technique due to the potential for an increased risk of infection at the site.
- The patient must receive the necessary tips and instructions in order to guarantee a continuity in the care process (for example, perform stretches or eccentric exercises) and in order to minimize the risks (such as letting 24 hours pass after the treatment before bathing in a pool or in public baths, due to the risk of infection).
- In the case of needling techniques performed on the trunk muscles, patients must be warned of pneumothorax symptoms, especially if they are going to be exposed to exercise and/or important changes in pressure, such as flying or scuba diving.
- Explain the use of indwelling needles (including tacks) and the procedures for their retention, removal and disposal.

1.5 INDICATIONS AND CONTRAINDICATIONS

1.5.1 Indications

The general indications of invasive physiotherapy techniques include the treatment of pain and other symptoms associated with dysfunction of the musculoskeletal, neurological and cardiovascular systems. Specifically, these are described in the chapters on dry needling, acupuncture, mesotherapy, intratissue percutaneous electrolysis (EPI® technique), PNT, high-volume image-guided injections and injection techniques (see chapters 8–19).

In any case, the physiotherapist must perform an assessment and physiotherapy diagnosis in order to determine the suitability of the invasive physiotherapy techniques for each individual patient.

KEY POINTS

Before applying any invasive physiotherapy technique it is essential that the physiotherapist performs an assessment and physiotherapy diagnosis.

1.5.2 Contraindications

Absolute contraindications

Invasive physiotherapy techniques must not be performed under the following circumstances[111,121]:

- extreme fear of needles (belonephobia).
- patients with coagulation alterations (deep punctures must be avoided).
- history of adverse reaction to needles (or intramuscular or intravenous injections).
- in a lower limb with lymphoedema, as this increases the likelihood of infection.
- patients who are hesitant to receive the treatment based on their own fears or beliefs.
- in cases when informed consent cannot be obtained due to difficulties regarding communication and comprehension or related to the age of the subject (underage).
- in situations of medical emergency. In these cases, first aid must be applied and transport must be arranged to a medical facility with emergency care.

When treatment is contraindicated, it is important for the physiotherapist to respect this circumstance and not become persuaded by an enthusiastic patient who demands one of the invasive techniques.

Relative contraindications

Once the absolute contraindications have been assessed, consider the relative contraindications. The professional must evaluate suitability according to the risk–benefit relation.

- disorders of the immune system: these patients are more susceptible to infection:
  - patients with immunodepression or immunosuppression illnesses (e.g. cancer, hepatitis, human immunodeficiency virus [HIV]).

- patients who have received immunosuppressive treatment or cancer therapy.
- weakened patients, or those with a chronic illness.
- acute immune system disorders (for example, acute states of rheumatoid arthrosis).

- coagulation disorders: the application of needles should be avoided in patients with haemorrhagic disorders or coagulation disorders, or in people who are receiving anticoagulation therapy or who take medicine that has an anticoagulant effect.
- vascular pathology, as these patients can be more susceptible to bleeding or infection.
- diabetes: the repair process of the tissues may be compromised and there may be worse peripheral circulation.
- pregnancy: especially during the first 3 months of pregnancy, and after this period, whenever the area to be treated may affect the fetus.
  - traditional acupuncture texts note a variety of points (LI4, SP6, GB21, BL32, BL60 and BL67) that are forbidden during early or midterm pregnancy, as they are believed to 'dispel the fetus'. However, there is no known published report linking acupuncture treatment with abortion or miscarriage.[142] There is evidence to indicate that acupuncture is effective in treating pregnancy-related back and pelvic pain, and should be considered as an arguably safer alternative to analgesic medication.[143,144]
- patients who have difficulty communicating their sensations properly.
- epilepsy, especially unstable epilepsy.
- allergy to metals (especially nickel): needles of other materials can be used or with a Teflon® coating.
- allergy to latex gloves: gloves made with another material can be used.
- areas with erosions or wounds.
- children: informed consent is necessary of the parents or guardian. It is recommended not to apply invasive physiotherapy techniques in children under 13 years of age.
- caution in the puncture of joints due to the risk of infection.
- prosthetic implants.
- implants and electrical devices.
- malignant tumours or in their proximity. However, acupuncture can be used as a complementary measure combined with other treatments for the relief of pain and other symptoms in order to reduce the side effects of chemotherapy and radiotherapy and therefore to improve quality of life.

1.6 COMPLICATIONS: ACCIDENTS AND ADVERSE REACTIONS

The potential risk of invasive techniques demands that the professional be knowledgeable regarding the complications and associated adverse effects, as well as preventive strategies and measures to take when these occur.

There are no references to date that have analysed the complications and adverse effects for most techniques that are encompassed under the term 'invasive physiotherapy', except for acupuncture,[145–150] dry needling[63] and infiltrations.[151,152] Although acupuncture differs from dry needling and percutaneous needle electrolysis in terms of the underlying foundations, objectives and clinical applications, all these techniques use a solid puncture needle and, therefore, the acupuncture studies on safety may help to establish a similar context. The adverse effects studied in the case of infiltrations are similar to those obtained with mesotherapy: both techniques use a hollow needle and are based on the injection of a drug (homeopathic or allopathic). The adverse effects may be termed side effects, when judged to be secondary to a main or therapeutic effect.

The Cochrane systematic review on acupuncture treatment for migraine[153] indicates that fewer adverse effects and fewer dropouts were found in patients treated with acupuncture compared to groups receiving pharmacological treatment.

It is important to classify and quantify the adverse effects associated with puncture techniques. Their severity can be classified as mild (minor), significant or serious (major), according to the following criteria:

- mild (minor): reversible, short-lived and do not seriously inconvenience the patient
- significant: requiring medical attention or interfering with the patient's normal activity
- serious (major): requiring hospital admission (or prolongation of current hospital stay) and resulting in persistent or significant disability/incapacity or death.

Several large-scale observational studies have provided convincing evidence that acupuncture is a safe intervention.[120,146,147,149,154] Reports of serious adverse effects (major) such as pneumothorax or breakage of the needle are extremely rare (0.1–1%).[148] However, 8–11% of patients report mild (minor) adverse effects such as pain throughout the puncture and postpuncture, bleeding and bruising, followed by vegetative symptoms.[130–135]

KEY POINTS

The most common adverse effects include post-needling soreness and minor haematomas.

Other complications or adverse effects, such as drowsiness, weakness, worsening of the pain, headache, nerve irritation, cellulite, needle allergy, anxiety, panic, euphoria, hyperaesthesia, difficulty talking, asthma attack, abortion, angina pectoris or damage to metal implants, are less common.[145–150]

KEY POINTS

The dangers are limited and the probability of these events occurring is rare. In most cases, provided safety measures are followed, they are mostly avoidable.

The most common adverse effects, complications and accidents are described in the following sections, together with those that are the most serious (table 1.1).

1.6.1 Pain

During needle insertion

The presence of pain during needle insertion is usually due to incorrect technique or poor handling skills on the part of the professional, or the use of inappropriate needles.[155] Pain can also be experienced by highly sensitive patients. In most patients, a skilful and rapid needle insertion into the skin is painfree.

It is important to distinguish between the 'acupuncture sensation' characterized by burning, tingling and heaviness, indicating the arrival of *De-Qi* to the point (see chapters 2 and 15) and reactions of actual pain.

Postinsertion

The pain that appears when the needle is deeply inserted within the tissues can be due to contact with nerve fibres that are pain receptors (see chapter 2). In this case the needle must be withdrawn until it lies immediately below the skin before being carefully reinserted again in another direction. This may also be due to the patient moving and causing the needle to move. After insertion, 'silence' must be sought. In other words, the feeling of pain must disappear, so that if patients are not directly observing the needle they would not realize that it was inserted into the skin. If the sensation persists, or if the pain is of a throbbing nature, or generates other symptoms, the needle must be withdrawn.

After needle withdrawal

This is often due to inexperienced manipulation or excessive stimulation. In techniques such as dry needling or PNE over myofascial trigger points, postneedling soreness is common during the first 24–48 hours, occasionally lasting up to 4 days.

Prevention strategies

- The correct insertion technique (see chapter 2) and the optimal degree of applied force must be perfected until the ultimate painfree technique is achieved.
- Use a guide tube to minimize pain during insertion (see chapter 2).
- Use silicone-coated needles or needles with a polished shaft and a cone-shaped tip in order to improve needle manipulation and reduce pain (see chapter 2).
- Apply pressure on the area after the needle approach. This can reduce the local sensitivity that appears after treatment.
- The patient's response must be closely monitored at both a verbal and non-verbal level.

Measures to be taken

- Apply cold locally and compress the area to minimize pain.

1.6.2 Bleeding

The bleeding provoked by invasive techniques consists of a minor blood effusion that occurs after the needle is withdrawn. This is one of the more frequent adverse reactions and is of minor importance. It usually involves a minimal amount of bleeding that is rapidly controlled.

Prevention strategies

- Carry out haemostasis.
- Take care in patients with an abnormal tendency for bleeding (e.g. treatment with anticoagulants, thrombocytopenia).
- Avoid varicose veins.

Measures to be taken

- Using cotton wool or a sterile gauze, apply pressure to the point where the minor bleeding appears in order to promote haemostasis.
- Apply cold locally and compress the area in order to minimize the bruising.

TABLE 1.1   **Summary of the most common complications and the most common (minor) and most serious (less frequent) adverse effects**

Adverse effects	Symptoms/signs	Prevention	Measures to be taken
Bleeding	Minor	Haemostasis Precaution in patients with an abnormal tendency for bleeding (e.g. treatment with anticoagulants, thrombocytopenia) Avoid varicose veins	Using sterile cotton wool, apply pressure to the point Local ice application to minimize bruising
Bruising	Minor		
Pain during insertion	Minor	Observe the patient's response: verbal and non-verbal communication	Avoid the sensation of acute pain and burning by immediately withdrawing the needle in these cases
Pain postinsertion	Minor Lasting from 1 hour to 2 days, but occasionally for up to 4 days	Haemostasis in the puncture region Combined stretch with the application of cold	Apply local cold and compression to the area to minimize the pain
Needle breakage	Significant	Always use single-use needles (never use the same needle repeatedly) The quality of the needles is important. All needle packaging should be CE-marked Leave approximately 1 cm of the needle shaft poking outside the skin	Advise the patient to stay calm and not move, to avoid the needle penetrating even deeper into the tissues Use a pen to mark around the insertion point to aid identification of the area If the broken fragment is visible, remove it with tweezers; if the broken fragment is not visible, the tissue should be softly pressed close to the insertion until it comes out and then it must be withdrawn using tweezers If the needle cannot be withdrawn at the time, medical assistance is necessary as the needle will need to be surgically removed
Pneumothorax	Serious Shortness of breath Chest pain Dry cough Decreased sounds under auscultation These symptoms may not appear until several hours posttreatment, therefore patients must be warned, especially if they are going to be exposed to exercise and/or important changes in pressure, such as flying or diving	Apply puncture techniques on one side of the chest only Have a perfect knowledge of the reference points of the pleura and the supraclavicular fossa The insertion of the needle through the wall of the thorax and into the lungs is extremely painful, much more so than the normal pain associated with puncturing the thoracic wall When this type of pain is generated during a puncture in the area of the thoracic wall, use a stethoscope to assess a possible decrease in the sound of the lung	If a possible pneumothorax is suspected, the patient must be immediately sent to the closest medical emergency room Instruct the patients to explain to the emergency personnel that they have been treated with invasive puncture techniques in the area of the thorax wall and that, therefore, an X-ray of the thorax may be necessary to rule out a possible pneumothorax

1.6.3 Bruising

Occasionally, after the puncture, and due to the perforation of small vessels, a minimal amount of bleeding will occur which causes immediate bruising in the area.

Prevention strategies

- Carry out haemostasis.
- Take care in patients with an abnormal tendency for bleeding.
- Avoid varicose veins.

Measures to be taken

- Apply immediate pressure to the area using cotton wool or a sterile gauze to facilitate haemostasis.
- Apply cold and compression over the area to minimize bruising.
- Advise patients of possible bruising (although this information will appear in the informed consent form that they will have previously signed).

1.6.4 Vegetative reactions

Mild vegetative reactions, such as paleness, sweating, goose bumps, coolness of the skin and visceral effects, are frequent, especially when a greater stimulus is used, such as a greater application time, a larger number of needles or associated with an electric current. This indicates a segmental response that activates the repair processes. This is what some authors describe as the organism's response to a threat.[156] These symptoms are usually short-lived (disappearing within 5–10 minutes).

At certain times, increased vegetative reactions are described along with a brief and reversible loss of consciousness (vasovagal episode) associated with a loss of elasticity in the muscles, signs of stiffness in the joints and a loss of range of motion (as if the joint were blocked). There is also a decrease in the activity of the organs and an alteration of peristalsis, resulting in spasm.

Prevention strategies

- Ask patients beforehand whether they have suffered from episodes of dizziness and fainting in similar situations (when giving blood or on removal of a tooth).
- Ask whether the person has a fear or phobia of needles.
- Some patients demonstrate a vegetative response due to visualization of the procedure on the ultrasound screen.

- Special attention is necessary when the needle application points can cause hypotension, such as LV3 (see chapter 15).
- Often, these reactions are due to nervousness, hunger, fatigue, weakness, an inappropriate position or excessive manipulation.

Measures to be taken

- Withdraw the needles immediately and place the patient in a horizontal position with the head lowered and the legs raised.
- Avoid the patient sitting up on the plinth.
- Ventilate the space (room, treatment cabin) where the patient is being treated.
- Offer a sweet, warm drink.
- The patient usually responds quickly to these measures, but if the symptoms persist, urgent medical assistance is required.
- If the person faints, use the fingernail to press energetically on DU26 or DU25 (tip of the nose) or any *Jing* 'starter' point (see chapter 15).
- The increased vegetative reactions require assessment on behalf of the emergency services to rule out any complications.

1.6.5 Bent needle

Occasionally, sudden movements made by the patient (avoidance movements) or involuntary movements (associated with intense local spasm responses) or poor technique can cause the needle to bend (figure 1.4).

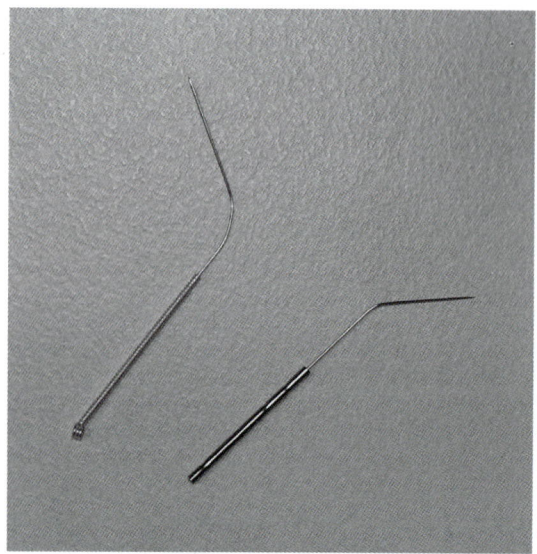

FIGURE 1.4 ■ Bent needles.

Prevention strategies

- Carefully examine each needle before using it. If a needle is bent, has a corroded shaft or a defective tip, dispose of it (see chapter 2). It is essential to check that the puncture material to be used has a CE stamp or equivalent (see chapter 2).
- Insert the needle with the patient relaxed and placed in an optimal position.
- Use the optimal puncture technique and avoid bending the needle during the invasive treatment.

Measures to be taken

- Change the needle for a new one and repeat the technique.

1.6.6 Stuck needle

After needle insertion and manipulation (frequently when twisting the needle), it may be difficult or impossible to sink it further or even withdraw it. This may be because the tissue fibres become interwoven with the needle shaft (see chapter 2), causing it to get stuck, or due to a muscle spasm around the needle or the patient moving.

Prevention strategies

- Avoid excessive needle twists to prevent the skin and the soft tissue getting stuck around the needle.

Measures to be taken

- Allow time for the patient to relax, then gently manoeuvre the needle out.
- If the needle is stuck due to excessive rotation in one direction, twist it in the opposite direction and try to withdraw it.
- If the needle is stuck due to a muscle spasm, leave it in place for a short time, gently massage around the needle to relax the muscle and gently reattempt removal. Alternatively, surround the stuck needle with four small needles, wait a few seconds then reattempt removal or apply a brief stimulus with an electric current.
- Another option would be to ask for a gentle isometric contraction of the antagonist, as this would help relax the target tissue (reciprocal inhibition).
- If the stuck needle is due to the patient having changed position, return the patient

to the original position and then withdraw the needle.
- If unsuccessful, seek medical help.

1.6.7 Broken needle

Broken needles can be due to poor-quality manufacture or a defect (such as erosion or cracks between the shaft and the handle) or due to inappropriate needle manipulation (such as the use of excessive force), a strong muscle spasm, a sudden and uncontrolled movement by the patient, the incorrect withdrawal of a stuck or bent needle or the prolonged use of galvanic current. The intersection point between the shaft and the handle (see chapter 2) is the most common point for breakage.

Prevention strategies

- Always use single-use needles (never use the same needle repeatedly).
- The expiry date on the box and on individual needle packaging should be checked by the physiotherapist before use. Needles should not be used if they have passed the expiry date.
- The quality of the needles is important. All needle packaging should be CE-marked.
- Leave approximately 1 cm of the needle shaft poking outside the skin.

Measures to be taken

- Advise the patient to stay calm and not move, to avoid the needle penetrating even deeper into the tissues.
- Use a pen to mark around the insertion point to aid identification of the area.
- If a part of the broken needle sticks out from the skin, the fragment should be removed with tweezers.
- If the broken fragment is at the level of the skin, the tissue should be softly pressed close to the insertion until the fragment comes out and then it must be withdrawn using tweezers.
- If it is completely below the skin, the patient is asked to return to the previous position, which is frequently when the end of the needle body appears.
- If the needle cannot be withdrawn at that time, seek medical assistance as the needle will need to be surgically removed. Biplanar fluoroscopy can locate and mark the foreign body (needle), allowing for a more straightforward surgical exploration.

- Depending on the area and the possible risk of infection or injury, the decision not to remove the needle may be taken. In scientific literature, reports have been published of needles or needle fragments being retained in all types of circumstances (e.g. breast biopsy, after giving birth, after insulin injection) in patients who are asymptomatic and without any changes being reported for over 11 or even 25 years.[157]

1.6.8 Losing a needle

It is easier to forget the needles in static puncture techniques, which is when the needle is left in the puncture area during a period of time or when several body parts are punctured, such as in acupuncture.

Prevention strategies

- All needles must be counted. A forgotten needle will cause pain in the tissue or may lead to serious complications, such as pneumothorax. In order to reduce the loss of needles it is useful to make a record and check the number of needles inserted and removed (figure 1.5). Another option is to use an electronic timer to count the number of needles and also to record the duration of treatment.
- In acupuncture treatment, pay special attention to the needles in the hairline because these are easier to forget.
- It is recommended that those qualified HCWs who insert the needles are the HCWs who remove them. Needle tasks should not be assigned to or carried out by an assistant (e.g. physiotherapy assistant).

Measures to be taken

- This depends on the possible damage inflicted.

1.6.9 Burns

In the case of moxibustion[158,159] or the application of electricity associated to the puncture, such as in percutaneous needle electrolysis or EA, it is possible to cause a burn to the patient.

Prevention strategies

- Apply the technique correctly.
- Pay special attention to patients with a reduced level of consciousness, sensory disorders, psychotic disorders and dermatitis, or in areas of altered circulation.

Measures to be taken

- Inform the patient.
- Refer to the medical team for treatment.

1.6.10 Local infection

Negligence in the use of strict aseptic technique can cause a local infection.[160,161]

Prevention strategies

- Always use a sterile needling technique.
- The skin in the region to be treated must be inspected to see if it presents any signs of infection, in which case the procedure is contraindicated. Avoid needling over thin, fragile or infected skin.
- Patients with an affected immune system, vascular illness or diabetes are at greater risk.
- Avoid puncture of acute inflammatory lesions or skin lesions, cysts, tumours, ganglion cysts and puncturing in the proximity of prosthetic implants.
- Disinfect the work surfaces before receiving a new patient in order to avoid infection via cross-contamination. For this reason it is important that the clinical furniture have flat surfaces with no junctions. The plinth must be cleaned with a cloth using a 1% bleach solution or with disinfectant wipes of 1% chlorhexidine digluconate and 70° ethanol.

Measures to be taken

- Refer the patient to the medical service for care.

1.6.11 Pneumothorax

Pneumothorax is one of the most serious but, also, less frequent adverse effects associated with puncture techniques (only nine cases have been described in the scientific literature over the last 20 years).[162–171] The most common symptoms are coughing, chest pain and dyspnoea. Commonly, the onset of symptoms due to pneumothorax induced via needle techniques does not occur until several hours after the treatment session. For this reason, patients must be warned of these symptoms, especially if they are going to be exposed to exercise and/or important changes in pressure, such as flying or scuba diving.

Prevention strategies

- In the posterior aspect of the thorax, the needle must be inserted superficially

PATIENT'S NAME	

DATE	ACUPUNCTURE TREATMENT	NEEDLES

		IN	OUT

Sign

		IN	OUT

Sign

(The form repeats with DATE lines on the left, ACUPUNCTURE TREATMENT lines in the center, and NEEDLES with IN and OUT checkboxes and Sign lines on the right, for ten entries.)

Therapist's name _____

Therapist's signature _____

FIGURE 1.5 ■ Record for counting needles. (Adapted from: Randal G, Collins R. *Clinical Guidelines for the use of Acupuncture within the Physiotherapy Service. Peninsula Community Health.* 2012. Available at: http://www.rcht.nhs.uk/DocumentsLibrary/PeninsulaCommunityHealth/OperationsAndServices/OTAndPhysio/AcupunctureInPhysio.pdf).

towards the midline, with an approximate length of 25 mm. Do not use deep needling techniques at the base of the neck.
- Apply puncture techniques on one side of the body only.

- A perfect knowledge of the reference points of the lung and pleura is necessary (see chapter 3).
- The insertion of the needle through the wall of the thorax and into the lungs is

extremely painful, much more so than the normal pain associated with puncturing the thoracic wall.

- When this type of pain is generated during a puncture in the area of the thoracic wall, use a stethoscope to assess a possible decrease in the sound of the lung.
- Special precautions are advised for long-term smokers, for those suffering from scoliosis and those with a thin frame.

Measures to be taken

- If a possible pneumothorax is suspected, the patient must be immediately sent to the closest medical emergency room.
- Instruct patients to explain to the emergency personnel that they have been treated with needling techniques in the area of the thorax wall and that, therefore, an X-ray of the thorax may be necessary to rule out a possible pneumothorax (figure 1.6).

1.6.12 Fainting and convulsions

On rare occasions, a patient may suffer from mild seizures after application of the invasive technique. The reason for this is unclear, although it may be due to a sudden vagal stimulation to the heart.

Prevention strategies

- Ask all patients who are going to receive a needling treatment whether they have a history of seizures. In the event of a positive response, keep a close watch on these patients during treatment.
- If patients have a history of unexplained seizures, needle techniques are not advised.
- On the first visit use gentle stimulation.

Measures to be taken

- If a patient feels faint or nauseous or is experiencing sudden sweating, remove all needles immediately. Lay the patient flat, maintaining a clear airway, and attempt to rouse the patient. If the situation does not stabilize rapidly or the seizures continue, the patient must be taken to the closest medical emergency room.

1.6.13 Injuries to organs

When applied correctly, invasive techniques should not damage any organ. However, if organ damage does occur, it can be serious. Accidents can happen during treatment due to the characteristics of the needles used, the precise application sites of the needles, the insertion depth of the needles, the manipulation techniques and the stimulation applied.

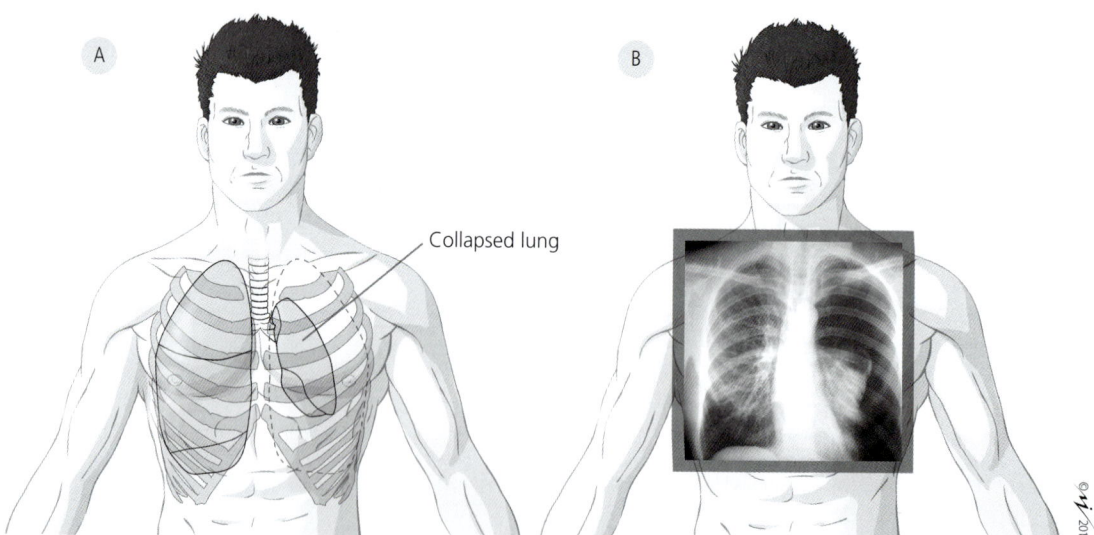

Collapsed lung

FIGURE 1.6 ■ Pneumothorax. (A) In a pneumothorax, air from a ruptured lung enters the pleural cavity with no means of escape. As air pressure builds up, the affected lung is compressed (collapsed lung) and all of the mediastinal structures are displaced to the opposite side of the chest, and the hemidiaphragm is depressed. (B) Chest X-ray shows a left-sided pneumothorax (right side of the figure) which is under tension, manifest as displacement of the heart and mediastinal tissues to the right and depression of the left hemidiaphragm. The left hemithorax is black due to air in the pleural cavity. (Colour version of figure is available online).

Prevention strategies

- The safest way to perform a deep puncture technique is to do so under echoguidance (see chapters 2, 4 and 7).
- Pay special attention to the application points that are close to vital organs or sensitive areas.
- Punctures on the thorax, the back and the abdomen should be performed with care. Special attention should be paid regarding the direction (if possible, in an oblique or horizontal direction) and the depth of the needle insertion.
- Perfect knowledge of the anatomical areas of interest is essential (see chapter 3).
- Avoid the area of the lungs and the pleura. An accidental puncture may cause traumatic pneumothorax (see section 1.6.11 and figure 1.6).
- Avoid the area of the liver and spleen. A puncture affecting these organs can cause haemorrhage and abnormal sensitivity to touch or pressure, as well as stiffness of the abdominal muscles.
- Avoid the kidney area. A puncture of the kidney can cause pain in the lumbar region and haematuria. If the damage is mild, the haemorrhage will stop spontaneously, but if the haemorrhage is serious, a state of shock will occur with a drop in blood pressure.
- Avoid deep invasive techniques over superior cervical vertebrae and surrounding areas, as these can reach the medulla oblongata, causing headaches, nausea, vomiting, a sudden decrease in the rhythm of breathing and disorientation, followed by seizures, paralysis or coma.
- Deep puncture techniques in the vertebral spine must be performed with caution. Above the first lumbar vertebra the spinal cord can be reached, producing immediate symptoms in the extremities or in the trunk below the puncture point.
- Certain areas, such as the external genitals, the nipples, the umbilicus and the eyeball, should not be touched with the needle.

Measures to be taken

- Accidental damage to an important organ requires urgent medical or surgical assistance.

1.6.14 Nerve damage

Nerve damage caused by direct puncture usually causes immediate symptoms, including acute and intense pain in the puncture area that irradiates towards the distal extremity. It may also be due to the compression produced by haematoma. In the ensuing days a sensation of tingling or 'electric shock' is frequent, which irradiates towards the distal extremity from the site of the puncture, when the tissue is subjected to compression, stretching, voluntary contraction or daily activities that involve the area. The symptoms continue for days, weeks, months and even, on rare occasions, permanently.

Prevention strategies

- Apply the deep puncture techniques guided by ultrasound.
- Have a perfect knowledge of the anatomical areas of interest.

Measures to be taken

- Refer to the medical team for assessment. A specific treatment does not exist. Usually, pharmacological treatment is commenced with vitamin complexes (B_1, B_6, B_{12}) such as neurobion®.

1.6.15 Needlestick injury

A sharps injury is an incident that causes a needle to penetrate the skin. This is sometimes called a percutaneous injury. This is usually due to malpractice, neglect or an unexpected sudden movement made by the patient.

Sharps injuries are a well-known risk in the health and social care sector. Sharps contaminated with an infected patient's blood can transmit more than 20 diseases, including hepatitis B and C and HIV.

The European Framework Directive on Prevention from Sharps Injuries in the hospital and healthcare sector (Directive 2010/32/EU)[172] signed by the European Public Services Union and the European Hospital and Healthcare Employers' Association on 17 July 2009 guarantees minimum safety and health requirements throughout Europe while Member States are allowed to maintain or establish more stringent measures:

Member States shall bring into force the laws, regulations and administrative provisions necessary to comply with this Directive or shall ensure that the social partners have introduced the necessary measures by agreement by 11 May 2013 at the latest. Moreover, Member States shall determine what penalties are applicable when national provisions enacted pursuant to this Directive are infringed.

Employers and workers' representatives must work together to eliminate and prevent risks, protect workers' health and safety, and create a safe working environment following the hierarchy of general principles of prevention via information and consultation. Thorough risk assessment should be carried out when injury, blood or other potentially infectious material is possible or present and should focus on how to eliminate these risks. Risk management measures are: specifying and implementing safe procedures (including safe disposal), eliminating unnecessary sharps use, providing safety-engineered medical devices, prohibition of recapping, coherent overall prevention policy, training and information, personal protective devices and offering vaccination. Workers should report any accident to the responsible person; any accident should be investigated and the victim treated.

Prevention strategies

- Follow practical steps prior to any procedure involving needles, as well as during and after the procedure (box 1.1).
- A large number of infectious diseases can be avoided with vaccinations that provide active immunity. Of these, the hepatitis B vaccine is the most important for all personnel who come into contact with blood or other objects contaminated with blood.
- Do not go past the 80% capacity of needle boxes or sharps containers (see section 1.7), which is marked on the containers as a safety line ('Warning: do not fill above the line'). This helps avoid needlesticks caused by used needles.
- Do not use other containers besides those approved for needle disposal.
- Do not store used sharps in an open container where they can be reused or cause needlestick injuries when dumped.
- If a guide tube is used during needle insertion, manipulate it correctly (figure 1.7). If a guide tube is used, the needle must be resheathed with the handle first.
- Do not recap needles. Recapping commonly leads to needlesticks. The needle containers are designed for storing needles without a plastic protector. If recapping is necessary, use a one-handed technique (figure 1.8). Establish a policy/procedure for safe recapping when necessary for the procedure being performed. Re-educate staff about disposal hazards and provide instruction on safe practices. Used needles and other sharps should not be recapped, bent, removed from disposable syringes or

---

BOX 1.1	Preventing needlestick injuries

Following proper work practice procedures will minimize the risk of needlestick injury. Here are practical steps you should take:

PRIOR TO PROCEDURE USING NEEDLES (✓)

✓ Ensure all equipment is available and within arm's reach
✓ Ensure lighting is adequate
✓ Place a sharps disposal container nearby and know where it is located
✓ Instruct patients to avoid sudden movements
✓ Do not expose sharps/needles until moment of use and keep pointed away from user

DURING PROCEDURE (✓)

✓ Maintain visual contact with needles during use
✓ Alert patient (and other staff) when placing or retrieving needles
✓ Remain aware of positioning of other staff to avoid accidental contact
✓ Do not pass needles by hand; place and retrieve from predetermined centralized location/tray

POSTPROCEDURE (✓)

✓ Ensure all needles are accounted for and visible
✓ Transport reusable sharps in a secured closed container
✓ Visually inspect the disposal container to ensure needle will fit
✓ Keep fingers away from the tip of the device when disposing, and avoid placing hands close to the opening of the container
✓ Check trays, linens and waste materials prior to handling for needles accidentally misplaced or left behind

Adapted from The American Nurses Association.[200]

---

manipulated either by hand or by any technique that involves directing the point of the needle towards any part of the body, unless the specific procedure requires recapping to be performed.

KEY POINTS

All professionals practising needle techniques must have been immunized against (or have immunity to) hepatitis B before practising. A review of hepatitis immunization is required in line with trust policy and the guidelines for safe practice.

Measures to be taken

- If you suffer an injury from a sharp which may be contaminated: encourage the wound

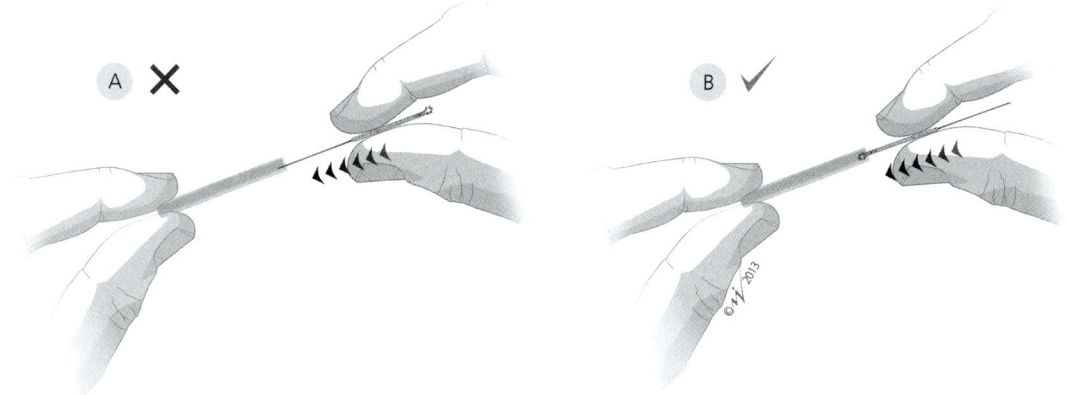

FIGURE 1.7 ■ Procedure for safe resheathing. (Colour version of figure is available online).

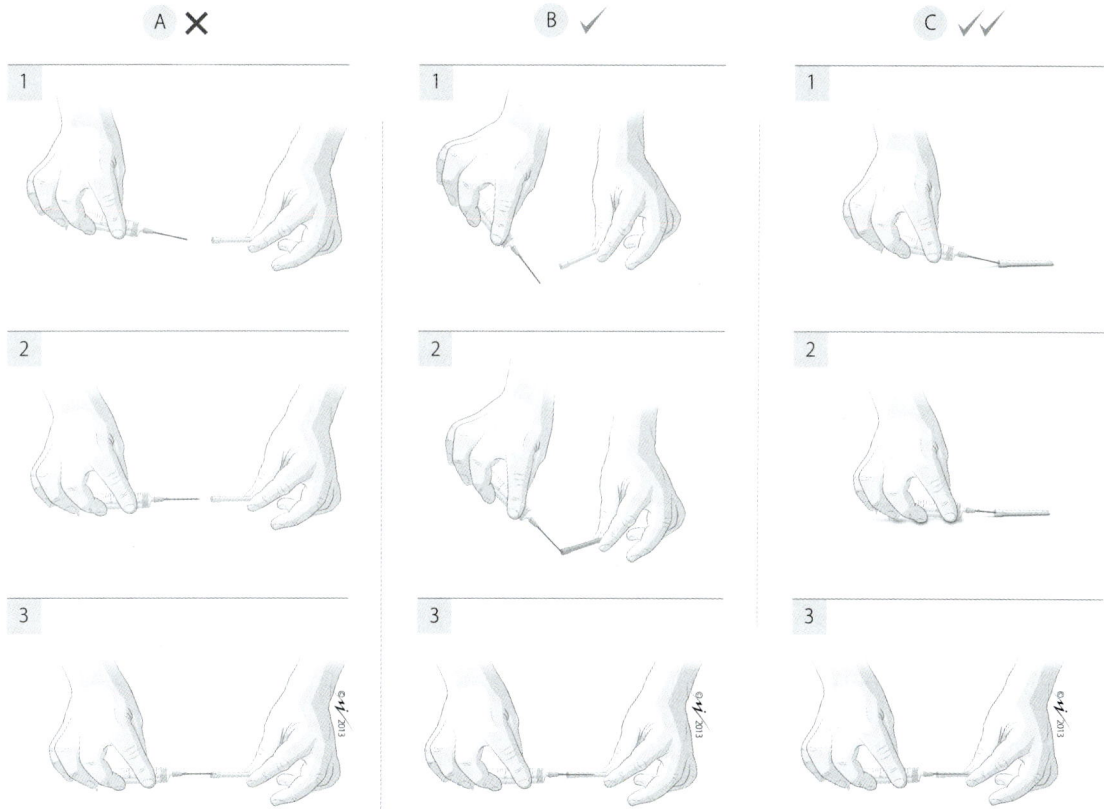

FIGURE 1.8 ■ Procedure for safe recapping. One-handed technique. (Colour version of figure is available online).

to bleed gently, ideally holding it under running water; wash the wound using running water and plenty of soap; don't scrub the wound whilst you are washing it; don't suck the wound, but dry it and cover with a waterproof plaster or dressing.

• Seek urgent medical advice (for example, from your Occupational Health Service) as effective prophylaxis (medicines to help fight infection) is available.

• Report the injury to your employer.

• Establish the need to administer postexposure prophylaxis for HIV and hepatitis B virus (HBV).[173] Postexposure prophylaxis for HCV is not indicated, as the administration of immunoglobulin and antiviral agents is not recommended for postexposure prophylaxis to blood that tests positive for HCV.

- In the case of exposure to HBV:
  - In non-vaccinated personnel: begin vaccination.
  - In vaccinated personnel (three doses): Appropriate antibody response (≥10 mIU/mL): vaccination not required. Non-appropriate antibody response (<10 mIU/mL): vaccination.
- The conventional anti-HB vaccine (Enger-ixB®) must be administered intramuscularly in the deltoid muscle as soon as possible within the first 24 hours. This must be administered together with anti-HB immunoglobulin but in different areas (deltoids: vaccine; gluteus: immunoglobulin).
- For exposure to HBV and HCV,[174] the professional does not need to take precautions to prevent secondary transmission during follow-up; however the affected clinician must avoid donating blood, semen, plasma, organs or tissues. The affected person does not need to modify sexual practices or avoid pregnancy. If a woman is breastfeeding, it is not necessary to stop.
- For exposure to HIV, antiretroviral pharmacological treatment must be administered as soon as possible, within the first 24 hours postexposure (ideally before the first 4 hours) and must be taken for 4 weeks if good tolerance is shown. Treatment should begin 48–72 hours after exposure.
- After exposure to HIV, the following measures must be practised,[175] especially in the first 6–12 weeks after exposure, when most people infected by HIV are expected to convert: sexual abstinence or use of condoms to prevent sexual transmission and avoidance of pregnancy, avoidance of the donation of blood, semen, organs, tissues and plasma. If a woman is breastfeeding, she should consider stopping due to the risk of transmission.
- Follow up the affected person on behalf of the service of preventive medicine or the corresponding specialist in infectious diseases.
- Investigate the circumstances of the accident and take measures to prevent recurrence. This may include a change in work practices, equipment and/or training of staff.

1.6.16 Allergic reactions

Allergic reactions are rare but may be related to the material of which the needles are made.

During the first treatment session, it is particularly important to observe the reaction around the needle insertion point.

Prevention strategies

- Check for known metal allergy, especially to stainless steel or nickel needles.
- Check for known silicone allergy if using silicone-coated needles, e.g. Seirin® (see chapter 2).

Measures to be taken

- If the skin becomes red, itchy and raised, remove the needles and review at a later date.
- If unsuccessful, seek medical help.

1.6.17 Anaphylactic shock

Anaphylactic shock is defined as a systemic type I hypersensitivity that occurs in individuals with specific immunological characteristics, resulting in mucocutaneous manifestations (hives, angio-oedema, itchiness, redness, conjunctivitis), cardiovascular manifestations (hypotension, vasodilation with secondary hypovolaemia, increase in capillary permeability which leads to the loss of intravascular volume, tachycardia, bradycardia, thoracic pain, syncope), respiratory manifestations (dyspnoea, laryngospasm, stridor, wheezing, rhinorrhoea, cough) and gastrointestinal manifestations (nausea, vomiting, dysphagia, diarrhoea, abdominal cramps) that may be life-threatening.

Of the five groups of allergens responsible for almost all cases of anaphylactic shock (anaesthetics and curares, *Hymenoptera* venom, antalgics, iodized products used for contrast and antibiotics), the most important for its use in infiltrations and mesotherapy is lidocaine.

Prevention strategies

- The clinical history must include questions directed at identifying previous anaphylactic episodes.
- In mesotherapy, homotoxicological drugs are recommended, as these are completely safe and do not cause potential anaphylactic shock responses.

Measures to be taken

- Patients who suffer from an anaphylactic reaction should be recognized and treated using the airway, breathing, circulation, disability, exposure (ABCDE) approach.[176]

- This represents a medical emergency. Treatment must be administered immediately.[177,178] Adrenaline is the medicine of first choice. Its properties correct the anomalies of the shock.
- Severe shock requires the use of adrenaline hydrochloride intravenously at a dose of 0.25–1 mg diluted in 10 mL of physiological solution applied very gradually.

Use of other medicines related to injection therapy practice

Adrenaline. There is provision within the Prescription Only Medicines (Human Use) Order 1997 (SI 1997/1830) – section 7[179] which allows any person to administer certain injectable medicines for the purpose of saving life in an emergency. There is therefore no need for a Patient Group Direction for the administration of adrenaline where a physiotherapist is employed by a Health Service Organization that has a formal written anaphylaxis policy in place, and the organization provides adrenaline for use by its staff in the event of an emergency.

1.6.18 Accidental cut

Accidental cuts can occur due to poor technique when opening a vial during the performance of infiltration or mesotherapy techniques.

Prevention strategies

- Do not open glass ampoules with bare hands. Protect fingers from cuts with a piece of gauze when opening ampoules.

Measures to be taken

- Disinfect the wound caused by the cut.
- Cover any cuts and put on non-sterile gloves before treatment.

1.6.19 Unexpected adverse reaction report form

Most published studies on adverse effects caused by invasive techniques are on the subject of acupuncture. For this reason, it is necessary to provide the professional with a tool (appendix 1) that can be used to document the complications, accidents and adverse effects as a consequence of treatment with invasive physiotherapy techniques.

In the international community, the Dry Needling Association in Switzerland or Seminarios Travell & Simons® (Spain) have a web-based registry for reporting adverse effects in dry needling, and MVClinic® (Spain) for PNE. Anonymous incident reports allow for the reporting of complications and serious adverse events.

1.7 MEDICAL WASTE MANAGEMENT

1.7.1 Concept

An infectious substance is a material known or reasonably expected to contain a pathogen. A pathogen is a microorganism (including bacteria, viruses, rickettsiae, parasites and fungi) or other agent, such as a proteinaceous infectious particle (prion), that can cause disease in humans or animals.

A dangerous waste product is any substance or object that is listed as a dangerous substance, as well as the containers in which they have been kept. It is the name given to products held to be dangerous by the local government according to what has been established in European bylaws or international agreements.

Regulated medical waste or clinical waste or (bio)medical waste means a waste or reusable material derived from the medical treatment of an animal or human, which includes diagnosis and immunization, or from biomedical research, which includes the production and testing of biological products.

According to current laws, used needles and sharp objects are considered regulated medical waste or clinical waste or (bio)medical waste and are potentially dangerous.

Sharps represent any object contaminated with a pathogen or that may become contaminated with a pathogen through handling or during transportation and that is also capable of cutting or penetrating the skin or the packaging material. Sharps includes needles, syringes (with or without the attached needles), scalpels, broken glass, culture slides, culture dishes, broken capillary tubes, broken rigid plastic and exposed ends of dental wire.

These products must abide by a series of safety measures during the processes of manipulation, collection, transport, treatment and elimination, as these represent risks for the professional, for public health and for the environment. The purpose of this process is to ensure the waste is disposed of appropriately, and this process is known as waste management.

Prior to managing waste, the authorization for producing biomedical waste is requested on behalf of the producer (e.g. centre, clinic, hospital) to the public administration.

1.7.2 Production authorizations

The performance of activities that produce biomedical waste products requires specific authorization on behalf of health authorities.

The producers of dangerous waste products are subject to the following standards:

- Waste products must be properly separated and dangerous waste products must not be mixed. Specifically, the mixing of products that may result in increased danger or handling difficulties must be avoided.
- The containers of dangerous waste products must be properly packaged and labelled according to the approved standards.
- A register of the dangerous waste products produced and imported must be maintained, as well as their final destination.
- Waste products must be delivered to a licensed medical waste company in order to manage the waste; the company must be supplied with the information necessary for the appropriate treatment and disposal of these waste products.
- Those who create waste are obliged to hand it over (if they cannot handle it themselves) to a waste management site for its assessment or disposal, and to sign a voluntary agreement or memorandum of understanding that lists these procedures. The organization is considered the medical waste generator and is responsible for the medical waste until it is destroyed, meaning that it must be stored in appropriate conditions of hygiene and safety.

Key Points

The abandonment, dumping or uncontrolled elimination of waste is prohibited, together with any mixing or dilution of the waste that impacts its handling.

The first point to consider regarding correct waste management is to reduce the amount of waste generated, i.e. waste minimization. Strict control of all that is acquired (and avoidance of the deterioration or expiry of the products or materials) should be practised, as, in the long term, this too will convert to waste.

1.7.3 Waste management

Waste management can be classified into two distinct processes:

1. Internal handling: this includes operations involving procedures such as manipulation, classification, packaging, labelling, collection, transport and storage within the workplace.
2. External handling: this involves collection, transport, treatment and disposal of the waste once it has been removed from the centre that generated the waste.

Handling

Below is a series of general instructions for the management of waste in order to guarantee safety and hygiene:

- Containers must always be kept closed and should only be opened for short periods, strictly for introducing the needles. Containers must have a safe access to the disposal opening.
- Containers should not be filled more than approximately 80% (three-quarters full) of capacity (the containers usually have a mark indicating the limit; figure 1.9). The containers should be checked routinely by staff and disposed of when they are three-quarters full. Once they are 80% full they must be closed and transported to the temporary storage space until they are collected.
- Containers that are in use must never be left in transit areas or places that can cause people to stumble, and must always be kept far away from any sources of heat.
- The sharps container must be accessible to professionals who use, maintain or dispose of sharps devices. There must be sufficient numbers of conveniently placed containers. A sharps container must be located in each procedure room.
- Proper selection (volume, number) and adequate use of sharps disposal containers are important to prevent needlestick injuries.
- Solid waste should never be compacted.
- General waste is defined as materials that have not been contaminated or visibly soiled with blood or other potentially infectious materials. General waste includes products such as paper towels used for drying hands and wrappers. General waste should be placed in a normal consumer bin bag, and the bag may be discarded in a regular waste receptacle.
- Medical waste is defined as materials that have been contaminated with blood or other potentially infectious materials. All used disposable sharp instruments, such as needles, syringes or broken glass, should be placed immediately in a sharps disposal container, despite the fact that sharps are now engineered with sharp injury

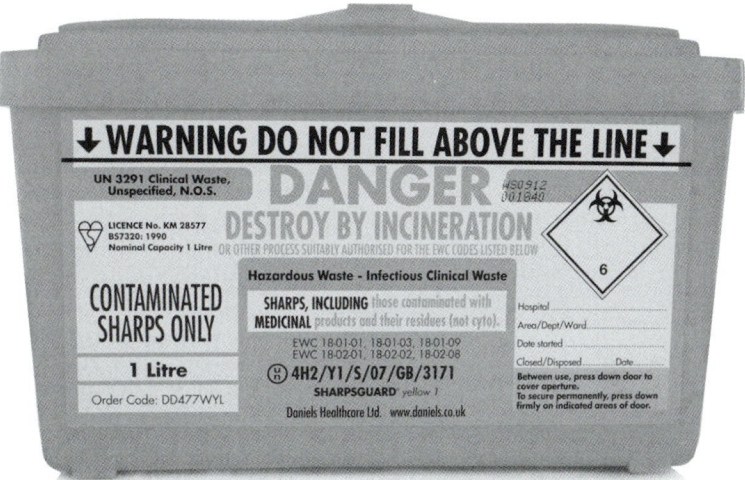

FIGURE 1.9 ■ Sharps container for the disposal of biosanitary waste. (Colour version of figure is available online).

protection features (safe syringes and needles) (see chapter 2). Medical waste, such as gloves, swabs, guide tubes, dressing, cotton wool or gauze used to clean the area, whether or not stained with blood, must be placed in a suitable clinical waste bag. Waste products must not be mixed together.

- The sharps container should be readily accessible and located as close as possible to the patient care or work area.
- Body fluids in small amounts, such as blood in a withdrawn syringe, may be discarded in a sharps container.

KEY POINTS

Used needles and sharp objects must be disposed of in a sharps container and the remaining medical waste in a clinical waste bag.

Medical waste disposal or sharps container

- Sharps containers must be made of rigid polypropylene (thermoplastic material). These are durable yellow containers that are impervious, leak-proof, puncture- and shock-resistant and resistant to solvents (figure 1.9) under all normal environmental conditions.
- When selecting the type of container, consider the volume of waste generated and the space available for temporary storage in the physiotherapy service within the clinic, centre or hospital. All containers must present the approved CE marking or licence.

Labelling

- Dangerous waste containers must be clearly labelled, with legible and indelible writing, at least in the official state language.
- The outer packaging must bear the company name of the manufacturer or distributor, a container ID number (or unique model number), a display of the international biohazard symbol with either a fluorescent orange or fluorescent red background, as shown in figure 1.9, and the words 'Regulated Medical Waste-Sharps, UN 3291 or Regulated Medical Waste, UN 3291' noted on the package.
- Also, the sharps container must include a tag that contains a complete identification of the sender and the destination, including an emergency phone number in case the package is damaged during transport.

Collection

The frequency of waste collection depends on the volume generated and is established based on local laws and regulations.

In centres that only generate sharps waste in quantities of less than 3 kg per month, the collection can be quarterly.

Transport of special biomedical waste

Transport will be performed in accordance with local jurisdictional policies and procedures. The handover of waste from the producer to the transporter must be accompanied by follow-up and control documents.

Whatever method is used, all final disposal methods should be made complying with the state and local regulations.

Destruction

Medical waste disposal or the sharps container should be incinerated via a licensed medical waste company or needle collection service, or disposed of according to local regulations.

1.8 INFORMED CONSENT

1.8.1 Concept

The WCPT within its Declaration of Principles (1995)[180] establishes informed consent as a standard of good practice, in the same way as the CSP[118] and the European region of the WCPT do in the document on *European Core Standards of Physiotherapy Practice*,[104] dating from 2005 and 2008, respectively.

This constitutes the recognition of the moral right that each person has to participate freely and validly, manifesting their approval of the attention received. This is a basic right of patients, together with the right to information and the recognition and confidentiality of health information regarding the patient.

1.8.2 Conditions

The key points to consider when seeking informed consent are as follows[181,182]:

- Informed consent must be voluntarily signed, without any pressure or influence exercised by the professional, family member or friend.
- It must be obtained *prior* to commencing treatment.
- The information regarding the technique must be provided in an appropriate format and language.
- Consider patients' age, emotional state and cognitive abilities. For example, in people aged under 18, consent must be provided by the father, mother or guardian, or in people with cognitive deficiencies such as Down's syndrome.
- The treatment options, including the benefits, risks and collateral effects, must be

explained to the patient. For example, in the application of PNE techniques, the patient must be informed of the effectiveness of the technique as well as the minimal risk of suffering an alkaline burn.

- Patients must be granted the opportunity to ask any questions they may have. The patient must be given enough time to read and understand the information and must be granted several opportunities to ask questions.
- Patients must be informed of their right to refuse the physiotherapy care at any time, without affecting their future care.
- If the patient refuses treatment, this must be registered in the patient's notes, together with the reasons for this, if known.
- In hospitals or university clinics, patients must be reminded that they may be treated by a student of physiotherapy or physiotherapy assistant, and they must be granted the possibility of refusing this option and being treated by a fully qualified physiotherapist.
- Patients must be informed that their treatment may be observed by a student, and they must be given the opportunity to refuse this option.
- The patient's consent for the treatment plan must be noted within the person's clinical records.
- When possible, patients must be provided with information leaflets regarding the technique, in order to help inform the consent process.
- All information provided to the patient must be filed in the person's clinical history. For example, a copy of the signed consent form and the leaflet describing the technique should be filed if these are used.

1.8.3 Informed consent form

The informed consent form and checklist (figure 1.10) are used in the consent process to help

INFORMED CONSENT CHECKLIST FORM FOR ACUPUNCTURE

PATIENT'S NAME	
DIAGNOSIS	
PREVIOUS TREATMENT	

INFORMED CONSENT CHECKLIST

EXPLANATION

Treatment procedure of needle insertion
Stimulation of needle (manual, electrical)
Transient symptoms (fatigue, faint, temporary aggravation)
Warned not to drive immediately after treatment if fatigued

CAUTIONS/CONTRA-INDICATIONS	Yes	No
Pregnant	☐	☐
Allergies	☐	☐
Systemic steroids	☐	☐
Anti-coagulants/blood clotting disorders	☐	☐
History of seizures	☐	☐
Diabetes	☐	☐
Low blood pressure	☐	☐
Swelling/tumour or infection (no needle)	☐	☐
Pacemaker (no electro-acupuncture)	☐	☐
Needle phobia	☐	☐
Exhibiting uncontrolled movement	☐	☐
Patient confused	☐	☐
Atrial fibrillation/heart	☐	☐
Has the patient eaten?	☐	☐

PARTICULAR NOTES

THERAPIST'S SIGNATURE   PRINT NAME   DATE

PATIENTS' CONSENT   PRINT NAME

FIGURE 1.10 ■ Checklist for acupuncture treatment. (Adapted from Randal G. & Collins R.[201]).

HCWs to inform patients and as a record of consent given. The completion of the form is just one part of the consent process and it should be completed only after an appropriate full explanation of the procedure is provided, with discussion and time for reflection by those consenting. All parts are equally important. In this sense, HCWs must be trained in how to obtain valid consent.

In the appendices, several examples of consent forms for invasive techniques are provided. These forms offer a suggested format and may be adapted as necessary for local needs, provided they comply with the local regulations, settings and codes of practice. If a standardized consent form already exists, that has been agreed on by the Department of Health Services and Public Safety or by associations, HCWs should use this.

1.9 COST-EFFECTIVENESS OF INVASIVE TECHNIQUES

The rationalization and optimization of health-care resources are among the most important aspects for the viability of health systems in the West. It is increasingly important for health interventions financed by the national health systems of different countries to consider the quality, effectiveness and cost derived from the use of these resources.

An increasing number of studies have analysed the cost-effectiveness of invasive techniques; mainly these are focused on acupuncture. Studies by Witt et al.[183,184] and Wonderling et al.[185] reached the conclusion that acupuncture it is an effective technique as far as costs are concerned. These authors found that acupuncture treatments required smaller amounts of analgesic and anti-inflammatory drugs during the following 6 months,[186] thus reducing referral to secondary care.[187] A study by Taylor et al.[188] concluded that, according to WHO cost-effectiveness threshold values, acupuncture is a cost-effective treatment strategy for patients with chronic low-back pain. In the same manner, a systematic review of cost-effectiveness analyses by Kim et al.[189] indicated that all cost–utility analyses showed that acupuncture with or without usual care was cost-effective compared with waiting-list control or usual care alone in dysmenorrhoea, allergic rhinitis, osteoarthritis and headache. In the cost-effectiveness analysis, acupuncture was beneficial at a relatively low cost in six European and Asian studies.

A recent systematic review of the literature[26] suggests that physiotherapists working in extended-scope practice roles within orthopaedic settings may be comparable with medical doctors in terms of clinical decision making, and may improve the efficiency of outpatient management pathways with higher levels of patient satisfaction.[190] Harrison et al.[191] in the UK and Morris et al.[192] in Australia reported the cost of an extended-scope practice by physiotherapists, resulting in a decrease in costs.

Specifically in the case of epicondylalgias,[193] carpal tunnel syndrome,[194,195] frozen shoulder,[196] subacromial impingement syndrome[197] and whiplash,[198] PNE, dry needling and injection therapy have been demonstrated to have a good cost-effectiveness relation in comparison to surgical intervention and other interventions.

In general, professionals who commonly use these techniques[199] agree that these are more effective and they reduce the number of sessions needed to improve patient functionality.

1.10 REFERENCES

1. World Confederation for Physical Therapy. WCPT guideline for physical therapist professional entry level education. London, UK: WCPT; 2011. Available at: <http://www.wcpt.org/guidelines/entry-level-education>; [Accessed 1 Jul 2014].
2. American Physical Therapy Association. Normative model of physical therapist professional education. Washington DC, USA: APTA; 2004.
3. European Region of the World Confederation for Physical Therapy. European physiotherapy benchmark statement. Brussels, Belgium: ER-WCPT; 2003. Available at: <http://www.physio-europe.org/index.php?action=80>; [Accessed 1 Jul 2014].
4. World Confederation for Physical Therapy. Policy statement: Physical therapist practice specialisation. London, UK: WCPT; 2011. Available at: <www.wcpt.org/policy/ps-specialisation>; [Accessed 1 Jul 2014].
5. World Confederation for Physical Therapy. WCPT guideline for qualifications of faculty for physical therapist professional entry level programmes. London, UK: WCPT; 2011. Available at: <www.wcpt.org/guidelines/faculty-qualifications>; [Accessed 1 Jul 2014].
6. Libro blanco del título de grado en fisioterapia. Available at <http://www.unex.es/unex/oficinas/oce/documentos/libroblanco/fisioterapia>; [Accessed 1 Jul 2014].
7. Chartered Society of Physiotherapy. Policy statement on continuing professional development (CPD). London, UK: CSP; 2007. Available at: <http://www.csp.org.uk/uploads/documents/csp_policy_statement_2007.pdf>; [Accessed 1 Jul 2014].
8. Hayhurst C. A vision to transform society. PT in Motion 2014;6(2):20–6.
9. World Confederation for Physical Therapy. Policy statement: Description of physical therapy. London, UK: WCPT; 2011. Available at: <http://www.wcpt.org/policy/ps-descriptionPT>; [Accessed 1 Jul 2014].
10. Mayoral O. Fisioterapia invasiva del síndrome de dolor miofascial. Fisioterapia 2005;27(2):69–75.
11. Valera-Garrido F, Minaya-Muñoz F. Fisioterapia Invasiva. Barcelona: Elsevier; 2013.
12. Melchart D, Linde K, Fischer P, et al. Acupuncture for idiopathic headache. Cochrane Database Syst Rev 2001;(1):CD001218, Review. Update in: Cochrane Database Syst Rev. 2009;(1):CD001218.
13. Kietrys DM, Palombaro KM, Azzaretto E, et al. Effectiveness of dry needling for upper-quarter myofascial pain: a systematic review and meta-analysis. J Orthop Sports Phys Ther 2013;43(9):620–34.
14. NIH Consensus Conference. Acupuncture. JAMA 1998;280(17):1518–24.
15. Furlan AD, van Tulder M, Cherkin D, et al. Acupuncture and dry-needling for low back pain: an updated systematic review within the framework of the cochrane collaboration. Spine (Phila Pa 1976) 2005;30(8):944–63.
16. Finocchio LJ, Dower CM, McMahon T, et al. Reforming Health Care Workforce Regulation: Policy Considerations for the 21st Century. San Francisco, CA: Pew Health Professions Commission; 1995.

17. Australian standards for physiotherapy. Canberra, ACT: Australian Physiotherapy Council; 2009.

18. Dean E. Physical Therapy Practice in the 21st Century: A New Evidence-informed Paradigm and Implications'. Foreword from the special issue editor. Physiother Theory Pract 2009;25(5–6):328–9.

19. Dean E. Physical therapy in the 21st century (Part I): toward practice informed by epidemiology and the crisis of lifestyle conditions. Physiother Theory Pract 2009;25(5–6):330–53.

20. Dean E. Physical therapy in the 21st century (Part II): evidence-based practice within the context of evidence-informed practice. Physiother Theory Pract 2009; 25(5–6):354–68.

21. Kersten P, McPherson K, Lattimer V, et al. Physiotherapy extended scope of practice – who is doing what and why? Physiotherapy 2007;93(4):235–42.

22. The Chartered Society of Physiotherapy. Chartered Physiotherapists Working as Extended Scope Practitioners (ESP): Guidance for members. London, UK: The Chartered Society of Physiotherapy; 2003.

23. Lowe J, Prior M. A systematic review of the literature on extended scope of practice physiotherapy. Canberra, Australia: ACT Government Health Directorate: ACT Government; 2008. Available at: <http://www.health .act.gov.au/c/health?a=sendfile&ft=p&fid=1378078168 &sid=>; [Accessed 1 Jul 2014].

24. Stanhope J, Beaton K, Grimmer-Somers K, et al. The role of extended scope physiotherapists in managing patients with inflammatory arthropathies: a systematic review. Open Access Rheumatology: Research and Reviews 2012;4:49–55. Available at: <http://www .dovepress.com/the-role-of-extended-scope-physio therapists-in-managing-patients-with–peer-reviewed -article-OARRR>; [Accessed 1 Jul 2014].

25. Morris J, Grimmer K, Gilmore L, et al. Principles to guide sustainable implementation of extended-scope-of-practice physiotherapy workforce redesign initiatives in Australia: stakeholder perspectives, barriers, supports, and incentives. J Multidiscip Healthc 2014;7: 249–58.

26. Stanhope J, Grimmer-Somers K, Milanese S, et al. Extended scope physiotherapy roles for orthopedic outpatients: an update systematic review of the literature. J Multidiscip Healthc 2012;5:37–45.

27. Suckley J. Core clinical competencies for extended-scope physiotherapists working in musculoskeletal (Msk) interface clinics based in primary care: a Delphi consensus study. PhD thesis. University of Salford, College of Health and Social Care School of Nursing, Midwifery and Social Work, UK; 2012.

28. Australian Physiotherapy Association (APA). Scope of Practice [position statement]. Victoria: Melbourne: Australian Physiotherapy Association; 2009. Available at: <http://www.physiotherapy.asn.au/Documents Folder/Advocacy_Position_Scope_of_Practice_2009 .pdf>; [Accessed 1 Jul 2014].

29. World Confederation for Physical Therapy. WCPT Glossary: Terms used in WCPT's policies and resources. London, UK: WCPT; 2014. Available at: <http://www.wcpt.org/sites/wcpt.org/files/files/ WCPT_glossary2014_version2_1.pdf>; [Accessed 20 Jul 2014].

30. Thompson M. The role of higher education in the career paths of board-certified clinical specialists in geriatric physical therapy: implications for professional and post professional education. J Phys Ther Educ 2001;15(2):10–16.

31. Smith LC. The decision to specialize: Accounts of nine board-certified specialists. PT Magazine 2001;9(6): 52–9.

32. Conrad S. Taking on the specialist certification exam – and winning. Perspectives for new professionals of the American Physical Therapy Association. 2013.

33. World Confederation for Physical Therapy. Policy statement: Specialisation. London, UK: WCPT; 2011. Available at: <www.wcpt.org/policy/ps-specialisation>; [Accessed 1 Jul 2014].

34. Sibbald B, Shen J, McBride A. Changing the skill-mix of the health care workforce. J Health Serv Res Policy 2004;9(Suppl. 1):28–38.

35. Atkins E. Physiotherapists' experience of implementing their injection therapy skills. Physiotherapy 2003;89(3): 145–57.

36. Canadian Physiotherapy Association. Scope of practice. Ontario, Canada: CPA Practice and Research Department; 2010 (Revised April 2012). Available at: <http:// www.physiotherapy.ca/getmedia/e2541bbc-f95d-4d8b -b689-98365bc4abbd/Scope-of-Practice_EN.pdf .aspx>; [Accessed 1 Jul 2014].

37. Canadian Alliance of Physiotherapy Regulators. Analysis of practice 2008: a report on physiotherapists' practice in Canada [Internet]. Toronto: The Alliance; 2008. Available from: <http://www.alliancept.org/pdfs/ AnalysisOfPractice2008.pdf>; [cited 2011 Mar 30].

38. The Chartered Society of Physiotherapy (CSP). Scope of physiotherapy practice. London, UK; 2008. Available at: <http://www.csp.org.uk/publications/scope -physiotherapy-practice-2008>; [Accessed 1 Jul 2014].

39. The Chartered Society of Physiotherapy. Royal Charter granted by King George V dated 9 Jun 1920.

40. Association of Social Work Boards (ASWB), Federation of State Boards of Physical Therapy (FSBPT), Federation of State Medical Boards (FSMB), National Board for Certification in Occupational Therapy (NBCOT), National Council of State Boards of Nursing (NCSBN) & National Association of Boards of Pharmacy (NABP). Changes in healthcare professions' scope of practice: Legislative considerations. 2006 (revised 2009). Available at: <https://www.ncsbn .org/ScopeofPractice_09.pdf>; [Accessed 1 Jul 2014].

41. Newhouse RP, Stanik-Hutt J, White KM, et al. Advanced practice nurse outcomes 1990–2008: a systematic review. Nurs Econ 2011;29(5):230–50, quiz 251.

42. Venning P, Durie A, Roland M, et al. Randomised controlled trial comparing cost effectiveness of general practitioners and nurse practitioners in primary care. BMJ 2000;320(7241):1048–53.

43. World Health Organization. WHO Nursing and Midwives Progress Report 2008-2012. 2013. Available at: <http://www.who.int/hrh/nursing_midwifery/ NursingMidwiferyProgressReport.pdf>; [Accessed 1 Jul 2014].

44. Iglehart JK. Expanding the role of advanced nurse practitioners–risks and rewards. N Engl J Med 2013; 368(20):1935–41.

45. Williams CD, Short B. ACR and ASRT development of the radiologist assistant: concept, roles, and responsibilities. J Am Coll Radiol 2004;1(6):392–7.

46. Needle JJ, Petchey R, Lawrenson JG. A survey of the scope of therapeutic practice by UK optometrists and their attitudes to an extended prescribing role. Ophthalmic Physiol Opt 2008;28(3):193–203.

47. Shankaran V, Brooks M, Mostow E. Advanced therapies for chronic wounds: NPWT, engineered skin, growth factors, extracellular matrices. Dermatol Ther 2013;26(3):215–21.

48. Desmeules F, Roy JS, MacDermid JC, et al. Advanced practice physiotherapy in patients with musculoskeletal disorders: a systematic review. BMC Musculoskelet Disord 2012;13:107.

49. American Physical Therapist Association. Guidelines: Physical Therapist Scope of Practice. 2014. Available at: <https://www.apta.org/uploadedFiles/APTAorg/About_Us/Policies/Practice/ScopePractice.pdf>; [Accessed 1 Jul 2014].

50. American Physical Therapist Association. Guide to Physical Therapist Practice. Second edition. Phys Ther 2001;81:9–744.

51. Australian Physiotherapy Council. Feedback on the Consultation Paper: Proposed Acupuncture Accreditation Standard (Stage 2) [Internet]. Melbourne; 2011. Available at: <http://www.physiotherapy.asn.au/APAWCM/Advocacy_P/Submissions/submission%20-%20stage%202%20proposed%20acupuncture%20accreditation.pdf>; [Accessed 1 Jul 2014].

52. Dommerholt J, Mayoral-del-Moral O, Gröbli C. Trigger point dry needling. J Man Manip Ther 2006;14(4):70E–87E.

53. Pan Devon PGD Development Group. Patient Group Direction 5.01 version 3.0 Administration of Botulinum Toxin A (Botox®) by Specialist Neurological Physiotherapists. 2014. Available at: <http://www.torbaycaretrust.nhs.uk/publications/TSDHC/PGD%20Botulinum%20Toxin%20(Botox).pdf>; [Accessed 1 Jul 2014] [Internet].

54. Convention on the Recognition of Qualifications concerning Higher Education in the European Region CETS No.: 165. [Internet]. Available at: <http://conventions.coe.int/Treaty/Commun/QueVoulezVous.asp?NT=165&CM=8&DF=10/17/2007&CL=ENG>; [Accessed 1 Jul 2014].

55. Lisbon Recognition Convention. Council of Europe. Convention on the recognition of qualifications concerning higher education in the European region. European Treaty Series – No. 165. Brussels, Belgium: Council of Europe; 1997.

56. Canadian Physiotherapy Association. Acupuncture and the Use of Dry Needling Techniques in Physiotherapy. [Internet]. Available at: <http://www.physiotherapy.ca/getmedia/531a0158-a8b0-4553-8dbf-b87d72082e58/Acupuncture-and-the-Use-of-Dry-Needling-Techniques-in-Physiotherapy_en-doc.pdf.aspx>; [Accessed 1 Jul 2014].

57. Araujo, João Eduardo de. About the rights of practicing acupuncture in Brazil. Rev Bras Fisioter 2012;16(4):V–VI.

58. World Health Organization. Guidelines on basic training and safety in acupuncture. 1999. Available online at: <http://whqlibdoc.who.int/hq/1999/WHO_EDM_TRM_99.1.pdf>.

59. Hopwood V, Lovesey M, Mokone S. Acupuncture and related techniques in physical therapy. Singapore: Churchill Livingstone; 1997.

60. International Association of Acupuncture of Physical Therapists (IAAPT). Standards of Safe Acupuncture Practice by Physiotherapists. 1999 (revised 2003). Available at: <http://www.wcpt.org/sites/wcpt.org/files/files/private/iaapt/IAAPT-secure-Safety_Standards_for_IAAPT-June_2003.pdf>; [Accessed 1 Jul 2014].

61. Australian Society of Acupuncture Physiotherapists (ASAP). Guidelines for Safe Acupuncture and Dry Needling Practice. 2013. Available at: <http://www.dryneedling.com.au/wp-content/uploads/2013/08/ASAP_Guidelines_2013.pdf>.

62. Paris SV. A history of manipulative therapy through the ages and up to the current controversy in the United States. J Manual Manip Ther 2000;8(2):66–77.

63. Mayor DF. Electroacupuncture: an introduction and its use for peripheral facial paralysis. J Chin Med 2007;84:52–63. Available at: <http://www.jcm.co.uk/media/cms/File/JCM84_electro.pdf>; [Accessed 1 Jul 2014].

64. Brady S, McEvoy J, Dommerholt J, et al. Adverse events following trigger point dry needling: a prospective survey of chartered physiotherapists. J Man Manip Ther 2014;22(3):134–40.

65. American Academy of Orthopaedic Manual Physical Therapists (AAOMPT). 'AAOMPT Position Statements – Dry Needling.' Retrieved 2/3/2011. 2009. Available at: <http://www.aaompt.org/about/statements.cfm>; [Accessed 1 Jul 2014].

66. Rainey CE. The use of trigger point dry needling and intramuscular electrical stimulation for a subject with chronic low back pain: a case report. Int J Sports Phys Ther 2013;8(2):145–61.

67. White PF, Craig WF, Vakharia AS, et al. Percutaneous neuromodulation therapy: does the location of electrical stimulation effect the acute analgesic response? Anesth Analg 2000;91(4):949–54.

68. Ghoname EA, Craig WF, White PF, et al. Percutaneous electrical nerve stimulation for low back pain: a randomized crossover study. JAMA 1999;281(9):818–23. Erratum in: JAMA 1999;281(19):1795.

69. Ghoname EA, White PF, Ahmed HE, et al. Percutaneous electrical nerve stimulation: an alternative to TENS in the management of sciatica. Pain 1999;83(2):193–9.

70. Nagraba Ł, Tuchalska J, Mitek T, et al. Dry needling as a method of tendinopathy treatment. Ortop Traumatol Rehabil 2013;15(2):109–16.

71. Rha DW, Park GY, Kim YK, et al. Comparison of the therapeutic effects of ultrasound-guided platelet-rich plasma injection and dry needling in rotator cuff disease: a randomized controlled trial. Clin Rehabil 2013;27(2):113–22.

72. Dragoo JL, Wasterlain AS, Braun HJ, et al. Platelet-rich plasma as a treatment for patellar tendinopathy: a double-blind, randomized controlled trial. Am J Sports Med 2014;42(3):610–18.

73. James SL, Ali K, Pocock C, et al. Ultrasound guided dry needling and autologous blood injection for patellar tendinosis. Br J Sports Med 2007;41(8):518–21, discussion 522.

74. Moraes VY, Lenza M, Tamaoki MJ, et al. Platelet-rich therapies for musculoskeletal soft tissue injuries. Cochrane Database Syst Rev 2014;4:CD010071.

75. McShane JM, Shah VN, Nazarian LN. Sonographically guided percutaneous needle tenotomy for treatment of common extensor tendinosis in the elbow: is a corticosteroid necessary? J Ultrasound Med 2008;27(8):1137–44.

76. Housner JA, Jacobson JA, Misko R. Sonographically guided percutaneous needle tenotomy for the treatment of chronic tendinosis. J Ultrasound Med 2009;28(9):1187–92.

77. American Physical Therapy Association. Physical Therapists and the performance of dry needling – An educational resource paper. Alexandria, VA: APTA; 2012. Available at: <http://www.apta.org/StateIssues/DryNeedling/ResourcePaper/>; [Accessed 1 Jul 2014].

78. American Physical Therapy Association. Clinical practice educational resource paper. Alexandria, VA: APTA; 2013. Available at: <http://www.apta.org/StateIssues/DryNeedling/ClinicalPracticeResourcePaper/>; [Accessed 1 Jul 2014].

79. Federation of State Boards of Physical Therapy (FSBPT). Dry needling resource paper (Intramuscular manual therapy). 4th ed. 2013. Available at: <https://www.fsbpt.org/download/DryNeedlingResourcePaper_4thEdition.pdf>; [Accessed 1 Jul 2014].

80. Dommerholt J, Fernández-de-las-Peñas C. Trigger point dry needling. An evidence and clinical-based approach. Edinburgh: Churchill Livingstone, Elsevier; 2013.

81. Hobbs V. Dry needling and acupuncture emerging professional issues, in Qi Unity Report. Sacramento: AAAOM; 2007.

82. American Physical Therapy Association. Manipulation Education Committee. Manipulation education manual for physical therapist professional degree programs. Alexandria, VA: APTA; 2004. Available at: <http://www.apta.org/uploadedFiles/APTAorg/Educators/Curriculum_Resources/APTA/Manipulation/ManipulationEducationManual.pdf>; [Accessed 1 Jul 2014].

83. Valera-Garrido F, Minaya-Muñoz F, Medina-Mirapeix F. Ultrasound-guided percutaneous needle electrolysis in chronic lateral epicondylitis: short-term and long-term results. Acupunct Med 2014;32(6):446–54. Available at: <http://aim.bmj.com/content/early/2014/08/13/acupmed-2014-010619.full?rss=1>; [Accessed 12 April 2015].

84. The Chartered Society of Physiotherapy (CSP). Clinical guideline for the use of injection therapy by physiotherapists. London, UK; 1999.

85. The Chartered Society of Physiotherapy (CSP). The use of medicines in physiotherapy injection-therapy in NHS settings. 3rd Edition (Formerly 'Mixing of medicines in physiotherapy practice.' Issued March 2008). London, UK: 2010. Available at: <http://www.acpom-it.co.uk/wp-content/uploads/2012/04/UseOfMedicinesInInjectionTherapy-CspGuidance.pdf>; [Accessed 1 Jul 2014].

86. Saunders S. Advanced in injection therapy for physiotherapist. The Chartered Society of Physiotherapy Annual Congress 2008. Manchester, UK; 2008.

87. Chambers I, Hide G, Bayliss N. An audit of accuracy and efficacy of injections for subacromial impingement comparing consultant, registrar and physiotherapist. J Bone Joint Surg Br Orthopaedic Proceedings 2005; 87-B:160.

88. Saunders S, Longworth S. Injection Techniques in Orthopaedics and Sports Medicine with CD-ROM: A practical manual for doctors and physiotherapists. 3rd ed. Oxford, UK: Churchill Livingstone; 2006.

89. Smith G. Review of steroid-only injection therapy clinics performed by a physiotherapist working in primary care. Int Musculoskelet Med 2011;33(2):61–3.

90. Birchall D, Ismail AM, Peat G. Clinical outcomes from a physiotherapist-led intra-articular hyaluronic acid injection clinic. Musculoskeletal Care 2008;6(3):135–49.

91. Kuipers K, Cox R, Doherty D, et al. The process of developing a non-medical (advanced allied health) botulinum toxin A prescribing and injecting model of care in a public rehabilitation setting. Aust Health Rev 2013;37(5):624–31.

92. Kim DS, Jeong TY, Kim YK, et al. Usefulness of a myofascial trigger point injection for groin pain in patients with chronic prostatitis/chronic pelvic pain syndrome: a pilot study. Arch Phys Med Rehabil 2013;94(5):930–6.

93. Lee SJ, Ahn DH, Jung JH, et al. Short-term change of handgrip strength after trigger point injection in women with muscular pain in the upper extremities. Ann Rehabil Med 2014;38(2):241–8.

94. Shin HJ, Shin JC, Kim WS, et al. Application of ultrasound-guided trigger point injection for myofascial trigger points in the subscapularis and pectoralis muscles to post-mastectomy patients: a pilot study. Yonsei Med J 2014;55(3):792–9.

95. Entry-to-Practice Physiotherapy Curriculum. Content Guidelines for Canadian University Programs. A Council of Canadian Physiotherapy University Programs publication©, produced by HealthQuest Consulting in association with the Canadian Physiotherapy Association, the Canadian Alliance of Physiotherapy Regulators, and the Accreditation Council of Canadian Physiotherapy Academic Programs. 2009.

96. The Chartered Society of Physiotherapy (CSP). Learning and development principles for CSP accreditation of qualifying programmes in physiotherapy. London, UK; 2012. Available at: <http://www.csp.org.uk/sites/files/csp/secure/ld_principles.pdf>; [Accessed 1 Jul 2014].

97. American Physical Therapy Association. A normative model of physical therapist professional education: Version 2000. Alexandria, VA: APTA; 2000.

98. Australian Health Practitioner Regulation Agency. Approved programs of study. 2013. Available at: <http://www.ahpra.gov.au/Education/Approved-Programs-of-Study.aspx?ref=Physiotherapist>; [Accessed 1 Jul 2014].

99. McMeeken JM. Celebrating a shared past, planning a shared future: physiotherapy in Australia and New Zealand. New Zealand J Physiother 2014;42(1):1–8.

100. European Region of the World Confederation for Physical Therapy. European physiotherapy benchmark statement. Barcelona, Spain; 2003. Available at: <http://www.physio-europe.org/download.php?document=51&downloadarea=6>; [Accessed 1 Jul 2014].

101. Physiotherapy in Clinical Specialties II. Universidad de San Jorge. [Internet]. Available at: <http://gdweb.usj.es/VRhtml.php?plan=13&idGuia=2089&idAsig=30387&nd=1&anyo=2013-14&version=4.0>; [Accessed 20 Jul 2014].

102. Entry-level physiotherapy program. Universidad San Pablo CEU. [Internet]. Available at: <http://www.uspceu.com/es/estudios/grado/medicina/fisioterapia/plan-de-estudios.php>; [Accessed 20 Jul 2014].

103. Health Professions Council (UK). Standards of Proficiency – Physiotherapists. 2003 (revised 2007, 2013). Available at: <https://www.hcpc-uk.org/assets/documents/10000DBCStandards_of_Proficiency_Physiotherapists.pdf>; [Accessed 20 Jul 2014].

104. European Region of World Confederation for Physical Therapy. European core standards of physiotherapy practice. Brussels, Belgium: ER-WCPT; 2008. Available at: <http://www.physio-europe.org/download.php?document=71&downloadarea=6>; [Accessed 20 Jul 2014].

105. American Physical Therapy Association. Standards of practice for physical therapy. Alexandria, VA: APTA; 2013. Available at: <https://www.apta.org/uploadedFiles/APTAorg/About_Us/Policies/Practice/StandardsPractice.pdf>; [Accessed 20 Jul 2014].

106. The Chartered Society of Physiotherapy (CSP). Quality Assurance Standards for physiotherapy service delivery. London, UK; 2013. Available at: <http://www.csp.org.uk/sites/files/csp/secure/csp_quality_assurance_standards.pdf>; [Accessed 1 Jul 2014].

107. World Confederation for Physical Therapy. WCPT guideline for standards of physical therapy practice. London, UK: WCPT; 2011. Available at: <http://www.wcpt.org/sites/wcpt.org/files/files/Guideline_standards_practice_complete.pdf>; [Accessed 1 Jul 2014].

108. New Zealand Society of Physiotherapists. Standards of physiotherapy practice. Wellington, New Zealand; 2006.

109. Consejo General de Colegios de Fisioterapeutas de España (CGCFE). Resolución 05/11. Punción Seca. Madrid, España; 2011. Available at: <http://www

.consejo-fisioterapia.org/images/Resolucin_05-2011 _Aprobado_AG_19-11-2011_Puncin_Seca.pdf>; [Accessed 1 Jul 2014].

110. Stephans EB. Manipulative therapy in physical therapy curricula. Phys Ther 1973;53:40–50.

111. Australian Society of Acupuncture Physiotherapist. Guidelines for safe acupuncture and dry needling practice. 2013. Available at: <http://www .dryneedling.com.au/wp-content/uploads/2013/08/ ASAP_Guidelines_2013.pdf>; [Accessed 1 Jul 2014].

112. World Confederation for Physical Therapy. Ethical principles. London, UK: WCPT; 2011. Available at: <http://www.wcpt.org/ethical-principles>; [Accessed 1 Jul 2014].

113. Tribunal Constitucional de España. Sentencia 187/ 1991, de 3 de octubre de 1991. Available at: <http:// hj.tribunalconstitucional.es/HJ/es-ES/Resolucion/ Show/SENTENCIA/1991/187>; [Accessed 1 Jul 2014].

114. Tribunal Constitucional de España. Sentencia 155/1997, de 29 de septiembre de 1997. Available at: <http://hj.tribunalconstitucional.es/HJ/es-ES/ Resolucion/Show/3420>; [Accessed 1 Jul 2014].

115. Bachmann S, Colla F, Gröbli C, et al. Swiss Guidelines for safe Dry Needling. 2014. Available at: <http://www .dryneedling.ch/fileadmin/documents/Richtlinien _fu__r_sicheres_Dry_Needling_Engl_1.6.pdf>; [Accessed 20 Jul 2014].

116. Torbay and Southern Devon Health and Care NHS Trust and South Devon Healthcare NHS Trust. Physiotherapy Acupuncture Policy. Guidelines for safe, effective, evidence based practice. UK; 2013. Available at: <http://www.torbaycaretrust.nhs.uk/publications/ TSDHC/Acupuncture%20Policy.pdf>; [Accessed 20 Jul 2014].

117. Association of Paediatric Chartered Physiotherapists. Evidence-based guidance for physiotherapists. The use of botulinum toxin in children with neurological conditions. Available at: <http://www.csp.org.uk/sites/files/ csp/secure/use_of_botulinum_toxin.pdf>; [Accessed 20 Jul 2014].

118. Chartered Society of Physiotherapy (CSP). Core standards of physiotherapy practice. London, UK: CSP; 2005. Available at: <http://www.csp.org.uk/sites/files/ csp/secure/csp_core_standards_2005.pdf>; [Accessed 20 Jul 2014].

119. Vincent C. The safety of acupuncture. BMJ 2001; 323(7311):467–8.

120. White A, Hayhoe S, Hart A, et al. Adverse events following acupuncture: prospective survey of 32.000 consultations with doctors and physiotherapists. BMJ 2001;323(7311):485–6.

121. White A, Cummings TM, Filshie J. An introduction to Western medical acupuncture. Edinburgh: Churchill Livingstone; 2008.

122. Thompson JW, Cummings M. Investigating the safety of electroacupuncture with a Picoscope. Acupunct Med 2008;26(3):133–9.

123. WHO. Guidelines on basic training and safety in acupuncture. World Health Organisation; 1999. p. 35.

124. Hoffman P. Skin disinfection and acupuncture. Acupunct Med 2001;19(2):112–16.

125. Hutin Y, Hauri A, Chiarello L, et al. Best infection control practices for intradermal, subcutaneous, and intramuscular needle injections. Bull World Health Organ 2003;81(7):491–500.

126. SARI. Guidelines for hand hygiene in Irish healthcare settings, The Strategy for the Control of Antimicrobial Resistance in Ireland (SARI) / Health Service Executive. 2005.

127. Albert RK, Condie F. Hand-washing patterns in medical intensive-care units. N Engl J Med 1981; 304(24):1465–6.

128. Graham M. Frequency and duration of handwashing in an intensive care unit. Am J Infect Control 1990;18(2): 77–81.

129. Dubbert PM, Dolce J, Richter W, et al. Increasing ICU staff handwashing: effects of education and group feedback. Infect Control Hosp Epidemiol 1990;11(4): 191–3.

130. Larson E, Killien M. Factors influencing handwashing behavior of patient care personnel. Am J Infect Control 1982;10(3):93–9.

131. Kim PW, Roghmann MC, Perencevich EN, et al. Rates of hand disinfection associated with glove use, patient isolation, and changes between exposure to various body sites. Am J Infect Control 2003;31(2): 97–103.

132. Thompson BL, Dwyer DM, Ussery XT, et al. Handwashing and glove use in a long-term-care facility. Infect Control Hosp Epidemiol 1997;18(2):97–103.

133. Girou E, Chai SH, Oppein F, et al. Misuse of gloves: the foundation for poor compliance with hand hygiene and potential for microbial transmission? J Hosp Infect 2004;57(2):162–9.

134. World Health Organization. WHO guidelines on hand hygiene in health care. 2009. Available at: <http:// whqlibdoc.who.int/publications/2009/9789241597906 _eng.pdf?ua=1>; [Accessed 20 Jul 2014].

135. Özkalp B, Aladağ MO, Turaçlar N, et al. In vitro effectiveness of alcohol based hand and skin disinfectants against various microorganisms. J Appl Biol Sci 2009; 3(1):67–9.

136. Özkalp B, Özcan MM, Koçak R, et al. In vitro effectiveness of 2-propanol based hand and skin disinfectants against various microorganisms. Asian J Chem 2011;23(10):4477–9.

137. Montville R, Schaffner DW. A meta-analysis of the published literature on the effectiveness of antimicrobial soaps. J Food Prot 2011;74(11):1875–82.

138. Paulson DS, Fendler EJ, Dolan MJ, et al. A close look at alcohol gel as an antimicrobial sanitizing agent. Am J Infect Control 1999;27(4):332–8.

139. United States Department of Labor, Occupational Safety and Health Administration. Occupational exposure to blood borne pathogens. Fed Regist 2001; 29CFR:1030.

140. Hughes KA, Cornwall J, Theis JC, et al. Bacterial contamination of unused, disposable non-sterile gloves on a hospital orthopaedic ward. Australas Med J 2013;6(6): 331–8.

141. White A, Cummings M, Barlas P, et al. Defining an adequate dose of acupuncture using a neurophysiological approach – a narrative review of the literature. Acupunct Med 2008;26(2):111–20.

142. Elden H, Ostgaard HC, Fagevik-Olsen M, et al. Treatments of pelvic girdle pain in pregnant women: adverse effects of standard treatment, acupuncture and stabilising exercises on the pregnancy, mother, delivery and the fetus/neonate. BMC Complement Altern Med 2008;8:34.

143. Ee CC, Manheimer E, Pirotta MV, et al. Acupuncture for pelvic and back pain in pregnancy: a systematic review. Am J Obstet Gynecol 2008;198(3):254–9.

144. Yuan J, Purepong N, Kerr DP, et al. Effectiveness of acupuncture for low back pain: a systematic review. Spine (Phila Pa 1976) 2008;33(23):E887–900.

145. MacPherson H, Thomas K, Walters S, et al. A prospective survey of adverse events and treatment reactions following 34,000 consultations with professional acupuncturists. Acupunct Med 2001;19(2):93–102.

146. MacPherson H, Thomas K, Walters S, et al. The York acupuncture safety study: prospective survey of 34,000 treatments by traditional acupuncturists. BMJ 2001; 323(7311):486–7.

147. Ernst E, White AR. Prospective studies of the safety of acupuncture: a systematic review. Am J Med 2001; 110(6):481–5.

148. Peuker E, Grönemeyer D. Rare but serious complications of acupuncture: traumatic lesions. Acupunct Med 2001;19(2):103–8.

149. Witt CM, Pach D, Brinkhaus B, et al. Safety of acupuncture: results of a prospective observational study with 229,230 patients and introduction of a medical information and consent form. Forsch Komplementmed 2009;16(2):91–7.

150. He W, Zhao X, Li Y, et al. Adverse events following acupuncture: a systematic review of the Chinese literature for the years 1956–2010. J Altern Complement Med 2012;18(10):892–901.

151. Saunders S. Injection therapy effective pain relief in physios hands – Congress article 6. London, UK: CSP; 2008. Available at: <http://www.csp.org.uk/frontline/article/injection-therapy-effective-pain-relief-physios-hands-congress-article-6>; [Accessed 20 Jul 2014].

152. The Chartered Society of Physiotherapists (CSP). CSP expectations of educational programmes in Injection Therapy for physiotherapists. Supporting good governance in neurological and musculoskeletal injection therapy. London, UK: CSP; 2011.

153. Linde K, Allais G, Brinkhaus B, et al. Acupuntura para la profilaxis de la migraña (Revision Cochrane traducida). En: Biblioteca Cochrane Plus 2009 Número 2. Oxford: Update Software Ltd. Available at: <http://www.update-software.com>; [Accessed 20 Jul 2014] (Traducida de The Cochrane Library, 2009 Issue 1 Art no. CD001218. Chichester, UK: John Wiley & Sons, Ltd.).

154. Capili B, Anastasi JK, Geiger JN. Adverse event reporting in acupuncture clinical trials focusing on pain. Clin J Pain 2010;26(1):43–8.

155. Weidenhammer W, Streng A, Linde K, et al. Acupuncture for chronic pain within the research program of 10 German Health Insurance Funds – basic results from an observational study. Complement Ther Med 2007;15(4):238–46.

156. Yun-Tao Ma, Ma M, Zang HC. Biomedical acupuncture for pain management: an integrative approach. St. Louis: Elsevier; 2005.

157. López-Olmos J. Cuerpo extraño perineal: aguja retenida tras el parto más de 25 años. Clin Invest Ginecol Obstet 2007;34(3):115–17.

158. Park JE, Lee SS, Lee MS, et al. Adverse events of moxibustion: a systematic review. Complement Ther Med 2010;18(5):215–23.

159. Yamashita H, Tsukayama H, Tanno Y, et al. Adverse events in acupuncture and moxibustion treatment: a six-year survey at a national clinic in Japan. J Altern Complement Med 1999;5(3):229–36.

160. Koh SJ, Song T, Kang YA, et al. An outbreak of skin and soft tissue infection caused by *Mycobacterium abscessus* following acupuncture. Clin Microbiol Infect 2010;16(7):895–901.

161. Roth M, Prigent F, Martinet C. Complication cutanée de la mésothérapie à propos de dix nouveaux cas. Nouv Dermatol 1994;13:694.

162. Whale C, Hallam C. Tension pneumothorax related to acupuncture. Acupunct Med 2004;22:101.

163. Peuker E. Case report of tension pneumothorax related to acupuncture. Acupunct Med 2004;22:40–3.

164. Kao CL, Chang JP. Bilateral pneumothorax after acupuncture. J Emerg Med 2002;22:101–2.

165. Jawahar D, Elapavaluru S, Leo PJ. Pneumothorax secondary to acupuncture. Am J Emerg Med 1999; 17:310.

166. Jones KS. Chest pain and breathlessness after acupuncture–again. Med J Aust 1998;169:344.

167. Olusanya O, Mansuri I. Pneumothorax following acupuncture. J Am Board Fam Pract 1997;10:296–7.

168. Vilke GM, Wulfert EA. Case reports of two patients with pneumothorax following acupuncture. J Emerg Med 1997;15:155–7.

169. Wright RS, Kupperman JL, Liebhaber MI. Bilateral tension pneumothoraces after acupuncture. West J Med 1991;154:102–3.

170. Gray R, Maharajh GS, Hyland R. Pneumothorax resulting from acupuncture. Can Assoc Radiol J 1991; 42:139–40.

171. Rotchford JK. Overview: adverse events of acupuncture. Medical Acupuncture 2000;11.

172. EUR-Lex. Council Directive 2010/32/EU of 10 May 2010 implementing the Framework Agreement on prevention from sharp injuries in the hospital and healthcare sector concluded by HOSPEEM and EPSU. Off J Eur Union 2010;L134:66–72. Available at: <http://eur-lex.europa.eu/legal-content/EN/TXT/PDF/?uri=CELEX:32010L0032&from=EN>.

173. Loscos LA, Colomer E, Marco MF, et al. Actitud a seguir en el caso de accidente biológico. Medifam 2002;12(9):16–35.

174. CDC. Recommendations for the prevention and control of hepatitis C virus (HCV) infection and HCV-related chronic disease. MMWR 1998;47(RR–19).

175. CDC. Public Health Service guidelines for the management of health-care workers exposures tio HIV and recommendations for postexposure prophylaxis. MMWR 1998;47(RR7):1–34.

176. Working Group of the Resuscitation Council (UK). Emergency treatment of anaphylactic reactions. Guidelines for healthcare providers. 2008. Available at: <www.resus.org.uk/pages/reaction.pdf>; [Accessed 20 Jul 2014].

177. Khan H. Treatment of anaphylactoid shock. N Engl J Med 1981;304(11):670.

178. Larard DG. Treatment of anaphylatic reactions. Anaesthesia 1980;35(10):1011–12.

179. The prescription only medicines (human use) order 1997 and shall come into force on 18th August 1997. Available at: <http://www.legislation.gov.uk/uksi/1997/1830/made>; [Accessed 20 Jul 2014].

180. World Confederation for Physical Therapy. WCPT Declaration of Principles and Position Statements. London, UK: WCPT; 1995. Available at: <http://www.wcpt.org/sites/wcpt.org/files/files/Ethical_principles_Sept2011.pdf>.

181. White A, Cummings M, Hopwood V, et al. Informed consent for acupuncture–an information leaflet developed by consensus. Acupunct Med 2001;19(2):123–9.

182. Council of International Organizations of Medical Science. Ethical guidelines for biomedical research involving human subjects. London, UK: CIOMS; 2008. Available at: <http://www.cioms.ch/frame_guidelines_nov_2002.htm>; [Accessed 20 Jul 2014].

183. Witt CM, Brinkhaus B, Reinhold T, et al. Efficacy, effectiveness, safety and costs of acupuncture for chronic pain – results of a large research initiative. Acupunct Med 2006;24(Suppl.):S33–9.

184. Witt CM, Reinhold T, Jena S, et al. Cost-effectiveness of acupuncture treatment in patients with headache. Cephalalgia 2008;28(4):334–45.

185. Wonderling D, Vickers AJ, Grieve R, et al. Cost effectiveness analysis of a randomised trial of acupuncture for chronic headache in primary care. BMJ 2004; 328(7442):744–9.

186. Myers CP. Acupuncture in general practice: effect on drug expenditure. Acupunct Med 1991;9:71–2.

187. Lindall S. Is acupuncture for pain relief in general practice cost-effective? Acupunct Med 1999;17(2): 97–100.

188. Taylor P, Pezzullo L, Grant SJ, et al. Cost-effectiveness of Acupuncture for Chronic Nonspecific Low Back Pain. Pain Pract 2013.

189. Kim SY, Lee H, Chae Y, et al. A systematic review of cost-effectiveness analyses alongside randomised controlled trials of acupuncture. Acupunct Med 2012; 30(4):273–85.

190. McClellan CM, Greenwood R, Benger JR. Effect of an extended scope physiotherapy service on patient satisfaction and the outcome of soft tissue injuries in an adult emergency department. Emerg Med J 2006;23(5): 384–7.

191. Harrison J, Rangan A, Shetty A, et al. Reducing waiting times: physiotherapy shoulder assessment clinic. Brit J Ther Rehabil 2001;8:57–9.

192. Morris J, Grimmer-Somers K, Kumar S, et al. Effectiveness of a physiotherapy-initiated telephone triage of orthopedic waitlist patients. Patient Relat Outcome Meas 2011;2:151–9.

193. Minaya-Muñoz F, Valera-Garrido F, Sánchez-Ibáñez JM, et al. Estudio de coste-efectividad de la electrólisis percutánea intratisular (EPI®) en las epicondialgias. Fisioterapia 2012;34(5):208–15.

194. Valera-Garrido F, Minaya-Muñoz F, Sánchez-Ibáñez JM. Cambios clínicos en el síndrome del túnel del carpo con la aplicación de la Electrólisis Percutánea Intratisular (EPI®). Fisioter calid vida 2011;14(1): 17–19. Available at: <www.colegiofisio-clm.org/docu mentos/fisioterapia_calidad_vida_7.pdf>; [Accessed 20 Jul 2014].

195. Makhlouf T, Emil NS, Sibbitt WL Jr, et al. Outcomes and cost-effectiveness of carpal tunnel injections using sonographic needle guidance. Clin Rheumatol 2013.

196. Bateman M, McClymont S, Hinchliffe SR. The effectiveness and cost of corticosteroid injection and physiotherapy in the treatment of frozen shoulder – a single-centre service evaluation. Clin Rheumatol 2014.

197. Jowett S, Crawshaw DP, Helliwell PS, et al. Cost-effectiveness of exercise therapy after corticosteroid injection for moderate to severe shoulder pain due to subacromial impingement syndrome: a trial-based analysis. Rheumatology (Oxford) 2013;52(8):1485–91.

198. Sterling M, Valentin S, Vicenzino B, et al. Dry needling and exercise for chronic whiplash – a randomised controlled trial. BMC Musculoskelet Disord 2009;10:160.

199. Valera-Garrido F, Minaya-Muñoz F, Sánchez-Ibañez JM, et al. Mitos y realidades en fisioterapia. Tendinitis vs. Tendinosis. En: I Congreso Internacional EPI®: Ponencias y Comunicaciones. Madrid; 2011. p. 100–1.

200. American Nurses Association's. Needlestick prevention guide. 2002. Available at: <http://www.nursingworld .org/MainMenuCategories/WorkplaceSafety/Healthy -Work-Environment/SafeNeedles/Needlestick Prevention.pdf>; [Accessed 20 Jul 2014].

201. Randal G, Collins R. Clinical Guidelines for the use of Acupuncture within the Physiotherapy Service. Peninsula Community Health. 2012. Available at: <http://www.rcht.nhs.uk/DocumentsLibrary/ PeninsulaCommunityHealth/OperationsAndServices/ OTAndPhysio/AcupunctureInPhysio.pdf>; [Accessed 20 Jul 2014].

1.11 APPENDIX

Appendix 1: Recording form for unexpected effects during invasive physiotherapy techniques

Fill in the information contained in this form by inserting ticks [✔] in the assigned boxes and writing your own responses.

Section I: Patient

1. Male ❑ Female ❑
2. Age: .... years
3. Medical diagnosis: ....
4. Other illnesses diagnosed: ....

Section II: Treatment

5. What invasive physiotherapy technique were you using? ....
   ....
6. For what reasons were you using this technique? ....
   ....
7. Is it the first time you were using this technique on this patient? Yes ❑ No ❑
8. List the other physiotherapy techniques you were using: ....
   ....
9. List all the medications that the patient was taking at the time, as far as you are aware: ....
   ....
10. List all the different treatments that the patient was receiving at the time, as far as you are aware: ....
    ....
11. What treatment dosage were you using?
    Device settings: ....
    Treatment duration: ....
12. Area of the body treated: ....
13. What machine version/model were you using? ....
    ....

Section III: Unexpected event

14. Describe the unexpected event that took place: ....
    ....
15. In your opinion the effect was Mild ❑ Moderate ❑ Serious ❑
16. How long after treatment did the adverse effect take place? ....
17. How long did the effect last? ....
18. Was treatment required for the effect?   Yes ❑   No ❑
19. Have you repeated the same treatment with this patient? Yes ❑   No ❑
    If the answer was yes, has the same effect occurred?   Yes ❑   No ❑

Section IV: The physiotherapist

20. Have you used this type of treatment before for this clinical problem? Yes ❑ No ❑
21. Describe any non -frequent effect that you may have observed associated with this type of treatment in the past with ANY patient:

EFFECT	SITUATION
1)	
2)	
3)	
4)	

22. List your thoughts regarding the effects that have occurred: ....
23. Can we get in touch with you in order to obtain further details?
    Yes ❑ No ❑ If the answer was yes, please give us a contact number, telephone number and/or email address:
    Name: ....
    Telephone N°: ....
    Email address: ....

Please forward this form via email to

Appendix 2: Informed consent form for dry needling

INFORMED CONSENT FOR DRY NEEDLING

Name and surname: .... Clinical History N°: ....
The purpose of the information in this form is not to alarm you or relinquish the physiotherapist treating you from any responsibility. This represents our effort to thoroughly inform you of the facts and enable you to take a considered and voluntary decision to authorize or reject this procedure.
It is obligatory for the physiotherapist to inform you and request your authorization.

AUTHORIZATION FOR TREATMENT OF MYOFASCCIAL TRIGGER POINTS (MTrPs) USING THE INVASIVE "DRY NEEDLING" TECHNIQUE

What is a myofascial trigger point (MTrP)?
A myofascial trigger point (MTrP), is a contracture area located within a taut bands of muscle that may cause local and referred pain as well as limit movement.

What does the treatment of myofascial trigger points using the "dry needling" invasive technique consist of?
The treatment is performed using an acupuncture needle, via which, once the skin of the area to be treated has been disinfected, the myofascial trigger point (MTrP) is reached, performing several approaches over this point without withdrawing the needle. A weekly session is established during a maximum of six sessions. If after the third session, no improvement is found, the treatment is suspended, and conservative physiotherapy treatment techniques are established as an alternative. Physical therapists who utilize dry needling as part of their physical therapy practice have received extensive training for the appropriate technique and use of dry needling. Dry needling IS NOT acupuncture.

What are the objectives of this technique?
The main objective of this technique is to overcome problems caused by acute or chronic pathologies derived from myofascial trigger points (MTrPs).

Am I likely to experience side effects or complications after being treated with this technique?
There are very few contraindications, and the same can be said for the dangers and the complications. The majority of the contraindications are relative.
- Regarding the complications, there is very little documentation on the subject, but the following are worth mentioning: contact dermatitis, muscle spasm or post puncture pain.
- The following contraindications are noteworthy: overwhelming fear of needles, patients receiving anticoagulant therapy, imunodepressed patients, lumphadenectomy and hypothyroidism. Puncture over areas of the skin that present any type of wound or scar; skin disorders such as psoriasis or infections, macules or tattoos. Allergy to metals (especially nickel). Furthermore, deep puncture is avoided in pregnant women, especially during the first three months of pregnancy, and after this period, as long as the area to be treated may affect the fetus. On the other hand, it is recommended to wait for at least 24 h after treatment before bathing in a pool or public baths, and to avoid this type of treatment in people who present generalized chronic pain, for example, in the case of fibromyalgia if the technique has previously been used without achieving any benefits.
- The dangers are limited and the probability of these occurring is minimal. If the appropriate precautions have been undertaken, these are mostly avoidable. These dangers are: pneumothorax, nerve injury, vasovagal syncope, muscular oedema, haemorrhage and risk of infection of the physiotherapist due to an accidental puncture with a contaminated needle.

PERSONALIZED RISK INFORMATION
The following risks are related to the previous health status of the patient, and the most significant are:
....
....

STATEMENT. I declare that:
- I have been informed of the risks of the treatment, and the possible alternatives have been explained to me. I know that I may revoke my consent at any time.
- I am satisfied with the information received, I have had the opportunity to ask any questions, and all of these have been answered.
- Consequently, I grant my consent

Name and signature of the patient   Name and signature of the physiotherapist
Date:..   Signature:..
                                                               Professional board licence number:.......................

Name of the legal representative in the case of handicap or in the case of a minor, indicating the relationship (father, mother, guardian, etc.)

Signature: .... ID N°..

WITHDRAWAL OF CONSENT
I have decided to revoke my prior authorization and will not continue forth with treatment, which I consider finalized on this date
Signature:.. ID N° ....
Date: ....

Appendix 3: Informed consent form for mesotherapy

INFORMED CONSENT FOR MESOTHERAPY

(Location) ...., (day) .... (month) .... (year) ....
Patient name... Date of birth...
Address.. Town...
Telephone N°.. IDN°..

I DECLARE
That via the present document I REQUEST AND AUTHORIZE the physiotherapist...
.... , graduated in physiotherapy with the professional
board licence N° .... and the rest of the team, to perform on me the treatment known as ....
....

BRIEF EXPLANATION OF THE INTERVENTION
Mesotherapy consists of the injection of small quantities of pharmacological and homeopathic substances into the intradermal space. The type of substances are chosen according to the problem to be treated. With this treatment painful processes, and inflammatory, degenerative and vascular disorders are improved.
The substances and devices used have been authorized for their use in medicine and cosmetic physiotherapy, medicine and sports physiotherapy, and bear the CE marking and the corresponding health register number.

RISKS INHERENT TO THE PATIENT AND THEIR PERSONAL CIRCUMSTANCES
I CONFIRM that the above mentioned treatment has been explained to me in detail by a physiotherapist in words that I could understand, together with an explanation of the typical risks, the undesired effects, any personalized risks, as well as the discomfort or, on occasion, the pains that may appear after the procedure. Other existing treatment options available on the market have been explained, as well as the pros and cons of each of these. Considering the above I have selected the previously described intervention.

I ACCEPT that RISKS AND COMPLICATIONS described by the medical science as inherent to this treatment may occur. The main risks that have been explained to me are as follows:
- Risks and complications common to any invasive physiotherapy treatment, among others: allergic reaction to the substance employed, bruising, and oedema that generally passes after a brief period with no need for treatment.
- Specific risks and complications related to this intervention that have been explained to me and that I acknowledge and accept. Specifically, small bruises or scabs may appear after the injection that disappear in a few days without further complications.
- Other risks and infectious complications that, although rare, are worth considering.

CONTRAINDICATIONS: patients that present coagulopathies or are under treatment with anticoagulants. Pregnant patients. Patients receiving treatment with immunosupressors.

I RECOGNIZE that in the course of the intervention, unforeseen circumstances can arise that force a change of plans and I give my specific authorization for the treatment of the same. In the case of complications during the intervention I authorize the centre to request the necessary help from other specialists, according to their best professional judgment.

I UNDERSTAND that medicine is not an exact science and that nobody can guarantee absolute perfection. I understand that the end result may not be what is expected by me, and I recognize that I have not been given a guarantee for this at all.

I HAVE BEEN INFORMED that the number of sessions and/or the amount of product necessary in order to achieve the desired effect has been communicated to me as an approximate guide, as it is impossible to previously know the exact amount of product or the number of sessions that are necessary, due to the different absorption/reaction responses of each patient.

I COMMIT TO faithfully follow, to the best of my abilities, the instructions of the physiotherapist for before, during and after the intervention previously mentioned.

I take responsibility for adhering to the measures recommended by the professional.

I CERTIFY that the information given in relation to my history and clinical surgical background is complete and correct, especially concerning allergies, diseases and personal risks.

I GRANT AUTHORIZATION for photos to be taken of the intervened area that may be used for a scientific, educational or medical purposes, understanding that their use does not constitute a violation of my right to privacy or confidentiality.

I AM AWARE that my information is going to be treated in an automated manner, which I grant authorization for, having been explained my rights according to the current data protection directive.

I have also been informed of my right to refuse the intervention or revoke this consent. I have been able to resolve all my questions regarding the above information and I have completely understood this CONSENT FORM (reaffirming each and every item and signing this document ON ALL THE PAGES AND THE DUPLICATE COPIES I reaffirm and consent the performance of this treatment.

The physiotherapist   Patient signature   Legal representative

I reject the treatment and have been extensively informed of the consequences of my decision.

The physiotherapist   Patient signature   Legal representative

Appendix 4: Informed consent form for percutaneous needle electrolysis (PNE)

INFORMED CONSENT FOR PERCUTANEOUS NEEDLE ELECTROLYSIS (PNE)

I declare that the physiotherapist (name) ....
has clearly explained the treatment that will be applied to the patient or in its case the legal representative (family
member or legal guardian): (name) ....
aged .... years old, with ID N° .... and address
.... Post Code................................... Town...
Telephone...

I have been informed:
1. That the therapeutic intervention consists in the physiotherapy treatment of the pathology using percutaneous needle electrolysis.
2. PNE techniques consists of the application of a galvanic current through an acupuncture needle placed directly in the lesion site of the degraded tissue, thus producing a destruction of the degraded fibrotic tendon tissue in order to subsequently produce an adequate inflammatory response for the regeneration, favouring the healing process.
3. That all physiotherapy therapeutic interventions, both due to the technique itself as well as the inherent characteristics of each patient (osteoporosis, arthrosis, prosthesis, pregnancy, endocrine problems, vascular problems, infections, tumours, congenital malformations, cardiopathy, pacemakers, etc.) entail a series of common complications which can be potentially serious.
4. That the complications that I may suffer have been explained and include:
    - Reduced joint mobility
    - Osteoarticular injuries
    - Vascular injuries
    - Nerve injuries
    - Musculotendinous injuries
    - Neurovegetative reactions, vasovagal shock (dizziness, nausea, vomiting, a decrease in the arterial tension, etc.).
    - Skin burns
    - Bruising
    - Increased pain
    - Other
5. That the technique shall be applied after precise assessment and diagnosis has been determined on behalf of a competent professional.

I have understood the explanations given to me in a clear and simple manner and the attending professional has allowed me to voice all my concerns and answered all my questions. I also understand that, at any time, and without the need for further explanations, I may revoke the consent given at this time.
For this purpose, I declare that I am satisfied with the information received and understand the aims and the risks of the treatment. Under these conditions,

I GRANT MY CONSENT

To receive the following treatment
....
Date:...

Signed: the physiotherapist   Signed: the patient

REVOCATION (WITHDRAWAL OF CONSENT)
Patient, or in its case, the legal representative (family or tutor) (name): ....
.... aged... years old,
with ID N° .... and address...
I revoke the consent given on (date).................................... and I do not wish to continue with the treatment, which
I consider finalized as of this date.

Signed: the physiotherapist   Signed: the patient

Appendix 5: Informed consent form for acupuncture

INFORMED CONSENT FOR ACUPUNCTURE

Patient name.. or in its defect,
(name)... with ID N° / Passport number ....
acting as legal guardian and or/tutor of the patient, and over the legal age, in full possession of my mental faculties
manifest that I have been satisfactorily informed by the physiotherapist (name)..
.... of the following points regarding the technique of ACUPUNCTURE,
MOXIBUSTION, CUPPING TECHNIQUE OR ELECTROACUPUNCTURE..
....

ACUPUNCTURE is a treatment modality based on Traditional Chinese Medicine (TCM).

ACUPUNCTURE consists of the introduction of fine sterile needles into acupuncture points producing a current-like
sensation around the needle and thus improving the metabolism, trophism and local circulation as well as producing
reflex responses in the nervous system.

Possible risks:

The complications associated with this technique are minimal, ranging from:
- Local discomfort in the puncture site, which passes in a few hours.
- Bruising in the areas of puncture and cupping.

Less frequently, the following may appear:
- Vasovagal syncope: (dizziness and vegetative response) occurring in select patients. This is accompanied by a
  sensation of heat, sweat, and fainting. This is not serious and passes in a few minutes.

I declare that I have been informed by the physiotherapist of the risks of the procedure and that I may revoke my
consent at any time.
I am satisfied with the information received, I have been able to ask any questions that I had and all my concerns have
been resolved.
Consequently, I grant my consent to receive ACUPUNCTURE, ELECTROACUPUNCTURE, NEEDLE + MOXIBUSTION AND
CUPPING treatment.

In (place)...on (day).................. of (month).................................... of (year)..........................

Signature of patient/legal representative and/or tutor   Signature of physiotherapist

REVOCATION (WITHDRAWAL) OF INFORMED CONSENT
As of (insert date).........................I revoke the consent granted for the performance of TCM and ACUPUNCTURE

Signature of the patient/representative and/or tutor   Physiotherapist signature

Appendix 6: Informed consent form for injection techniques

INJECTION CHECKLIST

Patient Name		Date of Birth	
NHS number		Date of injection	
Diagnosis		Time of injection	
Injection Site		Patient Consent	

CONTRA-INDICATIONS (Tick if absent)

Hypersensitivity to steroid/ LA		Prosthetic joint	
Patients under 18 years of age		Known latent/history of tuberculosis	
Systemic or local infection		Unstable joint	
Pregnancy or breast feeding		Myasthenia gravis	
Warfarin(administered under PGD)		Haemarthrosis	
3 Steroid injections in target joint in previous 12 months		Non coumain anticoagulants	
		Hypersensitivity to chlorhexidine (use alternative)	
		Low molecular weight heparin	

CAUTIONS (Tick if absent)

Drug interactions		Hepatic or severe renal impairment	
Oral steroid therapy		Respiratory impairment, - marked hypoxia	
Tendon rupture at site		Poorly controlled diabetes	
CHF/Cardiac conduction disturbances		Epilepsy	
Bleeding disorders		Immunosuppressed patients	
		Trauma of the area to be injected	

DRUGS/EQUIPMENT

STEROID		LOCAL ANAESTHETIC/ WATER/ SALINE		
Name		Name		
Batch No		Lot No		
Expiry Date		Expiry date		
Dose		Dose		
Checked		Checked		
Needle size/ gauge		Injected under	PGD	PSD

INJECTION PROCEDURE (tick if done)

EXPLANATION		TECHNIQUE	
Treatment options discussed		Site marked	
Side effects discussed - Subcutaneous atrophy		Hands washed	
- Depigmentation		Site cleaned	
- Infection		Bottles cleaned	
- Facial flushing		'No touch' technique	
allergic/anaphylactic reaction			
Post injection flare			
Information leaflet given		Aspiration check	
consent obtained		● Peppering ● Bolus	
Review arrangements (state)		Safe sharps disposal	
Advice to wait .... mins post injection			

OUTCOME MEASURES

Objective/subjective measures	Pre-injection	Post-injection	Review date
1.			
2.			
Adverse reaction			
Comments			
Therapist Name			
Therapist Signature			

CHAPTER 2

NEEDLING TECHNIQUES AND MODALITIES

Fermín Valera Garrido • Francisco Minaya Muñoz

We are all very ignorant, but not all ignorant of the same things.
ALBERT EINSTEIN

CHAPTER OUTLINE

KEYWORDS

needling techniques; invasive techniques; scope of practice, needle/s; needles coated/uncoated; tube introducer/guide; needle gauge; needle length; hypodermic needle; syringe; acupuncture; electroacupuncture; dry needling; percutaneous needle electrolysis; mesotherapy; injection therapy; percutaneous needle tenotomy; moxibustion; sharp pain; local twitch response; ultrasound-guided; palpation-guided.

2.1 PHYSIOTHERAPY AND NEEDLING TECHNIQUES

Physiotherapy is defined by the World Confederation for Physical Therapy (WCPT) as:

services to individuals and populations to develop, maintain and restore maximum movement and functional ability throughout the lifespan. This includes providing services in circumstances where movement and function are threatened by ageing, injury, disease or environmental factors. Functional movement is central to what it means to be healthy.[1]

Furthermore,

physical therapy is the service provided only by, or under the direction and supervision of, a physical therapist. It includes examination/ assessment, evaluation, diagnosis, prognosis/plan, intervention/treatment and re-examination.[1]

Needling techniques or invasive techniques (terms which may be used synonymously) are manual therapy interventions that use a filiform/ hollow needle to diagnose and treat neuromuscular pain and functional movement deficits. These techniques within the scope of physiotherapy practice can be referred to as invasive physiotherapy techniques.

In the nature of the physiotherapy process, the puncture needle (or acupuncture needle) can be considered as a specific assessment tool (or mechanical device), a prolongation of the physiotherapist's fingers, thanks to the so-called 'wand' phenomenon. This means that when you touch something with a wand held in one hand, the complex tactile and kinaesthetic mechanisms that are activated make it possible to 'feel' with the tip of the wand (needle), as if the nervous system had placed sensors there. Via this phenomenon, one may appreciate changes in the firmness of the tissues that the needle passes through. For example, a needle may be introduced into the proximal section of the patellar tendon and one is able to appreciate the superficial interphase, the intratendon area and the deep interphase until contact is made with the pole of the patella. Or, in the case of the rectus abdominis (see chapter 3, figure 3.3D), the physiotherapist can feel how the needle passes through the subcutaneous tissue from the superficial to deep level, as well as through the anterior lamina of the muscle sheath and the muscle tissue itself until the needle reaches the posterior lamina.

Needling techniques may form part of the physiotherapy treatment plan that is developed through the clinical reasoning process. Depending on the treatment goals, physiotherapists may use a range of different techniques and physical modalities, including manual therapy techniques, therapeutic exercise, electrotherapeutic modalities and physical agents.

The use of needles is within the scope of physiotherapy practice, specifically the use of mechanical modalities (mobilization/manipulation, vibration, pressure [acupuncture, dry needling]). These techniques may also be combined with physical agents (heat [moxibustion], light agents [infrared]) or electrotherapeutic modalities, including electrical stimulation for tissue repair (galvanic current [percutaneous needle electrolysis or PNE techniques], high-voltage pulsed current, microcurrent), for the purpose of analgesia (transcutaneous electrical nerve stimulation [electroacupuncture], percutaneous electrical nerve stimulation) or for neurofunctional electrical stimulation. Invasive techniques can be performed on their own or can be combined with regular physiotherapy treatment.

In this sense, the *WCPT Guideline for Physical Therapist Professional Entry Level Education*[2] provides a professional foundation whereby the use of needles can be legitimately incorporated into the physiotherapy practice. The interventions that may be used in curriculum development may include, but are not limited to, acupuncture and dry needling.[2] In our opinion, needle techniques are an advanced scope of practice and the physiotherapist performing needle techniques should: (1) have received additional education and appropriate training accredited by an educational organization; (2) have significant professional experience and competency development – we recommend 1 year of practice as a licensed physiotherapist prior to using the needling techniques; (3) perform in a manner that is consistent with generally accepted standards of practice (patient informed consent, clean-needle technique and universal precautions); (4) be covered by professional liability insurance cover, subject to the terms of the policy; and (5) limit the use of the modality to the treatment of generally accepted physical disorders within the scope of practice for physiotherapists (musculoskeletal, neuromuscular and cardiorespiratory systems).

The practice of injection therapy and other techniques involving injection of a substance into the tissue constitutes an extended scope of practice for physiotherapists. Over time, and due to changing professional roles, there are many examples of activities that have transferred from one professional group to another. Injection therapy is one example of this. Physiotherapists in the UK have performed this activity safely and effectively for many years (since 1997) and are an example for physiotherapists around the world.

Throughout this chapter, physiotherapists and other qualified professionals who have received training in invasive techniques will deepen their knowledge regarding the specific characteristics and classification of puncture needles. This is complemented by an in-depth description of the standard puncture needle, syringe and hypodermic needle, together with the various needling techniques and modalities available.

KEY POINTS

Needling techniques fall within the scope of physiotherapy practice.

2.2 BACKGROUND, CONCEPT AND CHARACTERISTICS OF PUNCTURE NEEDLES

2.2.1 Background

The first needles devised for healing, of which there is a record, date from the Stone Age (called *bian*) and were built from stone and flint – materials that were later substituted for bone, bamboo or jade. During the Bronze and Iron Age, metals began to be used: at first, the needles were made of copper, then bronze, and precious metals, such as silver and gold. This continued until the present time when these metals were replaced by stainless steel.

Traditionally, puncture needles are most commonly associated with acupuncture. The needles represent the most important tools of acupuncture practice and are, indeed, what gave this technique the name of 'acupuncture' itself, from *acus* = needle + puncture. The oldest medical text to appear in China is the *Huanghi Neijing* (over 2200 years ago). This work, which is divided into two parts, *Lingshu* and *Suwen*, describes the basic theories of traditional Chinese medicine, such as *ying* and *yang*, the five elements, the *De-Xi* (*Qi*) (vital energy) and the classical 'nine needles' used in acupuncture. These nine needles are comprised of the arrowhead needle (*Chan*), the sword-like needle, the round sharp needle (*Pi*), the millet grain (*Di*), prismatic (*Feng*), wide and rounded (*Yuan-li*), filiform (*Hao*), sharp-pointed (*Chang*) and round-body (*Da*) needles. Currently, filiform needles are used (*Hao*).[3,4]

More recently, other needling techniques have been used, such as dry needling, introduced in the 1970s by Travell, Simons and Lewit, or intratissue percutaneous electrolysis (EPI®), developed in the year 2000 by the Spanish physiotherapist José Manuel Sánchez Ibáñez.

2.2.2 Concept

The needle is a filament made from metal or another hard material, of a relatively small size, generally straight and sharp at one end, while at the other end there is an eye or loop for inserting a thread. It has been used since prehistoric times for sewing.

The needles used in techniques such as dry needling, acupuncture or PNE are straight and solid. These differ from those used in injection techniques or mesotherapy, which are hollow in order to administer the medication.

2.2.3 Characteristics

The needles used in puncture techniques, in general, must meet a series of characteristics in order to be considered adequate:

- Penetration: the needle must penetrate with ease, but it must cause the least trauma possible. Also, it must resist several insertions without losing sharpness or penetration capacity. From the professional point of view, the ideal is a needle with strong penetration power. The profile or shape of the tip will determine the power of penetration.
- Resistance: the needle must not bend in use. This is achieved by using highly resistant steel alloys that allow for the application of increasingly high forces without the needle bending.
- Ductility: the needle must bend before breaking. This is usually contradictory to being resistant, as the more resistant a material, the more fragile it usually is. To avoid this, alloys are used with a relatively low iron content that combine greater resistance with high flexibility.
- Flexibility: if the needle accidentally bends, it must be possible to bend it back to its

original shape. If the needle does not comply (i.e. if it bends during manipulation), there would be a risk of rupture. Technology has supported the design of needles in order to achieve needles that are less painful, as well as safe and easily manipulated.

2.3 DESCRIPTION OF THE STANDARD PUNCTURE NEEDLE

2.3.1 Tail

The tail of the puncture needle is usually round, and is the element that precedes the handle or holder (figure 2.1). Its purpose is to facilitate manipulation of the needle itself, together with the handle. The tail is characteristic of the Chinese-type needle and is the most commonly used in acupuncture techniques. It is formed by a rolled-up thread and presents an eye that is not useful, in contrast to solid sewing or surgical-type needles.

At present, it is an optional element and there are Korean-type metallic needles with no tail on the market used for acupuncture, although these are mostly used in dry needling techniques. In this case companies such as Agu-punt® have developed specific needles for dry needling with no tail (figure 2.1). Also, the needles that have a plastic handle do not have a tail.

2.3.2 Handle

The handle is a long element around which the needle is held and manipulated (figure 2.1). The

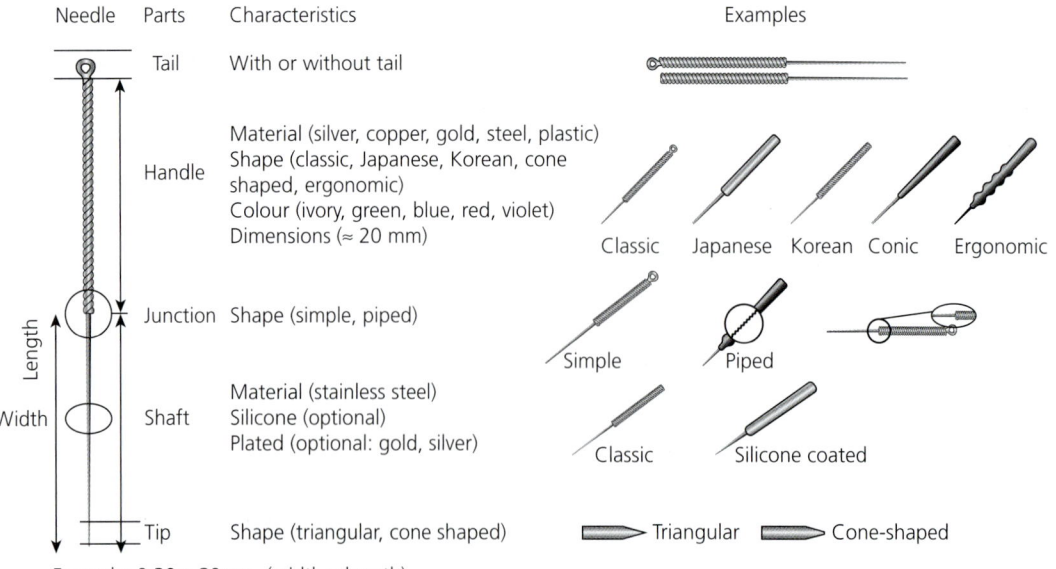

Needle	Parts	Characteristics	Examples
	Tail	With or without tail	
	Handle	Material (silver, copper, gold, steel, plastic) Shape (classic, Japanese, Korean, cone shaped, ergonomic) Colour (ivory, green, blue, red, violet) Dimensions (≈ 20 mm)	Classic Japanese Korean Conic Ergonomic
	Junction	Shape (simple, piped)	Simple Piped
	Shaft	Material (stainless steel) Silicone (optional) Plated (optional: gold, silver)	Classic Silicone coated
	Tip	Shape (triangular, cone shaped)	Triangular Cone-shaped

Example: 0,30 × 30mm. (width × length)

FIGURE 2.1 ■ Standard needle. Parts, characteristics and examples.

characteristics of the handle must allow for safe and comfortable manipulation.

It is important to consider four aspects in relation to the needle handle: the materials from which it is made, the shape, the colour and the dimensions (length and width). The materials and shape are quite variable depending on the needs and preferences of the professional, whereas the dimensions are usually similar.

Materials

The materials most frequently used are copper, silver, gold, stainless steel and plastic. Since ancestral times a healing property has always been attributed per se to noble metals such as gold, silver or copper. These metal materials are excellent conductors of heat and electricity, and thus very suitable for all electroacupuncture or moxibustion treatments. Furthermore, each noble metal has specific healing properties according to traditional Chinese medicine.[3,4]

Besides the use of metal, the handle or holder can be made of plastic; in this case polypropylene is generally used. Polypropylene is extremely light and compatible with both the skin and the environment.

As regards a plastic handle, its colour (e.g. brown, ivory, green, blue, red, purple) is determined by the width (diameter) of the needle shaft (e.g. 0.18 mm, 0.25 mm).

For the techniques of electroacupuncture, electrolipolysis, PNE or moxibustion, the handle must be metallic in order to favour conduction of the electric current and heat, respectively. Needles with a plastic handle cannot be used with these techniques. However, a new design of acupuncture needle with conductive plastic handle has been developed recently which provides electrical conductivity (JiaJian® company). Plastic handles are not suitable for moxibustion, as they are damaged by heat.

KEY POINTS

The needle handle must be metallic for the application of electroacupuncture, PNE, electrolipolysis or moxibustion.

Shape

With regard to the shape of the handle, most frequently this is linear, although it may also be cone-shaped. The classical shape is a thread braid (Chinese or Korean), although it may also be smooth (Japanese type) or more ergonomic, with a concave–convex design with different indentations to favour correct needle grip and manipulation (figure 2.1).

Size

The size of the handle in most acupuncture needles is approximately 20 mm depending on the different commercial brands. Some models designed for dry needling have a handle of greater width and length (25 mm) in order to facilitate needle manipulation. It is important to consider that the width of the needle shaft generally used to describe the product (for example, 0.30 mm × 25 mm) may not coincide with the width of the handle.

2.3.3 Root

The root or junction is the intersection point between the handle and the needle body. This is a critical needle zone, although there is a risk of rupture if it is manipulated excessively or inappropriately, or if there is a defect in the manufacture that could weaken this part of the needle. For application safety it is recommended that the depth of the puncture should not reach the junction point of the needle. That is, this area must not come into contact with the skin (figure 2.2).

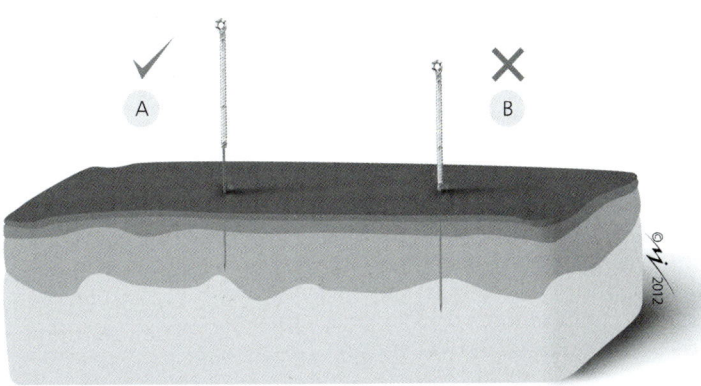

FIGURE 2.2 ■ Insertion of the needle into the skin. (A) Correct. (B) Incorrect. (Colour version of figure is available online).

This will facilitate extraction of the needle in the hypothetical case of rupture of the needle at this level.

At present, there are needles with reinforcements in the junction or intersection area. In these cases the needle and handle are joined with a special system to avoid separating one from the other. The needle profile has indentations or 'pipe'-style indentations in its junction with the handle so that this stays well inserted and it is impossible to separate the needle and handle (extra-firm union) (figure 2.1). The Cloud & Dragon® company were pioneers of this design in 2011.

Some commercial brands have patented systems for placing the needle shaft in the handle (proprietary tip design), so that the needle shaft is located at the precise centre of the handle. Theoretically this allows for reduced pain experience during the insertion, as the needle shaft is better positioned in relation to the handle used to manipulate the needle.

KEY POINTS

During puncture techniques, for safety reasons, it is recommended to avoid introducing the needle as far as the junction point.

2.3.4 Shaft

The shaft or body of the needle is the length of the needle from the intersection point with the handle to the tip (figure 2.1). The needle shaft of the puncture needle is straight and is the active element, together with the tip.

Materials and options

Currently, the material most frequently used is stainless steel, which can present as either a gold or silver coating and be covered with lubricating medical silicone (silicone-coated needles).

Stainless steel is the material of choice as it is resistant to corrosion (it does not rust) and to mechanical fatigue at high temperatures and it is biocompatible. The types of stainless steel used in the manufacture of puncture needles are those of the 300 series, known as authentic stainless steel and formed mainly by chromium-nickel alloys (with more than 7%). The most frequently used are the 304 (18-8) (chemical composition: 0.18% max. carbon, 18% chromium, 8% nickel, 2% max. manganese, 1% max. silicone, 0.0045% max. phosphorus, 0.03% max. sulphur), and 316 (chemical composition: 0.12% max. carbon, 16–18% chromium, 10–14% nickel, 2% max.

manganese, 1% max. silicone, 0.0045% max. phosphorus, 0.03% max. sulphur, 2–3% molybdenum), as these are the alloys that best resist corrosion, are not magnetic, have a high mechanical resistance and resist high temperatures better. A small percentage of molybdenum type 316 compared to 304 enables an improved resistance to corrosion due to chloride. Also used, but less commonly, is highly resistant surgical stainless steel 17-4 (chemical composition: 0.07% max. carbon, 17% chromium, 4% nickel, 4% copper, 1% max. manganese, 1% max. silicone, 0.0045% max. phosphorus, 0.03% max. sulphur), which gives the needle greater robustness, thus increasing the resistance to the needle sharpness and its durability.

Despite the multiple benefits, the metallic material of needles is not exempt from problems, as it can cause contact allergy, which consists of an exaggerated reaction of an organism when it comes into contact with the material and, consequently, causes eczema and/or irritation in the puncture area[5–8] (see chapter 1). In such cases it is recommended to change the needle material and send the patient to a specialist to identifiy the element responsible for this reaction. However, the prevalence and incidence of contact allergy are very low.[9]

The needle shaft can be coated, which means that it is covered with lubricating medical silicone. This reduces the resistance of the needle when it is inserted into the skin, and therefore reduces the amount of force necessary for penetration, resulting in a less painful puncture for the patient. The needle can be covered by one or several microscopic coatings of lubricant (for example, a triple lubricant coating).

KEY POINTS

Silicone-coated needles decrease the resistance of the needle in its insertion into the skin, achieving a less painful puncture.

Needles with a silicone coating in the shaft enable almost painfree application in dry needling and acupuncture techniques. However, they are not recommended for the application of PNE, electroacupuncture, electrolipolysis or moxibustion, as this decreases the electric current and the heat, respectively.

KEY POINTS

Silicone-coated needles are not appropriate for use with electroacupuncture, percutaneous needle electrolysis, electrolipolysis and moxibustion techniques.

Besides this, it is important to bear in mind a couple of aspects concerning the needle shaft:

- Smoothness of the needle: the small fragments that remain from the sharpening process can be a cause of painful punctures. In order to eliminate these particles, needles are subjected to a polishing process that smooths the surface and significantly reduces the amount of force necessary for the puncture. The needle is treated with one or several polishing processes (for example, double polishing, triple polishing). On occasion, as a final finish, the needles pass through an electromagnetic bath that smooths the surface and eliminates any remaining metal fragments. This results in an excellent sharpness that can perforate the skin with ease.
- Bending rigidity: the flexibility of the shaft facilitates the needle manipulation.

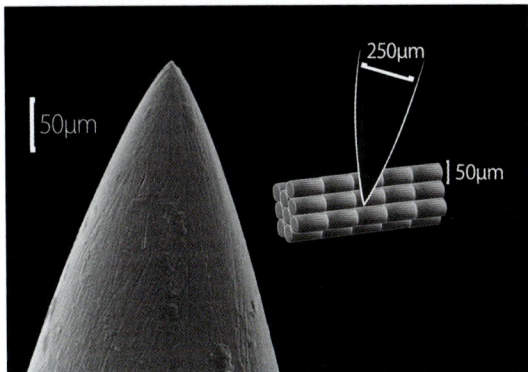

FIGURE 2.3 ■ Needle tip. Cone-shaped. Electron microscopic image. (Colour version of figure is available online).

KEY POINTS

Needle polishing helps eliminate irregularities, resulting in a puncture with reduced pain.

There are special needles with a Teflon-coated body available on the market that leave only the metallic tip free. These are commonly used in electromyography studies, but can also be used in dry needling techniques.

2.3.5 Tip

The tip is the pointed end of the needle and the element that penetrates the subject's skin. The tip is measured from the most distant point of the needle until where the needle shaft reaches its greatest width (figure 2.1).

Characteristics

The tip of the dry needling needle is flexible and not sharp, which differs from injectable needles, which are more rigid and sharper (figure 2.1).

The sharpening and polishing of the needle tip are determining factors regarding any pain the patient may experience during insertion into the dermis. Traditionally, the needle tip has been triangular (figure 2.1), although currently a cone-shaped tip is replacing this design (figure 2.3).

2.3.6 Dimensions

In the West, needle dimensions are expressed via two parameters: the width or diameter of the shaft (Ø) and the total needle length, both measured in millimetres or inches (equivalent to *tsun*). These dimensions correspond with the Japanese and Chinese measures. For example:

- Western measure (diameter [Ø] × length): 0.16 × 13 mm.
- Japanese gauge: 1.
- Chinese gauge: 40.

KEY POINTS

1 mm = 0.04 inches.

13 mm = 0.5 inches.

25 mm = 1 inch.

40 mm = 1.5 inches.

50 mm = 2 inches.

The dimensions of the puncture needle depend on the technique (for example, auriculotherapy compared to dry needling), on the depth of the tissue to be treated and the localization (i.e. in the hands and the face, the diameter is smaller so that the puncture is less painful).

The diameter (width) varies from 0.12 to 0.50 mm (the most often used are 0.25 and 0.30 mm) and these can be classified depending on the type of puncture technique performed:

- Body acupuncture: 0.25–0.40 mm.
- Auricular acupuncture: 0.14, 0.16, 0.17 and 0.18 mm.
- Cosmetic acupuncture: 0.14, 0.16, 0.17 and 0.18 mm.
- Paediatric acupuncture: 0.12, 0.14 and 0.16 mm.
- Dry needling: 0.25–0.30 mm.
- PNE: 0.30–0.32 mm.

The length is variable, ranging from 7 mm to 150 mm: the most frequently used are 25 and 30 mm. Over 75 mm these are called extra-long needles or special-length needles (75 mm, 100 mm, 125 mm and 150 mm). The longer needles are used when the area has quite a lot of muscle mass or adipose layer (for example, in the technique of dry needling over the gluteus medius), when the target tissue is deep (for example, the psoas iliacus or the soleus) or for performing needle-threading techniques, which is when two points that are on opposites sides of the same body part are joined with the needle (for example, in acupuncture 5TR and 6MC), or for specific techniques such as electrolipolysis.

Over a length of 75 mm, the needle width should be at least 0.30 mm, otherwise there is a risk of the needle bending.

In table 2.1 a summary of the needles available on the market is shown, in order of length and width, as well as the name of the commercial brand supplier.

KEY POINTS

The most commonly used needles in puncture techniques are 0.25 × 25 mm and 0.30 × 25 mm. The most frequently used needles in China for acupuncture are 0.25 × 40 mm.

2.3.7 Guide tube

The guide tube or simply the guide or introducer (figure 2.4) is a tube designed to minimize discomfort during needle insertion. The guide tube enables quick insertion of the needle through the epidermis. The material from which it is made is usually disposable sterile plastic, but it can also be made of metal (figure 2.4D) and the edges are straight or rounded; this is more pleasant when placed in contact with the skin.

Method of attachment of the needle to the guide

If the guide is made of plastic it can be secured to the needle in the following ways:

- Conventional attachment: the needle is secured to the guide via a plastic stopper of a more or less triangular shape, which is frequently blue or white (figure 2.4). The advantage of this type of system is that it is usually more economical, but it requires the stopper to be disposed of. This is the only fixation possible with needles with a metallic handle.
- Ultrasonic attachment: the needle handle is secured via ultrasonic welding.[10] With the application of mechanical high-frequency vibrations the molecules of both thermoplastic materials (handle and guide) can be moved, causing them to weld together

without reaching fusion point. The main advantage of this type of fixation is that, with simple pressure of the fingers over the handle and the guide, the needle is freed single-handedly. Currently, the only commercial brand that has developed this system is Seirin®, with the patented Light Touch Insertion™ system (figure 2.4B).

Presentation in the container

The guide tube is normally incorporated into the needle (unit) (figure 2.4E) or needles (5 units) in each blister pack (figure 2.4F), but it can separately accompany a pack of five or more needles (figure 2.4G) (pro-pack system, developed by Seirin®).

2.3.8 Protective cover

There are several different means of presentation (blister packs) for needles, depending on the materials employed (paper or aluminium) (figure 2.5A, B), the disposition (simple or double) (figure 2.5C) and the individuality (or not) of the needle in the blister compartment itself. Blister packs made with paper backings allow for fast and easy extraction as compared to aluminium, which requires the packaging to be opened with the fingernail. In the case of smaller needles, double blister packs made with paper can be used. Normally the needles are individually enclosed in each blister compartment, but they can also be found in numbers of five or 10 and associated, or not, with the guide tube.

The number of units in a blister pack varies between five, six and 10 needles (figure 2.5D, E) with a total of 100, 200 or 1000 units in each box.

The reverse aspect of the blister includes information relating to the size, expiry (use-by date), the manufacturer's code (lot number) and CE stamp.

2.3.9 Safety and manufacture

The Japanese company Seirin® was the first to produce disposable acupuncture needles in 1978. Since then, different brands have automated the production of needles so that the needles do not enter into contact with the hands and have also installed verification devices that guarantee continuous control during the manufacturing process. Currently all needles are sterilized in ethanol. It is important to ensure that the product has the CE marking or equivalent.

Another aspect related to safety is the product expiry date. The needle boxes usually indicate the expiry date, just like any other product.

TABLE 2.1 Puncture needles available according to length, width and commercial brand

Width (mm)	Length (mm)																
	7	9	10	12	13	15	16	20	25	30	40	50	60	75	100	125	150
0.12	–	–	–	–	–	Seirin	–	–	–	Seirin	–	–	–	–	–	–	–
0.14	–	–	–	–	C&D	Seirin C&D	–	–	–	Seirin	–	–	–	–	–	–	–
0.16	Huan-Qiu	–	TeWa	Ener-Q Huan-Qiu	–	Seirin TeWa	–	–	AG-P	Seirin TeWa	Seirin	–	–	–	–	–	–
0.17	AG-P	Acimud	–	–	–	–	–	–	–	–	–	–	–	–	–	–	–
0.18	Acimud	–	–	–	TeWa AG-P Hwato Ener-Q	TeWa	–	–	AG-P	Seirin TeWa AG-P Hwato Acimud	Seirin TeWa	–	–	–	–	–	–
0.20	Ener-Q	–	–	–	TeWa Hwato Ener-Q Acimut	Asiamed Seirin TeWa Acimud	–	–	Asiamed TeWa AG-P Ener-Q Acimut	Seirin TeWa AG-P Hwato Acimud	Seirin TeWa Hwato	Seirin TeWa Hwato	–	–	–	–	–
0.22	–	–	–	–	TeWa Hwato Ener-Q Acimut	–	–	–	–	Hwato	TeWa Hwato	Hwato	–	–	–	–	–
+0.25	–	–	–	–	TeWa AG-P Ener-Q Acimut	TeWa AG-P Acimud	–	Asiamed TeWa	Asiamed TeWa AG-P Ener-Q Acimut	Seirin TeWa AG-P Hwato Acimud	Asiamed Seirin TeWa AG-P Hwato Ener-Q Acimut	Seirin TeWa Hwato	Seirin C&D Hwato	Hwato	AG-P	–	–
0.26	–	–	–	–	Ener-Q Huan-Qiu Acimut TeWa	–	Ener-Q	–	Ener-Q Huan-Qiu Acimut	–	Ener-Q Huan-Qiu Acimut	Ener-Q Huan-Qiu	–	Ener-Q	–	–	–
0.30	–	–	Asiamed	–	TeWa	TeWa AG-P	Ener-Q	TeWa	TeWa AG-P Ener-Q Acimut	Asiamed Seirin TeWa AG-P Hwato Ener-Q Acimut	Seirin TeWa AG-P Hwato Acimut	Seirin TeWa AG-P Hwato	Seirin C&D AG-P Hwato	C&D AG-P Hwato Ener-Q	TeWa C&D Hwato	AG-P	–
0.32	–	–	–	–	Ener-Q	–	–	–	AG-P Ener-Q Huan-Qiu Acimut Ener-Q	–	AG-P Ener-Q Huan-Qiu Acimut	Ener-Q	–	Ener-Q	Ener-Q	Ener-Q	Ener-Q
0.35	–	–	–	–	–	–	–	–	Ener-Q	Hwato Ener-Q	Hwato Ener-Q	Asiamed TeWa Hwato	C&D	TeWa C&D Hwato	TeWa C&D	–	–
0.40	–	–	–	–	–	TeWa	–	TeWa	–	AG-P	AG-P	–	–	–	–	–	–
0.50	–	–	–	–	–	–	–	–	–	–	–	–	–	–	–	–	–

AG-P, Agu-punt; C&D, Cloud & Dragon.

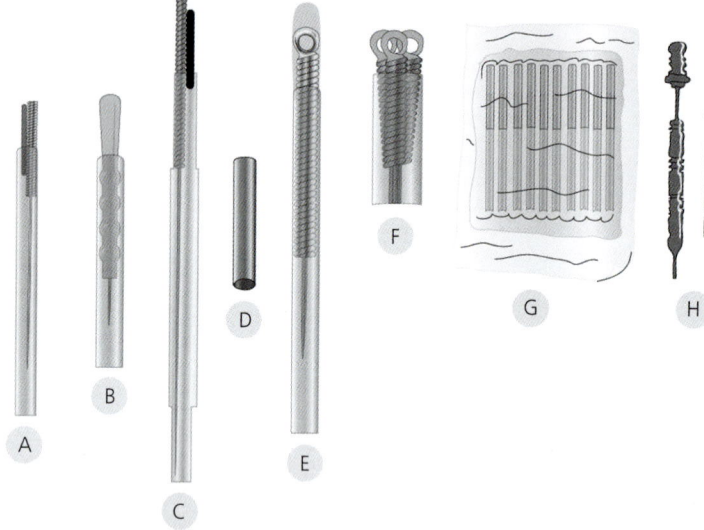

FIGURE 2.4 ■ Guide tube. (A) Guide tube: conventional attachment. (B) Guide tube: ultrasonic attachment. (C) Double guide tube. (D) Metallic guide tube. (E) Guide tube with individual needle. (F) Guide tube with five needles. (G) Individual guide tube with pack of 10 needles. (H) Injectors. (Colour version of figure is available online).

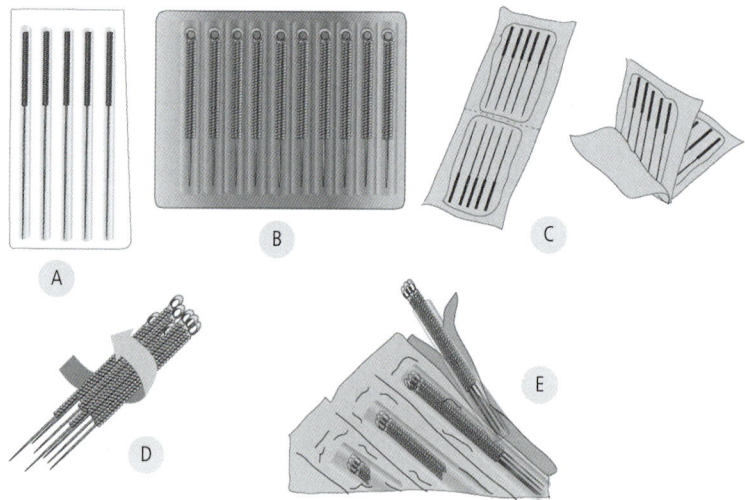

FIGURE 2.5 ■ Packaging. (A) Paper packaging. (B) Metallic packaging. (C) Double packaging. (D) 10-needle blister back. (E) 5-needle blister pack. (Colour version of figure is available online).

Depending on the amount of use one gets from the needles, the professional must choose between boxes of 100, 200 or 1000 units, considering that it takes approximately 2 years for them to expire.

Most puncture needles are manufactured in China and Japan.

2.3.10 Recommendations

The choice of the most appropriate needle greatly depends on the professional purpose (whether it is to be used for body acupuncture, dry needling, PNE or electroacupuncture) and, in any case, one must demand a needle that is safe to handle (determined largely by the safety of the production process) and that behaves optimally during puncture. This will depend on several factors:

- needle manipulation (ergonomics of the handle).
- sharpness of the tip and smoothness of the shaft.
- sensation of pain during application and sliding.
- bending rigidity.

Lastly it is important to consider the quality–price relation.

2.4 DESCRIPTION OF THE STANDARD SYRINGE AND HYPODERMIC NEEDLE (INJECTION EQUIPMENT) AND PROCEDURES

In infiltration and mesotherapy techniques, hollow needles are used that allow for the

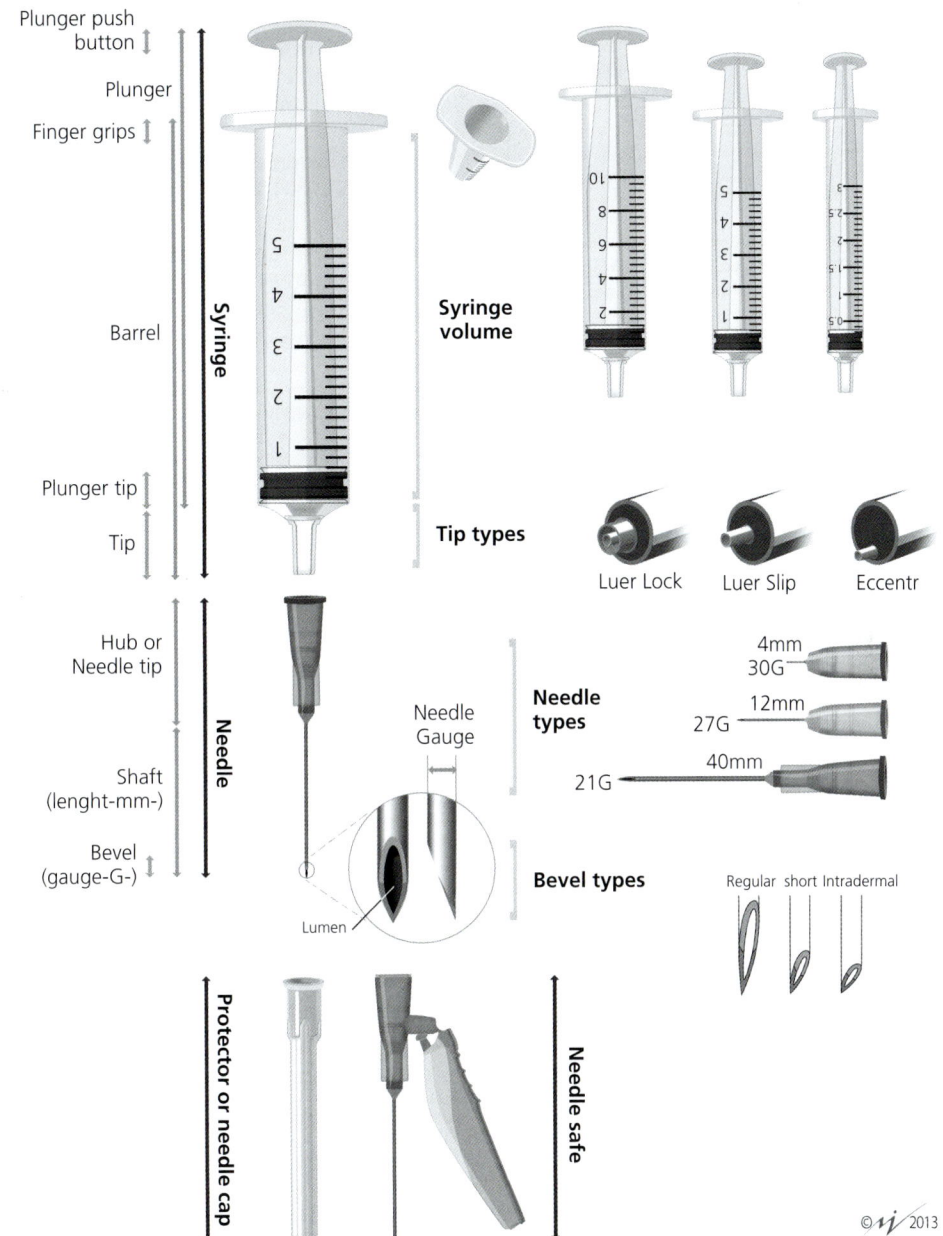

FIGURE 2.6 ■ Standard syringe and hypodermic needle. Parts, characteristics and examples. (Colour version of figure is available online).

injection of pharmacological substances. The injection equipment includes a syringe, a needle and the needle's protective cover (figure 2.6).

2.4.1 Syringe

The word 'syringe' is derived from *syrinx*, which means 'tube'. A syringe is a simple pump consisting of a plunger that fits tightly within a tube. Syringes can differ in type and size, and are selected according to their intended purpose. An international standard for the design of syringes has existed since 1993.[11] The ISO standard specifies a series of requirements (limits of acidity, cleanliness and alkalinity, limits of extractable metals, lubricant, graduated capacity, graduated scale, barrel, piston/plunger assembly, nozzle, performance, packaging, labelling) for sterile single-use hypodermic syringes made from plastic materials and used to aspirate fluids or to inject fluids immediately after filling. This excludes syringes such as those used with insulin and single-use glass syringes. These specifications ensure a degree of quality, guarantee effectiveness and provide safety.

All parts of a syringe that come into contact with the body must be kept free of contamination.

Parts of a syringe (figure 2.6)

A conventional syringe is composed of three parts: the barrel, the tip and the piston/plunger.

Barrel. The barrel is the part of the syringe that contains the fluid, whether it is medication, blood or a solution drawn from the body. It is sufficiently transparent for the user to see through it and usually graduated in millilitres to allow for precise measurements of the quantity of the fluid to be extracted or administered. The graduations are clear, concise and indelible. The barrel can range in size from 0.5 mL to 50 mL; the most frequent sizes used in injection techniques are 3 mL, 5 mL and 10 mL. When selecting a syringe, ensure that the amount of fluid or medicine that you are required to draw up will fit into the syringe.

Syringes are labelled according to how much liquid they can hold (syringe volume). For example, the packaging may specify '3 mL', meaning that the syringe can measure up to 3 mL of fluid.

The barrel has a finger grip located on the proximal end of the syringe by a snap-on motion to facilitate manipulation of the syringe or cartridge during injection or withdrawal of medical fluid into or from a site. The ISO specification requires that the finger grips must be of adequate size, shape and strength for the intended purpose and should enable the syringe to be securely held when in use.

Tip. The tip or termination is the interface, or connection, between the syringe barrel and the needle. The choice is made according to the application. Each manufacturer has its own specifications. The types of tips (figure 2.6) are:

- Luer slip and Luer lock syringes: a Luer slip syringe enables needle fixation on to the tip of the syringe by push slip. Luer lock syringe guarantees a more secure needle fixation as the needles are screwed on to the tip of the syringe.
- Concentric and eccentric syringes: concentric and eccentric refer to the location of the tip in relation to the body of the syringe. A concentric syringe has the tip centrally located. An eccentric syringe tip is offset towards the edge of the body.

Plunger. The plunger or piston is situated at the end of the syringe. Its purpose is to fill or empty the barrel. The plunger is pulled back to fill the barrel and pushed forward to empty the barrel.

Another important design criterion specified in the ISO standard is the plunger push button to finger grip length when the piston coincides with the zero graduation line. This optimal length guarantees that there is no unwanted increase in pressure during the injection of the last few millilitres of solution.

Safety syringes

The USA was the first country to adopt and actively enforce legislation on healthcare facilities in the use of safety syringes, when it passed the Federal Needlestick Prevention Act in 2000. Other healthcare markets are now following the USA, including Canada and the European Union, towards the mandatory protection of healthcare workers from needlestick injury and other unsafe injection practices.

Overall, safety syringes have the same components as standard needles. The most noteworthy difference between a safety syringe and its standard counterpart is the existence of a plastic shield which surrounds the needle and locks into place once the needle has been used.

Safety syringes are designed to prevent needlestick injuries.

2.4.2 Needle

The hypodermic needle was invented independently by Charles Gabriel Pravaz in France and by Alexander Wood in England in 1853. A hypodermic needle is a hollow needle generally used to inject substances into the body with a syringe or to extract fluids from it. The characteristics are that it is made of stainless steel, and is sharp and shiny. The word hypodermic translates to 'under skin'. The needle comprises the hub, shaft, lumen and bevel. Needles vary considerably in length, size of the shaft and size of the lumen. The length of the needle determines how deeply the injection can be placed. The diameter of the needle determines what types of solution can be pushed through the needle and the degree of pain elicited when the needle enters the skin. The diameter of the needle is associated with the needle gauge (G), with higher-gauge needles having a smaller diameter, i.e. 30G. Needle gauge has been proven to affect the frequency of pain and bleeding significantly during needle insertion into skin.

In general, the gauge, length and needle angle for injection techniques is 21–25G, 25–50 mm and 90° insertion to the skin (perpendicular approach to the skin with appropriate redirecting once the skin has been punctured), and 27–32G, 4 mm/12 mm and 45° insertion to the skin for mesotherapy, respectively.

KEY POINTS

The first number (in front of the G) indicates the gauge of the needle. The higher the number, the thinner the needle.

Parts of a needle (figure 2.6)

A needle consists of four parts: the hub, shaft, lumen and bevel.

Hub. The lower end of the syringe, opposite the plunger, terminates in a needle hub. This hub consists of a needle adapter that permits the needle to be attached to the syringe. The purpose of the hub is also to lock the needle in place while the syringe is being used for its desired function.

Shaft. The shaft or cannula is the length of the metal and is generally chosen according to the route and site of administration, the physical mass of the client and the thickness of the medication.

Lumen. The lumen, also known as the bore, is the hollow space within the needle. The diameter of the lumen is known by the gauge number of the needle. The lumen is selected with the same specifications as the shaft.

Bevel. The last part of the needle, the bevel, is the pointed end that determines the sharpness of the needle. There are three common bevel types: regular, intradermal and short. The regular bevel is the most commonly used bevel in injection techniques and mesotherapy. The needle is designed to pierce the skin with low penetration force and minimal drag as it is being inserted, thus reducing any discomfort to the patient.

Safety needles

Safety needles are needle-based safety devices that protect the healthcare worker from accidental needlestick injuries. The robust safety shield and easy one-handed design ensure that the clinician is protected against any exposure from sharps injury.

2.4.3 Protective cover/cap

The protective cover/cap is provided to maintain the sterility of the needle. Needlesticks are a common way of carrying infections between healthcare providers and patients. The needle bevel is covered in order to limit accidents and to ensure that only the intended patient is the recipient of the needlestick. In an attempt to reduce contamination and to increase safety, most needles are disposable and are discarded after a single use.

2.4.4 Product packaging and labelling

Adequate packaging (a hard plastic container or flexible wrapper) and labelling are regulatory requirements. For syringes and needles, in general, the packaging must retain the sterility of the content. Labelling serves to communicate safety and performance-related information to patients and users as well as to identify individual devices.

2.4.5 Procedures

Assembling a needle on to a syringe

A review of how to assemble a needle and syringe properly is presented in table 2.2. A thorough inspection of the equipment before use is very important to ensure that the materials are free from contamination and/or deterioration. The plastic caps on needles and syringes should not have been opened prior to use. In the event that needle or syringe covers appear to be loose, they should be discarded and replaced.

It is important to maintain an aseptic technique to prevent contamination of the needle and/or the syringe and to minimize the risk of infection.

Drawing medication (ampoule or vial)

See table 2.3.

KEY POINTS

Anyone accidentally pricked by a needle must immediately follow the infection control protocol for needlesticks.

TABLE 2.2 **Review of proper assembly methods for the needle and syringe**

Step by step	Condition	Caution
1. Remove the syringe from the package without contaminating the sterile parts	(a) If the syringe is packaged in a flexible wrapper, peel the sides of the wrapper away in order to expose the rear end of the syringe barrel (b) If the syringe is packaged in a hard plastic container, press down and twist the cap until there is a distinct 'pop' sound (c) If the 'pop' is not heard, the seal has been previously broken, and the equipment must be discarded	Check for water spots, tears and signs of deterioration or contamination in the wrappers. If any of these signs are noted, discard, and replace
2. Ensure that the plunger of the syringe moves freely by grasping the flared end of the syringe and pulling the plunger back and forth. If the syringe does not move freely, replace it with another sterile syringe		The shaft of the plunger must be sterile. Contamination could cause infection of the patient. Touch only the end of the plunger when testing for free movement
3. Remove the needle from the package ensuring that the sterile parts (needle hub or shaft) are not contaminated	(a) If the needle is packaged in a flexible wrapper, peel the sides of the wrapper away in order to expose the needle hub (b) If the needle is packaged in a hard plastic container, twist the cap until you hear a 'pop'. Remove the cap to expose the needle hub (c) If the 'pop' is not heard, the seal has been previously broken, and the equipment must be discarded	All parts of the needle are sterile Be careful not to touch the hub in order to prevent contamination. Only the outside of the needle cover may be touched
4. Join the needle and syringe by inserting the needle adapter of the syringe into the needle hub, being sure not to contaminate either part. Tighten the needle by turning one-fourth of a turn to ensure that it is securely attached. If the syringe has threads, you may need to turn more than the quarter turn		
5. Hold the needle and syringe upright and remove the protective cover from the needle by pulling it straight off		Do not twist the protective cover as this may pull the needle off the hub (a) Visually inspect the needle for burrs, barbs, damage and contamination (b) If the needle displays any defects or damage, replace the needle with another sterile needle
6. Place the protective cover back on the needle, ensuring that you do not stick yourself or to contaminate the needle. Place the assembled needle and syringe on the work surface		
7. When you assemble a needle and syringe, you are responsible for maintaining the total sterility and security of the equipment		

TABLE 2.3 Drawing medication

Step by step (ampoule and vial)	Condition	Caution
1. Ampoule. Lightly tap the upright ampoule to force any trapped medication from the ampoule neck and top 1. Vial. Remove the protective cap. If this is a multidose vial, the metal cap may have been removed already	If any of the following defects are noted on an ampoule or vial, return to pharmacy: (1) Examine the rubber stopper carefully for defects, such as small holes resulting from wear and tear (2) Hold the vial to the light to check for the existence of foreign particles and changes in colour and consistency of medication to be drawn (3) Check the expiration date and the date medication was opened on a multidose vial	Check the expiration date on medication container
2. Ampoule. Clean the neck of the ampoule with an antiseptic swab, using plenty of friction, and wrap the neck of ampoule with the same swab 2. Vial. Clean the rubber stopper with an antiseptic swab		Allow it to dry
3. Grasp the ampoule carefully with both hands, snap the neck by bending it away from the break line (the narrowest portion of ampoule neck is the weakest point and breaks easily) and break off the top of the ampoule, pressing away from you		Hold ampoule to light and carefully check for minute glass particles. If glass is present, discard and replace Opening ampoules is a particularly high-risk event for sharps injuries
4. Ampoule. Pick up the assembled needle and syringe in the dominant hand, remove the protective cover with your free hand and insert the needle into the opening of the ampoule, while holding the ampoule in your other hand 4. Vial. Pick up the vial with your free hand and insert the needle into the rubber stopper. Ensure that the needle tip completely passes through		
5. Ampoule. Pull back on the syringe plunger to draw up the solution from the ampoule into the syringe 5. Vial. Pull the plunger back to the desired cc mark, withdrawing the prescribed medication		Maintain the tip of the needle in the solution so you don't draw up air
6. Keep drawing back until you have a little more than the correct amount of liquid in the syringe. Then you can withdraw the needle out of the ampoule/vial and set the ampoule/vial down		Be careful not to touch the outside edge or bottom of the ampoule/vial with the needle
7. Both. Hold the syringe with the needle straight up, and push any air bubbles out of the syringe through the needle		
8. Both. Verify the correct dosage		

2.5 CLASSIFICATION OF PUNCTURE NEEDLES

Puncture needles can be classified in several ways: by their length and width, by the material they are made of and by the application time (short, semipermanent, permanent). From a clinical point of view, what is most interesting is the integration of all this information with the technique towards which it is directed (e.g. acupuncture, dry needling, PNE).

2.5.1 Body acupuncture needles

These are generally called filiform needles. Traditionally, three types of acupuncture needles are described (Chinese, Japanese and Korean): this is determined mainly by the material (metallic), the shape of the handle (pipe handle or smooth) and the presence, or absence, of a tail:

- Chinese needle: the Chinese-type needle has a piped handle with silver or copper thread with a rounded tail (figure 2.1). This is the most popular in acupuncture techniques.
- Korean needle: the Korean-type needle has a piped handle made of stainless steel with no tail (figure 2.1).
- Japanese needle: the Japanese-type needle has a smooth metallic handle made of stainless steel with a few indentations on it, with no tail (figure 2.1).

Besides the classic acupuncture needles it is important to add those that are made with a plastic handle.

Most frequent dimensions are 0.25×25 mm, 0.25×30 mm, 0.20×25 mm and 0.30×40 mm.

Acupuncture needles can be used for other puncture techniques, such as PNE or dry needling. However, recently, needles have been developed that are specifically made for these techniques.

In body acupuncture the plum blossom needle is also used. This is a group of seven filiform needles (seven-star) that form the shape of a flower fixed to the head of a hammer with a long and flexible handle. These can be disposable or may have a detachable head for sterilization. These needles are used to stimulate a channel or a specific point or in cupping therapy.

KEY POINTS

The most frequently used needle in acupuncture is the Chinese-type needle.

2.5.2 Electroacupuncture needles

The needles used for electroacupuncture must be metallic (handle and shaft) and non-coated (no silicone covering) in order to facilitate electric conduction.

Most frequent dimensions are 0.25×25 mm, 0.25×30 mm and 0.30×40 mm.

2.5.3 Auriculotherapy needles (auricular needles)

Auriculotherapy is a technique based on the treatment of pain, problems and illnesses via the stimulation of reflex points in the external ear. The reflex points can be stimulated both invasively and non-invasively.

Invasive treatments

- specific auriculotherapy acupuncture needles
- semipermanent needles
- intradermal needles
- needles for prolonged use.

Non-invasive treatments

- magnetic balls
- seeds
- laser.

Specific acupuncture needles for auriculotherapy

Acupuncture needles for auriculotherapy are characterized by being shorter and thinner than conventional needles

Typical dimensions are 0.14×7 mm, 0.14×10 mm, 0.16×7 mm and 0.16×10 mm.

In the case of small needles, stainless-steel injectors with a spring are available that enable depth adjustment in order to facilitate application (figure 2.4H).

TeWa® has developed a different model of auriculotherapy needle named Detox®, with the following characteristics:

- plastic handles that are wider and longer
- fluorescent handles
- double blister packs.

Most common dimensions are 0.16×7 mm, 0.20×7 mm, 0.20×13 mm, 0.22×7 mm and 0.22×13 mm.

Semipermanent needles or ASP ear needles

In auriculotherapy another type of needle is used – the ASP ear needle. ASP ear needles are usually made of stainless steel and are presented with, or without, an antiallergic textile adhesive plaster (transparent or opaque), which can be placed on one side or both, along with a third antiallergic adhesive for added support. These can come with a magnetic injector that facilitates use and provides an additional magnetic stimulation on top of that provided by the needle itself. These are semipermanent needles, as they can be inserted and left in place until the following session.

Dimensions are 0.2×1.5 mm with 2.5 mm diameter and 0.22×1.5 mm with a 4-mm diameter.

Intradermal needles

Intradermal needles are also applied in auriculotherapy. These measure less than 1 cm in length (between 3, 5 and 7 mm), are very fine (0.16 mm width) and with a minute tail shaped like a tennis racket on one side which prevents the needle penetrating completely into the skin. This is, therefore, a completely safe acupuncture technique (*Hinaishin-Ho*), which was first created in Japan by Dr Kobei Akebane more than 30 years ago. The needle is protected with waterproof tape and left in place for 3–7 days.

Most common dimensions are 0.16×3 mm, 0.16×5 mm and 0.16×7 mm.

These are usually presented as one needle per blister pack compartment with a protective cover or five needles per blister compartment in foam beddings.

Permanent needles or needles for prolonged use

Prolonged-use needles consist of a circular handle with a press needle mounted on a sterile adhesive plaster. These needles are small and work by maintaining pressure upon the desired point. They are left on the point for a long period of time (generally until they fall out on their own). A variant of this exists – a metallic ball or seed which is fixed to the point via an adhesive patch. They do not penetrate into the epidermis, but just provide pressure. This type of treatment is frequent in auriculotherapy and is beginning to be used to stimulate acupuncture points on the body.

Dimensions are 0.16×3 mm, 0.16×5 mm and 0.16×7 mm.

2.5.4 Hand acupuncture needles and needles used in other microsystems (for example, nose acupuncture)

Acupuncture needles used for the hand (and other microsystems) are characterized by being shorter and finer than conventional needles.

Most common dimensions are 0.18×7 mm and 0.18×8 mm.

2.5.5 Needles for dry needling

The boom in use of dry needling techniques has caused several commercial brands to centre their efforts on creating specific needles with the collaboration of notable professionals (such as Agupunt®). The characteristics that define these needles and differentiate them from acupuncture needles are shown in table 2.4.

Most common dimensions are 0.25×25 mm and 0.30×25 mm.

However, the needles most used in dry needling are body acupuncture needles. Monopolar needles are used less frequently in dry needling (figure 2.7), and are used more commonly in electromyography and characterized by having a central sharpened point that improves skin penetration, as well as a soft coating to reduce friction during insertion (Teflon needles). They are electrically treated in order to guarantee the recording of extremely low noise (a crucial aspect in electromyography studies). The most common sizes are 25, 37 and 45 mm. The width of these needles is expressed in gauges (G), which is equivalent to the diameter in millimetres: 0.50 mm = 25G, 0.45 mm = 26G, 0.40 mm = 27G, 0.36 mm = 28G, 0.33 mm = 29G, 0.30 mm = 30G and 0.25 mm = 31G.

Several electromyography studies have shown that these needles can help detect the presence of myofascial trigger points (MTrP), which can be treated with the same needles. Therefore these needles have both a diagnostic and therapeutic value.

2.5.6 Needles for percutaneous electrolysis

The needles used in percutaneous electrolysis techniques are metallic (needle body and handle) in order to favour transmission of the electric current. The width and length of the needle are determined by the depth and type of tissue treated.

Most common dimensions are 0.30×25 mm, 0.30×30 mm, 0.30×40 mm and 0.32×40 mm.

2.5.7 Electrolipolysis needles

The needles used in electrolipolysis are metallic (body and handle), and identical to those used in body acupuncture, although longer.

Most common dimensions are 0.35×40 mm, 0.35×50 mm, 0.30×100 mm, 0.32×100 mm and 0.35×100 mm.

TABLE 2.4   Characteristics of needles used for dry needling

Characteristics	Advantages	Differences	
		Acupuncture	Dry needling
Needle with no tail	Greater precision during punctures		
Wider and more rigid handle	Improved manipulation and control during the whole treatment		
Surgical stainless steel	Stronger material, allowing for improved sharpening and maintenance during the multiple insertions		
Triple lubricant coating	The lubrication reduces the pain during the insertion		
Triple polish	Eliminates irregularities, achieving a less painful insertion		

Adapted from Agu-punt®. Nuevas agujas APS® para punción seca. Barcelona: Agu-punt®; 2012.

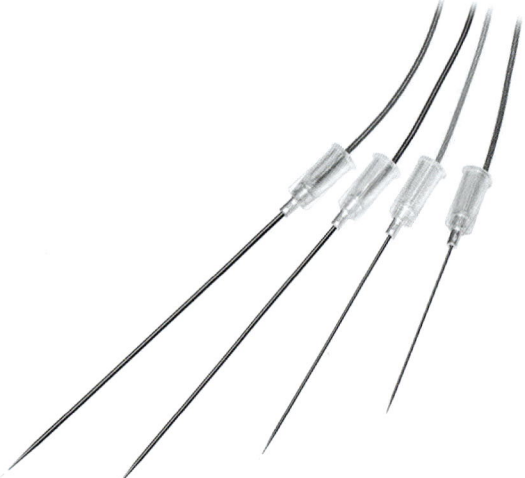

FIGURE 2.7 ■ Monopolar needles. (Colour version of figure is available online).

2.5.8 Mesotherapy needles

The needles used in mesotherapy are hollow, with a bevel, and small. The most frequent diameter is 27–32G (see chapter 14) and the length is 4–12 mm.

2.5.9 Injection needles

The needles used in injection techniques are hollow, with a bevel, and the most frequent diameter is 19–25G. The appropriate needle gauge and length are determined by a number of factors, including target tissue, drug formulation and patient population.

2.5.10 Contact needles

Contact needles are made of gold, silver or stainless steel and have rounded tips that are applied upon the acupuncture points. They come into contact with the skin (touching it) but without penetrating into the patient's body. Traditional Chinese philosophy establishes that an energetic flow is created through the properties of different metals in touch with the skin with the energy of the specific meridian points. Examples of contact needles are the Maeda, Zanshin and Teishin needles.

2.6 LOCATING THE PUNCTURE SITE

The target tissue for the puncture can be very diverse (figure 2.8) and will be determined by the therapy goal and the specific puncture technique.

2.6.1 Local stimulation

The structures that are most frequently stimulated are at the level of the muscle, the classic location over the taut band and MTrP, although the motor point can also be stimulated. Occasionally, the location of both these points (myofascial and motor) coincides with the acupuncture

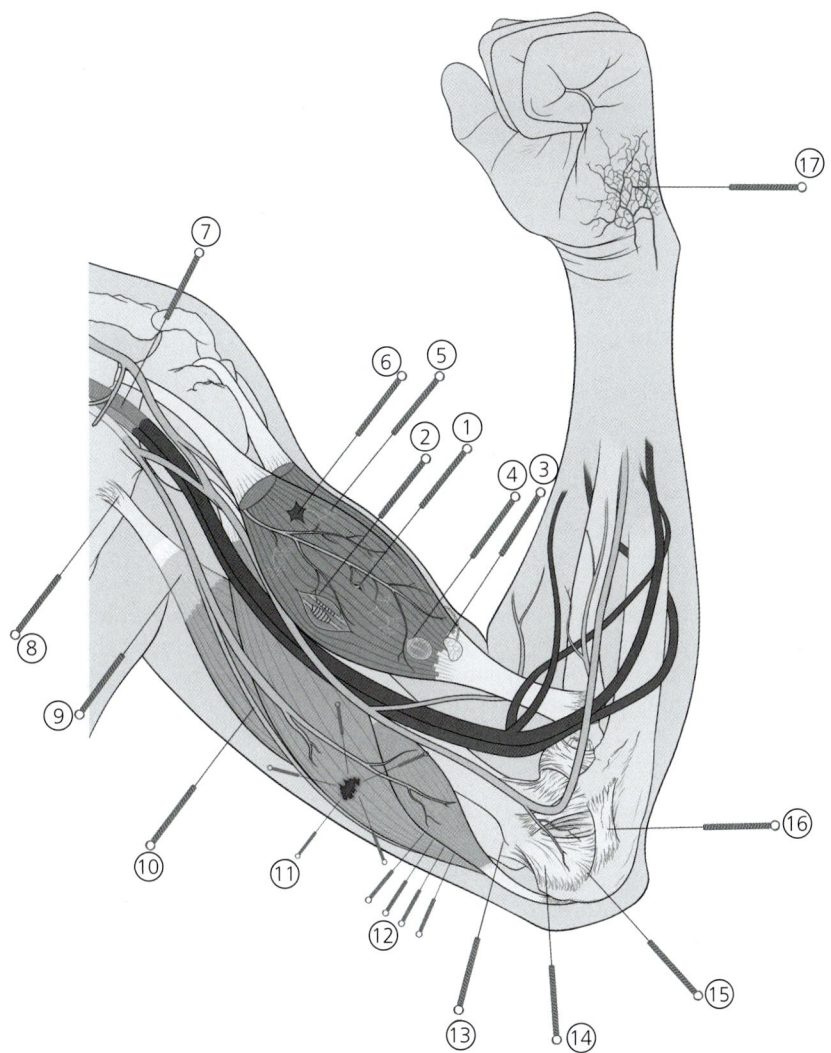

FIGURE 2.8 ■ Local stimulation. 1, Motor point (motor nerve trunk at hilum); 2, muscle belly (muscle spindles); 3, musculotendinous junction (Golgi tendon organs); 4, muscle belly (paciniform corpuscles near musculotendinous junction); 5, muscle belly (free nerve terminals: A-delta fibers, C fibers); 6, muscular trigger point (neuromuscular junction and other loci); 7, neurovascular bundle (nerve, artery, vein and/or lymphatics); 8, tenoperiosteal junction; 9, deep fascia; 10, peripheral nerve trunk (motor and sensory nerves); 11, healthy tissue around injury or unhealthy tissue; 12, fascial plane (between muscles) or tight band (within muscle); 13, periosteum; 14, joint capsule; 15, intra-articular insertion (synovial membrane); 16, ligament; 17, distal arteriolar network. (Courtesy of Dr. Alejandro Elorriaga Claraco). (Colour version of figure is available online).

points (see chapters 3 and 15). At the level of the tendon, it is usually the tendon itself while, over the nervous tissue, it is possible to stimulate the proximity of the peripheral nerve branches with techniques such as electroacupuncture or liberate their entrapment using PNE.

2.6.2 Segmental stimulation

Segmental symptoms may be located on the dermatome, the myotome, the sclerotome (table 2.5) or the viscerotome (table 2.6) of a segment (or related segments) (figure 2.9). For example,

TABLE 2.5 Sclerotome and sites used for stimulation

Sclerotome	Target stimulation
C1	Occiput
C4	Acromion
C4, C5	Spine of scapula
C5	Greater tubercle of humerus
C6, C7	Lateral epicondyle
T1–L5	Spinous process
L2	Iliac crest
L3, L4	Medial aspect of tibial plateau
L5	Greater trochanter

TABLE 2.6   Viscerotome: segmental levels of the autonomic innervations of the body

Part or organ of body	Sympathetic	Parasympathetic
Sublingual and submandibular salivary glands	T1–T4	Facial nerve
Parotid salivary glands	T1–T4	Glossopharyngeal nerve
Heart	T1–T4	Vagus nerve
Lung	T1–T4	Vagus nerve
Kidney	T5–T9	Vagus nerve
Gastrointestinal tract		
Oesophagus	T5–T6	Vagus nerve
Stomach	T6–T10	Vagus nerve
Small intestine	T9–T10	Vagus nerve
Large intestine: to splenic flexure	T11–L1	Vagus nerve
Large intestine: to splenic flexure to rectum	L1–L2	S2–S4
Urinary bladder	T12–L2	S2–S4
Reproductive system (male and female)	T12–L2	S2–S4

a superficial pain at the shoulder (dermatome) can be generated by an alteration at C4 or a trigger point with referred pain to the deltoid muscle (myotome) can be related to a segmental C5–6 alteration; similarly, pain on the lateral elbow epicondyle (sclerotome) can be associated with dysfunction of C6, and problems in the stomach (viscerotome) can be related to an alteration at T6.

KEY POINTS

During puncture techniques, it is important to distinguish between those symptoms or signs with a local origin and those that are the result of a segmental dysfunction. Functional assessment is essential.

2.7 NEEDLING TECHNIQUES

2.7.1 Insertion-based techniques

Insertion-based techniques are simple but require practice so that they can be performed skilfully, causing less pain. The most commonly performed techniques are:
- Holding the needle: the needle must be held with the tips of the thumb and index finger of the hand that is performing the puncture (currently the dominant hand). The tip of the middle finger protects the needle and helps guide it. The other hand can stabilize the puncture area or help guide the needle.
- Flat palpation: the non-dominant hand fixes the affected area and tenses or stretches the skin surrounding the target tissue with the help of the index and middle finger or the index and thumb or the middle finger

and thumb. The dominant hand inserts the needle between both fingers (figure 2.10).
- Pincer palpation: with the thumb and index finger of the non-dominant hand the tissue is pinched at the level of the selected point while, with the other hand, the needle is inserted. In acupuncture this technique is adequate for points with lesser subcutaneous tissue located directly upon the bony structures and, in dry needling, for the muscles where a pincer grip can be applied, such as the sternocleidomastoid muscle or the biceps brachii (figure 2.11).
- Puncture with a guide tube: a puncture using a guide tube is employed for performing a fast puncture with painfree insertion. The application procedure varies depending on the size of the needle.
  - Application procedure for a standard needle using a guide tube (figure 2.12): the application procedure consists of placing the guide tube (which comes with the needle) in contact with the site where the needle is inserted. The needle protrudes above the tube, so that between the top of the handle of the acupuncture needle and the upper end of the guide tube there is typically 3–5 mm clearance. Afterwards, a blunt tap is applied with the index finger on to the needle while supporting it with the other hand in order to insert it 3–5 mm through the skin into the acupuncture point. The blow can be performed with the distal or middle phalanx (in which case the tap must be firmer and must achieve insertion of the needle into the first skin barrier in a more effective manner).
  - Application procedure for longer needles using a guide tube (figure 2.13): the

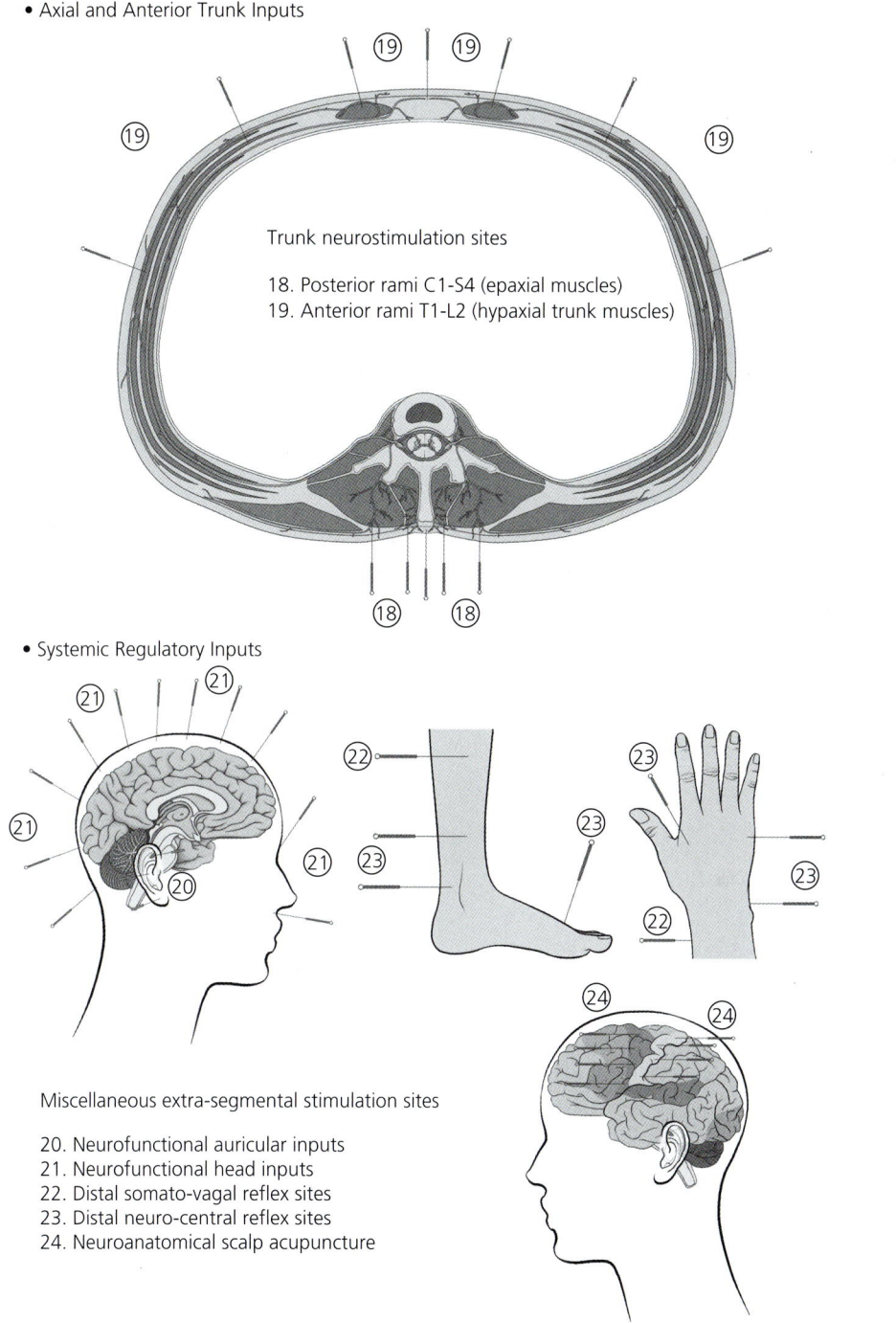

• Axial and Anterior Trunk Inputs

Trunk neurostimulation sites

18. Posterior rami C1-S4 (epaxial muscles)
19. Anterior rami T1-L2 (hypaxial trunk muscles)

• Systemic Regulatory Inputs

Miscellaneous extra-segmental stimulation sites

20. Neurofunctional auricular inputs
21. Neurofunctional head inputs
22. Distal somato-vagal reflex sites
23. Distal neuro-central reflex sites
24. Neuroanatomical scalp acupuncture

FIGURE 2.9 ■ **Segmental stimulation.** (Courtesy of Dr. Alejandro Elorriaga Claraco). (Colour version of figure is available online).

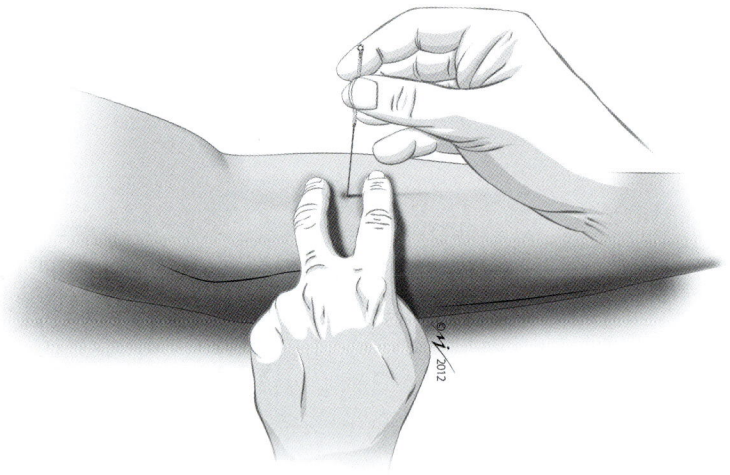

FIGURE 2.10 ■ Flat palpation. (Colour version of figure is available online).

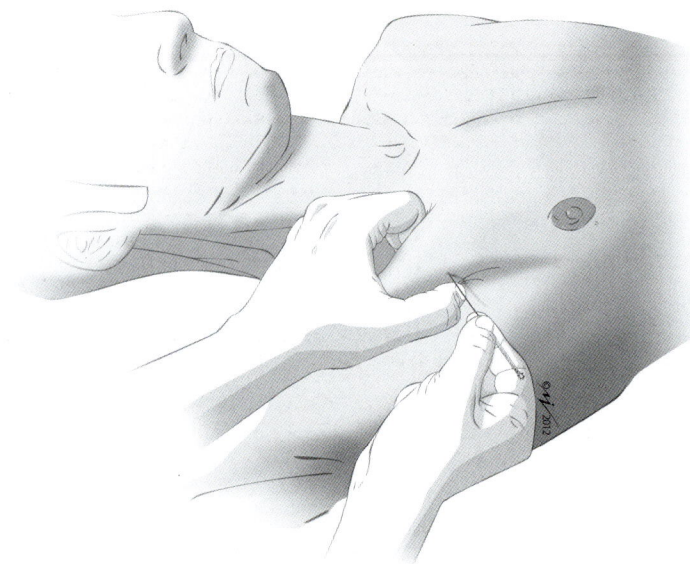

FIGURE 2.11 ■ Pincer palpation. (Colour version of figure is available online).

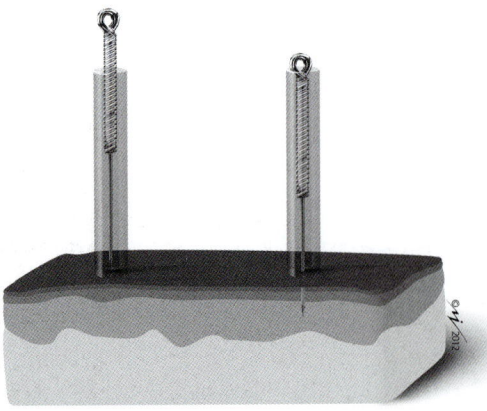

FIGURE 2.12 ■ Application procedure using a standard needle and a guide tube. (Colour version of figure is available online).

TeWa® acupuncture brand has been a pioneer in the development of the Safe-T sleeve (figure 2.4C) in order to ensure a correct and safe application of longer needles. In this case, each needle comes with a guide tube, one of which is the same as the conventional guide, which is called the insertion tube, as it allows the professional to insert the needle into the dermis (in the manner described in the previous point) and a second, shorter guide, called a guide sleeve, which is on the outside of the insertion tube, is used after withdrawing the conventional guide tube. The sleeve enables completion of the insertion and manipulation of the

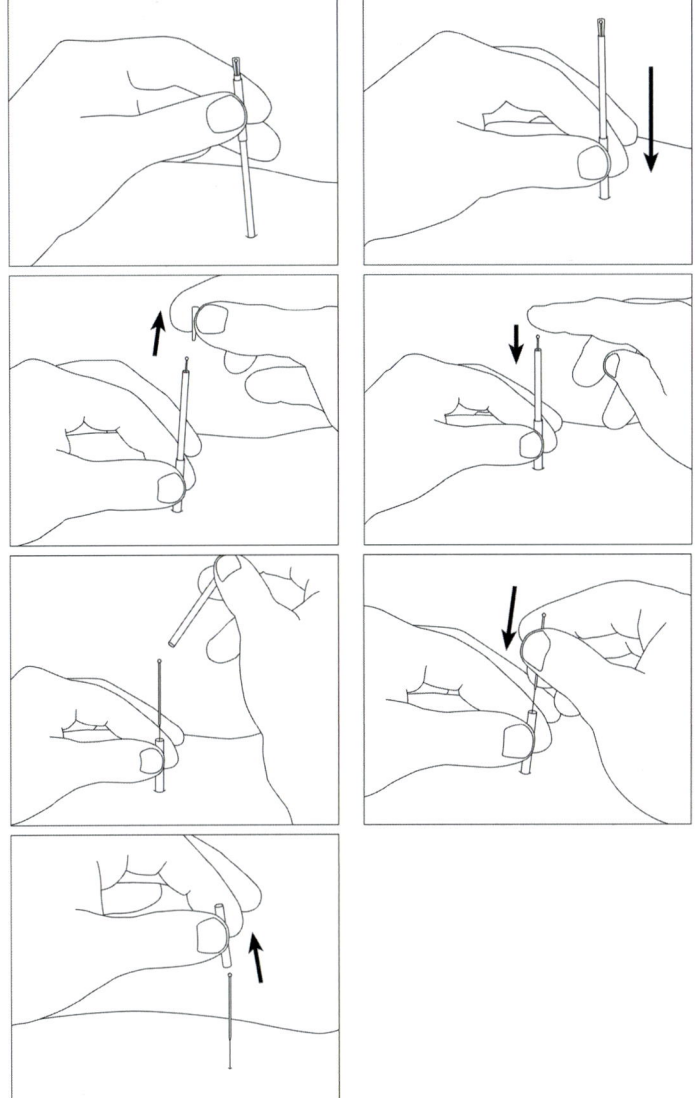

FIGURE 2.13 ■ Application procedure for longer needles using a guide tube. (Courtesy of TeWa®).

needle without compromising sterility, as this system enables needle insertion without having to touch the needle shaft.

- Puncture guiding the needle with the other hand: in puncture of the deeper points, longer needles are used. In order to avoid the needle deviating from the intended direction, or to avoid the needle bending, it is guided with the other hand, which holds it using sterile cotton wool (figure 2.14). Currently, there are double guide tube systems that guarantee safe and correct insertion of longer needles (TeWa® system).

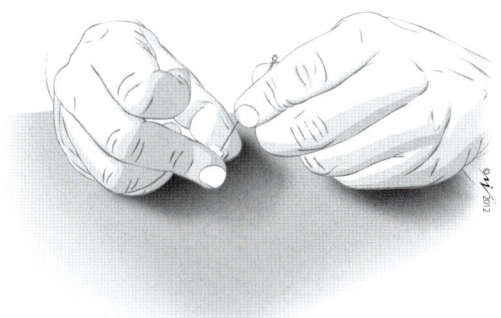

FIGURE 2.14 ■ Invasive technique using the other hand as a guide. (Colour version of figure is available online).

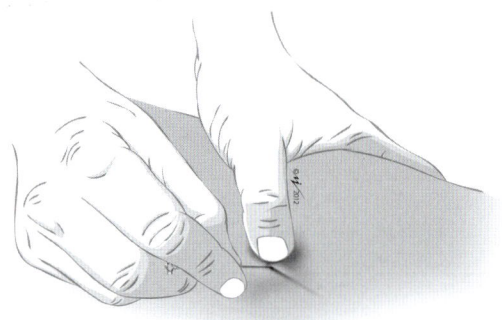

FIGURE 2.15 ■ Invasive technique using nail pressure. (Colour version of figure is available online).

- Puncture applying pressure with the nail: the nail of the thumb or index finger applies slight pressure upon the area that is to be punctured. The puncture takes place alongside the nail, so that the nail acts as a guide for the insertion of the needle whilst securing the point (figure 2.15).

Once the first skin barrier is crossed, it is recommended to perform small movements with the needle in order to facilitate insertion, especially when the needle remains 'stuck' in the facial tissue.

It is possible to decrease the painful sensation that accompanies needle insertion by using a distraction strategy:
- Complete the procedure using a guide tube.
- Verbal-cognitive distraction: start a relaxed conversation with the patient on a pleasant topic (e.g. holidays, travel, sports), which will help distract the person's attention away from the needle.
- Progressive contact: place the needle tip for a moment on the subject's skin to provoke a minimal pain and then introduce the needle 1–2 mm before the final insertion. Do this with care, as the opposite effect can be observed in patients who are apprehensive of needles.
- Skin pinch: give a small pinch of the skin to desensitize the mechanoreceptors and then immediately perform the puncture.
- Respiratory cycle: insert the needle while the patient is exhaling.

2.7.2 Mobilization/manipulation techniques

The needle mobilization and manipulation techniques are the different procedures performed by the professional to reach the puncture target. The most commonly used manipulation techniques are as follows.

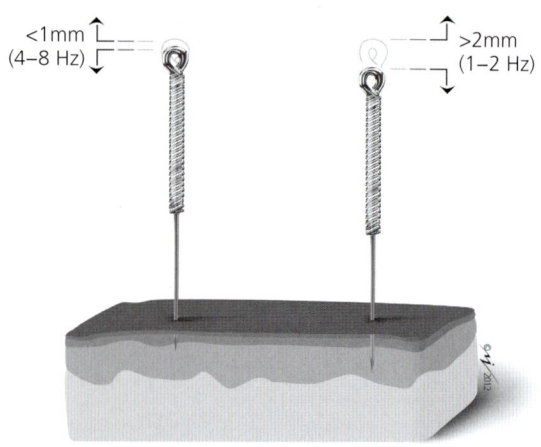

FIGURE 2.16 ■ Lifting and thrusting. (Colour version of figure is available online).

Insertion

The needle is introduced to the desired depth and then immediately withdrawn without twisting or stimulating the tissue in any way.

Lifting and thrusting

The needle is lifted upwards and thrust downwards. A low-amplitude movement is used (<1 mm) combined with high frequency (approx. 4–8 Hz) or high amplitude (>2 mm) and low frequency (approx. 1–2 Hz) over different planes (figure 2.16). This can be performed on a single plane or on multiple tissue planes (fan-like application).

Sparrow pecking

This is a method of rapid lifting and thrusting. Once the needle is introduced to the desired depth, it is partly withdrawn, thrust and rotated rapidly various times like a bird pecking food (figure 2.17). This technique must be avoided in areas of the plexus. This is the technique of choice for stimulating the periosteum and the corresponding sclerotome, and is called periosteal pecking. For example, it is used over the acromion in order to stimulate C4 or the lateral epicondyle to stimulate C6–7.

Scraping

This technique consists of using the nail of the index finger to scrape the needle handle while the needle is inserted in the target region (figure 2.18).

Swaying

This technique consists of holding the handle of the needle and gently swaying it from left to right (figure 2.19).

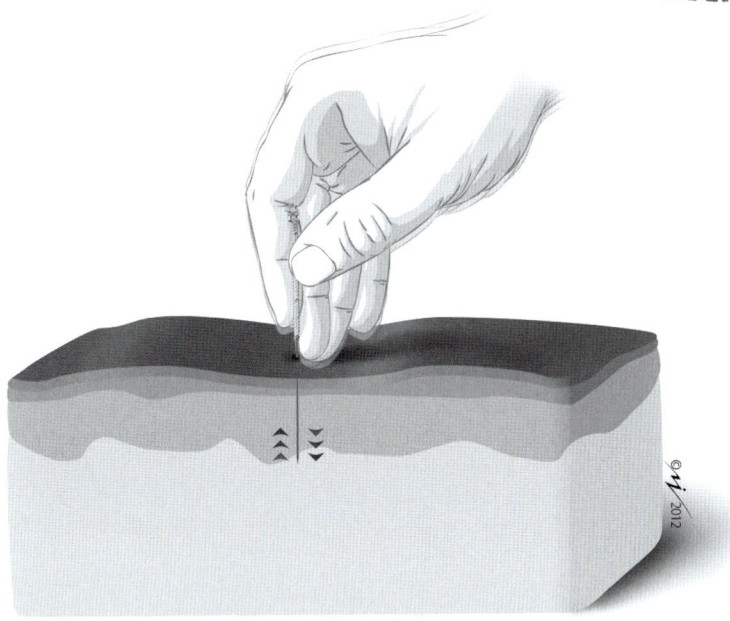

FIGURE 2.17 ■ Sparrow pecking. (Colour version of figure is available online).

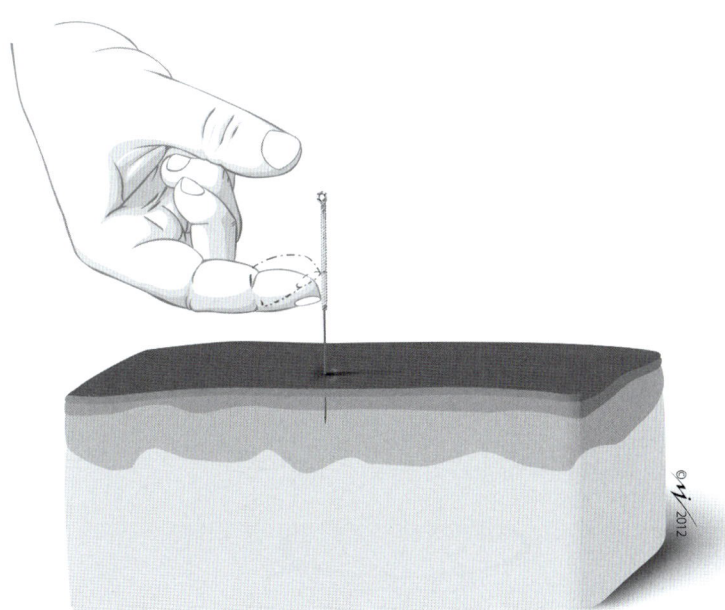

FIGURE 2.18 ■ Scraping. (Colour version of figure is available online).

Flicking

This consists of flicking the needle handle or tail with the index finger to shake the needle slightly (figure 2.20).

Rotation

Together with simple puncture, rotation is the most frequently applied needle movement. Four main components to the needle twist are described: (1) the width (small–large); (2) the frequency (high–low); (3) the direction (unidirectional–bidirectional); and (4) the number of rotations.

- Width: reduced width (rotation of the needle with a rotation angle of <90°) or greater (rotation angle >180°) (figure 2.21).
- Frequency: rotations of a high frequency (approx. 4–8 Hz) and low frequency (approx. 1–2 Hz) are both considered.
- Direction: unidirectional or bidirectional; in other words, twisting one way or the other. In this case, the studies performed[12–14] conclude that the unidirectional or bidirectional twist generated by the needle can

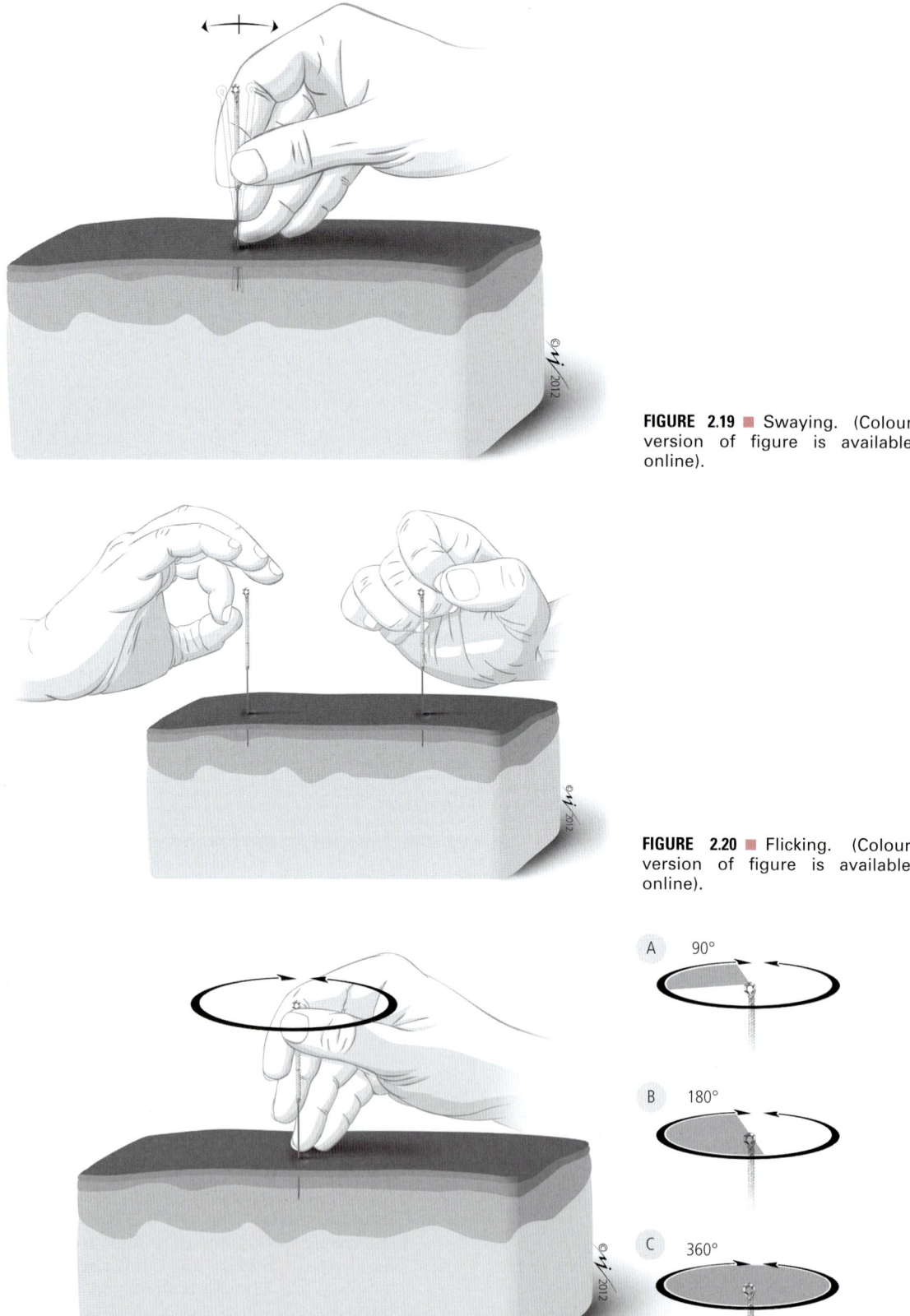

FIGURE 2.19 ■ Swaying. (Colour version of figure is available online).

FIGURE 2.20 ■ Flicking. (Colour version of figure is available online).

FIGURE 2.21 ■ Needle rotation angle. (A) 90°. (B) 180°. (C) 360°. (Colour version of figure is available online).

induce an active response of fibroblasts (figure 2.22). There are several possible combinations for stimulating the tissue via the mechanotransduction mechanism.[15–17] With rotation this is in a single direction (unidirectional) and a conceptual model can be established[12–14] that is reproducible in clinical practice. When the needle is given a few twists, the connective tissue is tensed and this causes the needle to become 'blocked' or 'stalled' (called 'needle grasp') (figure 2.23). In this case, additional rotation causes large amounts of connective tissue to remain rolled around the needle forming a spiral or, presumably, generating a strong mechanical stimulus. It is not clear what happens with the stimulus generated by the needle in a bidirectional twist, when the needle is twisted slightly one way and then twisted in the same manner in the opposite way.

- Number of rotations: several possible combinations are available in order to obtain a stimulus over the fibroblasts. It is thought that an optimal response is obtained with two or three turns.[12–15]

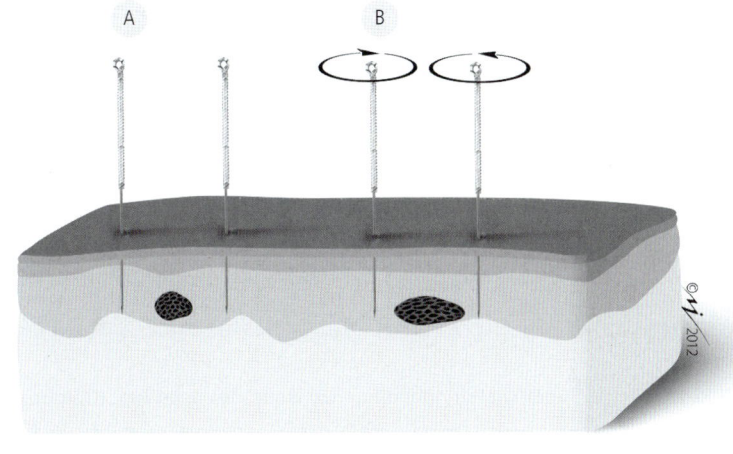

FIGURE 2.22 ■ Effect of rotating the needle. (A) Insertion into points close to the target tissue. (B) The twist causes a mechanical stimulus on the target tissue. (Colour version of figure is available online).

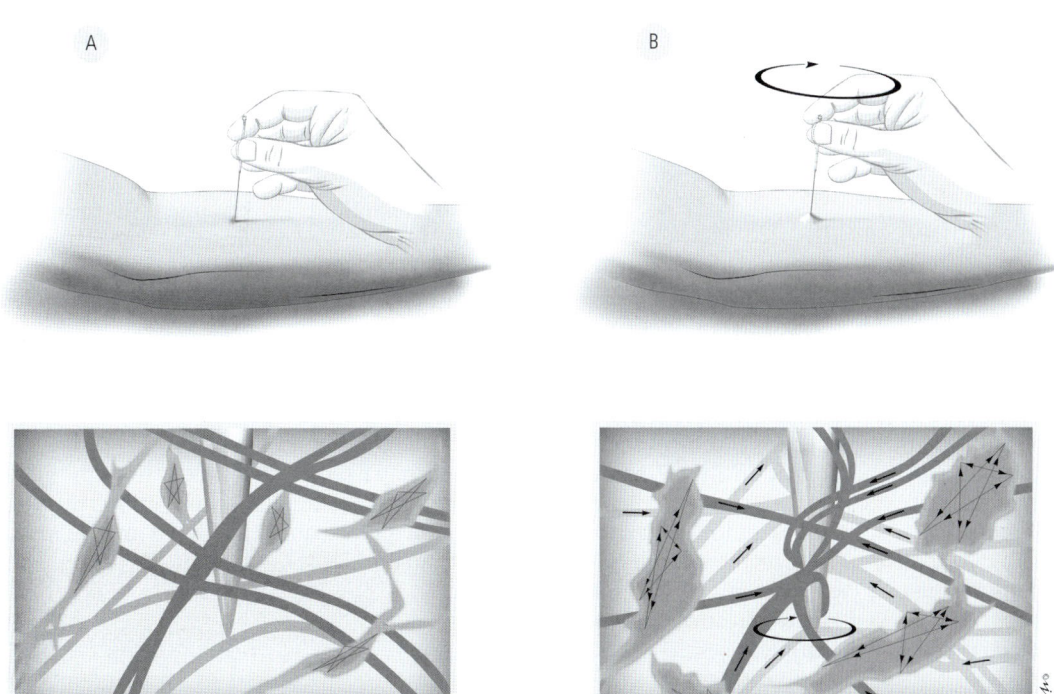

FIGURE 2.23 ■ Effect of rotating the needle upon the soft tissue: needle grasp. (A) Insertion. (B) Rotation. (Adapted from: Langevin HM, Konofagou EE, Badger GJ, et al. Tissue displacements during acupuncture using ultrasound elastography techniques. Ultrasound Med Biol. 2004 Sep;30(9):1173–1183). (Colour version of figure is available online).

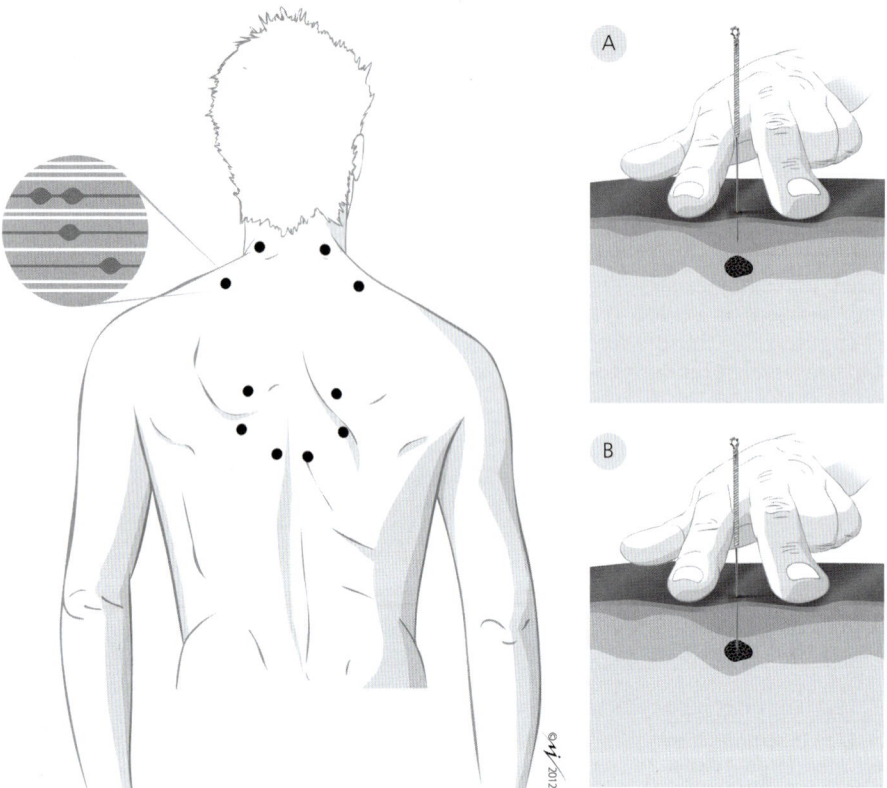

FIGURE 2.24 ■ (A) Superficial dry needling. (B) Deep dry needling. (Colour version of figure is available online).

KEY POINTS

The most common needle manipulation techniques are lifting and thrusting of the needle, together with rotation.

2.7.3 Applied techniques

Acupuncture

The most commonly applied techniques in acupuncture are insertion with rotation and sparrow pecking. Traditional Chinese medicine distinguishes between tonification (stimulation) techniques and sedation (dispersion). High-frequency techniques, with short rotation in the sense of the meridian, are considered to be tonifying, and low-frequency techniques, with longer rotations and in the opposite sense of the meridian, are sedating techniques (see chapter 15). The scraping technique is used as a tonification technique in selected points for chronic cases.

Dry needling

Dry needling techniques can be classified according to whether the needle reaches the MTrP and the taut band. In this manner, one can differentiate between superficial dry needling techniques, when the needle is inserted about 5–10 mm into the tissue above the MTrP (figure 2.24A) (simple insertion), and deep dry needling techniques when the needle passes through the MTrP (figure 2.24B) (technique of sinking and raising the needle in a fan-like application) (see chapter 8).

Percutaneous needle tenotomy

Percutaneous (across/through the skin) needle tenotomy (cutting or making an incision in a tendon) is a common procedure in the treatment of chronic tendon problems. In this technique, a hypodermic needle is advanced through the skin in order to make small incisions and slices within a tendon (approximately 20–30 needle passes) (see chapter 11).

Percutaneous needle electrolysis

Regarding the treatment of the tendon tissue, PNE techniques such as EPI®, EPTE® or MEP® are targeted at different interphases (superficial interphase, intratendon and deep interphase) (figure 2.25) while, in the case of the

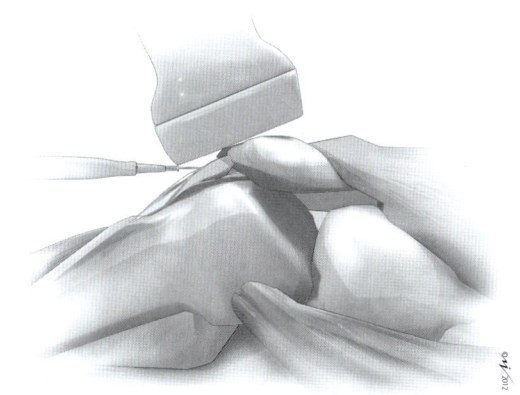

FIGURE 2.25 ■ Percutaneous needle electrolysis. (Colour version of figure is available online).

muscle tissue, the approach to the MTrPs consists of lifting and thrusting the needle into different planes in the taut band and MTrP (see chapters 8 and 14). These techniques are often associated with needle rotation to reinforce the mechanotransduction effect.[15–17]

Mesotherapy

The most commonly used techniques in mesotherapy are epidermal and intradermal injection, intradermal nappage and intradermal papule (see chapter 17). In these cases, the medication is applied at a local level in small but repeated quantities. In addition, application without medication can be performed ('dry mesotherapy'), as the cutaneous stimulation of the needle itself (approximately 4 mm) generates a local response (increased circulation and metabolism at the local level) and constitutes a segmental stimulus at the dermatome level.

Injection therapy

Injection techniques can be divided into single-injection techniques and 'peppering' or 'fan' techniques. The single-injection technique consists of depositing the solution in a single flow (the bolus technique) at the identified area of maximal tenderness. The entire contents of the syringe are deposited at the site, after which the needle is withdrawn. This technique is most often used for the treatment of bursae and joint cavities.

The 'peppering' or 'fan' technique involves a fanning in-and-out motion of the needle while injecting the affected tissue (several small droplets). Three-dimensional imaging of the target structure is an important adjunct to this technique as the needle tip must be introduced into different parts of the structure via half-withdrawals and redirections in order to be able to infiltrate the solution both deeply and more superficially. This technique is probably the most commonly used method for tendons and ligaments.

2.8 APPLICATION MODALITIES

A series of different application modalities exist with regard to needle puncture techniques. These are the application at a greater or lesser depth, or the use of a greater or lesser tilt with a manually guided application (or with the use of ultrasound guidance), the use of local anaesthesia or not, depending on the application time and, finally, whether these are associated with other physical agents such as heat (moxibustion) or electricity (e.g. electroacupuncture, electrolipolysis, PNE).

2.8.1 Palpation-guided versus ultrasound-guided

Invasive techniques can be applied using palpation (conventional anatomical landmark palpation-guided interventions) or musculoskeletal ultrasound (ultrasound-guided interventions) (see chapter 7).

Traditionally, invasive techniques have been palpation-guided, and are an intrinsic part of the technique, such as in the case of acupuncture, where there is a thousand-year-old representation of the meridians and acupuncture points along with their corresponding anatomical and topographical relations.

The main advantage of ultrasound-guided interventions is that they enable a completely safe technique, reducing the risks of complications, and increasing the effectiveness of the technique, as these applications allow identification of the affected tissue and, therefore, treatment is specifically targeted at the area. This is especially important in techniques such as PNE or dry needling where deep tissues are treated.

The main difficulties associated with the application of ultrasound-guided techniques are the technical problems of managing the ultrasound probe and the needle bimanually and the impossibility of performing the application in select small areas with conventional probes, as there is not enough space.

In any case, musculoskeletal ultrasound enables analysis of the tissue and, therefore, the presence of a vasculonervous element can be ruled out and a follow-up of the treated area is possible.

2.8.2 Depth of the puncture

The depth of the puncture depends on the location of the target body structure that one intends to stimulate, the constitution of the patient (thin, athletic or stocky patients) and the invasive technique to be applied. Besides this, in traditional Chinese medicine the overall symptoms are considered. For example, when the process is mild or acute a more superficial puncture is performed whereas, in severe or chronic pathologies, needles are generally introduced at a greater depth.

From a neurophysiological point of view, the puncture depth is an essential element to achieve segmental stimulus of the different structures, and depending on whether one wishes to stimulate at the level of the dermatome, myotome, sclerotome or viscerotome (figure 2.26) (see chapter 10). According to this concept, the deeper the application, the greater the stimulus.

Scientific evidence suggests that a greater puncture depth achieves a greater local response (greater superficial blood flow in the skin and the muscle).[18-21]

Depending on the invasive technique, the following approximate tissue depths can be stimulated:

- Mesotherapy uses subcutaneous applications at 3–4 mm.
- In acupuncture most punctures are performed at a maximum depth of 1 cm.
- In electrolipolysis the applications are performed on the fat tissue from 1 cm to 4–5 cm depth.
- Dry needling and PNE techniques use punctures at various depths; the most common range from 1 cm to 7 cm deep, depending on the target tissue.

2.8.3 Direction of the puncture

The puncture angle depends on the topographic characteristics of the selected point and its target structures (figure 2.27).

Perpendicular puncture

A perpendicular puncture is performed in areas of muscle or fat tissues. In this case, the needle is introduced perpendicularly to the skin surface.

Oblique puncture

The needle is inserted at an angle of 30–50° in relation to the skin surface. This technique is used when the target tissue must be accessed obliquely in relation to the puncture point. It is appropriate in points with scarce soft tissue, for example in an approach on the thorax in order to avoid a pneumothorax or when treating the head area. It is also used in techniques of zoned acupuncture,[22] when the needle is inserted at 30° to the skin and introduced until it remains flat upon the skin.

Transverse/horizontal puncture

The needle is introduced at a 5–15° angle in relation to the skin surface. This technique is used in points located below a very thin layer of soft tissue, such as, for example, in the case of acupuncture points found on the skull.

2.8.4 Number of needles

The number of needles used in the same session depends on the technique. In acupuncture and

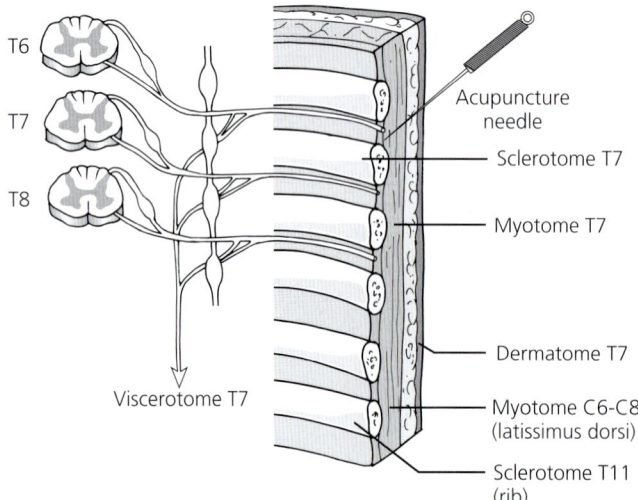

FIGURE 2.26 ■ Puncture depth. Topographic relations among the different structures in the T7 segment. Depending on the depth of puncture, different segments can be influenced. (Adapted from: Ma YT, Ma M, Cho ZH. Biomedical Acupuncture for Pain Management. An Integrative Approach. St Louis, MO: Elsevier; 2005). (Colour version of figure is available online).

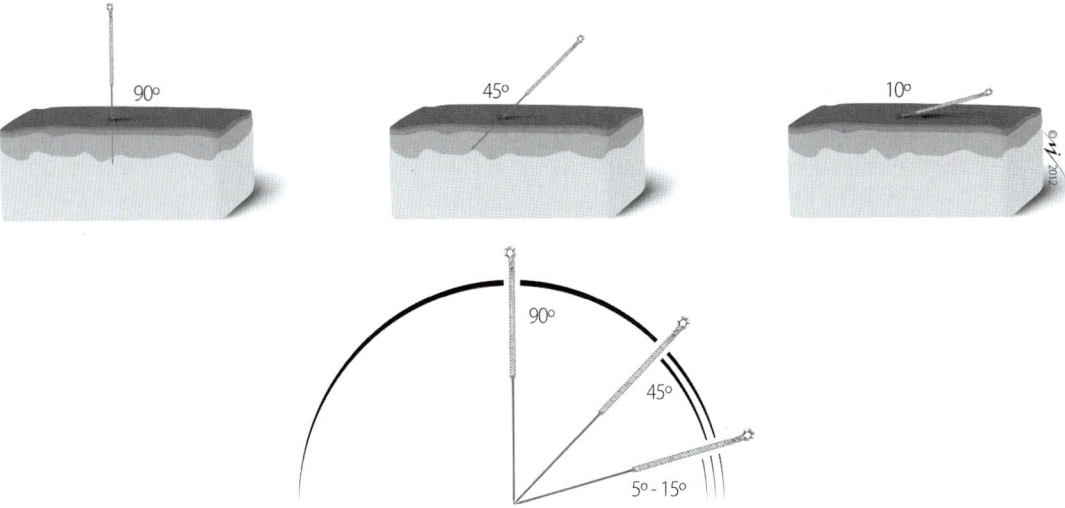

FIGURE 2.27 ■ Direction of the puncture. (Colour version of figure is available online).

TABLE 2.7	Factors involved in the strength of sensory stimulation (–/+) that may affect the dose of a treatment	
Treatment variable	**–**	**+**
Number of points	Minimum treatment involves one point only; usual treatment involves 4–10 points	More points
Needle type	Highly polished surface reduces effect	Larger diameter may have greater effect
Number of needle insertions	Minimum one needle insertion	More insertions
Depth of insertion	Superficially	From superficial to deep
Needle stimulation	Only manual (mechanical) stimulation	Increasing from manual, such as the addition of electrical or heat stimulation after needle insertion
Type of electrical stimulation	Transcutaneous electrical nerve stimulation (TENS), microcurrent	Galvanic current, high-volt pulsed galvanic stimulation
Needle retention time	10 mi (acupuncture)	Longer is generally considered to be stronger, up to about 30 minutes maximum (acupuncture)
Treatment frequency	Usually weekly	Twice weekly

mesotherapy, the number of punctures is greater than in dry needling or PNE. In clinical acupuncture practice, 8–10 punctures are used on average in each session (up to a maximum of 30), and the number of sessions per week is usually one or two. The recommendation is to increase the dose gradually once you know how the patient responds. Table 2.7 shows the factors involved in the strength of sensory stimulation that may affect the dose of a treatment.

Similarly, it is important to assess the clinical state of the patient, especially in the presence of disorders such as fibromyalgia, which can react with episodes of intense pain if the system is overstimulated by a large number of punctures. Likewise this is true where the immune system is depressed, or in illnesses such as diabetes, when the inflammatory response is altered.

KEY POINTS

The greater the number of needles, the greater the stimulus to the system.

2.8.5 Local anaesthetic measures

Invasive techniques can be applied with the help of local anaesthetics in order to reduce pain and increase patient comfort. They are especially useful in sensitive areas, such as the sole of the foot; however they reduce the possibility of patients being able to correlate the pain (that motivated the consultation in the first place) with the area that the needle is stimulating. The most commonly used measures are topical EMLA™-type creams and sprays or cold systems such as Coolsense®:

- EMLA™: this is a local anaesthetic composed of lidocaine and prilocaine, which is indicated for alleviating pain on the skin prior to interventions such as punctures. The common dose in adults for puncture techniques is approximately 2 g (1 g of EMLA™ is approximately 3.5 cm). For this purpose, the cream must be applied to the area and covered with an occlusive dressing (for example, transparent plastic) for a minimum of 1 hour and a maximum of 5 hours.[23] This is commonly used in applications over the perineal muscles.
- Cold sprays: a local anaesthetic effect is achieved with the application of a cold spray to the skin surface. The procedure consists of applying a spray over the skin for 2–4 seconds at a minimal distance of 20 cm, with an approximate angle of 30°, and a small and uniform spraying with two or three applications. It is advisable to avoid spraying a single point, as this can produce acute pain. The first time cold spray is applied it is advisable to demonstrate the technique to the patient first by applying the cold spray on the physiotherapist's hand, and then using the spray on the patient's hand to avoid a shock or muscle spasm in the area to be treated. These products are particularly used in mesotherapy applications (figure 2.28A).
- Coolsense®: this is a recently developed system consisting of a local anaesthesic that, when it comes into contact with skin, makes it cold. In this case anaesthesia is achieved by contact of the instrument with the target area of the skin at a temperature of between 0 and –4°C for 4–5 seconds. Prior to the application, the instrument is kept in the freezer for a minimum of 1 hour (figure 2.28B).

The main advantage of the cold systems (sprays and Coolsense®) in comparison to EMLA™ is the time needed to achieve local anaesthesia.

2.8.6 Needle retention time

We can distinguish between immediate, semipermanent and permanent punctures. There is no evidence to show that immediate punctures are superior to semipermanent or permanent punctures.

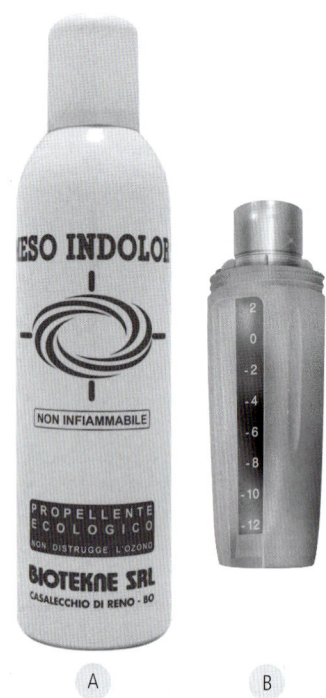

FIGURE 2.28 ■ (A) Cold spray. (B) Coolsense®.

- Immediate punctures are kept in place during the session.
- Semipermanent punctures are kept in place until the following session.
- Permanent punctures are left in for a long time (generally until they fall away by themselves). They are usually implanted in the outer ear. The technique consists of introducing the needle and stabilizing it with surgical tape until it falls out on its own.

2.8.7 Associated physical agents

The mechanical effect of the needle (associated with the puncture) can be combined with other physical agents and electrotherapeutic modalities, such as:

- Heat: the application of heat via the needle (known as 'hot-needle acupuncture') is used in moxibustion techniques (figure 2.29).
- Light: infrared light may be used with acupuncture applications as an associated measure to promote relaxation.
- Electricity: there are several possibilities for combining the mechanical effect of the needle with the electric current (transcutaneous electrical nerve stimulation [TENS]-type current [acuTENS] or microcurrents) (see chapter 16) (figure 2.30).

- Vibration: with a tuning fork or manual 'vibration' techniques, whereby the needle is grasped and vibrated.

2.9 OBJECTIVES OF THE NEEDLING TECHNIQUES

Six main objectives are associated with the invasive techniques: (1) *De-Xi* (*Qi*) sensation; (2) local twitch response (LTR); (3) reproduction of the pain pattern; (4) tissue elasticity; (5) needle effect; and (6) muscle contraction.

2.9.1 *De-Xi* (*Qi*) sensation

According to acupuncture technique, if the acupuncture point has been correctly located as regards direction and depth, the patient may describe sensations such as: 'dull pressure',

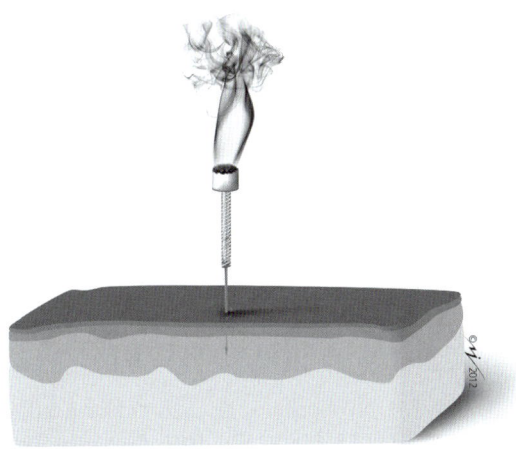

FIGURE 2.29 ■ Moxibustion. (Colour version of figure is available online).

'electric tingling', 'tension', 'heaviness' and 'heat', all of which last for milliseconds,[24] and which are different from the simple pain associated with the puncture. This phenomenon is known in Chinese literature as *De-Xi* or *Qi* (which represents the arrival of *Xi* or *Qi* energy). The goal is to trigger the *De-Xi* and orient it towards the preferred direction. In other words, once *De-Xi* is elicited, the needle must be directed towards the area of interest. For example, in the TH23 point (located upon the tail of the eyebrow) the *De-Xi* is sought and the needle is oriented outwards in the case of temporal headaches, or inwards in the case of eye pathology or tear duct disorders. If the *De-Xi* sensation irradiates along the course of the meridian, the phenomenon of propagated sensation along channels occurs. This is most frequent when muscle points are stimulated. In the same manner, the professional must perceive the *De-Xi* as a resistance to the movement of the needle, which is known as 'needle grasp'.

Most acupuncture specialists consider the provocation of *De-Xi* during puncture as a sign of a positive clinical result.[24–29] Recently, however, the influence of *De-Xi* in the result of acupuncture treatments was studied for patients with osteoarthritis of the knee and hip.[30] The results showed that there was no significant correlation between the strength of the *De-Xi* and the improvement of the pain and, also, that there were no significant differences in pain relief for those who felt *De-Xi* and those who did not. The study concluded that the presence and intensity of *De-Xi* have no effect on the pain relief obtained in patients with osteoarthritis. The *De-Xi* effect can be reinforced when associated with the stimulus of the needle with electric current (electroacupuncture) or the vibration (tuning fork or manual 'vibration').

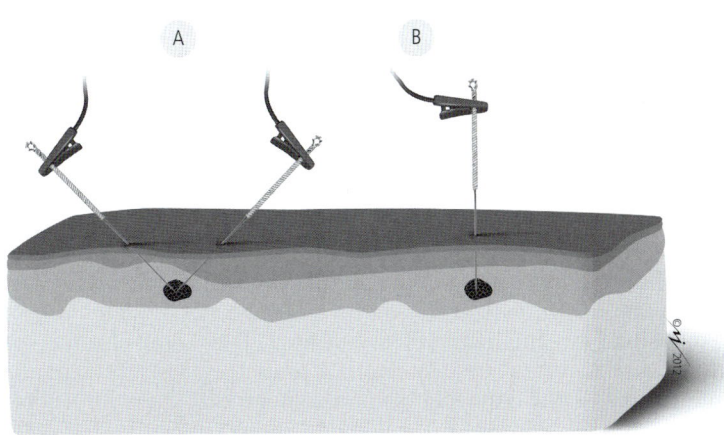

FIGURE 2.30 ■ Electroacupuncture. (A) *Ashi* points. (B) Intramuscular. (Colour version of figure is available online).

2.9.2 Local twitch response

The LTR is an involuntary muscle contraction associated with puncture on an MTrP or neighbouring area. This response has a diagnostic character, as it confirms the existence of a myofascial dysfunction and a therapeutic dysfunction, as elicitation of an LTR is associated with greater effectiveness of the puncture technique (see chapter 8). There appears to be a correlation between the high velocity with which the needle is inserted and the possibility of obtaining an LTR.[31–33]

2.9.3 Reproduction of the pain pattern

The reproduction of the patient's symptomatic pain (the reason for the consultation) can be achieved by a mechanical deformation of the affected tissue (compression, traction, stretching, contraction or puncture). In the case of stimulation with MTrPs via dry needling or PNE it is possible to reproduce the patient's referred pain pattern or, in the case of a tendinopathy, trigger the pain pattern that the subject experiences after a sports activity, although this is usually of less intensity. For example, needle stimulation of the MTrP found on the infraspinatus muscle can cause pain in the patient's anterior shoulder. Also, stimulation in the inferior pole of the patella in relation to the deep fibres of the patellar tendon and Hoffa's fat pad can reproduce the symptoms of patellar tendinopathy.

2.9.4 Tissue elasticity

During the application of puncture techniques, changes in tissue texture are perceived by the therapist, and often a significant reduction in tissue resistance is felt. This is described by the authors as a 'softening' effect of the involved collagen tissue. It can also be a useful criterion for the physiotherapist, indicating the need to finish the application of the technique. In this sense, the needle or needle holder acts as an extension of the therapist's hands through which this change is perceived.

2.9.5 Needle effect

The needle effect, described by Lewit,[33] is the immediate analgesic effect of the puncture when the needle manages to reach the precise point responsible for the patient's symptoms. The improvement in real time is referred to as the summation of the immediate improvement of

the pain as well as the function (e.g. mobility, force, stability).

2.9.6 Muscle contraction

In the stimulation of the motor point and the peripheral nervous branch, the objective is to achieve a rhythmic non-painful contraction. On occasion, the initial contraction is irregular and of poor quality, and this is indicative of muscular dysfunction.

In any of these circumstances, the effectiveness of the puncture technique is greater.

2.10 SENSATIONS PRODUCED BY THE NEEDLE PUNCTURE

2.10.1 Provoked sensations

The biological mechanisms associated with the puncture will determine the characteristics of the different sensations that the patient describes during the treatment.

The puncture per se is considered to be a process of nociceptive stimulation that causes mechanical and biochemical effects. The mechanical effects are the pressure of the needle on the skin, the target area and the alteration of the nociceptors. The biochemical effects include the neurogenic inflammation induced by the needle and the liberation of neuropeptides from the nociceptors and the different tissues, substance P, bradykinin, prostaglandins, serotonin, somatostatin and calcitonin gene-related peptide.[34–39]

When the physiotherapist inserts the needle into the patient's body, the first effect is loss of continuity of the skin (first defensive barrier of the immune system) and of the superficial fascia. The puncture produces a 'microtrauma' or 'microlesion' in the whole of the soft tissue that it passes through, including muscle fibres, nerve terminals, blood vessels, fascias, tendons, ligaments and periosteum. It also activates the self-repairing processes of the tissue. These 'microlesions' are understood to be a mechanical and neurophysiological stimulus of the soft tissue via a physical agent such as the needle. They remain active when the needle is extracted, which makes the biological system activate both the physiopathological repair systems of the soft tissue, as well as the neurobiological systems of pain in order to normalize the acute or chronic dysfunction of the soft tissue. This process requires coordination of the nervous, immunoendocrine and cardiovascular systems, via control that is determined both by peripheral mechanisms (e.g. nociceptors and the liberation of neuropeptides) as well as central mechanisms.

Once the needle touches the patient's skin and passes through it, the response of the nociceptors of the sensitive cutaneous nerves is quite varied (especially type III fibres or type Aδ) (table 2.8 and figure 2.31). Therefore the sensation the patient feels can range from a nervous current that extends from proximal to distal (equivalent to *De-Xi* or *Qi* described in acupuncture), to shooting pain, tingling and even, at times, a feeling of burning. Once the needle

TABLE 2.8 Neurophysiology of needling

Sensory fibre ABC type	Sensory fibre I–IV type	Diameter (μm)	Velocity (m/s)	Function	Role in analgesia	Response elicited
Aα	1a	15–20	70–120	Annulospiral muscle spindles (length)		
	1b			Golgi tendon organ (load)		
Aβ	II	5–12	30–70	Touch		
Aγ	II	3–6	15–30	Flower spray muscle spindles (length)	+	Numbness
Aδ	III	2–5	12–30	Pinprick sensation (=first or fast pain)	+	Aching, distension, heaviness
C	IV	0.4–1,2	0.5–2	Aching pain (=second or slow pain)		Soreness

Adapted from Guyton and Hall.[42]

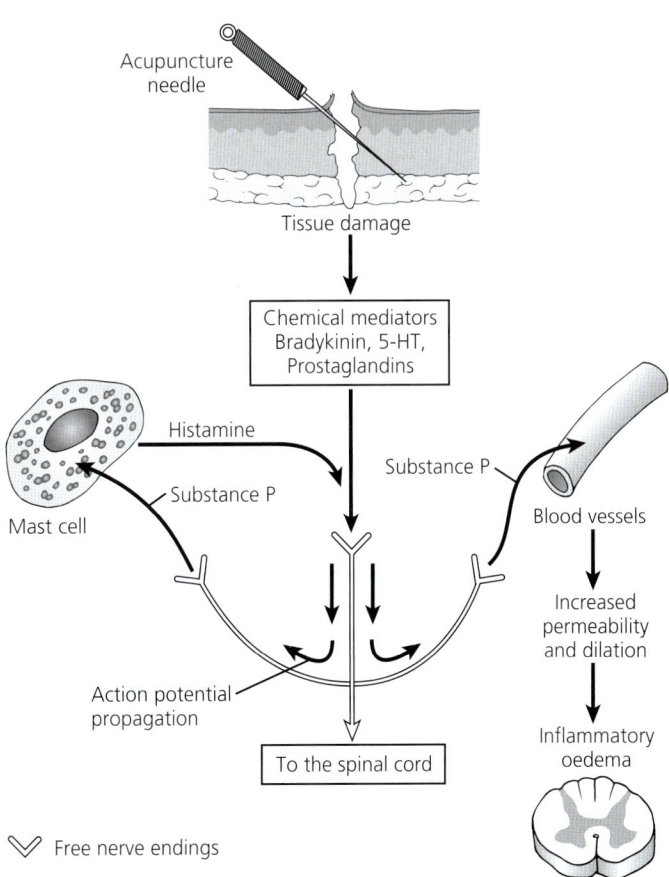

FIGURE 2.31 ■ Tissue damage and microbiological injury created by the needle. (Adapted from: Watson T. Electrotherapy: Evidence Based Practice. 12th edn. Edinburgh, Churchill Livingstone Elsevier; 2008).

reaches deep tissues, stimulation occurs, mainly over nerve terminals that innervate the muscle tissue and unmyelinated nervous sensitive terminals (type IV or type C fibres) which innervate the blood vessels and other soft tissues.

Commonly, an acute shooting pain appears when a blood vessel has been penetrated, but it may be associated with other signs, such as dull ache, a feeling of pressure, heaviness, residual pain, tingling, dysaesthesias. In summary, the sensation depends on the type of nervous fibre that has been stimulated via the needle and the physiological conditions of the neighbouring tissue (for example, the possible presence of inflammation mediators). It is important to warn patients that some sensations caused by the puncture, such as a heaviness, pressure or dull ache, can remain for 1–2 days (this is something that occasionally coincides with the peak of maximal pain, followed by a decrease over the following 2–3 days).

KEY POINTS

A feeling of shooting pain when the needle is inserted is usually indicative of having reached a blood vessel.

On the other hand, when a puncture is performed over points on the patient's upper or lower extremities, the patient may experience a slight sensation of a current ascending or descending along the length of the stimulated extremity. This is equivalent to the phenomenon of propagated sensations along the channel (described in acupuncture). When punctures are performed on the trunk, the sensation that a patient experiences may be local. Some patients refer to experiencing an odd sensation, similar to energy circulating from the needle, towards the head and towards the feet. This could be due to the convergence of cutaneous and muscular afferents.

Immediately after introducing the needle into the skin and reaching the target tissue, the painful sensation felt by the patient decreases considerably or totally disappears until needle manipulation commences. This phenomenon is known as the 'silence of the painful sensation'. If, once the needle is inserted, the pain persists, is acute, or generates discomfort in the patient, it is appropriate to withdraw the needle and reinsert it in an adjacent point. Once the needles are inserted, the patient should also experience a cool sensation, especially in applications that remain for longer periods, such as acupuncture. In this case it is possible to combine the puncture with measures of superficial heat, such as infrared.

Although the most common sensations patients report caused by puncture are produced via peripheral mechanisms, central mechanisms also have a role in the clinical presentation of the patient and the effectiveness of the invasive techniques. The central nervous system controls and coordinates the peripheral mechanisms when the needle penetrates the skin and reaches a deep tissue. From the peripheral receptors, the information passes upwards along the spinothalamic tract, the brainstem, the thalamus and the hypothalamus until it reaches the somatosensory cortex and the limbic system. These are areas of the central nervous system that perform important tasks, such as nociceptive processing and perception of the pain experienced by the patient. In clinical daily practice, reactions such as sweating, tachycardia or goose bumps (piloerection) are symptoms that the patient experiences and which are also key in the effectiveness of puncture techniques.

2.10.2 Response patterns

Regarding the response elicited by the invasive techniques, different patterns can be described among the subjects that are important for clinical practice.

Strong responders

These are the patients who respond surprisingly fast to the invasive techniques, immediately after the application of a small stimulation. This response may be of relaxation, euphoria, drowsiness or crying and, in any case, they describe a feeling of feeling 'well'. These are patients who require little treatment and few sessions and who will rapidly improve. They respond far better than normal.

Weak responders

In these cases the invasive techniques require a greater stimulation (for example, a greater number of needles, needles with a larger diameter and the use of manipulation techniques) in order to achieve an effect. They do not have an immediate response and it is harder to provoke stimulus, such as *De-Xi*. These patients require a greater number of sessions.

Between both of these extremes are the so-called 'mid-responders', who respond more in the mid-range. In other words, they are perceived as being average, given that approximately half respond below this value (mid-low responders), while the other half respond above (mid-high responders).

Non-responders

These patients do not display a therapeutic response to invasive treatment. However, although some patients may not display an immediate local or general reaction to the treatment, it does not necessarily mean that they are 'non-responders'. This must be assessed in the mid to long term. Non-responders are usually associated with changes in the immune system, such as diabetes, or associated with the consumption of steroids or corticosteroids.

Clinically, it is important to distinguish between strong and weak responders when planning a therapeutic intervention. In the case of patients who are weak responders, a treatment that is below their dosage will not cause relief of symptoms. However, for strong responders, a dosage above the necessary could even worsen their symptoms, at least temporarily. This reaction is equivalent in pharmacology to the therapeutic dosage above the necessary.

2.11 PHYSIOLOGICAL REACTIONS TO THE NEEDLE PUNCTURE

2.11.1 Skin

The skin is the first defence barrier of the human body. When a puncture breaks the skin, a cascade of physiological events are triggered as a response to the mechanical aggression.

When the patient presents a musculoskeletal disorder, and during clinical study, the physiotherapist identifies a sensitive area susceptible to treatment via a needle puncture. Often, the electric conductivity of the skin is increased around this area while its resistance is decreased due to the presence of liquid in the interstitial space and the presence of ions as a result of inflammation. The introduction of a needle at this point will provoke a local acute inflammatory response of all skin components. As a consequence, the first objective sign is redness of the skin around the puncture (dilation of the arterial and venous networks) followed by the appearance of oedema. This vasodilation of the autonomous nervous system is mediated by substance P, triggering an immune reaction due to stimulation of the mast cells, which liberates histamine, a platelet-activating factor and leukotrienes.[39,40]

2.11.2 Connective tissue

When the needle is inserted into the tissue, an initial coupling occurs between the metallic body of the tissue and the collagen fibres. This affinity is caused by superficial tension and attraction between the needle metal and the electric charge of the connective tissue. Once this coupling has occurred, the friction force becomes the leading element. At this point, needle rotation increases tension in the fibres due to the fact that they wind around the needle, which in turn causes traction and realignment of the network of connective tissue fibres.[12–14] Clinically, the physiotherapist perceives needle resistance, not just with regard to the rotation, but also frequently occurring when the needle penetrates the skin and, at the same time, the patient feels a sensation of rigidity. According to clinical evidence, the liberation response of this resistance that the patient experiences is greater and faster when the application of a galvanic current is associated with the mechanical needle stimulus, as occurs in PNE techniques.

This mechanical stimulus affects the extracellular matrix, the fibroblasts, the cross-bridges between collagen fibres and, according to various authors, the capillary endothelial cells. As a response to this physical deformation, the cells initiate a cascade of cellular and molecular events, such as the reorganization of the intracellular cytoskeleton, migration and cellular contraction, autocrine liberation of growth factors and the activation of intracellular information tracts and nuclear binding proteins that promote the transcription of specific genes. This physiological phenomenon is known as mechanotransduction.[15–17]

For clinicians, it is important to have a clear understanding of the immediate effect of the puncture. Although it is known that the success of the puncture techniques does not solely lie in manipulation of the needle, in daily clinical practice, the physiotherapist may benefit from the effect that this mechanical stimulus provokes over the resistance of the soft tissue.

2.11.3 Muscle tissue

The puncture produces a decrease in local muscle tension referred by the patient as a consequence of a myofascial dysfunction. As we have already explained, the needle manipulation and the puncture per se have an effect of mechanical deformation on the fibres of collagen tissue. According to clinical evidence, the mechanical stimulus also helps to stretch the muscle, blocking, on the one hand, the process of energetic crisis (described by Simons[41]) that currently sustains the pathophysiology of the MTrPs as well as the reflex points of the acupuncture system.

These aforementioned mechanisms have been demonstrated to be effective for muscular relaxation, the re-establishment of local blood circulation, and the promotion of tissue repair, without any side effects. Furthermore, if the patient presents a myofascial acute and localized pain, muscle relaxation can be achieved immediately. In other clinical situations ongoing treatment is required.

Conflict of interest declaration

The authors declare that they have no conflicts of interest.

2.12 REFERENCES

1. World Confederation for Physical Therapy. Policy statement: description of physical therapy. London, UK: WCPT; 2011. Available at: <http://www.wcpt.org/policy/ps-descriptionPT>; [Accessed 20 Jul 2012].
2. World Confederation for Physical Therapy. WCPT guideline for physical therapist professional entry level education. London, UK: WCPT; 2011. Available at: <http://www.wcpt.org/guidelines/entry-level-education>; [Accessed 20 Jul 2012].
3. Baldry P. Acupuncture, trigger points and musculoskeletal pain, 3rd ed. Edinburgh: Elsevier; 2005.
4. Ma YT, Ma M, Cho ZH. Biomedical acupuncture for pain management. An integrative approach. St Louis, MO: Elsevier; 2005.
5. Rietschel RL, Fowler JF. Fisher's contact dermatitis. 6th ed. Hamilton, Ontario: BC Decker; 2008.
6. Lilly E, Kundu RV. Dermatoses secondary to Asian cultural practices. Int J Dermatol 2012;51:372–9.
7. Tanii T, Kono T, Katoh J, et al. A case of prurigo pigmentosa considered to be contact allergy to chromium in an acupuncture needle. Acta Derm Venereol 1991;71: 66–7.
8. Romaguera C, Grimalt F. Contact dermatitis from a permanent acupuncture needle. Contact Dermatitis 1981;7:156–7.
9. Yamashita H, Tsukayama H, Tanno Y, et al. Adverse events in acupuncture and moxibustion treatment: a six-year survey at a national clinic in Japan. J Altern Complement Med 1999;5:229–36.
10. Fernández Villegas I, Bersee HEN. Ultrasonic welding of advanced thermoplastic composites: an investigation on energy-directing surfaces. Adv Polym Tech 2010;29: 112–21.
11. ISO 7886-1. Sterile hypodermic syringes for single use – part 1. Syringes for manual use. Geneva; 1993.
12. Langevin HM, Konofagou EE, Badger GJ, et al. Tissue displacements during acupuncture using ultrasound elastography techniques. Ultrasound Med Biol 2004;30: 1173–83.
13. Langevin HM, Bouffard NA, Badger GJ, et al. Subcutaneous tissue fibroblast cytoskeletal remodeling induced by acupuncture: evidence for a mechanotransduction-based mechanism. J Cell Physiol 2006;207:767–74.
14. Langevin HM, Churchill DL, Cipolla MJ. Mechanical signaling through connective tissue: a mechanism for the therapeutic effect of acupuncture. FASEB J 2001;15: 2275–82.
15. O'Toole M, Lamoureux P, Miller KE. A physical model of axonal elongation: force, viscosity, and adhesions govern the mode of outgrowth. Biophys J 2008;94:2610–20.
16. Ingber DE. Tensegrity: the architectural basis of cellular mechanotransduction. Annu Rev Physiol 1997;59: 575–99.
17. Konofagou EE, Langevin HM. Using ultrasound to understand acupuncture. Acupuncture needle manipulation and its effect on connective tissue. IEEE Eng Med Biol Mag 2005;24:41–6.
18. Sandberg M, Lundeberg T, Lindberg LG, et al. Effects of acupuncture on skin and muscle blood flow in healthy subjects. Eur J Appl Physiol 2003;90:114–19.
19. Vincent CA, Richardson PH, Black JJ, et al. The significance of needle placement site in acupuncture. J Psychosom Res 1989;33:489–96.
20. Haker E, Egekvist H, Bjerring P. Effect of sensory stimulation (acupuncture) on sympathetic and parasympathetic activities in healthy subjects. J Auton Nerv Syst 2000;79:52–9.
21. Sandberg M, Lindberg LG, Gerdle B. Peripheral effects of needle stimulation (acupuncture) on skin and muscle blood flow in fibromyalgia. Eur J Pain 2004;8: 163–71.
22. Carrión J. Acupuntura zonal. Barcelona: Hispano Europea; 2011.
23. Prospecto: información para el usuario EMLA™ 25 mg/g + 25 mg /g crema. Agencia Española de medicamentos y productos sanitarios. Available at: <http://www.aemps.gob.es/cima/especialidad.do?metodo=verFichaWordPdf&codigo=61096&formato=pdf&formulario=PROSPECTOS>; [Accessed 20 Jul 2012].
24. White P, Bishop F, Hardy H, et al. Southampton needle sensation questionnaire: development and validation of a measure to gauge acupuncture needle sensation. J Altern Complement Med 2008;14:373–9.
25. Ezzo J, Berman B, Hadhazy VA, et al. Is acupuncture effective for the treatment of chronic pain? A systematic review. Pain 2000;86:217–25.
26. White AR, Ernst E. A trial method for assessing the adequacy of acupuncture treatments. Altern Ther Health Med 1998;4:66–71.
27. MacPherson H, Asghar A. Acupuncture needle sensations associated with De Qi: a classification based on experts' ratings. J Altern Complement Med 2006;12: 633–7.
28. Mao JJ, Farrar JT, Armstrong K, et al. De qi: Chinese acupuncture patients' experiences and beliefs regarding acupuncture needling sensation – an exploratory survey. Acupunct Med 2007;25:158–65.
29. Park JJ, Akazawa M, Ahn J, et al. Acupuncture sensation during ultrasound guided acupuncture needling. Acupunct Med 2011;29:257–65.
30. White P, Prescott P, Lewith G. Does needling sensation (de qi) affect treatment outcome in pain? Analysis of data from a larger single-blind, randomised controlled trial. Acupunct Med 2010;28:120–5.
31. Hong CZ. Lidocaine injection versus dry needling to myofascial trigger point. The importance of the local twitch response. Am J Phys Med Rehabil 1994;73: 256–63.
32. Baldry P. Superficial versus deep dry needling. Acupunct Med 2002;20:78–81.
33. Lewit K. The needle effect in the relief of myofascial pain. Pain 1979;6:83–90.
34. Levine JD, Fields HL, Basbaum AI. Peptides and the primary afferent nociceptor. J Neurosci 1993;13: 2273–86.
35. Cheng RS, Pomeranz BH. Electroacupuncture analgesia is mediated by stereospecific opiate receptors and is reversed by antagonists of type I receptors. Life Sci 1980;26:631–8.
36. Kwon S, Lee B, Yeom M, et al. Modulatory effects of acupuncture on murine depression-like behavior following chronic systemic inflammation. Brain Res 2012;1472:149–60.
37. Li M, Tjen-A-Looi SC, et al. Repetitive electroacupuncture causes prolonged increased met-enkephalin expression in the rVLM of conscious rats. Auton Neurosci 2012;170:30–5.

38. Zhang Y, Meng X, Li A, et al. Acupuncture alleviates the affective dimension of pain in a rat model of inflammatory hyperalgesia. Neurochem Res 2011;36:2104–10.

39. Xu GY, Winston JH, Chen JD. Electroacupuncture attenuates visceral hyperalgesia and inhibits the enhanced excitability of colon specific sensory neurons in a rat model of irritable bowel syndrome. Neurogastroenterol Motil 2009;21(12):1302–e125.

40. Becker O, Reichmanis M, Marino AA, et al. Electro-physiological correlates of acupuncture points and meridians. Psychoenerg Syst 1976;1:195–212.

41. Simons DG. New views of myofascial trigger points: etiology and diagnosis. Arch Phys Med Rehabil 2008; 89:157–9.

42. Guyton AC, Hall E. Textbook of medical physiology. 12th ed. Philadelphia: Elsevier Saunders; 2011.

PART **II**

CADAVER-BASED APPROACHES IN PHYSIOTHERAPY

CHAPTER 3

Cadaver-Based Approaches in Physiotherapy

Francisco J. Valderrama Canales • Francisco Minaya Muñoz • Fermín Valera Garrido

We may learn a great deal from books, but we learn much more from the contemplation of nature – the reason and occasion for all books.
SANTIAGO RAMÓN Y CAJAL

CHAPTER OUTLINE

KEYWORDS

cadaver-based approaches; lung; pleura;
pneumothorax; kidney; interface;
vasculonervous bundle; needle
techniques; dry needling; acupuncture;
clinical points.

3.1 INTRODUCTION

Physiotherapy, intrinsically, requires a thorough knowledge of the superficial anatomy of the human body and an extremely accurate interpretation of the relations between the anatomical structures of the deep planes. The incorporation of new therapeutic procedures from a percutaneous approach which are minimally invasive, such as dry needling or percutaneous needle electrolysis (PNE), makes it essential for physiotherapists to broaden their knowledge of the relations that the muscles, tendons and ligaments have with regard to the vasculonervous paths and the various organs in each region. In other words, one must fully appreciate the topographic anatomy, in order to be able to 'scrutinize' from the skin's surface the location of the deep structures that need to be avoided during the praxis of invasive physiotherapy techniques, and, on the other hand, in order to assess properly the different soft tissues, thereby improving the application of these techniques.

These premises determine the main objective of this chapter, which consists of presenting the most relevant anatomical relations for the clinical practice of minimally invasive physiotherapy, according to the common therapeutic approach in the anatomical regions of interest.

The chapter is organized in order to address the large body regions, without an exhaustive description of all the subdivided areas (although these may be cited from time to time). Each section presents the main relations between the anatomical structures in the different planes of each region, the territories of vasculonervous conflict (which need to be considered in order to contemplate minimally invasive therapies in musculoskeletal medicine and physiotherapy), and the methods for approaching clinically relevant structures using puncture techniques. This information must be considered in order to study the minimally invasive techniques and to access clinically relevant structures using puncture techniques. An exception is the shoulder, one of the most common regions from the point of view of these therapies. The connections between the numerous muscles that act on the articular complex of the shoulder are described, even though these represent the muscles that reach the area from regions pertaining to the trunk, the neck or the head. This singularity is taken into consideration within this evidently clear functional relation, and therefore is also reasonable from a therapeutic point of view. With regard to the veins and nerves that are found in the superficial fascia, subcutaneous or epifascial tissues, only those that arc highly relevant are mentioned.

Regarding the landmarks cited pertaining to the position of the structures, the professional should be aware that these are merely a guide, and that all of them, naturally, are indicated in relation to the norm established by the anatomical position. Thus, these cannot be considered exact patterns, as many correspond to the descriptions of cadaver dissections and this already implies differences and variations as regards the living individual, as interindividual differences are vast depending on individual constitution, age, height and distinctive anatomy. One mustn't forget that, in human anatomy, variation is the norm. Thus, caution should be exercised when coming across expressions such as 'two finger widths' or similar, and even with measurement references in centimetres.

In all the descriptions, the most current anatomical terminology is used,[1,2] as published by the Federative International Committee on Anatomical Terminology in 1998[3-4] and reprinted in 2011[5] by its successor, the Federative International Program for Anatomical Terminology. Occasionally, in the text some terms appear that are not included in the *Terminologia Anatómica*,[1] but that are indelibly incorporated into clinical jargon: these terms are shown in brackets the first time they are cited in the text, e.g. calcaneus tendon (Achilles tendon).

3.2 TOPOGRAPHICAL ANATOMY OF THE HEAD

3.2.1 Regions

There are many regions that can be described in the head, but it is not practical for the purpose of minimally invasive therapies to enumerate them all, and their boundaries, in detail. Nevertheless, abundant descriptions are to be found in the bibliography on topographical anatomy.[6,7] These descriptions will focus on the main anatomical relations, in order to approach the muscles of mastication and the facial muscles (mimic muscles).

3.2.2 Anatomical relations of interest

The facial musculature is epifascial and, therefore, is found embedded within the subcutaneous tissue of the head. This characteristic means that the sensitive branches of the trigeminal nerve and the motor branches of the facial nerve are the nervous structures that can be accidentally encountered during muscular approaches. In the same way, profuse vascularization of the face makes it probable that a vessel will be reached, although the main ones can be avoided with adequate knowledge of their pathways (figure 3.1).

The muscles of mastication comprise the temporal, masseter, medial and lateral pterygoid muscles. The temporal muscle lies in the fossa of the same name, above the zygomatic arch, and is covered by the temporal fascia, which is very

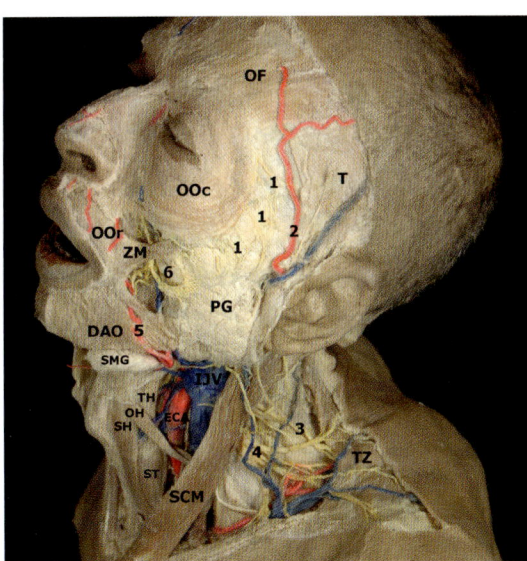

FIGURE 3.1 ■ Left lateral view of a dissection of the face and neck regions. Facial muscles (DAO, depressor anguli oris; OF, frontal belly of the occipitofrontalis muscle; OOc, orbicularis oculi; OOr, orbicularis oris; ZM, zygomaticus major), motor branches of the facial nerve (1), facial artery (5), submandibular gland (SMG), parotid gland (PG) and the masseter muscle; parotid duct (6). In the temporal region the temporal fascia and the temporal muscle (T) are observed; the frontal branch of the superficial temporal artery (2). Structures of the anterior triangle of the neck: sternocleidomastoid muscle (SCM), infrahyoid muscles (SH, sternohyoid; OH, omohyoid; ST, sternothyroid; TH, thyrohyoid), the external carotid artery (ECA) and the internal jugular vein (IJV). In the posterior triangle of the neck, between the posterior border of the sternocleidomastoid (SCM), the clavicle (C) and the border of the trapezius (TZ), spinal nerve (3) and the supraclavicular branches of the cervical plexus (4). (Courtesy of Drs. JR. Sañudo, T. Vázquez and E. Maranillo).

strong (figure 3.1). The superficial temporal artery ascends vertically and anterior to the tragus and divides, 2 or 3 cm above the zygomatic arch, into the parietal branch, which ascends in the same direction, and into the frontal branch, which is directed softly upwards and forwards. The masseter muscle extends between the angle of the mandible and the zygomatic arch. It is partially covered in its posterior border by the parotid duct (duct of Stenon), which is directed horizontally towards the cheek to perforate the buccinator muscle and access the vestibule of the oral cavity (figure 3.1). Also surfacing from the parotid parenchyma, the zygomatic and buccal branches of the facial nerve pass superficially in a posteroanterior direction over the masseter (figure 3.1). The pterygoid muscles are found in the infratemporal fossa (figure 3.2), which is medial to the ramus of the mandible and inferior to the horizontal plane marked by the zygomatic arch. The maxillary artery passes deep to the ramus of the mandible and is directed anteriorly over the lateral aspect of the lateral pterygoid muscle (30–40% of the time it does so medially).[8,9] As well as the maxillary artery, the inferior alveolar and lingual branches of the mandibular branch of the trigeminal nerve pass by the interstitium created by the two pterygoid muscles, in the direction of the mandible and lateral to the medial pterygoid muscle (figure 3.2).

3.2.3 Areas of vasculonervous conflict and anatomical landmarks

The maxillary artery and the lingual and inferior alveolar nerve pass through the infratemporal fossa, where the pterygoid muscles lie. The masseter muscle, located in the parotid region, relates to the parotid gland, the parotid duct and the facial nerve. In the temporal region, from where the temporal muscle is approached, the superficial temporal artery and its branches, frontal and parietal, are the anatomical structures that are related to the muscle.

The main anatomical references concern the position of the parotid gland, the facial artery and vein, and the temporal artery and its two terminal branches.[10,11] The superior border of the parotid gland corresponds with the posterior two-thirds of the inferior border of the zygomatic arch. The posterior border is delimited by the anterior part of the external auditory foramen, the mastoid process and the anterior border of the sternocleidomastoid muscle, and the inferior border corresponds with an imaginary line that unites the vertex of the mastoid process with the root of the greater horn of the

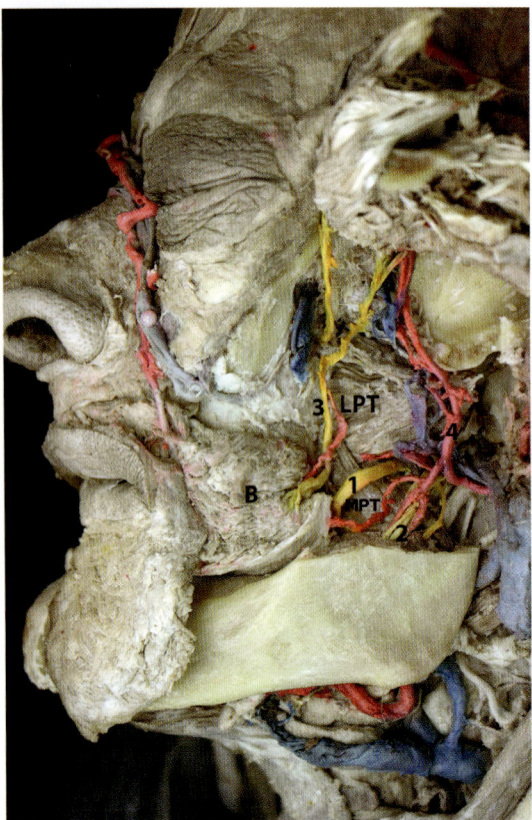

FIGURE 3.2 ■ Infratemporal region. Left lateral view of a dissection of the infratemporal region. The ramus of the mandible has been removed and the temporal muscle displaced upwards in order to access the fossa. In the infratemporal fossa, the lateral pterygoid muscle (LPT) and medial pterygoid muscle (MPT) are found; the lingual nerve (1), the inferior alveolar nerve (2) and the buccal nerve (3), which is headed towards the buccinator muscle (B), and the maxillary artery (4) are also observed. (Courtesy of Drs. JR. Sañudo, T. Vázquez and E. Maranillo).

the frontal branch, which is directed obliquely anteriorly and slightly upwards.

3.2.4 Approaches for structures and key sites used during puncture techniques

Next, the approaches are described for puncturing the most relevant anatomical structures and/or those that present the most difficulty during minimally invasive procedures of daily clinical practice.

- Masseter muscle:
  - position: supine.
  - location: different points along the muscle.
  - procedure: puncture using a flat palpation technique, insert the needle in a cranial direction, searching for the myofascial trigger point (MTrP) or the motor point.
- Temporal muscle:
  - position: supine.
  - location: different points in the anterior, intermediate and posterior parts of the muscle.
  - procedure: puncture using a flat palpation technique, insert the needle in a cranial direction, searching for the MTrP or the motor point.
- Lateral pterygoid muscle:
  - position: supine.
  - location: usually the central part of the inferior division of the muscle.
  - procedure: puncture using a flat palpation technique, insert the needle in a cranial direction, through the infratemporal fossa, searching for the MTrP or the motor point.

3.3 TOPOGRAPHICAL ANATOMY OF THE NECK

3.3.1 Regions

For increased simplicity, the following regions are described: anterior cervical (anterior triangle of the neck), sternocleidomastoid, lateral cervical (posterior triangle of the neck) and posterior cervical (nape).[10] The anterior and lateral regions of the neck are subdivided into several more triangles.[6]

The anterior cervical region or anterior triangle of the neck falls within the anterior midline of the neck, the anterior border of the sternocleidomastoid muscle and the base of the

hyoid bone. The anterior border of the gland extends in a variable manner over the surface of the masseter. The parotid duct is found approximately one finger width below the inferior border of the zygomatic arch. The trajectory of the facial artery, together with the facial vein, can be indicated by a line which begins from the antegonial notch, just anterior of the angle of the mandible, in the anterior border of the masseter, to a point located 1 cm lateral to the oral commissure. From there, the vessels head towards the nasogenian sulcus, passing through to the medial palpebral commissure. The superficial temporal artery ascends in a vertical line that passes just in front of the tragus and divides, 2 or 3 cm above, in the parietal branch, which continues in the same vertical direction, and in mandible. The sternocleidomastoid region corresponds on the surface with the prominence of the muscle itself, from the mastoid process to sternal and clavicular insertions.

The lateral region of the neck falls between the posterior border of the sternocleidomastoid muscle, the anterior border of the trapezius muscle and the clavicle.

The posterior cervical region includes the area delimited by the anterior border of both trapezius muscles, while the superior and inferior limits correspond with the limits of the neck. The external occipital protuberance, of which the most prominent point is the cephalometric union point, can be used as a reference for the superior boundary, and the spinous process of the prominent vertebra, C7, for the inferior boundary.

3.3.2 Anatomical relations of interest

It is vital to take into account that, in approaches to the trapezius or the scalene muscles in the neck, the apex of the pleural cavity and the lung is much closer, so it is easier to puncture these structures.

Anterior region of the neck

In the anterior cervical triangle the platysma muscle is found; this is subcutaneous, together with the hyoid muscles (except for the geniohyoid and the inferior belly of the omohyoid), which are situated deep to the cervical fascia, and the prevertebral muscles, which are also placed deep in relation to the visceral tract of the neck. Epifascially, the anterior jugular vein is found parallel to the anterior border of the sternocleidomastoid, and deep to the muscles, to the thyroid gland distally, and to the visceral tract of the neck, which, along its course, covers the prevertebral muscles. Additionally, next to the anterior border of the sternocleidomastoid muscle, and above the horizontal plane (marked by the superior border of the thyroid cartilage), the carotid artery is found with its two terminal branches, external and internal, as well as the internal jugular vein, the vagus nerve and the superficial branch of the ansa cervicalis (figure 3.1).

Sternocleidomastoid region

Running through this region epifascially is the external jugular vein. On a deep plane, next to the insertion on the clavicle, the clavicular belly of the sternocleidomastoid muscle partially covers the jugular venous arch. On a more superficial level, the muscle covers the carotid sheath with the common carotid artery, the internal jugular vein and the vagus nerve (figure 3.3C). More cranially, and from anterior to posterior, the scalene muscles are found together with the levator scapulae muscle. The phrenic nerve passes in front of the anterior scalene muscle while, between the anterior and middle scalene, the anterior branches of the cervical nerves C2–C4 emerge. Over the levator scapulae the lesser occipital nerve descends anterior and inferiorly (and later becomes superficial to the sternocleidomastoid) and, posteriorly and more cranially, the accessory nerve is found (approximately 4 cm distal to the mastoid process).

Lateral region of the neck

In the posterior cervical triangle there is continuity with the anatomical structures described in the sternocleidomastoid region. Between the anterior and middle scalene, over the first rib, the subclavian artery passes and, above this, the three trunks of the brachial plexus. Dorsal to the group formed by the scalenes, the levator scapulae muscle is found with the accessory nerve descending over it and, as a more posterior muscle, the splenius capitis. Inferiorly, the region is crossed by the posterior belly of the omohyoid muscle, with an anteroposterior direction that is almost horizontal. Lateral to it, the brachial plexus produces the supraclavicular branches and crosses the transverse cervical artery (figure 3.2).

Posterior region of the neck

This region is comprised of the posterior territory of the neck or the nape region. Deep to the descending part of the trapezius muscle, the muscles of the back proper corresponding to the neck and the head are found. In the first place, these are the splenius of the neck and the head, followed by the longissimus of the head and the semispinalis of the neck and the head (figure 3.4) and, on a deeper plane, the group formed by the suboccipital muscles: rectus capitis posterior minor, rectus capitis posterior major, obliquus capitis superior and obliquus capitis inferior (figure 3.5). The deep cervical artery and vein ascend along the deep aspect of the semispinalis of the head, which is perforated by the greater occipital nerve very close to the superior nuchal line. In the depths of the region, the obliquus capitis inferior and superior of the head

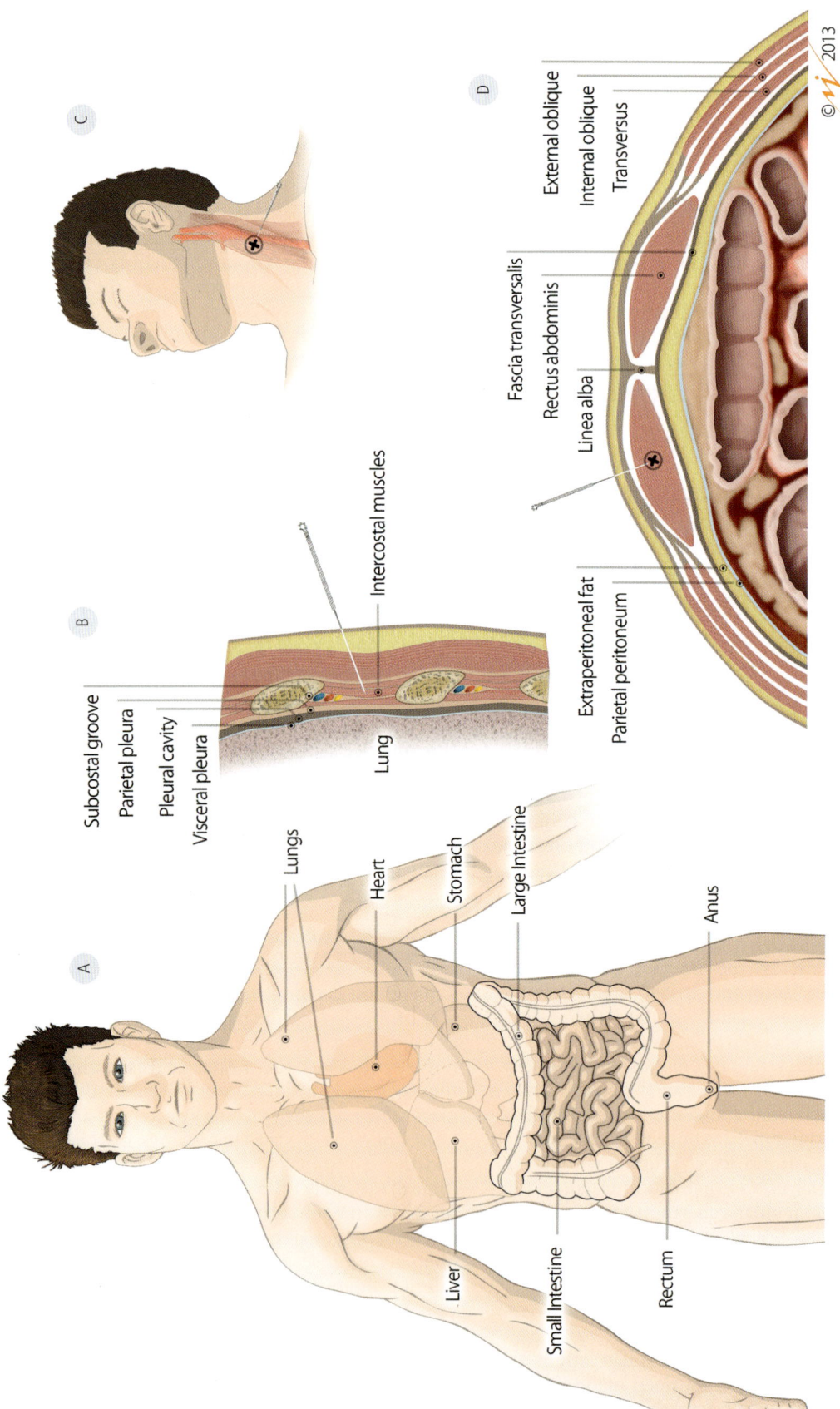

FIGURE 3.3 ■ (A) Surface projections of the organs on to the anterior wall of the trunk. (B) Sagittal cross-section of the intercostal muscles. Clinical points: The needle target for the intercostal muscles is below the rib on the midpoint of the intercostal space. Avoid damaging the vasculonervous bundle that runs in the costal groove on the inferior surface of each rib, and the collateral branches of the intercostal nerve and vessels that run along the superior surface of each rib. (C) Surface projections of the common carotid artery on to the sternocleidomastoid muscle. Clinical points: The needle target is from lateral to medial in the direction of the myofascial trigger point or the motor point. (D) Axial cross-section of the abdominal wall below the umbilicus. The aponeuroses of the external oblique, internal oblique and the transversus abdominis muscles pass anteriorly to the rectus abdominis muscle, leaving only the transversalis fascia posteriorly. Clinical points: The needle target for rectus abdominis is in the middle of the muscle. Avoid damaging the parietal peritoneum.

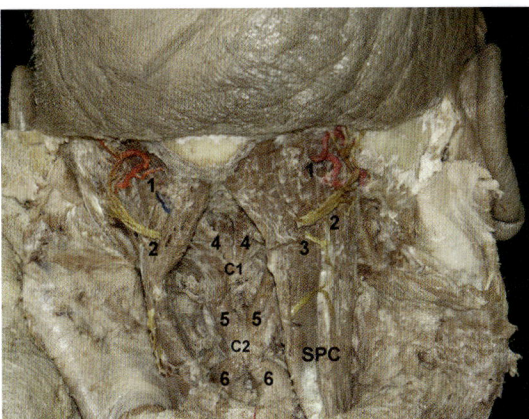

FIGURE 3.4 ■ View of a dissection of the posterior neck region. The planes of the trapezius and splenius muscles are dissected and have been laterally displaced, therefore both semispinalis capitis muscles (SPC) can be seen. The vasculonervous structures are the occipital artery (1), the greater occipital nerve (2) and the third occipital nerve (3), for which, on the right side, its communications with other posterior branches are conserved. (Courtesy of Drs. JR. Sañudo, F. Valderrama, T. Vázquez and E. Maranillo).

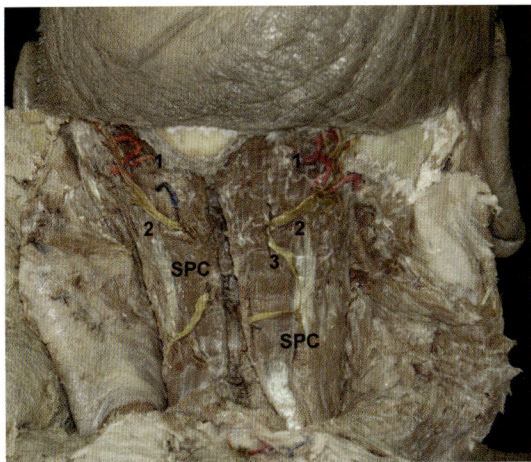

FIGURE 3.5 ■ View of the same dissection as figure 3.4, in which the left semispinalis capitis (SPC) is displaced laterally; the SPC on the right side remains in place, in order to allow a view of the suboccipital muscles rectus capitis posterior minor (4) and rectus capitis posterior major (5). The SPC (6) is also identified. The position of the spinous process of the atlas (C1) and of the axis (C2) is also identifiable. The vasculonervous structures are the occipital artery (1), the greater occipital nerve (2) and the third occipital nerve (3). (Courtesy of Drs. JR. Sañudo, F. Valderrama, T. Vázquez and E. Maranillo).

and the rectus capitis posterior major muscles delimit the suboccipital triangle, in which the vertebral artery is found. The greater occipital nerve passes, from inferior, superficially over the obliquus capitis inferior, approximately one

finger width from the vertex of the transverse process of the axis.

3.3.3 Areas of vasculonervous conflict and anatomical landmarks

The four regions described in the neck, being an area of passage between the head and the trunk and the upper limb, can be considered as areas of vasculonervous conflict. In the anterior triangle of the neck, there are structures such as the thyroid gland, the common carotid artery, the external carotid artery, the superior thyroid artery, the internal jugular vein and the vagus nerve. In the sternocleidomastoid region, the common carotid artery is included, together with the external carotid artery, the internal carotid artery, the vagus nerve, the phrenic nerve, the anterior rami of the C2–C4 nerves, the superior trunk of the brachial plexus, the lesser occipital nerve, the great auricular nerve and the transverse cervical nerve. In the posterior triangle of the neck, the external jugular vein, the transverse cervical vein, the subclavian artery, the transverse cervical artery, the superior trunk of the brachial plexus, the supraclavicular branches of the brachial plexus, the accessory nerve and the supraclavicular nerves are found. In the posterior region of the neck, the suboccipital muscles delimit the suboccipital triangle, within which we can find the vertebral artery, whereas the greater occipital nerve goes around the inferior oblique muscle, crossing the triangle from below upwards.

Several basic landmarks are described in order to position diverse structures in the neck.[11] The position of the common carotid artery is indicated by the anterior border of the sternocleidomastoid muscle (figure 3.3C). From the clavicle up to the superior border of the thyroid cartilage is a line which overlaps with the common carotid artery and, from this point, with the external carotid artery, which falls slightly anterior to the border of the muscle. The internal jugular vein is slightly lateral to the common carotid artery. Within the carotid sheath, and common to both vessels, the vagus nerve can be found, lateral to them in the pathway of the common carotid and medially from the carotid division towards cranial. The subclavian artery can be traced from the surface by a curved line, convex upwards, which extends from the sternoclavicular joint to the middle point of the clavicle, with the highest point of the convexity 1–3 cm above the clavicle. The external jugular vein is revealed by a line traced from the angle of the mandible to the middle point of the clavicle. The facial nerve, at its exit from the stylomastoid foramen, is found approximately 2.5 cm deep from the middle point of the anterior border of the mastoid process.

In order to define the course of the accessory nerve, a line is traced from the angle of the mandible to the middle point of the anterior border of the sternocleidomastoid muscle (approximately 3–5 cm from the vertex of the mastoid process). The projection of the line to the anterior border of the trapezius muscle, crossing the posterior triangle of the neck, indicates the course of the accessory nerve in this triangle. The cutaneous branches of the cervical plexus are grouped together around the emergence of the accessory nerve and can be identified as follows: the lesser occipital nerve comes out above the accessory nerve and continues upwards to the posterior border of the sternocleidomastoid muscle towards the mastoid process. The great auricular nerve and the transverse cervical nerve emerge immediately below the accessory nerve, with the great auricular nerve heading towards the angle of the mandible, whereas the transverse cervical nerve crosses the belly of the sternocleidomastoid horizontally. The supraclavicular nerves emerge caudally from these last two and heads in the direction of the clavicle. The superior border of the brachial plexus can be delimited by a line traced from the middle point of the inferior border of the arch of cricoid cartilage to the centre point of the clavicle.

For the approaches within the suboccipital region, the landmark described for the puncture and extraction of cerebrospinal fluid from the posterior cerebellomedullary cistern can be used. In this technique, the needle is inserted into the middle point between the external occipital protuberance and the spinous process of the axis, and directed towards the nasion cephalometric point, passing in between the rectus capitis posterior minor muscles. When approaching the cistern, the needle must never exceed a depth of 4–5 cm, with the muscle plane found at 2–3 cm depth. On the other hand, the rectus capitis posterior major muscle originates in the spinous process of the axis, and, external to the rectus capitis posterior minor muscle, it also follows the inferior nuchal line, one finger width above the line that unites the spinous process of the axis with the transverse process of the atlas. The obliquus capitis inferior muscle extends between the spinous processes of the axis and the transverse process of the atlas, whereas the obliquus capitis superior muscle originates from the transverse process of the axis and is headed towards the cranium, vertically and

external to the rectus capitis posterior major muscle.

3.3.4 Approaches for structures and key sites used during puncture techniques

We shall continue with a description of the puncture approaches of the most relevant anatomical structures and those that present the most difficulty during the minimally invasive procedures of daily clinical practice.

- Scalene muscles:
  - position: supine.
  - location: different points.
  - procedure: puncture using a flat palpation technique, inserting the needle perpendicular to the muscle, searching for MTrP or the motor point.
- Sternocleidomastoid muscle:
  - position: supine.
  - location: different points along the muscle.
  - procedure: puncture using a pincer grip palpation technique, inserting the needle from lateral to medial in the direction of the MTrP or the motor point (figure 3.3C).
- Obliquus capitis inferior muscle:
  - position: prone.
  - location: central part of the muscle.
  - procedure: using the reference of the projection of the transverse process of C1 and the spinous process of C2, puncture using a flat palpation technique, inserting the needle in a medial, posterior and caudal direction, searching for a hard end-feel (bone) with the tip of the needle (figure 3.6A and A1).

3.4 TOPOGRAPHICAL ANATOMY OF THE TRUNK

3.4.1 Regions

This section describes the constitution and the main anatomical relations of the abdominal wall and the vertebral region, which covers the cutaneous area that lies within the transverse processes, in a horizontal direction, and from the level of the lumbosacral joint to the beginning of the neck, or until it meets the posterior cervical region, vertically.[6,7] Because of their clinical relevance (figures 3.7 and 3.8 and table 3.1), the acupuncture points and the most important MTrPs are shown in relation to possible zones of conflict.

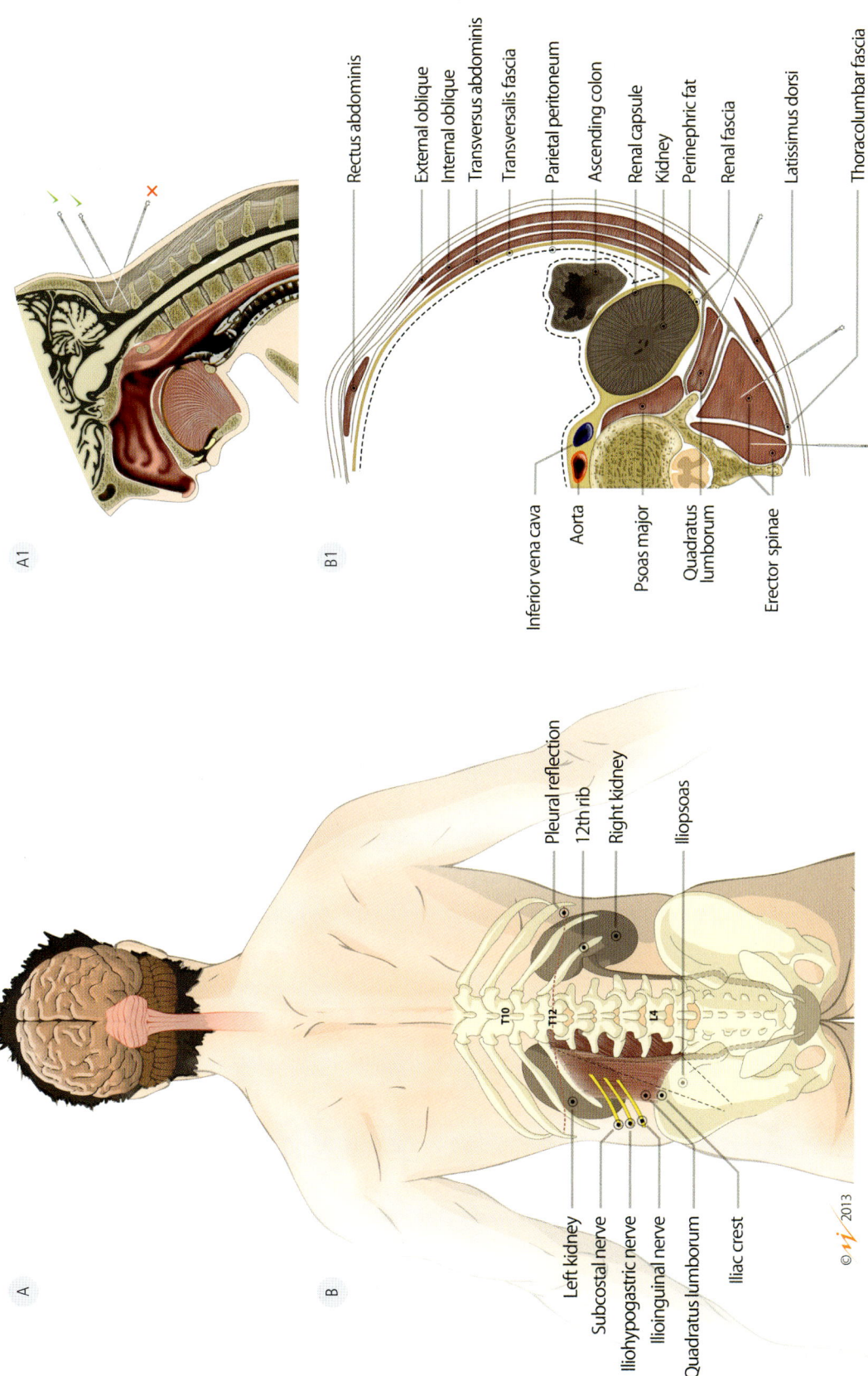

FIGURE 3.6 ■ (A) Surface projections of the brain, cerebellum and spinal cord. (A1) Sagittal cross-section of the head. Clinical points: Avoid using a proximal oblique direction due to the risk of nerve damage. (B) Surface projections of the kidneys on to the posterior wall of the trunk. (B1) Axial cross-section of the abdomen at L1. Clinical points: Puncture of the paravertebral muscles must be performed perpendicular to the same or from lateral to medial. Due to the risk of pneumothorax the puncture should not be performed from medial to lateral. The puncture of the quadratus lumborum is performed with the needle parallel to the plane of the back (or in a slightly oblique direction). Take particular care due to the proximity of the kidney.

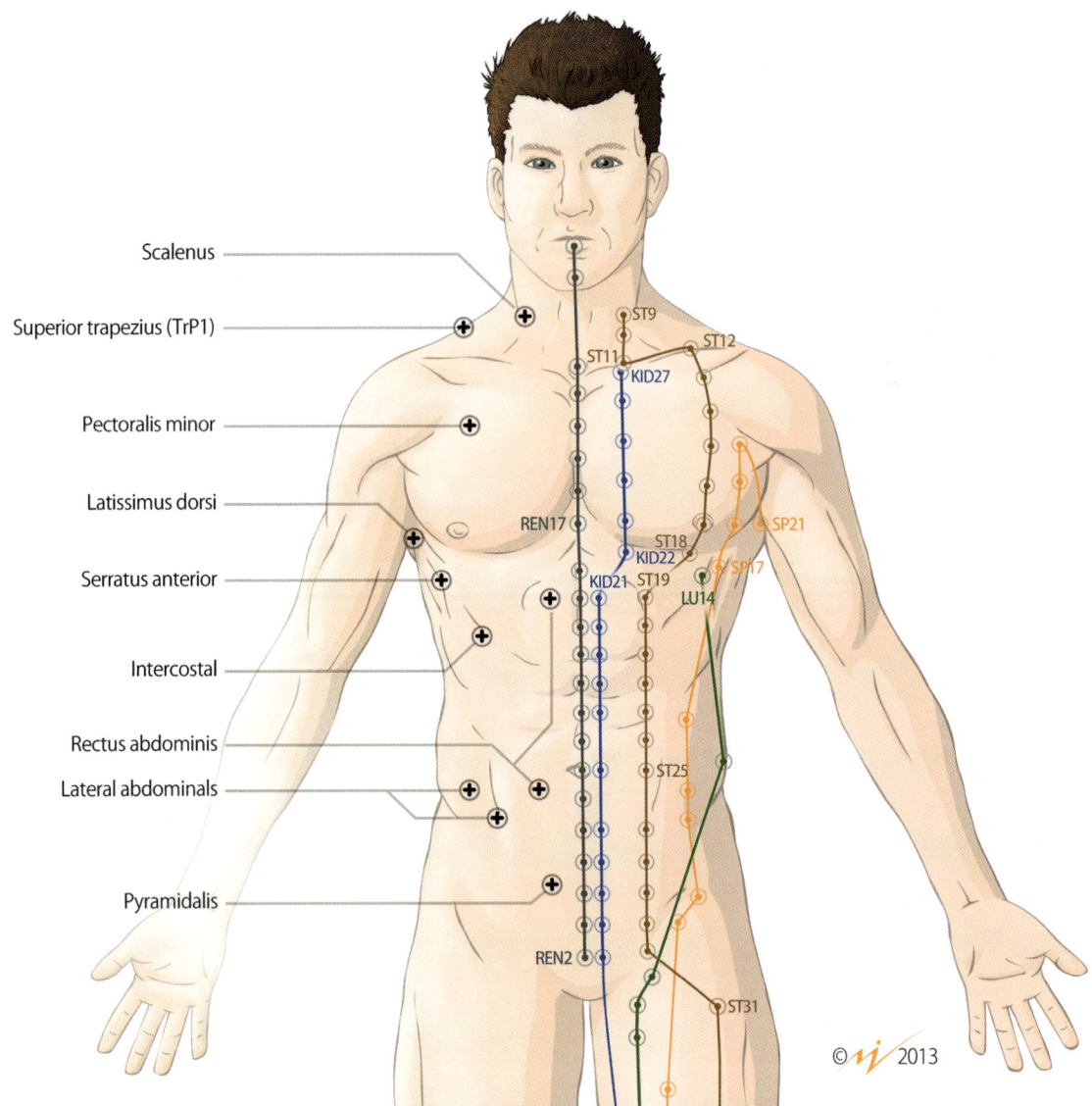

Scalenus

Superior trapezius (TrP1)

Pectoralis minor

Latissimus dorsi

Serratus anterior

Intercostal

Rectus abdominis

Lateral abdominals

Pyramidalis

ST9
ST12
ST11
KID27
REN17
ST18
KID22
KID21 ST19
SP17
LU14
SP21
ST25
REN2
ST31

© rj 2013

FIGURE 3.7 ■ The most important acupuncture and myofascial trigger points and their relation to possible risk zones on the anterior trunk wall.

3.4.2 Anatomical relations of interest

Anterior wall

The main relations of the muscles found in the anterior wall of the thorax (figure 3.3A), pectoralis major and minor and serratus anterior, are described in the section on the upper limb. The anterior abdominal wall contains the rectus abdominis, external oblique, internal oblique and transversus abdominis muscles (figure 3.3D). This is a group of thin muscles, deeply lined by the transversalis fascia (or fascia of the transversus abdominis), which separates them from the preperitoneal fat layer and, at the same time, from the parietal peritoneum and the intraperitoneal viscera. Between the transversus abdominis and the internal oblique muscles, the subcostal, iliohypogastric and ilioinguinal nerves pass, following a path from posterior to anterior above the iliac crest.[9,12] The inguinal canal is found above the inguinal ligament, which contains the spermatic cord in males and the round ligament of the uterus in females. In relation to the rectus abdominis are the anterior epigastric artery and the superior epigastric artery, with its satellite veins, along all the craniocaudal length of the muscle. These arteries are found deep between the muscle and the transverse fascia caudally

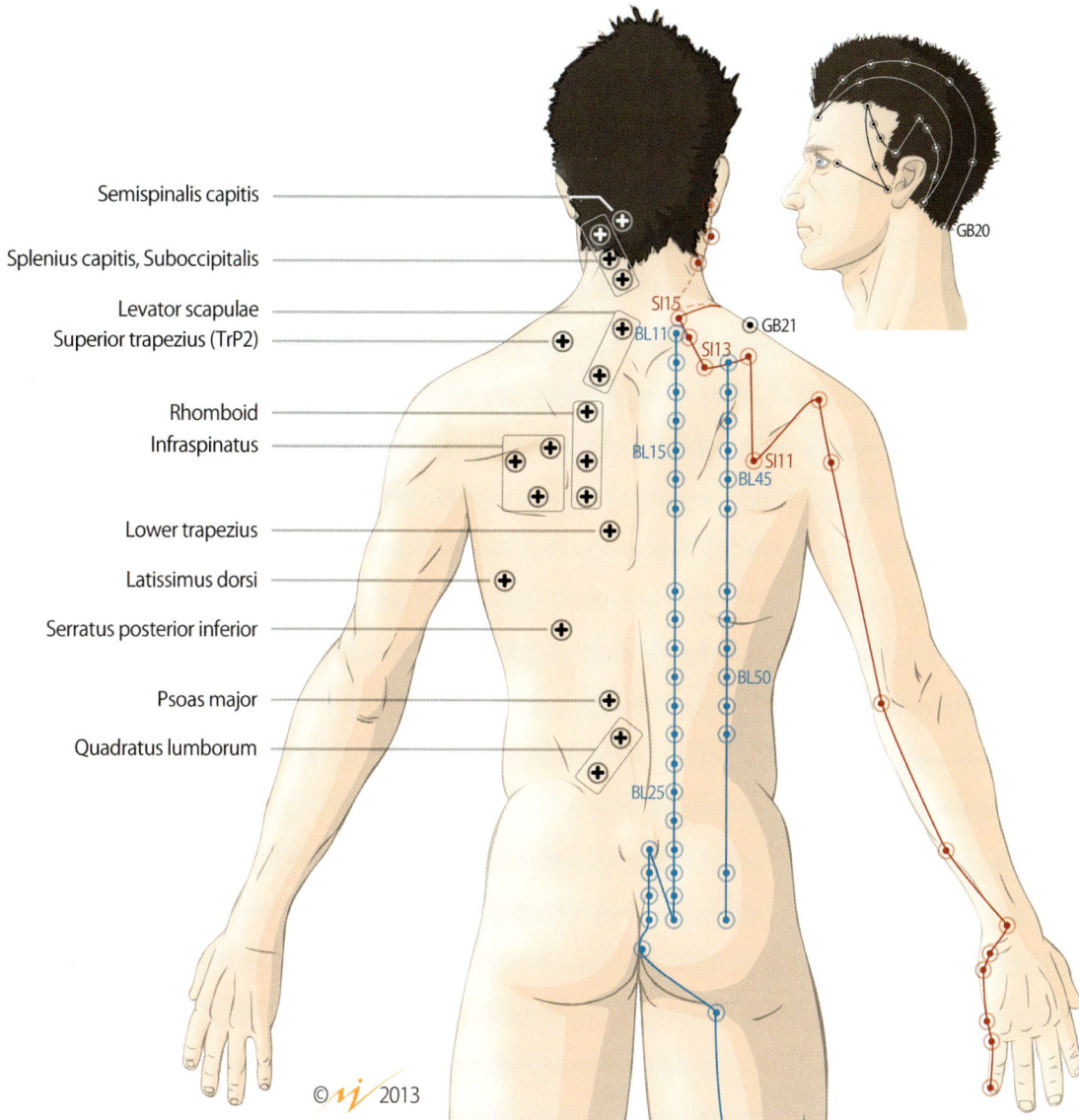

Semispinalis capitis

Splenius capitis, Suboccipitalis

Levator scapulae
Superior trapezius (TrP2)

Rhomboid
Infraspinatus

Lower trapezius

Latissimus dorsi

Serratus posterior inferior

Psoas major

Quadratus lumborum

GB20

SI15
BL11
GB21
SI13

BL15
SI11
BL45

BL50

BL25

© rj 2013

FIGURE 3.8 ■ The most important acupuncture and myofascial trigger points and their relation to possible risk zones on the posterior trunk wall.

to the arcuate line and between the muscle and the rectus sheath cranial to the arcuate line. Epifascially, the superficial epigastric vein passes close to the semilunar line.

Posterior wall

The serratus posterior muscles are found to be superficial to the posterior lamina, or superficial lamina, of the thoracolumbar fascia (figure 3.6B1). In other words, they are superficial to the dorsal muscles (a group formed by the erector spinae, among others). The serratus posterior superior is deep in relation to the trapezius and

the rhomboids and the serratus posterior inferior is deep in relation to the lattisimus dorsi. The quadratus lumborum muscle is the dorsal muscle of the flat muscles of the abdomen and, as such, it is related to the obliques and transversus abdominis due to its origin and functions. The relations of the quadratus lumborum are many and highly relevant (table 3.1), as they form a bed upon which the kidneys lie, and from which the kidneys are separated by the fascia of the quadratus lumborum (or anterior lamina, or deep lamina, of the thoracolumbar fascia), the pararenal fat, the renal fascia, the adipose capsule and the fibrous capsule (figure 3.6B and B1).

TABLE 3.1 **Relevant anatomy for needle insertion and location of acupuncture points and myofascial trigger points (MTrPs)**

Anatomical viscera/ structure	Risk	Recommended puncture depth to reach viscera/structure (length)	High-risk points
Thoracic viscera			
Heart	Cardiac tamponade	10–20 mm	REN17
Lung	Pneumothorax	Supraclavicular (10–25 mm)	GB21 DDN MTrPs in superior trapezius and anterior scalene
		Midclavicular line (10–20 mm)	ST11–ST18 LU2 KID22–KID27
		Medial scapular line (15–20 mm)	BL41–BL54 DDN MTrPs in rhomboids, serratus posterior superior and levator scapulae
		Posterior wall of the trunk (10–25 mm)	DDN MTrPs in illiocostalis thoracis, longissimus thoracis, semispinalis thoracis, cervicus and capitus
Abdominal viscera			
Anterior area	Minimal risk of intestinal perforation	20–40 mm	Mainly any ST, SP, KID, REN points on the front of the body
Kidney	Minimal risk of damage tissue	25–60 mm	DDN MTrPs in quadratus lumborum and psoas major
Peripheral nerves			
Suprascapular	Nerve injury	40 mm	LI16
Median		10–15 mm	P5–P7
Ulnar		0.5 mm	HE4–HE7
Radial		0.5 mm	LU8, LU9
Posterior interosseous		10–20 mm	TB5, TB6 DDN MTrPs in supinator and common wrist extensors
Deep fibular nerve		20–30 mm	GB34, BL39, BL40
Tibial nerve		20–30 mm	KID6, KID6
Central nervous system			
Spinal cord and spinal nerve roots	Nerve injury	25–45 mm	BL11–BL20
Medulla oblongata	Brainstem injuries	40–60mm	DU16
Blood vessels			
Radial vessels		0.5 mm	LU8, LU9
Popliteal vessels	Pseudoaneurysm	20–30 mm	BL40
Dorsalis pedis artery		10–13 mm	ST42

REN, Ren Mai meridian; HE, heart meridian; LU; lung meridian; ST, stomach meridian; KID, kidney meridian; BL, bladder meridian; P, pericardium meridian; SP, spleen meridian; LI, large intestine meridian; GB, gall bladder meridian; TB, triple burner meridian; DU, Du Mai meridian; DDN MTrPs, deep dry needling of myofascial trigger points.

Additionally, the subcostal, iliohypogastric and ilioinguinal nerves cross the kidneys obliquely from a medial and cranial aspect in a lateral and caudal direction (figure 3.6B).

Vertebral region

The vertebral region contains the muscles of the back proper, which extend paravertebrally from the sacrum to the base of the cranium in a succession of lumbar, thoracic, cervical and cranial segments. The erector spinae is the most superficial of the muscles of the back proper, although it is covered by the lattisimus dorsi muscle and the serratus posterior inferior muscle caudally, and the trapezius, rhomboids and serratus posterior superior muscles cranially. It is formed by the three parallel tracts that, from medial to lateral, are the spinalis, the longissimus and the iliocostalis. The thoracic segment from the spinalis is the only one that has an appreciable development and extends between the spinous processes of T2 to L3. The thoracic component of the longissimus (which also has segments in the neck and the head) extends from the sacrum to the first rib, whereas the lumbar and thoracic iliocostalis (also with segments in the neck and the head) reaches the first rib over the angles of the ribs, where it inserts, and this constitutes a good landmark for its approach. Deep to the erector spinae is the transversospinalis muscle group, with muscular fascicles between the transverse and spinous processes, including the so-called multifidus and rotator muscles. It is important to consider the anatomical relation of all the musculature in this region with the lungs and its pleural cavity (the virtual space between the visceral and parietal pleura) (figure 3.9).

The pleura is a delicate serous membrane that folds back on to itself to form a double-layered membranous structure, wrapping each lung in the form of a closed invaginated sac. The potential space between both layers is known as the pleural cavity (figures 3.3B and 3.9). The sheath of pleura that adheres to the surface of the lungs and dips into the fissures between their lobes is known as the visceral pleura. The parietal pleura, on the other hand, lines the inner surface of the chest wall and the diaphragm, and is reflected over the pulmonary hilum as visceral pleura. The parietal pleura goes by different names as it covers diverse territories: the costal pleura, which lines the inner surface of the ribs and intercostal muscles (video 3.1; figure 3.10A and D); the diaphragmatic pleura, lining the convex surface of the diaphragm; the mediastinal pleura, which borders the mediastinum; and the cervical pleura (cupula of the pleura) which rises

into the neck, to coat the apex of the lungs (figure 3.9C). On the surface of the body, the boundaries of the pleural sac can be marked out as lines, which indicate the limits of the parietal pleura and are referred to as the lines of pleural reflection (figure 3.6B and 3.9).

The dome of the pleura (cervical pleura) can be marked out on the surface by a curved line drawn from the sternoclavicular joint to the junction of the medial and middle thirds of the clavicle; the apex of the pleura is found about 2.5 cm (1 inch) above the level of the upper surface of the clavicle. This structure is important, as the pleura can be injured (with consequent pneumothorax) above the clavicle when needling the descending fibres of the superior trapezius muscle (figure 3.10A), the anterior scalene muscle (figure 3.7) or the gall bladder 21 (GB21) acupuncture point (figure 3.8 and table 3.1).

On each side, the lines of pleural reflection pass from behind the sternoclavicular joint. On the right side, the anterior border of the pleura descends, almost reaching the midline behind the sternal angle, and continues downward until it reaches the xiphisternal joint. On the left side, the pleura has a similar course, but at the level of the fourth costal cartilage it deviates and extends to the lateral margin of the sternum to form the cardiac notch (figure 3.9A). This is important because in 5–8% of individuals congenital foramina exist due to incomplete ossification and fusion of the sternal plate,[13–16] which most commonly occurs at the level of the fourth intercostal plate (figure 3.10C). For this reason cardiac tamponade due to injury of the heart or pericardium could occur when needling the Ren Mai 17 (REN17) acupuncture point (figure 3.7). Needling should be performed superficially (table 3.1) and obliquely over the sternum.[13]

The lower margins of the pleura on both sides follow a curved line, which crosses the eighth, 10th and 12th ribs at the midclavicular lines, the midaxillary lines and the sides of the vertebral column; that is, at the lateral border of the erector spinae muscle (video 3.2). The lower margins of the lungs cross, at the same point, the sixth, eighth and 10th ribs, at the midclavicular lines, the midaxillary lines and the sides of the vertebral column, respectively. The distance between the two borders corresponds to the costodiaphragmatic recess (figure 3.9).

The importance of knowing the surface projections of the lungs and pleura is strongly emphasized (box 3.1), as needling techniques that involve the cervical, thoracic and lumbar regions can be associated with potential risk of pneumothorax.

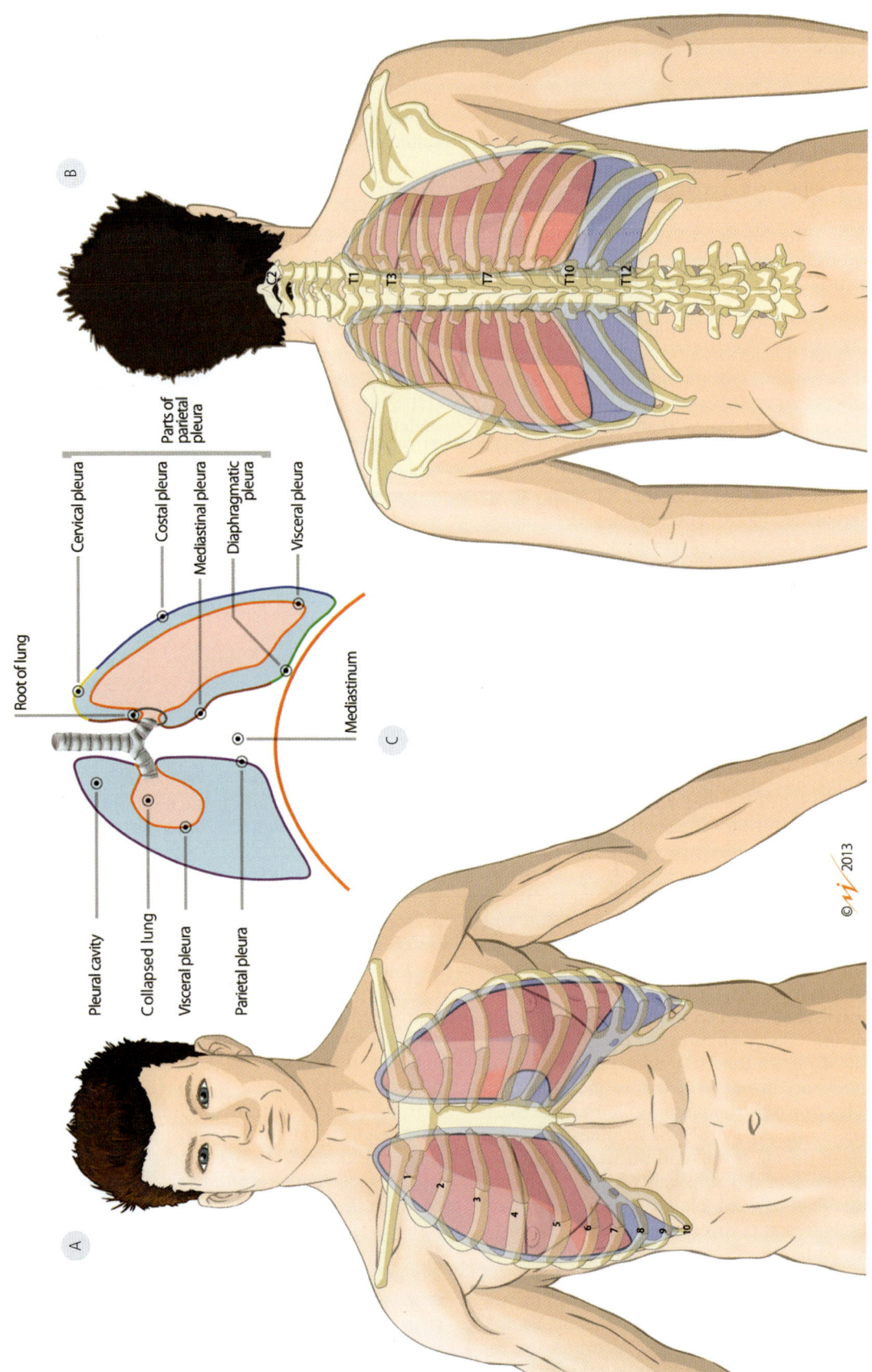

FIGURE 3.9 ■ Surface projections of the lungs and the pleura: (A) on to the anterior thoracic wall; (B) on to the posterior thoracic wall. (C) Parts of the parietal pleura. Clinical points: Important vertebral landmarks to avoid the risk of pneumothorax. Pleura in blue; lungs in purple.

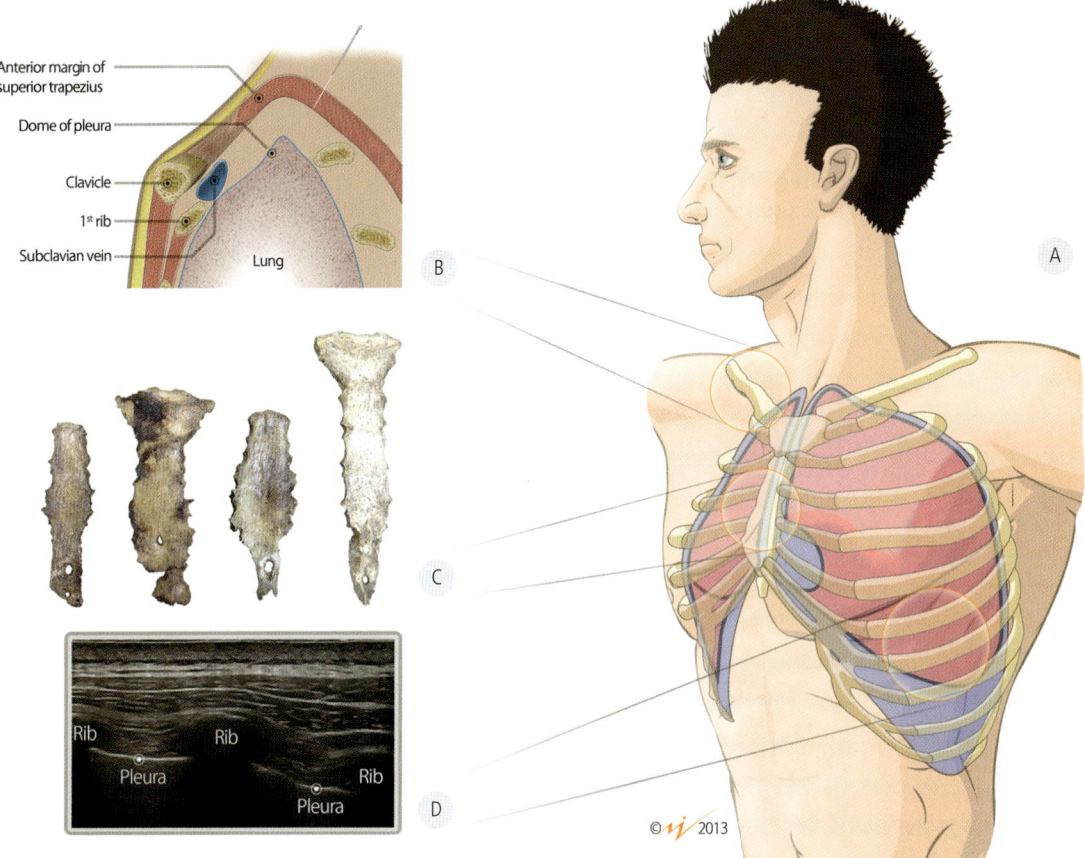

Anterior margin of superior trapezius

Dome of pleura

Clavicle

1st rib

Subclavian vein

Lung

B

A

C

Rib

Rib

Pleura

Rib

Pleura

D

© *rj* 2013

FIGURE 3.10 ■ (A) Surface projections of the lungs and the pleura on to the lateral thoracic wall. (B) Sagittal cross-section of the superior trapezius muscle. Clinical points: Caution due to the proximity of the dome of the pleura and risk of pneumothorax. (C) Congenital sternal foramen. (D) Ultrasound imaging of the muscles of the thoracic cage. Caution due to the proximity of the pleura.

BOX 3.1	**Surface projections of the pleura: risk of pneumothorax with needle techniques**

1 inch (2.5 cm) above the level of the upper surface of the clavicle.
Eighth rib anteriorly at the midclavicular line.
On the left side, at fourth costal cartilage to the lateral margin of the sternum.
Tenth rib laterally at the midaxillary line.
Twelfth rib posteriorly.

The regions associated with possible pneumothorax following needle techniques are subclavicular, paraspinal and medial scapular.

3.4.3 Areas of vasculonervous conflict and anatomical landmarks

Anterior wall

There is an approximate rule for locating the inferior epigastric vessels which traces a curved line, laterally concave, from the middle point of the inguinal ligament to the umbilicus, although publications related to the lesion of the epigastric vessels in abdominal laparoscopies indicate that this rule is not altogether reliable.[17] The superficial epigastric artery is located above the inguinal ligament and is directed from medial to lateral. The superficial epigastric vein lies close to the semilunar line, lying on the inner aspect of the line in its pathway to the umbilicus, and close to it, but on the external side, from the umbilicus upwards.

Posterior wall

The serratus posterior superior muscle extends from the spinal processes of C6 to T2 until the angles of the second to the fifth ribs, therefore, it is oblique laterally and upwards, and the dorsal scapular nerve passes superficially and slightly lateral to the transverse processes. The serratus posterior inferior muscle extends from the spinous processes of T11 to L2 to the last four ribs; therefore it is oblique laterally and upwards.

The quadratus lumborum muscle extends between the 12th rib, the iliac crest and the costal processes of the lumbar vertebrae.

Vertebral region

The spinalis muscle is located immediately above the lateral surface of the spinous processes of the thoracic vertebrae; the iliocostalis muscle passes over the costal angles and, between these and the spinalis, the longissimus can be found.

3.4.4 Approaches for structures and key sites used during puncture techniques

We will continue with a description of the puncture approaches of the most relevant anatomical structures and those that present the most difficulty during the minimally invasive procedures of daily clinical practice.

- Quadratus lumborum muscle:
  - position: contralateral decubitus.
  - location: multiple points in the muscle from the 12th rib to the iliac crest.
  - procedure: puncture using a flat palpation technique, inserting the needle parallel to the plane of the back (or in a slightly oblique direction), anterior to the paravertebral muscles (figure 3.6B and B1).
- Pubic symphysis:
  - position: supine.
  - location: fibrocartilage and expansions from the insertions of the rectus abdominis muscle.
  - procedure: puncture using a flat palpation technique, inserting the needle perpendicular to the symphysis, searching for the area of fibrotic tissue.
- Intercostal muscles:
  - position: supine or side-lying position.
  - location: multiple points in the different rib interspaces.
  - procedure: puncture with the guide hand placed on the patient's chest, placing a finger on the rib on each side of the MTrP and inserting the needle angled no more than 45° from the skin surface.
    An ultrasound-guided puncture is recommended, whereby the needle is inserted into the middle of the muscle, avoiding the inferior border of the rib where the vasculonervous bundle is located (figure 3.3B).

3.5 TOPOGRAPHICAL ANATOMY OF THE UPPER LIMB

3.5.1 Regions

The upper limb is formed of six large regions: shoulder, arm, elbow, forearm, wrist and hand.[6,7]

Shoulder

Cranially, the shoulder is limited by the clavicle and the superior border of the scapula, and inferiorly by a plane that is at a tangent to the inferior border of the pectoralis major and, anteromedially, the mammary region. For description purposes, the shoulder is subdivided into the deltoid, axillar and scapular regions.

- The deltoid region corresponds with the prominence of the deltoid muscle.
- The axillary region can be described as a pyramid of four sides with a truncated vertex. The base, on an inferior plane, corresponds with the common definition of axilla and is made up of the cutaneous lining and the axillary fascia and extends between the proximal and medial part of the arm and the lateral surface of the thorax. The anterior wall includes the subclavius muscle, part of the pectoralis major and minor muscles, and the clavipectoral fascia. The medial wall contains part of the serratus anterior muscle, which is included both in the wall of the axilla as well as in the thoracic wall. The posterior wall is also formed by the subscapularis muscle, teres major and lattisimus dorsi. The definition of the lateral wall of the axilla varies depending on the descriptions provided by different authors. Some describe this as being located within the intertubercular sulcus (bicipital groove of humerus) and others describe it as formed by the muscles of the arm. In any case, what is relevant is that the axilla communicates with the arm through the lateral aspect, and it is here that the vasculonervous elements between the shoulder and the arm pass through.
- The scapular region corresponds to the territory situated dorsal to the scapula and the posterior aspect of the axilla.

Arm

The arm extends between the shoulder and the elbow, from a circular imaginary line inferior to the tendons of pectoralis major and the lattisimus dorsi until two finger widths above the cubital fossa or, in other words, above the elbow pit. It includes the anterior brachial region and the posterior brachial region, or the anterior and posterior regions of the arm.

Elbow

This is the segment that lies between the arm and the forearm, from which it is separated by a virtual circular line that passes two finger widths below the elbow pit. It is comprised of the anterior elbow region, or anterior cubital region or cubital fossa, and the posterior cubital region or posterior elbow region.

Forearm

The forearm spans from its proximal limit, in the elbow, to a circular line, distally, that passes over the head of the ulna, which separates it from the wrist.

Wrist

In the wrist, which extends distally until the virtual limit marked by a circular line that passes over the scaphoid tubercle and the distal limit marked by the pisiform bone, there are anterior and posterior carpal regions, where the carpal tunnel and ulnar canal (Guyon's canal) are found ventrally, and the six carpal tendinous sheaths of the extensor muscles, dorsally.

Hand

In the hand we can distinguish a palmar, or volar, surface and a dorsal surface. In the palmar region we can distinguish, apart from the palmar concavity, the thenar and hypothenar eminences, which correspond to the intrinsic musculature of the thumb and the little finger, respectively.

3.5.2 Anatomical relations of interest

Shoulder

The common pathway of the axillary nerve and the posterior humeral circumflex artery, which winds around the surgical neck of the humerus in a lateral direction and from posterior towards anterior, is related to the spinal and acromial parts of the deltoid. The clavicular part of the deltoid relates to the pathway of the anterior humeral circumflex artery which, on a deeper level to the deltoid, passes from medial to lateral over the surgical neck of the humerus and crosses superficially the intertubercular groove in order to ascend towards the joint capsule parallel to

the crest of the greater tubercle. The rotator interval is a triangular space between the tendons of the subscapularis and supraspinatus muscles and the base of the coracoid process and covered by the coracohumeral ligament, containing the tendon of the long head of the biceps brachii muscle and the superior glenohumeral ligament,[18–20] and that has no vasculonervous relations of interest.

The clavipectoral fascia, through which the thoracoacromial artery crosses, spans between the subclavius muscle and the superior border of the pectoralis minor muscle. Also, the medial and lateral pectoral nerves pierce the clavipectoral fascia, distributing their terminal branches in the plane between the pectoralis major and minor muscles. Behind the clavipectoral fascia, the pectoralis minor in the acromial insertion and the subclavius muscle, the axilla is found with the axillary vein, the axillary artery and, deeper still, the infraclavicular part of the brachial plexus. Between the pectoralis major and deltoid muscles, the deltopectoral triangle is found which, superficially, corresponds with the infraclavicular fossa (Mohrenheim fossa). This contains the proximal segment of the cephalic vein before becoming perforating and accessing into the axilla, where it empties into the axillary vein. A large portion of the pectoralis major and minor muscles are found in the pectoral region, which is thoracic, and therefore, separated from the pleural cavity and the lung by one to two finger widths.

The intercostal vasculonervous bundle is located in the costal groove, found in the inferior border of each rib (figure 3.3B). The serratus anterior muscle is involved both in the wall of the axilla and that of the thorax, and extends, also, towards the scapular and lateral pectoral regions, partially covering the first to ninth ribs, or the 10th, and the corresponding intercostal spaces, with the long thoracic nerve, and the lateral thoracic artery (external mammary artery) descending superficial to it (figure 3.11). The subscapularis muscle forms the largest part of the posterior wall of the axilla and therefore relates to the fascicles of the brachial plexus, the axillary vein and artery, the thoracodorsal nerve and the long thoracic nerve. The teres minor and teres major muscles relate to the circumflex scapular artery in the upper triangular space (medial triangular space, medial axillary space or foramen omotricipitale) and the axillary nerve and the posterior humeral circumflex artery in the quadrangular space (quadrilateral space [of Velpeau] or foramen humerotricipital) (figure 3.12). The lattisimus dorsi muscle relates to the thoracic wall, the corresponding intercostal spaces and the thoracodorsal nerve.

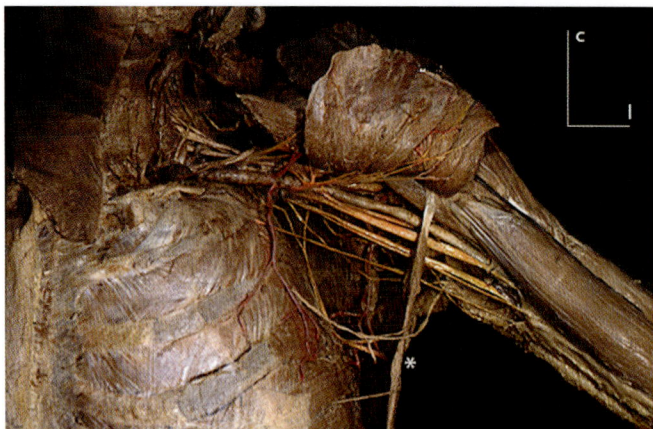

FIGURE 3.11 ■ Panoramic view displaying a dissection of the ventral aspect of the left shoulder. The axillary artery and the terminal branches of the brachial plexus head towards the arm. The cadaver presented an axillary arch (*), an anatomical variation which is found in 5–7% of the population, and which consists of a muscle fascicle which, passing in front of the plexus and the artery, extends between the latissimus dorsi and, in this case, the coracobrachialis muscle (it can also be found within the pectoralis major muscle or the fascia of the biceps brachii). Orientation: c, cranial; I, lateral. (Courtesy of Drs. JR. Sañudo, F. Valderrama, T. Vázquez and E. Maranillo).

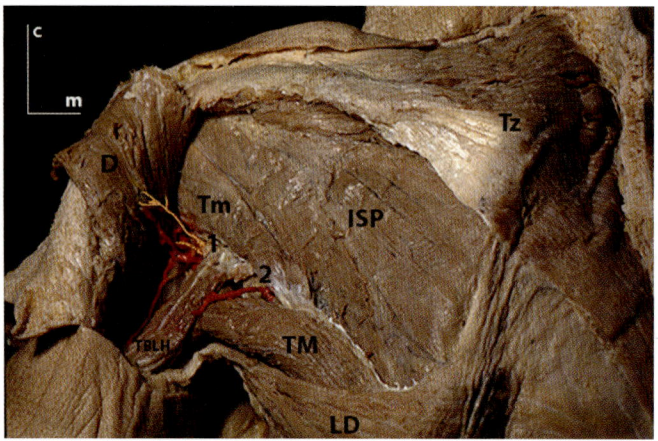

FIGURE 3.12 ■ Panoramic view of dissection of the posterior aspect of the left shoulder. The following muscles can be identified: deltoid (D), teres minor (Tm), infraspinatus (ISP), trapezius (Tz), long head of triceps brachii (TBLH), teres major (TM) and latissimus dorsi (LD). The axillary nerve and posterior humeral circumflex artery can be observed (1) as they pass by the quadrangular space, whereas the circumflex scapular artery (2) crosses the triangular space. Orientation: c, cranial; m, medial. (Courtesy of Drs. JR. Sañudo, F. Valderrama, T. Vázquez and E. Maranillo).

The trapezius muscle is comprised of three parts: the descending, transverse and ascending parts (superior [upper], intermediate [middle] and inferior [lower] parts). In the case of the descending part, a large portion of its course lies within the posterior neck region, crossing the suprascapular region, and reaching the clavicle, passing by the lateral neck region. The transverse part extends from the vertebral region, crosses the interscapular and scapular region and reaches the acromion in the deltoid region. The ascending part also begins in the vertebral region and crosses the interscapular region, reaching the spine of the scapula within the scapular region. The accessory nerve runs its course on the deep aspect of the trapezius, in the descending part after having crossed, from upwards to downwards and from front to behind, the levator scapulae muscle in order to continue descending vertically until it reaches the interior border of the ascending part. The levator scapulae muscle also relates to the accessory nerve and, on the deeper aspect, with the dorsal scapular nerve. The rhomboid minor and major muscles are related in their superficial aspect to the accessory nerve and, on the deeper aspect, with the dorsal scapular nerve. The dorsal scapular artery runs parallel to the medial border of the scapula. The

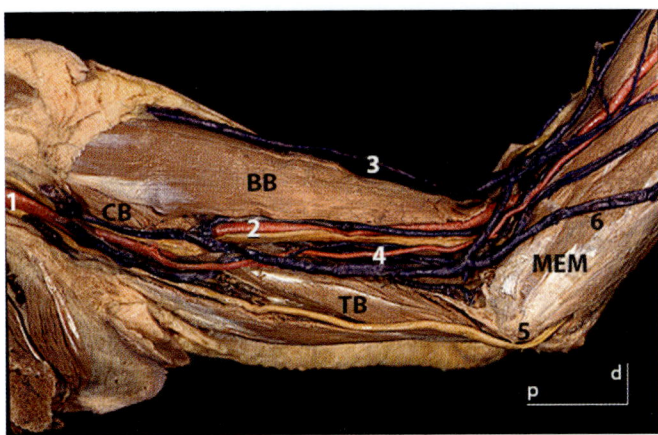

FIGURE 3.13 ■ Medial view of a dissection of the left arm. The following muscles can be observed: biceps brachii (BB), coracobrachialis (CB), triceps brachii (TB) and, from the medial epicondyle of the elbow towards the forearm, the medial epicondyle muscles (MEM). The vasculonervous elements are the axillary artery (1), the brachial artery and the median nerve (2), the cephalic vein (3), a brachioulnar artery (4) (an anatomical variation consisting of the presence of an ulnar artery from the arm) and the ulnar nerve (5) (at the point where it passes by the cubital canal posterior to the medial epicondyle) and the basilar vein (6). Orientation: p, proximal; d, distal. (Courtesy of Drs. JR. Sañudo, T. Vázquez and E. Maranillo).

supraspinatus muscle is found in the supraspinatus fossa of the scapula, in the depths of the descending and middle parts of the trapezius, relating to the suprascapular nerve and artery which pass through the depth of the supraspinatus fossa, laterally, from the scapular notch until entering the infraspinatus fossa, in relation to the scapular neck.

In the supraspinous fossa the existence of foramina has been described.[21,22] This is an anatomical variation of relevance for needling techniques, as there is a risk of pneumothorax when puncturing the supraspinatus muscle. The infraspinatus muscle occupies the infraspinatus fossa and relates to the suprascapular nerve and artery that come from the supraspinatus fossa. In the infraspinous fossa congenital foramina of the scapula have also been described, measuring up to 2–5 mm in diameter in 0.8–5.4% of individuals.[21] This is important as case studies have been reported describing iatrogenic pneumothorax resulting from needling the small intestine 11 (SI11) acupuncture point (figure 3.8).

There are areas in the upper quarter and thoracic cage in which congenital anomalies have been described that are of relevance for needling techniques (the foramina in the infraspinous fossa, the foramina in the supraspinous fossa and incomplete ossification and fusion of the sternal plate).

Arm

The coracobrachialis, biceps brachii, brachialis and triceps brachii are muscles that all belong to the arm, although the proximal portion of the long head of the biceps brachii and the coracobrachialis muscle belong to the axilla, and the distal portions of the biceps brachii and the brachialis reach the elbow region. In almost 90% of cases, the coracobrachialis muscle is pierced by the musculocutaneous nerve, which reaches it from a proximal and medial direction.[23] In the inner aspect of the arm, within the anterior compartment, over the medial intermuscular septum, the brachial canal can be found, containing the median nerve, the ulnar nerve and the brachial artery as main elements (figure 3.13). Further distal, the ulnar nerve leaves the canal and is found in the posterior compartment of the arm. In 8–18% of individuals,[8,24] the biceps brachii muscle can have accessory bellies. In posterior approaches of the arm, over the triceps brachii, it is important to consider the helical path of the radial nerve, together with the deep brachial artery, which both run from a proximal and medial direction towards distal and lateral, so that in the middle third of the arm they are found over the radial sulcus in the posterior aspect of the humerus. Finally, the musculocutaneous nerve runs distal to the biceps brachii and the brachialis muscles in a direction from proximal and medial towards distal and lateral. Epifascially two veins are, in general, clearly visible: the cephalic vein of the arm on the lateral aspect and the basilic vein of the arm on the medial aspect (figure 3.13).

Elbow

In the cubital fossa, the presence of vasculonervous elements is highly relevant, and thus, for better systematization, the medial and lateral bicipital grooves are described. The insertion tendon of the biceps brachii muscle is the common element to both grooves, and from the tendon to the pronator teres muscle the medial bicipital groove is found, whereas between the tendon and the brachioradialis muscle the lateral bicipital groove is found. From medial to lateral, the medial bicipital groove contains the inferior ulnar collateral artery, the median nerve and the brachial artery (figure 3.14).

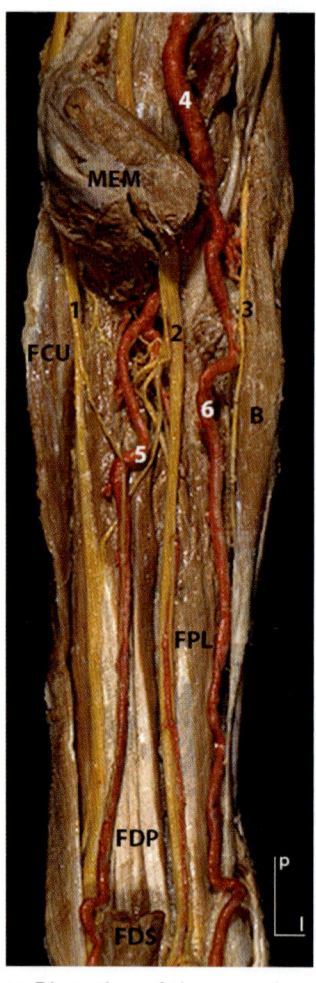

FIGURE 3.14 ■ Dissection of the ventral region of the left forearm. The medial epicondyle muscles (MEM) have been sectioned and proximally displaced, including the flexor digitorum superficialis (FDS), which is seen distally. Flexor carpi ulnaris muscle (FCU), flexor digitorum profundus muscle (FDP), flexor hallucis longus muscle (FPL) and brachioradialis muscle (B). The vasculonervous structures are: the ulnar nerve (1), the median nerve (2), the superficial branch of the radial nerve (3), the brachial artery (4), the ulnar artery (5) and the radial artery (6). Orientation: p, proximal; l, lateral. (Courtesy of Drs. JR. Sañudo, F. Valderrama, T. Vázquez and E. Maranillo).

Approximately 2 cm distal to the crease of the elbow, in most cases, a terminal division occurs of the brachial artery into the radial artery and the ulnar artery; however, it is important to bear in mind that, in 8% of cases, a superficial ulnar artery can be found located superficially to the pronator teres muscle.[8,25] If present, it can be identified by its superficial pulse which can be seen with the naked eye (figure 3.14). The lateral bicipital groove contains, deep to the brachioradialis muscle, the division of the radial nerve into its terminal branches (superficial and deep branches), the musculocutaneous nerve, which immediately becomes epifascial and continues as the lateral cutaneous nerve of the forearm (sensitive), and the anastomosis between the deep brachial artery and the radial recurrent artery.

The anatomical relation between the branches of the radial nerve and the humeroradial joint is important as the superficial branch is anterior to the joint, and, laterally, the deep branch is found running between the two planes of the supinator muscle. Over the lateral epicondyle there is a common extensor tendon that gives origin to the extensor carpi ulnaris, the extensor digiti minimi, the extensor digitorum and the extensor carpi radialis brevis, which is the deepest in origin and has fibres that originate directly from the radial collateral ligament and the annular ligament.[26,27] Therefore, it has a very significant relation with the humeroradial joint.

In the posterior elbow region, the cubital tunnel is found dorsal to the medial epicondyle; it is an osteofibrous passage through which the ulnar nerve passes. Between the lateral epicondyle and the olecranon, the anconeus muscle is found, which receives its innervation on the deep aspect, from proximal and medial to distal and lateral, a plane through which the interosseous recurrent artery also passes in a near-vertical path. Subcutaneous to this region, the subcutaneous bursa of the olecranon is found.

Forearm

The muscles of the anterior compartment of the forearm are distributed in four layers. From medial to lateral these are: the superficial layer, formed by the flexor carpi ulnaris, the palmaris longus (a muscle which is absent in 10–20% of the population[28]), the flexor carpi radialis and the pronator teres muscles. The second layer is formed by the flexor digitorum superficialis muscle; the third layer includes the flexor digitorum profundus and the flexor pollicis longus muscles, and the pronator quadratus muscle, which is found in the distal third of the forearm, forms the deepest, or fourth, layer. The median, ulnar and superficial branch of the radial nerve, and the radial and ulnar arteries, are the main vasculonervous structures of the anterior forearm region, and their anatomical relations change according to their proximal or distal position along the forearm (figure 3.14). The median nerve enters the forearm through the humeral and ulnar heads of the pronator teres muscle although, occasionally, it can pass superficially, or deep, to both, or pierce the humeral head.[26]

The median nerve in its distal trajectory is found in the deep aspect of the flexor digitorum superficialis muscle, surrounded by the same fascia as the muscle, although, in very exceptional circumstances, it can travel on the superficial aspect of the same muscle. Approximately 5 cm proximal to the flexor retinaculum (transverse carpal ligament, or anterior annular ligament), the median nerve becomes superficial and is located medial to the tendon of the flexor carpi radialis muscle (figure 3.15). The ulnar nerve can be located throughout all of its forearm length

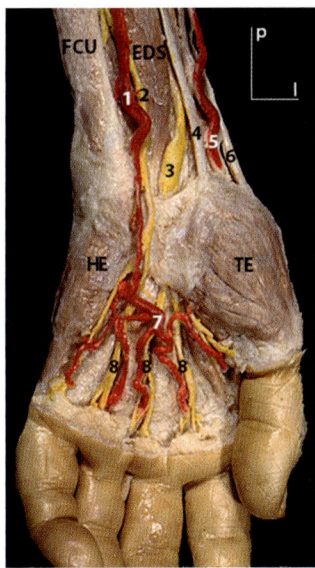

FIGURE 3.15 ■ Dissection of the palmar region of the left hand, including the carpus and the distal forearm. The following muscles are shown: flexor carpi ulnaris (FCU), extensor digitorum superficialis (EDS), the tendon of the flexor carpi radialis (4) and the tendon of the brachioradialis (6). In the hand we observe the hypothenar eminence (HE) and thenar eminence (TE). The vasculonervous elements are the ulnar artery (1) and the ulnar nerve (2) (the relation between both has been accidentally modified), the median nerve at its entrance to the carpal tunnel (3), the radial artery (5), the superficial palmar arch (7) and the common palmar digital branches of the nerves and arteries (8). Orientation: p, proximal; l, lateral. (Courtesy of Drs. JR. Sañudo, F. Valderrama, T. Vázquez and E. Maranillo).

over the flexor digitorum profundus. Proximally, it is covered by the palmaris longus muscle, if it is present, and the flexor carpi radialis muscle, at the surface, and the flexor digitorum superficialis at a deeper level whereas, from the union of the proximal third and the middle third of the forearm, a site where the ulnar artery becomes lateral to the nerve, it is covered exclusively by the flexor carpi ulnaris muscle.

Before following a common course with the ulnar nerve, the ulnar artery is first deep to the ulnar head of the pronator teres muscle in order to pass deep to the median nerve as soon as this is crossed and continue its course, from proximal and median to distal and medial, over the belly of the flexor digitorum profundus until it becomes lateral to the ulnar nerve. The radial artery is covered, from the cubital fossa distalward, by the belly of the brachioradial muscle, passing anterior to the insertion of the pronator teres muscle and, from the myotendinous junction of the brachioradialis muscle, it lies medial to the tendon in all its length within the pulse groove, which is subfascial, and where it rests proximal to the flexor pollicis longus, and, distally, to the pronator quadratus muscle (figure 3.14). The arterial common pattern of the forearm, with one ulnar artery and one radial artery, occurs in 84% of individuals, but it is important to consider the possible presence of a median artery (8%) or a superficial ulnar artery (8%).[24,29] The anterior interosseous nerve and artery are the deepest vasculonervous structures of the anterior compartment of the forearm and they run, over the anterior aspect of the interosseous membrane, deep to the flexor digitorum profundus and the flexor pollicis longus muscles.

In the posterior forearm region there are two muscular planes which contain on the superficial layer, and from lateral to medial, the brachioradialis, the extensor carpi radialis longus, the extensor carpi radialis brevis, the extensor digitorum, the extensor digiti minimi and the extensor carpi ulnaris muscles. On the deep plane, from proximal to distal and from lateral to medial, the following muscles are found: the supinator, the abductor pollicis longus, the extensor pollicis brevis, the extensor pollicis longus and the extensor indicis muscles (figure 3.16). Proximally, the deep branch of the radial nerve is found deep to the superficial belly of the supinator muscle (supinator arch: arcade of Frohse) and runs all along this belly and the deep belly, emerging distally, as the posterior interosseous nerve, in the interstitium between the supinator and abductor pollicis longus muscles. The nerve continues distally, innervating the

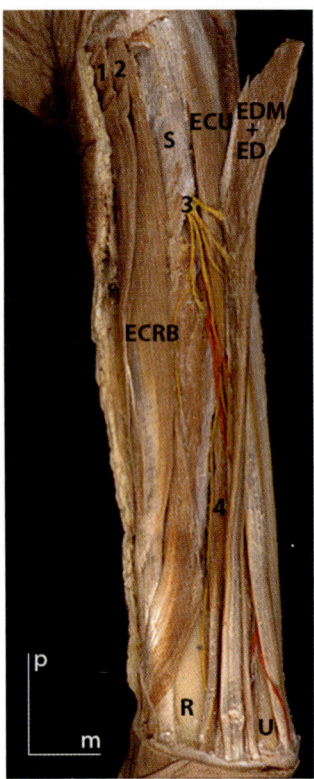

FIGURE 3.16 ■ Dorsal view of a dissection of the left forearm. The extensor digiti minimi (EDM) and extensor digitorum (ED) muscles have been sectioned and displaced medially in order to observe the course of the posterior interosseous nerve (3) after exiting from between the two layers of the supinator muscle (S). The brachioradialis (1), extensor carpi radialis longus (2), extensor carpi radialis brevis (ECRB), extensor carpi ulnaris (ECU) and the extensor indicis (4) muscles are visible, as well as the radius (R) and the ulna (U). Orientation: p, proximal; m, medial. (Courtesy of Drs. JR. Sañudo, F. Valderrama, T. Vázquez and E. Maranillo).

remaining muscles of the compartment (figure 3.16). The superficial branch of the radial nerve, which is sensitive, runs from proximal to distal firstly deep to the brachioradialis muscle and lateral to the radial artery (figure 3.14), to the segment between the middle and distal third of the forearm, which is where the nerve separates from the artery and heads dorsally in order to become epifascial, two finger widths proximal to the styloid process of the radius.

Wrist

In the anterior wrist region, the presence of the carpal tunnel is highlighted as an osteofibrous tunnel formed dorsally by a canal limited by the carpal bones and ventrally by the flexor retinaculum, within which are contained the four tendons of the flexor digitorum superficialis muscle, covered by their synovial sheaths, and the median nerve on the superficial plane, and the four tendons of the flexor digitorum profundus muscle plus the tendon of the flexor pollicis longus, in a deeper plane. Some German authors, or those with a Germanic influence, also include the tendon of the flexor carpi radialis muscle among the structures crossing the carpal tunnel, based on the fact that, although the tendon passes within an independent fibrous compartment to the common compartment of the flexor digitorum tendons and the median nerve, it is covered by the flexor retinaculum.[9,12] The median nerve passes the carpal tunnel lateral to the flexor tendons. The ulnar canal (Guyon's canal) is the subfascial space, medial to the carpus (figure 3.13), within which the ulnar nerve and artery access the hand, with the nerve located medial to the artery.[30]

In the dorsal carpal region, six osteofibrous compartments are found, through which the tendons of the muscles that extend the hand and the fingers enter the hand surrounded by their synovial sheaths.[31] From radial to ulnar, these correspond with the tendons of the following muscles: the abductor pollicis longus and extensor pollicis brevis, the extensor carpi radialis longus and brevis, the extensor pollicis longus, the extensor digitorum and the extensor indicis, the extensor digiti minimi and, finally, the extensor carpi ulnaris. The tendon of the abductor pollicis longus muscle is double in almost all individuals.[31]

Hand

The thenar eminence is formed by the following muscles, from superficial to deep: the abductor hallucis brevis, the opponens pollicis, the flexor pollicis brevis and the adductor pollicis. Both the thenar branch and the lateral branch of the median nerve pass through the medial aspect of the eminence. Also, within the medial aspect of the thenar eminence, but at a deeper level, the deep branch of the ulnar nerve passes. In the palmar concavity, that contains the lumbrical muscles and the palmar and dorsal interossei muscles in the deepest layer, the superficial palmar arch of the ulnar artery and the deep palmar arch of the radial artery are found, both of which can present variations such as the non-formation of the arch,[8,9,12] together with the common digital palmar arteries and nerves (figure 3.15), and the superficial branch of the ulnar nerve and the palmar common branches of the median nerve. The intrinsic musculature of the little finger forms the hypothenar eminence composed of the abductor, flexor and opponens digiti minimi muscles, which are listed from superficial to deep, with the superficial and deep branches of the ulnar nerve running lateral to these structures.

In the dorsal aspect of the hand, the dorsal metacarpal arteries and the dorsal digital branches of the radial and ulnar nerves run parallel to the metacarpals in the interosseous spaces.

3.5.3 Areas of vasculonervous conflict and anatomical landmarks

The axillary nerve and the posterior circumflex humeral artery wind around the humerus approximately 2 cm above the central point of a line which unites the tip of the acromion with the inferior border of the deltoid tuberosity.[11] Both elements access the deltoid region from the axilla through a quadrangular space, which is delimited from above by the belly of the teres minor muscle, medially by the belly of the long head of the triceps brachii muscle, inferiorly by the muscle belly of the teres major, and laterally, by the humerus itself. However, in 16% of cases, the artery does so from the triangular interval (lower triangular space or triceps hiatus),[9,10,12] a space found within the following boundaries: the teres major superiorly, the body of the humerus laterally and the long head of the triceps brachii muscle medially. The triangular space contains the scapular circumflex artery and is delimited superiorly by the muscle belly of the teres minor, inferiorly by the belly of the teres major and laterally, by the long head of the triceps brachii muscle.[6,10]

The axilla is an area of communication between the neck and the upper limb, which contains the brachial plexus, the axillary artery and vein and five groups of lymphatic nodules. The course of the axillary artery can be observed upon abduction of the arm to a square angle, drawing a line from the centre of the clavicle to the point where the tendon of the pectoralis major muscle crosses the prominence of the coracobrachialis muscle.[11] This reference is also useful for indicating the posterior, lateral and medial fascicles of the brachial plexus, as they run in relation to the artery.

The axillary vein is at first anterior to the artery, and then becomes medial, as it goes distal. The origin of the thoracoacromial artery corresponds with a point where the axillary artery crosses the superior border of the pectoralis minor muscle. The communication between the axilla and the arm occurs on the lateral aspect of the axilla, which leads into the medial aspect of

the arm. Thus, upon exiting the axilla, the brachial artery and the median and ulnar nerves run along the medial aspect of the arm. The long thoracic nerve descends superficially to the serratus anterior, approximately over the midaxillary line, and the lateral thoracic artery is slightly anterior to it.

The accessory nerve runs over the deep aspect of the trapezius, in the descending part, after having crossed from upwards to downwards and from the front backwards, the levator scapulae muscle. The nerve then continues its vertical descent (with an approximate reference being along the free aspect of the transverse processes) deep to the medial and ascending fibres, until it almost reaches the inferior extent of the ascending part. The dorsal nerve of the scapula courses vertically, over the deep aspect of the rhomboid muscles, laterally located in relation to the costotransverse joints. The nerve and the suprascapular artery pass along the bottom of the supraspinatus fossa in a lateral direction, passing behind the neck of the scapula through the scapular notch, located in the middle third between the root of the spine of the scapula and the lateral border of the acromion, until it enters the infraspinatus fossa.

In the arm, the brachial artery and the median nerve continue together to the medial bicipital groove, in which the nerve is medial to the artery. The ulnar nerve is approximately located in the middle third of the arm, within the posterior compartment and courses towards the posterior aspect of the medial epicondyle. The course of the radial nerve can be indicated by a line which passes just below the posterior axillary fold towards the lateral aspect of the humerus in the union between its middle and inferior third and, from there, it passes vertically distally, ventral to the lateral epicondyle. Approximately 2 cm distal to this epicondyle, the articular interline of the humeroradial joint is found.[11]

The position of the radial artery in the forearm is represented by a line that goes from the lateral border of the biceps brachii tendon to the medial part of the anterior aspect of the radial styloid process. Due to the curved course of the ulnar artery, two lines have to be traced in order to indicate its progression. One line extends from the ventral aspect of the medial epicondyle to the radial aspect of the pisiform bone, in which the middle and distal thirds of this line represent the distal course of the artery. The proximal third of the artery corresponds with a line that goes from the centre of the cubital fossa to the union of the upper and middle thirds of the first line. The course of the median nerve in the forearm is marked proximally by the middle point of the line that joins both epicondyles on the ventral aspect of the arm, and distally, by the point along the medial border of the flexor carpi radialis tendon when it crosses deep to the flexor retinaculum. The ulnar nerve is found over a line that goes from the anterior aspect of the medial epicondyle to the lateral border of the pisiform bone. The superficial branch of the radial nerve continues the trajectory of the radial nerve after the lateral epicondyle, situated deep to the brachioradialis muscle and lateral to the radial artery, to the point between the middle and distal thirds of the forearm, where it separates from the artery and heads dorsally, becoming epifascial two finger widths proximal to the styloid process of the radius.[11]

The median nerve passes the carpal tunnel that lies lateral to the tendon of the middle finger of the flexor digitorum superficialis muscle and superficial to the tendon of the index finger of the flexor digitorum superficialis muscle medially, and the flexor pollicis longus laterally.[31] In the ulnar canal, the ulnar nerve and artery access the hand laterally to the tendon of the flexor carpi ulnaris muscle and the pisiform bone and medial to the hook of the hamate, with the nerve situated medial to the artery.[30]

The tendons of the extensor carpi muscles and the extensors of the fingers are situated as follows within the osteofibrous compartments: the first compartment contains the tendons of the abductor pollicis longus and the extensor pollicis brevis,[32] which, distally, forms the ventral limit of the radial fossa, in the depth of which the scaphoid bone is found proximally, and the trapezium bone distally, with the radial artery passing above the latter; the tendon of the abductor pollicis longus is double in almost all individuals. The second compartment is found immediately lateral to the dorsal tubercle of the radius and contains the tendons of the extensor carpi radialis longus and brevis. Immediately medial to the dorsal tubercle of the radius, the third compartment contains the tendon of the extensor hallucis longus, which distally forms the dorsal limit of the anatomical snuffbox. Slightly medial to the third compartment, the fourth compartment contains the four tendons of the extensor digitorum superficially, and the tendon of the extensor indicis and the distal portion of the posterior interosseous nerve on the deep plane. The fifth compartment, for the extensor digiti minimi, is found over the head of the ulna and marks the interline of the distal radioulnar joint. The sixth compartment is formed by the tendon of the extensor carpi ulnaris and is lateral to the styloid process of the ulna.[11,31]

3.5.4 Approaches for structures and key sites used during puncture techniques

Next, the approaches are described for puncturing the most relevant anatomical structures and those that present the most difficulty during the minimally invasive procedures of daily clinical practice.

- Infraspinatus muscle:
  - position: prone.
  - location: central part of the muscle.
  - procedure: puncture using a flat palpation technique, inserting the needle in a perpendicular direction and searching for the MTrP or the motor point.
- Pectoralis major muscle – sternal part:
  - position: supine with the arm in slight abduction.
  - location: central part of the muscle.
  - procedure: puncture using a pincer grip and inserting the needle in a medial and cranial direction, searching for the MTrP or the motor point.
- Subscapularis muscle:
  - position: supine with the arm in abduction and external rotation (in order to separate the scapula from the ribcage and therefore reveal the muscle easier).
  - location: anterior aspect of the scapula.
  - procedure: the therapist places the dorsal aspect of his or her triphalangeal fingers of the medial hand over the ribcage (in order to delimit the approach and avoid accessing into the ribcage); with the lateral hand, the needle is inserted from the lateral border of the scapula towards the subscapular fossa in a medial, posterior and cranial direction.
- Deltoid muscle – anterior, medial and posterior part:
  - position: contralateral decubitus.
  - location: middle one-third of the muscle.
  - procedure: using a pincer grip, puncture the specified area by inserting the needle in a perpendicular sense, to reach the MTrP or motor point.
- Descending trapezius muscle:
  - position: prone.
  - location: central portion of the more vertical muscle fibres.
  - procedure: pincer grip of the specified area; for the descending part a needle is inserted in an anterior and cranial direction, searching for the MTrP or motor point; for the transverse part, the needle

is inserted perpendicularly, searching for the MTrP or the motor point (figure 3.10-A).

- Levator scapulae muscle:
  - position: contralateral decubitus.
  - location: at the level of the beginning of the neck, just in front of the anterior border of the descending part of the trapezius.
  - procedure: puncture using a flat palpation technique, inserting the needle in a posterior and caudal direction, searching for the MTrP or the motor point.
- Rotator interval:
  - position: supine with the arm in a neutral position or in internal rotation in order to anteriorize the insertion fibres of the supraspinatus which form the rotator interval.
  - location: area formed by the anchor points of the long head of the biceps brachii (caudal), fibres of the supraspinatus tendon (cranial) and the subscapularis (medial).
  - procedure: two approaches: puncture from cranial to caudal, perpendicular to the structure (figure 3.17) or from medial to lateral, or from lateral to medial depending on the affected tissue.

- Tendon of the supraspinatus muscle – articular part and enthesis:
  - position: supine with the arm against the body in neutral rotation.
  - location: width of the tendon and enthesis in the greater tubercle of the humerus.
  - procedure: for the articular part, a needle is inserted from a lateral approach beneath the anterolateral border of the acromion, searching for the area of the tendon with signs of degeneration; for the enthesis, the needle is inserted from an anterosuperior approach with an orientation of 40° in a lateral and caudal direction.
- Brachioradialis muscle:
  - position: supine, with the patient's forearm in neutral prone supination.
  - location: central part of the muscle in the posterior antebrachial (forearm) region, before the elbow crease.
  - procedure: puncture using a pincer grip, inserting the needle from lateral to medial directed to the MTrP or motor point.
- Anconeus muscle:
  - position: supine, patient's elbow slightly flexed and forearm pronated.

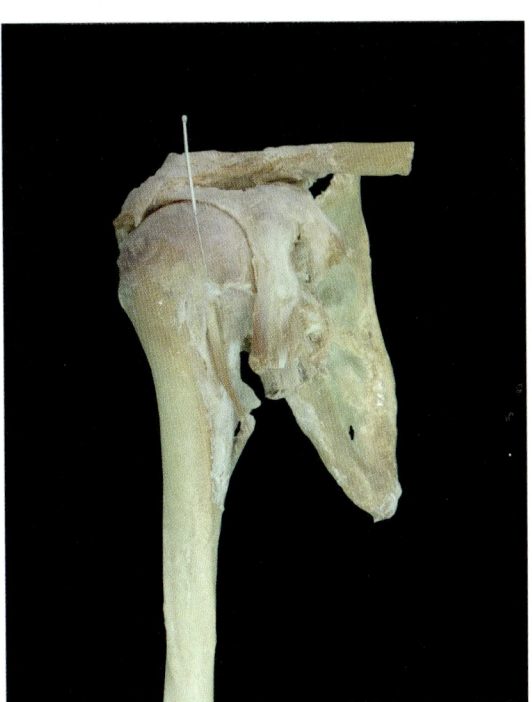
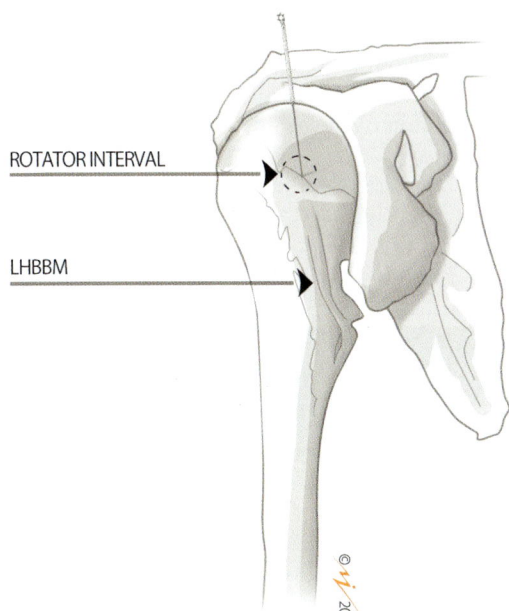

ROTATOR INTERVAL

LHBBM

FIGURE 3.17 ■ Rotator interval: craniocaudal approach on the structure. LHBBM, long head of the biceps brachii muscle.

- location: central part of the muscle and in depth.
- procedure: puncture using a flat palpation technique, inserting the needle one finger width from the posterior border of the lateral epicondyle and in a medial, anterior and craniocaudal direction, searching for the MTrP or motor point.
- Extensor carpi radialis longus muscle:
  - position: supine, with the patient's forearm in neutral pronosupination.
  - location: superior one-third of the muscle belly in the posterior antebrachial (forearm) region before crossing the elbow crease.
  - procedure: puncture using a pincer grip and inserting the needle from lateral to medial directed at the MTrP or motor point.
- Extensor carpi radialis brevis muscle:
  - position: supine, with the patient's forearm pronated.
  - location: central part of the muscle.
  - procedure: flat puncture of the muscle belly, inserting the needle in a perpendicular direction towards the MTrP or motor point.
- Common extensor tendon of the lateral epicondyle muscles:
  - position: supine, with the patient's elbow slightly flexed and forearm pronated.
  - location: insertion of the common tendon on the lateral epicondyle.
  - procedure: the needle is inserted with a 30° orientation from caudal to cranial searching for the insertion of the tendon on the lateral epicondyle (figure 3.18).
- Tendon of the extensor carpi radialis brevis muscle:
  - position: supine, with the patient's elbow slightly flexed and the forearm pronated.

- location: insertion of the tendon in the deepest plane of the lateral epicondyle.
- procedure: the needle is inserted in a 45–60° orientation from caudal to cranial and slightly from anterior to posterior, searching for the insertion of the deep fascicle of the tendon in the lateral epicondyle.
- Extensor carpi radialis brevis – capsule of the humeroradial joint:
  - position: supine, with the patient's elbow in slight extension and the forearm in neutral prone supination (in this manner, more articular space is created in order to facilitate the insertion of the needle).
  - location: through the extensor digitorum and the extensor carpi radialis brevis muscles until greater resistance is met; this corresponds with the capsuloligamentous complex of the joint and the deepest fascicle of the extensor carpi radialis brevis (which lines the joint).
  - procedure: puncture using a flat puncture technique, inserting the needle perpendicular to the joint (figure 3.19).
- Arcade of Frohse (supinator arch):
  - position: supine, the patient's arm slightly flexed and the forearm supinated.
  - location: the fibrotic connective tissue which can compromise the radial nerve when it meets the arch, or the connective tissue which surrounds the nerve.
  - procedure: using the landmark represented by the projection of the humeroradial articulation in the anterior aspect of the forearm (2 cm lateral to the biceps brachii tendon), puncture using a flat palpation technique, inserting the needle in a posterior and slightly lateral and cranial direction.

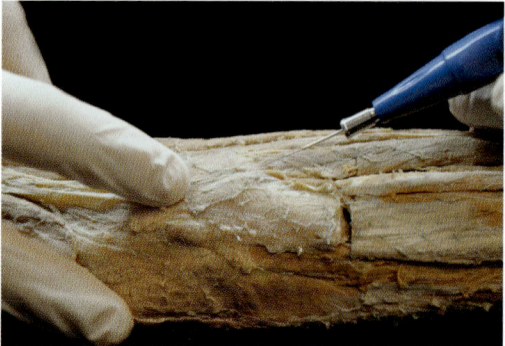
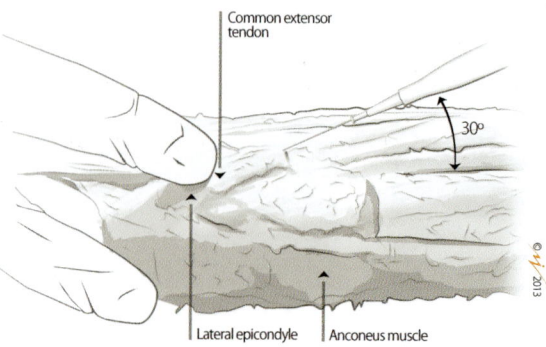

Common extensor tendon

30°

Lateral epicondyle | Anconeus muscle

FIGURE 3.18 ■ Common extensor tendon: enthesis approach.

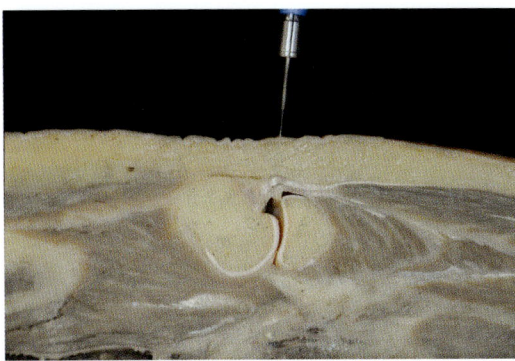
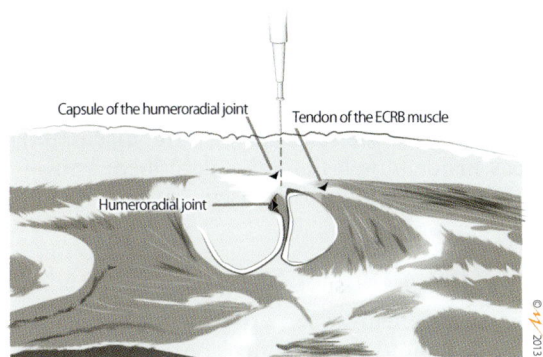

FIGURE 3.19 ■ Extensor carpi radialis brevis (ECRB) – capsule of the humeroradial joint: therapeutic approach over the deep fascicle of the tendon and joint capsular ligamentous complex.

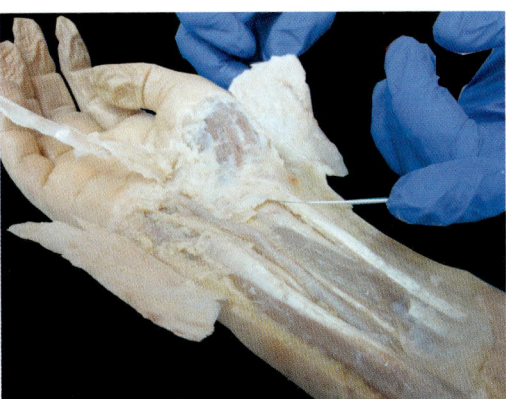
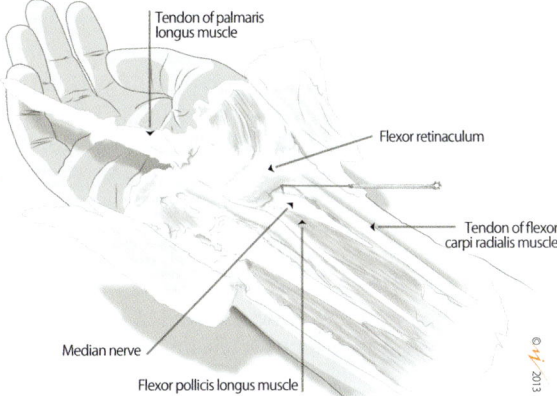

FIGURE 3.20 ■ Median nerve: carpal tunnel approach.

- Carpal tunnel:
  - position: supine; the patient's arm is extended and the forearm is supinated. The space between the tendons is located.
  - location: fibrotic connective tissue which can compromise the median nerve when it meets the carpal tunnel, in relation to the flexor retinaculum or the flexor tendons, or the connective tissue which surrounds the nerve (see video 3.3).
  - procedure: in order to release the interface between the nerve and the flexor tendons, the space between the tendons of the palmaris longus and the flexor carpi radialis is located (with the median nerve lying in between both of these), and approximately 2–3 cm above the wrist crease, the needle is inserted just beside the ulnar border of the tendon of the flexor carpi radialis with a 30–40° orientation and following a caudal and posterior direction. In order to release

the interface between the flexor retinaculum and the nerve, a needle is inserted in the same location with a 15° orientation, following a caudal and slightly posterior direction (figure 3.20).

3.6 TOPOGRAPHICAL ANATOMY OF THE LOWER LIMB

3.6.1 Regions

Six regions are described in the lower limb: the gluteal region, the thigh, the knee, the leg, the ankle and the foot. However, not all authors regionalize the lower limb with these demarcations.[6,7]

Gluteal region

This is limited inferiorly by the gluteal fold, anterolaterally by a line which connects the anterior superior iliac spine with the greater trochanter, superiorly by a prominence of the iliac crest and medially by the intergluteal cleft. According to functional criteria and topographic proximity, together with the muscles of the gluteal region, the relations with the iliacus and psoas major muscles are also described, known together as the iliopsoas muscle.

The thigh

Several systematizations exist for the thigh (or femoral region), but the division into anterior, femoral triangle (triangle of Scarpa) and posterior is both simple and practical. The anterior region corresponds with the ventral aspect of the thigh, which is found lateral to the prominence of the sartorius muscle, to an imaginary line between the greater trochanter and the lateral femoral condyle, which coincides approximately with the iliotibial tract, and ends distally with an imaginary line that passes two finger widths above the base of the patella, which demarcates with the region of the knee. The femoral triangle, which lies between the inguinal ligament superiorly, the sartorius muscle laterally and the adductor longus muscle medially, has a muscle floor formed laterally by the iliopsoas muscle and medially by the pectineus muscle. The posterior thigh region extends from the gluteal fold with medial and lateral boundaries that coincide with the anterior region and distally with the circular line that passes two finger widths above the patella, and separates it from the knee.

The knee

The proximal boundary of the knee region corresponds with a horizontal line which passes two finger widths above the base of the patella, and caudally by another horizontal line that passes by the inferior limit of the tibial tuberosity. For descriptive reasons, the anterior knee and the posterior knee regions are considered, with the popliteal fossa found within their depth.

The leg

The crural region, or the leg region, extends from its proximal boundary with the knee to an imaginary circular line that passes above the malleoli. In the leg, both an anterior and a posterior region are described.

The ankle

The talocrural region, or ankle region, contains the territories corresponding to the talocrural

joint, the malleoli and the heel, although other systems exist.

The foot

In the foot we can distinguish a dorsal area, or the dorsum of the foot, and a plantar area, or the sole of the foot.

3.6.2 Anatomical relations of interest

Gluteal region

The sciatic nerve is the main related structure in this region (figure 3.21), although the superior and inferior gluteal vessels and nerves are also relevant. The sciatic nerve is flat and normally reaches 1.5 cm width; it exits the pelvis by the greater sciatic foramen, inferior to the piriformis muscle in 85% of cases, but in almost 15% of

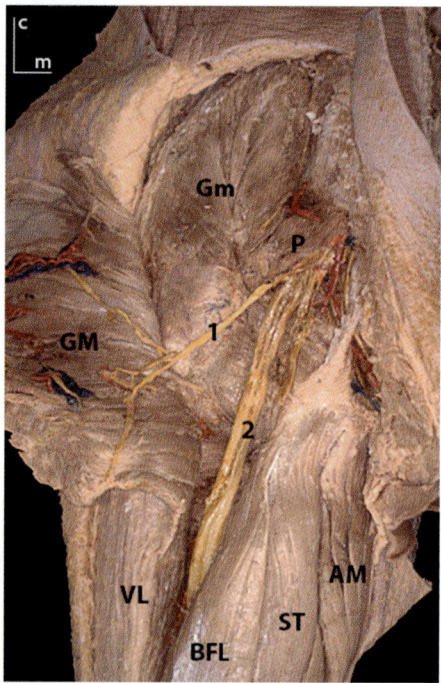

FIGURE 3.21 ■ Dissection of the left gluteal region. The medial margin of the gluteus maximus has been sectioned (GM) in order to displace the muscle laterally and visualize the gluteus medius muscle (Gm) and the piriformis muscle (P), under which the inferior gluteal nerve (1) and the sciatic nerve (2) are visible. In the posterior femoral region, the following muscles are visible: vastus lateralis (VL), long head of the biceps femoris (BFL), semitendinosus (ST) and adductor magnus (AM). Orientation: c, cranial; m, medial. (Courtesy of Drs. JR. Sañudo, F. Valderrama, T. Vázquez and E. Maranillo).

cases, the common fibular nerve component pierces the piriformis muscle belly.[12] In less than 1% of cases, the common fibular nerve exits the pelvis passing above the piriformis muscle belly.[12] In all cases the tibial nerve, the other terminal branch of the sciatic nerve, passes caudal to the piriformis. Once the sciatic nerve exits the pelvis, it becomes ventral to the superior gemellus muscle, the internal obturator, the inferior gemellus and the quadratus femoris, continuing vertically along the thigh over the adductor magnus. The superior gluteal vasculonervous bundle exits the pelvis from above the piriformis muscle, and then passes between the gluteus medius and minor muscles, reaching the tensor fascia latae muscle (figure 3.21).

The anatomical relations with the psoas major and iliacus muscle, together known as the iliopsoas muscle, are also described in this section (although they do not belong to the gluteal region), due to functional and topographic proximity. A greater portion of the muscle bellies pertaining to the psoas major and the iliacus course within the abdominal cavity, covered by the iliac fascia or the iliopsoas fascia, the extra-peritoneal fat and the parietal layer of the peritoneum.[33] The psoas major and iliacus are related to the peritoneum, the intestinal loops and the lateral femoral cutaneous, obturator and femoral nerves. Additionally, the psoas major is related to the kidneys, the anterior branches of the lumbar spinal nerves and the subcostal, iliohypogastric, ilioinguinal and genitofemoral nerves. The iliacus muscle also relates to the deep circumflex iliac artery which, in the depth of the transversalis fascia, extends in a posterior direction along the iliac crest.

Thigh

In the anterior thigh region, the vasculonervous relations of the quadriceps femoris muscle, formed by the rectus femoris, and the vastus lateralis, medialis and intermedius, and those of the sartorius and tensor fascia latae muscles are limited to those of the lateral femoral cutaneous nerve and the cutaneous and motor branches of the femoral nerve (figure 3.22). Notwithstanding, distally, in the vertex of the femoral triangle, it is important to consider the presence of the adductor canal (Hunter's canal), as it contains the femoral vessels, the descending genicular artery, the saphenous nerve and the nerve for the vastus medialis.

The presence of the femoral vasculonervous bundle marks the relations in the femoral triangle (figure 3.22). The most lateral element is the nerve, followed by the artery, and finally the

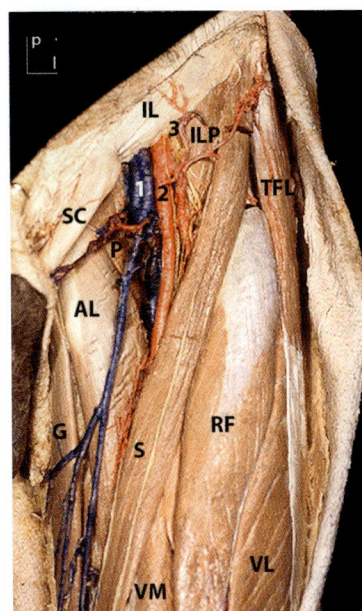

FIGURE 3.22 ■ Dissection of the left anterior thigh region. The borders of the femoral triangle are observed: the inguinal ligament (IL), the adductor longus (AL) and the sartorius muscle (S); the muscle 'floor' of the triangle is formed by the pectineus muscle (P) medially and the iliopsoas (ILP) laterally. The triangle contains the femoral vein (1), the femoral artery (2) and the femoral nerve (3). Other muscles: gracilis (G), vastus medialis (VM), rectus femoris (RF), vastus lateralis (VL) and the tensor fascia latae (TFL) are observed. It is also possible to observe the spermatic cord (SC). Orientation: p, proximal; l, lateral. (Courtesy of Drs. JR. Sañudo, F. Valderrama, T. Vázquez and E. Maranillo).

vein, although even more medial, an important lymphatic nodule obliterates the femoral canal (node of Cloquet; node of Rosenmüller). The arterial vessels worth consideration (all of which are branches of the femoral artery) are the external pudendal arteries, which are directed towards medial, and the external iliac circumflex artery, which heads laterally in parallel and below the inguinal ligament. The deep lymph nodes are also important and found over the area of the femoral triangle. Finally, as an epifascial structure, the great saphenous vein ends its course, accompanied by important superficial lymph nodes, draining the femoral vein through the saphenous hiatus of the fascia latae.

The posterior region of the thigh contains the so-called ischiocrural muscle group, formed by the biceps femoris, the semimembranosus and semitendinosus muscles (figure 3.21). In the deeper plane the adductor magnus is found, and between this and the biceps femoris, and lateral to the semimembranosus, the sciatic nerve lies,

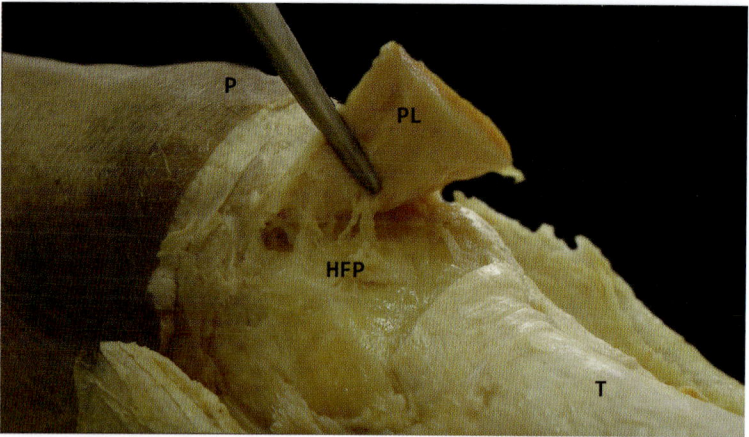

FIGURE 3.23 ■ Dissection of the left knee. Anatomic relation of Hoffa's fat pad (HFP) with the deep portion of the patellar ligament (PL). P, patella; T, tibia.

passing laterally to the ischial tuberosity to enter the thigh. Distally, on the medial aspect, the popliteal vessels cross the adductor hiatus formed by the tendon of the adductor magnus and run lateral to the muscle belly of the semimembranosus. Epifascially, the posterior femoral cutaneous nerve enters the thigh from the lateral third of the gluteal fold, and within the proximal third of the thigh it is found superficial to the biceps femoris muscle whereas, from the distal third, it is found superficial to the muscle belly of the semitendinosus muscle.

At the origin of the adductor muscles, over the body of the pubic bone and its inferior branch, the spermatic cord is relevant in male subjects (figure 3.22) and, in any case, the obturator foramen with the obturator nerve and artery and the root of the cavernous bodies surrounded by the ischiocavernosus muscles. In the territory of the pubic symphysis, important relations are established in the subpubic angle with the dorsal nerve and artery of the penis or the clitoris.

Knee

In the anterior knee region the relation between the patellar ligament[34] and the infrapatellar fat pad (fat pad of Hoffa) (figures 3.23 and 3.24) is particularly noteworthy. Other structures with interesting relations in the anterior knee region are the superficial pes anserinus, which superficially lines the medial collateral ligament and the lateral collateral ligament, which has a very relevant anatomical relation, both with the insertion of the iliotibial tract over the lateral condyle of the tibia, and especially with the popliteus muscle tendon,[35] which passes deep to the ligament in order to enter the joint capsule and insert in the lateral femoral condyle (figure 3.25).

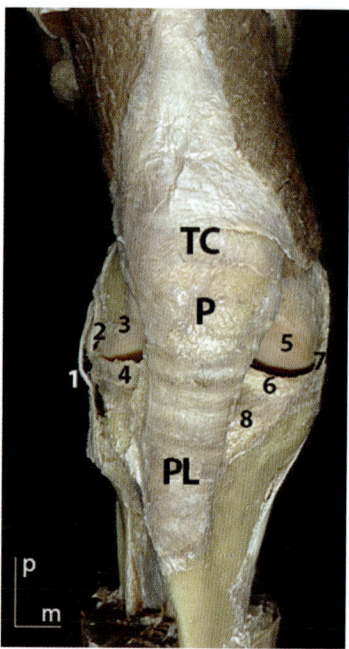

FIGURE 3.24 ■ Dissection of a left knee. The quadriceps tendon (TC) continues over the patella (P) and then follows towards the tibia as the patellar ligament (PL). From lateral to medial: fibular collateral ligament (1), crossed in depth by the popliteus muscle tendon (2) which inserts in the lateral femoral condyle (3); the lateral meniscus is also visible (4). In the medial compartment: the medial femoral condyle (5), the medial meniscus (6) and the collateral tibial ligament (7) are shown. The infrapatellar fat pad (Hoffa's fat pad) is also visible (8). Orientation: p, proximal; m, medial. (Courtesy of Drs. JR Sañudo, F. Valderrama, T. Vázquez and E. Maranillo).

The posterior knee region contains the distal portions of the ischiocrural muscles and the proximal extent of the triceps surae, which define the limits of the popliteal fossa, and the proximal part of the popliteus muscle (figures 3.25 and

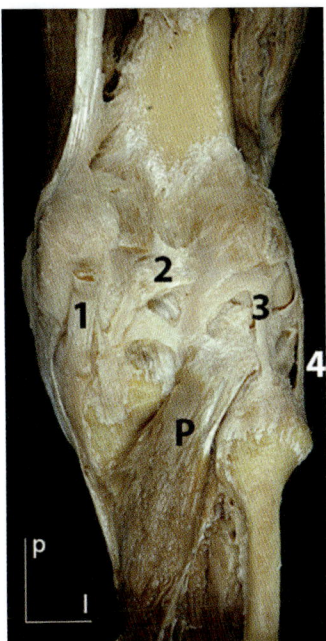

FIGURE 3.25 ■ Dissection of the posterior articular plane of a left knee. The tendon of the semimembranosus muscle (1), the oblique popliteal ligament (2), the arcuate popliteal ligament (3) and the fibular collateral ligament (4) are identified. Deep to this ligament, the tendon of the popliteus muscle (P) passes towards the lateral femoral condyle. Orientation: p, proximal; l, lateral. (Courtesy of Drs. JR. Sañudo, F. Valderrama, T. Vázquez and E. Maranillo).

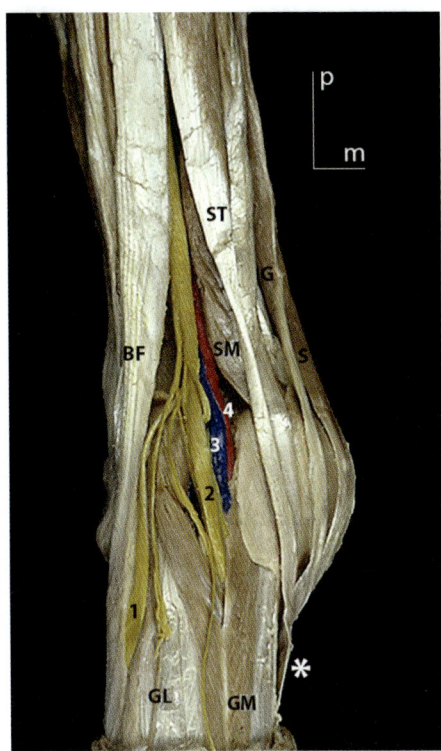

FIGURE 3.26 ■ Image of a dissection of the posterior region of a left knee. The common fibular nerve (1) is observed over the border of the biceps femoris muscle tendon (BF), the tibial nerve (2), the popliteal vein (3) and the popliteal artery (4). The semimembranosus muscle (SM) extends its tendon, forming the deep pes anserinus, and the tendons of the muscles that form the superficial pes anserinus (*), semitendinosus (ST), gracilis (G) and sartorius (S). The gastrocnemius is also distinguished, with its lateral (GL) and medial (GM) heads. Orientation: p, proximal; m, medial. (Courtesy of Drs. JR. Sañudo, F. Valderrama, T. Vázquez and E. Maranillo).

3.26). The fossa, which contains an abundance of fat and lymph nodes, has a diamond-like shape and is superiorly and laterally limited by the biceps femoris, superiorly and medially by the semimembranosus and inferiorly by the medial and lateral heads of the gastrocnemius and the lateral aspect of the plantaris muscle (this muscle is absent 5–10% of the time and its presence on one side does not necessarily indicate that it is present on the other).[8] The popliteal vascular bundle crosses the area vertically, with the vein located lateral to the artery during its proximal course and, as it becomes more distal, it becomes dorsal to it, accompanied by the tibial nerve, which is superficial to the vessels (figure 3.26). The common fibular nerve passes over the medial border of the belly of the biceps femoris muscle. Most of the time, the small saphenous vein perforates the popliteal fascia and drains into the popliteal vein.

Leg

In the anterior leg region, the medial aspect has a lack of muscles, as this corresponds with the medial surface of the tibia, whereas anterolaterally an anterior and a lateral compartment are described. The muscles of the anterior compartment are tibialis anterior, extensor hallucis longus and extensor digitorum longus, and their main anatomical relations are with the anterior tibial artery and the deep fibular nerve, which have a common course, immediately ventral to the interosseous membrane of the leg, in the interstitium that is found between the tibialis anterior muscle and the extensor digitorum longus proximally, and the tibialis anterior and the extensor hallucis longus from the middle third of the leg towards distal.

Apart from the three muscles already described, 90% of the population also present the fibularis tertius, which is found lateral to the extensor digitorum longus.[8] The lateral compartment contains the fibularis longus and brevis muscles. The muscle belly of the fibularis longus occupies the proximal two-thirds of the compartment, whereas the fibularis brevis, which is found deep to the longus, occupies the two distal thirds. Between both muscles and the anterior crural intermuscular septum, the superficial fibular nerve is found. This runs approximately until the confluence of the middle and distal third of the leg, where it becomes epifascial and heads towards the dorsum of the foot. At this point the nerve finally divides into its terminal branches, the medial and intermediate dorsal cutaneous nerves. The lateral compartment is separated from the deep plane of the posterior leg muscles only by the posterior crural intermuscular septum.

The muscles of the posterior compartment of the leg are divided into a superficial and a deep plane (figure 3.27). The superficial plane is made up of the triceps surae muscle, constituted of the medial and lateral gastrocnemius and the soleus, as well as the plantaris muscle. The deep plane, from medial to lateral, contains the flexor digitorum longus, the tibialis posterior and the flexor hallucis longus. Between both muscle planes runs the vasculonervous bundle, which is formed by the posterior tibial artery and the fibular artery, together with the tibial nerve. The posterior tibial artery and the tibial nerve, after having ventrally crossed the popliteal muscle, pass deep to the tendinous arch of the soleus and then run ventral to it over the tibialis posterior muscle, in the proximal third, and just between the flexor digitorum longus and the flexor hallucis longus muscles in the two distal thirds. The fibular artery, a branch from the posterior tibial artery, lies laterally over the tibialis posterior muscle and is covered by the flexor hallucis longus muscle. Epifascially, in the posterior aspect of the leg, the small saphenous vein courses vertically along the posterior midline on the surface of the leg, and is accompanied proximally by the medial sural cutaneous nerve and distally by the sural nerve; medially, the great saphenous vein ascends accompanied by the saphenous nerve.

Ankle

The anterior ankle region contains all the tendons of the extensor muscles which head towards their insertions covered by their synovial sheaths and which pass under the inferior retinaculum of the extensor muscles. From medial to lateral are the tendon of the tibialis anterior, the tendon of the extensor hallucis longus, the four tendons of the extensor digitorum longus, and, most often, the tendon of the fibularis tertius as the most lateral structure. Between the tendon of the extensor hallucis longus and the tendon for the second toe of the extensor digitorum longus runs the dorsal artery of the foot (dorsalis pedis artery), accompanied by the medial terminal branch of the deep fibular nerve. The anterolateral malleolar artery passes in front of the lateral malleolus, over the territories that correspond with the anterior talofibular ligament and the lateral aspect of the tarsal sinus. The saphenous veins run epifascially; the great saphenous vein is highly visible, ventral to the medial malleolus, whereas the small saphenous vein is observed behind the lateral malleolus.

The posterior ankle region contains the malleolar regions, or retromalleolar regions, and the calcaneal tendon (Achilles tendon). The medial retromalleolar region contains the so-called tarsal tunnel (in analogy with the carpal tunnel, as it is an osteofibrous canal), formed by the flexor retinaculum and the tibia, talus and calcaneus bones. Immediately behind the tibial malleolus, the tibialis posterior muscle tendon is found, followed by the tendon of the flexor digitorum longus, and the posterior tibial artery with its comitans veins, the tibial nerve, and, the most

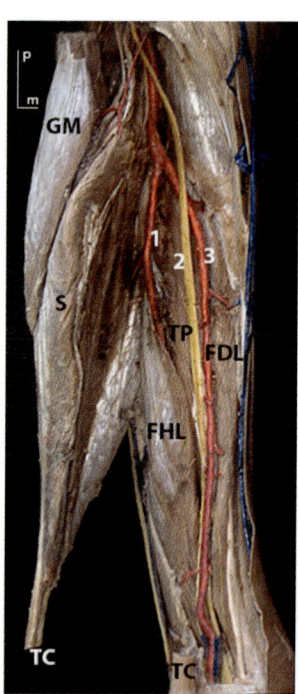

FIGURE 3.27 ■ Image of a dissection of the posterior region of a left leg. The calcaneal tendon (TC) has been dissected in order to displace the superficial muscles: medial gastrocnemius (GM) and soleus (S), distinguishing: the fibular artery (1), deep to the flexor hallucis longus (FHL), the tibial nerve (2) over the tibialis posterior muscle (TP) and the posterior tibial artery (3) and the flexor digitorum longus (FDL). Orientation: p, proximal; m, medial. (Courtesy of Drs. JR. Sañudo, F. Valderrama, T. Vázquez and E. Maranillo).

posterior element, the tendon of the flexor hallucis longus.[36] All the tendons are found within their synovial sheaths.

The content of the lateral retromalleolar region includes the tendons of the fibularis longus and brevis muscles, each with its respective synovial sheaths, that of the longus covering the brevis proximally, and becoming posterior to it as it goes distal. In the posterior ankle region, the prominence of the calcaneal tendon stands out, covered by the skin, the leg fascia and its epitenon.[37] The space between the tendon and the articular plane is filled distally with a fat pad (Kager's fat pad), in a way that is similar to the infrapatellar fat pad. In the enthesis with the calcaneus the calcaneal synovial bursa is found.

Foot

In the foot, two regions are distinguished: a dorsal region, or dorsum of the foot, and a plantar region, or sole. Epifascially, in the dorsum of the foot it is fairly easy to visualize the dorsal venous network, with the dorsal venous arch. This is continued with the medial and lateral marginal veins, origin of the great and small saphenous veins, respectively. On a subfascial layer, the dorsal artery of the foot (dorsalis pedis artery) is palpable between the tendon of the extensor hallucis and the tendon for the second toe of the extensor digitorum longus. From a muscular point of view, the dorsum is composed of a single muscle, the extensor digitorum brevis and hallucis brevis, deep to which pass the lateral tarsal artery and the branches of the deep fibular nerve which innervates it. On a deep plane we also find the dorsal metatarsal arteries in all the interosseous spaces, together with the cutaneous branch of the deep fibular nerve in the first space.

The sole of the foot presents a thick skin which is firmly joined to the subcutaneous layers (as occurs with the palm of the hand) and a unique subcutaneous structure with fat tissue found within cells of very dense and firm connective tissue that extends from the dermis to the plantar fascia. These fat cells are extremely vascularized and are particularly thick in order to absorb the pressures of the body weight adequately. On the superficial plane the plantar fascia is found; this is a dense and strong structure over which numerous superficial vascular and nervous branches of the medial and lateral plantar arteries and nerves surface, especially over the lateral border of the abductor hallucis muscle and its tendon, the medial plantar nerve and the superficial branch of the medial plantar artery.

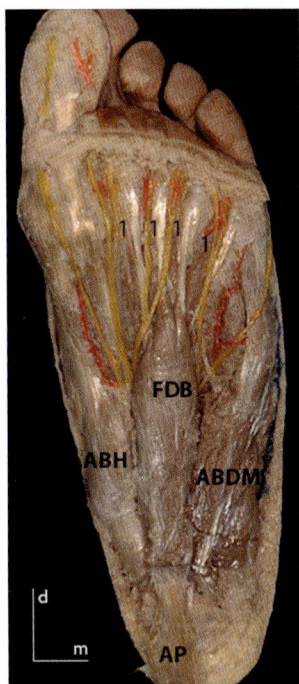

FIGURE 3.28 ■ Plantar view of the dissection of a left foot. The plantar aponeurosis (AP) has been distally sectioned and removed to allow a view of the first muscle plane, which contains the abductor hallucis (ABH), the flexor digitorum brevis (FDB) and the abductor digiti minimi (ABDM). The common plantar digital nerves and arteries (1) can be distinguished. Orientation: d, distal; m, medial. (Courtesy of Drs. JR. Sañudo, F. Valderrama, T. Vázquez and E. Maranillo).

Deep to the plantar fascia there are four muscular planes. The most superficial contains the flexor digitorum brevis (figure 3.28). The second plane contains the abductor hallucis medially and, laterally, the abductor digiti minimi, and between both muscles the quadratus plantae or flexor accessorius is found and, distal to this, the tendons of the flexor digitorum longus with the lumbrical muscles lying in between. Between this second plane and the first, from medial and posterior towards lateral and anterior, the lateral plantar vasculonervous bundle courses in relation to the medial border of the abductor digiti minimi. The contents of the third plane, from medial to lateral are: the flexor hallucis brevis, with its medial and lateral heads, and between these, the tendon of the flexor hallucis longus; the adductor hallucis, with its oblique head, parallel to the second metatarsal and the transverse head, found immediately plantar to the heads of the second to fifth metatarsal; and, finally, the flexor digiti minimi, the most lateral of all, over which the superficial branch of the lateral plantar nerve courses. The fourth and deepest plane contains the plantar and dorsal interossei muscles and the opponens digiti minimi muscle. The deep plantar vasculonervous bundle passes over the plantar interossei muscles, and divides into the plantar metatarsal arteries.[38]

3.6.3 Areas of vasculonervous conflict and anatomical landmarks

In order to locate the exact path of the sciatic nerve in the gluteal region accurately, we must first identify three bony landmarks: the posterior superior iliac spine, the ischial tuberosity and the greater trochanter. A line joins the posterior superior iliac spine with the ischial tuberosity; another line joins the greater trochanter and the ischial tuberosity. The bisection of both lines upon the surface of the gluteal region represents the course of the sciatic nerve and is oblique from proximal and medial to distal and lateral. The emergence of the superior gluteal vasculonervous bundle, above the piriformis muscle, can be found reasonably well in the confluence of the superior third and the middle third of the line that joins the posterior superior iliac spine with the ischial tuberosity. From this point, it is distributed between the gluteus medius and minor, reaching to the tensor fascia latae muscle. An important reference in this region is the ventrogluteal area (von Hochstetter triangle), which is considered a security area for intramuscular injections.[9]

The pathway of the sciatic nerve along the thigh is indicated by vertically prolonging the point of exit of the nerve from the gluteal region, and tracing a line to the superior angle of the popliteal fossa. The continuation of this vertical line through the centre of the popliteal fossa represents the position of the tibial nerve, whereas the common fibular nerve continues the line of the biceps femoris tendon. In the tarsal tunnel, immediately behind the tibial malleolus, the tendon of the tibialis posterior muscle is found, followed by the tendon of the flexor digitorum longus and, in turn, followed by the posterior tibial artery, the tibial nerve and the tendon of the flexor hallucis longus muscle, which is the most posterior and deep element. The lines for the deep fibular nerve and the anterior tibial artery go from the medial aspect of the head of the fibula to a midpoint between both malleoli. The dorsal artery of the foot is palpable between the tendon of the extensor hallucis and the tendon of the second toe of the extensor digitorum longus.[11]

The femoral artery in the femoral triangle is found in the midpoint between the anterior superior iliac spine and the pubic tubercle. One finger width on each side of the artery location, the femoral nerve is found laterally while the femoral vein is found medially.[11]

3.6.4 Approaches for structures and key sites used during puncture techniques

We shall continue with a description of the puncture approaches of the most relevant anatomical structures and those that present the most difficulty during the minimally invasive procedures of daily clinical practice.

- Gluteus medius and minor:
  - position: contralateral decubitus, 80° hip flexion and 90° knee flexion.
  - location: beneath the iliac crest (three finger widths, approximately) along its length.
  - procedure: puncture using a flat palpation technique, inserting the needle perpendicular to the muscle, in the direction of the crest and searching for the MTrP or the motor point.
- Psoas major and iliacus muscle:
  - position: supine, slight hip and knee flexion to relax the muscle (a component of maximal external rotation is added for the approach to the psoas major tendon in order to improve its accessibility for the insertion).
  - location: psoas major: pathway in the muscle towards the lesser trochanter; tendon of the iliopsoas: lesser trochanter; iliacus: pathway from the proximity of the anterior superior iliac spine towards cranial.
  - procedure: puncture using a flat palpation technique, inserting the needle lateral to the vasculonervous bundle located in the femoral triangle (one finger width lateral to the femoral artery) and medial to the sartorius muscle, perpendicular to the thigh, searching for the MTrP or motor point, or the insertion of the tendon on to the lesser trochanter.
- Pectineus muscle:
  - position: supine, slight abduction, flexion and external rotation of the hip.
  - localization: superior one-third of the muscle, deep to the femoral triangle.
  - procedure: puncture using a flat palpation technique, inserting the needle medial to the vasculonervous bundle found in the femoral triangle (one finger width medial to the femoral artery) and lateral to the adductor longus muscle,

perpendicular to the thigh, searching for the MTrP or motor point.

- Vastus medialis muscle:
  - position: supine.
  - location: along the muscle length, normally in the proximal and medial portions (four finger widths cranial to the base of the patella and two finger widths towards medial).
  - procedure: puncture using a flat palpation technique, inserting the needle perpendicular to the thigh, searching for the MTrP or motor point.
- Vastus lateralis muscle:
  - position: supine.
  - location: multiple points in the muscle along the lateral margin of the thigh.
  - procedure: puncture using a flat palpation technique, inserting the needle perpendicular to the thigh, but with a slight tilt towards anterior in order to avoid entering into the ischiocrural musculature, searching for the MTrP or motor point.
- Rectus femoris muscle:
  - position: supine.
  - location: superior one-third of the muscle, close to the anterior inferior iliac spine.
  - procedure: puncture using a flat palpation technique, inserting the needle perpendicular to the muscle, searching for the MTrP or motor point.
- Tendon of the adductor longus muscle:
  - position: supine, slight abduction, flexion and external rotation of the hip.
  - location: insertion on to the pubic ramus.
  - procedure: puncture using a flat palpation technique (although a pincer grip can also be used), inserting the needle in a medial and cranial direction, searching for the enthesis (feel a hard bony

end with the tip of the needle). An intra-tendon trajectory is recommended in order to avoid accessing delicate areas (e.g. pudendal canal, spermatic cord).

- Femoral nerve:
  - position: supine, slight hip abduction, flexion and external rotation.
  - location: connective tissue that surrounds the nerve.
  - procedure: puncture using a flat palpation technique, approximately 2 cm lateral to the artery, inserting the needle with a 30–45° orientation in the cranial direction.
- Medial collateral ligament:
  - position: supine, slight abduction, flexion and external rotation of the hip with the knee slightly flexed (alternatively, knee and hip flexed at 90° and foot supported on the plinth).
  - location: proximal attachment of the deep medial collateral ligament.[39]
  - procedure: puncture using a flat palpation technique, inserting the needle perpendicular to the femoral condyle, searching for the area of interest.
- Patellar ligament:
  - position: supine, knee slightly flexed (wedge underneath the knee).
  - location: intra-tendon at the proximal level together with the deep interphase – Hoffa's fat pad and body of the tendon; distal insertion on the tibia. The superficial interphase is not usually affected.
  - procedure: proximal intratendon approach on the inferior patellar pole or tendon body, inserting the needle with a 45° orientation from caudal to cranial (figure 3.29); deep interphase – Hoffa's fat pad: lateral approach (to avoid the saphenous nerve), inserting the needle perpendicular to the tendon below it (figure 3.30). Distally, the approach is

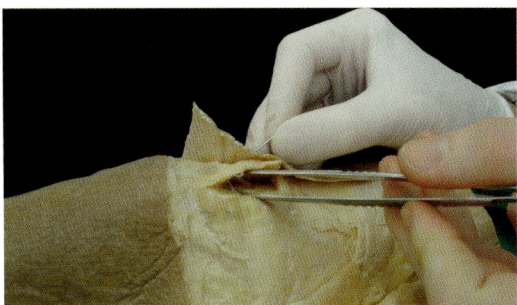
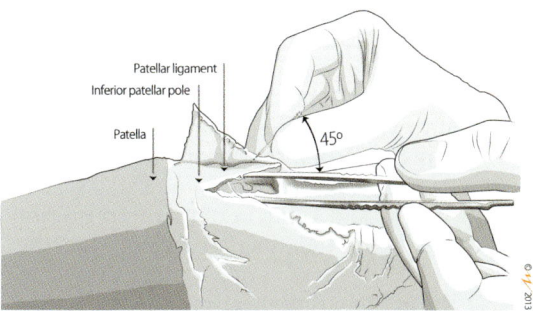

FIGURE 3.29 ■ Patellar ligament: proximal approach over the tendon.

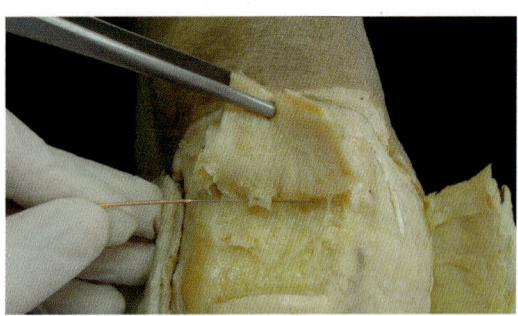
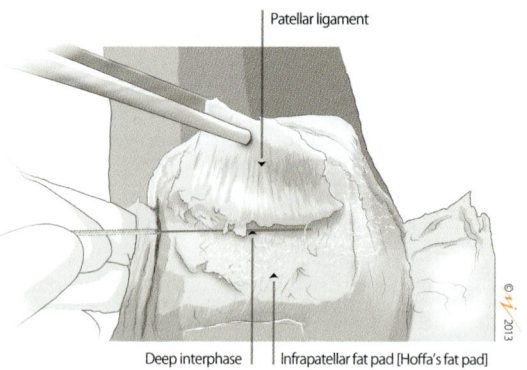

Patellar ligament

Deep interphase | Infrapatellar fat pad [Hoffa's fat pad]

FIGURE 3.30 ■ Patellar ligament: lateral approach over the deep interphase (deep paratendon – Hoffa's fat pad).

performed over the most degenerated point, with a 45° orientation from cranial to caudal.

- Gastrocnemius muscle:
  - position: prone, knee slightly flexed (wedge underneath leg).
  - location: normally in the proximal one-third of the medial gastrocnemius.
  - procedure: puncture using a flat palpation technique, inserting the needle perpendicular to the muscle, searching for the MTrP or the motor point.
- Soleus muscle:
  - position: contralateral decubitus (cranial location), knee slightly flexed; homolateral decubitus (caudal location), knee slightly flexed; or in prone.
  - location: cranial-lateral one-third and caudal-medial.
  - procedure: puncture using a flat palpation technique, inserting the needle parallel to the muscle (medial approach – caudal location; lateral approach – cranial location) searching for the MTrP or the motor point. If performed in prone, insertion of the needle is performed with the needle perpendicular to the muscle.
- Popliteus muscle:
  - position: homolateral decubitus, knee slightly flexed; or in prone.
  - location: central part of the muscle.
  - procedure: using one hand, the therapist displaces the medial gastrocnemius laterally; with the other hand a flat puncture is performed, inserting the needle parallel to the leg, deep to the medial gastrocnemius and right next to the posterior border of the tibia, searching for the MTrP or motor point. If performed in the prone position, a flat puncture is performed, inserting the needle in the most

lateral part of the medial gastrocnemius, perpendicular to the muscle.

- Achilles tendon:
  - position: prone.
  - location: superficial interphase – superficial fascia – epitenon; tendon body; deep interphase – Kager's fat pad.
  - procedure: superficial interphase: the therapist uses one hand to hold the skin using a pincer grip, and with the other hand the needle is inserted almost parallel to the leg; body of the tendon: intra-tendon approach, inserting the needle with a 40–45° orientation, searching for the degenerative or fibrous tissue; deep interphase: medial approach (to avoid the sural nerve in a lateral approach), inserting the needle perpendicular to the tendon from medial to lateral, searching for the degenerative or fibrotic tissue.
- Plantar fascia:
  - position: prone or homolateral decubitus.
  - location: insertion in the medial calcaneal process, subcalcaneal bursa and medial and lateral periostic zone of the calcaneus.
  - procedure: enthesis: the needle is inserted with a 45° inclination in a lateral, posterior and cranial direction, searching for the affected tissue (figure 3.31). The subcalcaneal bursa is approached perpendicular to the calcaneus in its central part. The medial and lateral periostic zone is reached with a 30° needle insertion over the painful area.
- Adductor hallucis muscle:
  - position: homolateral decubitus.
  - location: different points of the muscle along its medial border.
  - procedure: puncture using a flat palpation technique, inserting the needle with

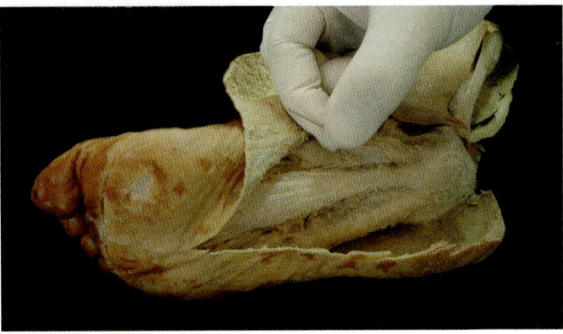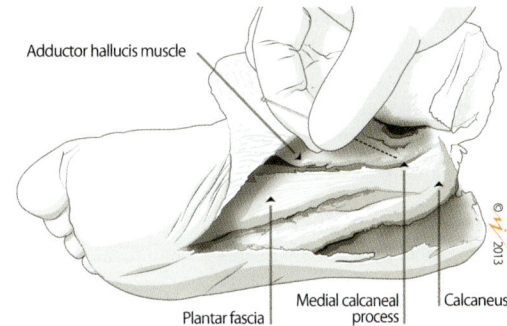

FIGURE 3.31 ■ Plantar fascia: lateral approach over enthesis.

a 45° orientation from medial to lateral and from dorsal to plantar, searching for the MTrP or motor point.

- Talocrural joint:
  - position: prone (posterolateral approach), supine, with the knee flexed to 90° and the foot supported on the stretcher (antero-medial and anterolateral approaches).
  - location: anterior capsule, anterolateral capsular recess – anterolateral ligament complex, posterior capsule.
  - procedure: posterolateral approach: next to the lateral border of the Achilles, in the triangular space between the Achilles tendon and the tendons of the fibularis muscles, the needle is inserted in an anterior and medial direction in search of the fibrotic tissue; anteromedial approach: 5 mm distal to the joint, just medial to the tendon of the tibialis anterior muscle, the needle is inserted perpendicular to the leg; anterolateral approach; 5 mm beneath the joint line, just lateral to the tendons of the extensor digitorum muscle, inserting the needle in a medial, posterior and cranial direction, searching for the fibrotic tissue.

3.7 Acknowledgements

Grateful thanks to Professor Jose R. Sañudo, and Dr. Teresa Vázquez and Dr. Eva Maranillo, for all they have taught me (Francisco J. Valderrama-Canales) and for what they represent to me both as professionals in their field and as friends.

To the many students over the last decade from the Department of Human Anatomy and Embryology, the Faculty of Medicine and the Faculty of Physical Therapy of the Complutense University of Madrid, who have inspired us with their enthusiasm and dedication in the study of human anatomy and the techniques of dissection.

This chapter is dedicated to Celia Moya, Manuel Ariza, Juan Nieto, Javi Rello, Paco Herranz, Antonio González, Ana Fogued and Lucho Leiva for their love, friendship, and support.

3.8 REFERENCES

1. Federative International Committee on Anatomical Terminology, Sociedad Anatómica Española. Terminología anatómica: terminología anatómica internacional. Madrid: Médica Panamericana; 2001.
2. Dauber W. Pocket atlas of human anatomy: founded by Heinz Feneis. Stuttgart: Thieme; 2011.
3. Federative Committee on Anatomical Terminology. Terminologia anatomica: international anatomical terminology. New York: Thieme; 1998.
4. Federative International Programme on Anatomical Terminologies. English tree view of Terminologia Anatomica, version 1998 [on-line], http://www.unifr.ch/ifaa/Public/EntryPage/ShowTA98EN.html [accessed 12 April 2015].
5. Whitmore I. Terminologia anatomica. International Anatomical Terminology; FIPAT, Federative International Programme on Anatomical Terminolgies. 2nd ed. Stuttgart New York: Thieme; 2011.
6. Rouviere H, Delmas A. Anatomía humana descriptiva, topográfica y funcional. 11th ed. Barcelona: Masson; 2005.
7. Testut L. Tratado de anatomía topográfica con aplicaciones medicoquirúrgicas. 8th ed. Barcelona: Salvat; 1972.
8. Bergman RA, Thompson SA, Afifi AK. Catalog of human variation. Munich: Urban & Schwarzenberg; 1984.
9. Paulsen F, Waschke J. Sobotta atlas of human anatomy. 15th ed. Amsterdam: Elsevier; 2013.
10. Standring S. Gray's anatomy. The anatomical basis of clinical practice. 40th ed. London: Elsevier.; 2008.
11. Gray H. Anatomy of the human body. 20th ed. Philadelphia: Lea & Febiger; 1918. New York: Bartleby; 2000. Available at: <http://www.bartleby.com/107/>; [accessed 9 Oct 2012].
12. Schünke M, Schulte E, Schumacher U, et al. Thieme Atlas of Anatomy. 6th ed. Stuttgart: Thieme; 2006.
13. McCutcheon L, Yelland M. Iatrogenic pneumothorax safety concerns when using acupuncture or dry needling in the thoracic region. Phys Ther Rev 2011;16(2):126–32.
14. Schratter M, Bijak M, Nissel H, et al. The foramen sternale: a minor anomaly – great relevance. Rofo 1997;166(1):69–71.

15. Peuker E, Cummings M. Anatomy for the acupuncturist – facts and fiction 2: The chest, abdomen, and back. Acupunct Med 2003;21(3):72–9.

16. Stark P. Midline sternal foramen: CT demonstration. J Comput Assist Tomogr 1985;9(3):489–90.

17. Epstein J, Arora A, Ellis H. Surface anatomy of the inferior epigastric artery in relation to laparoscopic injury. Clin Anat 2004;17:400–8.

18. Krief OP. MRI of the rotator interval capsule. Am J Roentgenol 2005;184:1490–4.

19. Gaskill TR, Braun S, Millett PJ. Multimedia article. The rotator interval: pathology and management. Arthroscopy 2011;27:556–67.

20. Morag Y, Bedi A, Jamadar DA. The rotator interval and long head biceps tendon: anatomy, function, pathology, and magnetic resonance imaging. Magn Reson Imaging Clin N Am 2012;20:229–59.

21. Gray DJ. Variations in human scapulae. Am J Phys Anthropol 1942;29(1):57–72.

22. Juss JK, Speed CA, Warrington J, et al. Acupuncture induced pneumothorax – a case report. Acupunct Med 2008;26(3):193–6.

23. Choi D, Rodríguez-Niedenführ M, Vázquez T, et al. Patterns of connections between the musculocutaneous and median nerves in the axilla and arm. Clin Anat 2002;15:11–17.

24. Rodríguez-Niedenführ M, Vázquez T, Choi D, et al. Supernumerary humeral heads of the biceps brachii muscle revisited. Clin Anat 2003;16:197–203.

25. Rodríguez-Niedenführ M, Vázquez T, Nearn L, et al. Variations of the arterial pattern in the upper limb revisited: a morphological and statistical study, with a review of the literature. J Anat 2001;199:547–66.

26. Platzer W. Color atlas of human anatomy, vol. 1. 6th ed. Stuttgart: Thieme; 2011.

27. Nayak SR, Ramanathan L, Krishnamurthy A, et al. Extensor carpi radialis brevis origin, nerve supply and its role in lateral epicondylitis. Surg Radiol Anat 2010;32:207–11.

28. Stecco C, Lancerotto L, Porzionato A, et al. The palmaris longus muscle and its relations with the antebrachial fascia and the palmar aponeurosis. Clin Anat 2009;22:221–9.

29. Rodríguez-Niedenführ M, Sañudo JR, Vázquez T, et al. Median artery revisited. J Anat 1999;195:57–63.

30. García-de-Lucas F, Valderrama-Canales FJ. Síndrome del Canal de Guyon. In: Neuropatías compresivas y de atrapamiento. Madrid: Momento Médico Iberoamericano; 2007. p. 121–34.

31. García-de-Lucas F, Valderrama-Canales FJ, Guillén-Vicente M. Tendinitis de la muñeca y de la mano. In: Ferrández Portal L director, editor. Actualizaciones SECOT 7. Barcelona: Elsevier-Masson; 2009. p. 49–61.

32. Robson AJ, See MS, Ellis H. Applied anatomy of the superficial branch of the radial nerve. Clin Anat 2008;21:38–45.

33. Alpert JM, Kozanek M, Li G, et al. Cross-sectional analysis of the iliopsoas tendon and its relationship to the acetabular labrum: an anatomic study. Am J Sports Med 2009;37:1594–8.

34. Pang J, Shen S, Pan WR, et al. The arterial supply of the patellar tendon: anatomical study with clinical implications for knee surgery. Clin Anat 2009;22:371–6.

35. Nyland J, Lachman N, Kocabey Y, et al. Anatomy, function, and rehabilitation of the popliteus musculotendinous complex. J Orthop Sports Phys Ther 2005;35:165–79.

36. Hopper MA, Robinson P. Ankle impingement syndromes. Radiol Clin North Am 2008;46:957–71.

37. Chen TM, Rozen WM, Pan WR, et al. The arterial anatomy of the Achilles tendon: anatomical study and clinical implications. Clin Anat 2009;22:377–85.

38. Vázquez MT, Maceira E, Valderrama-Canales FJ, et al. Anatomía quirúrgica del pie. Madrid: Acción Médica; 2004.

39. Narvani A, Mahmud T, Lavelle J, et al. Injury to the proximal deep medial collateral ligament: a problematical subgroup of injuries. J Bone Joint Surg Br 2010;92(7):949–53.

PART III

MUSCULOSKELETAL ULTRASOUND

CHAPTER 4

MUSCULOSKELETAL ULTRASOUND IN PHYSIOTHERAPY

Francisco Minaya Muñoz • Fermín Valera Garrido • Adrián Benito Domingo

Dare to be wise. Dare to think.
HORACE

KEYWORDS

International Classification of Functioning, Disability and Health (ICF); impairment; disability; musculoskeletal ultrasound; structure; function; ultrasound-guided intervention; activity limitation.

4.1 PHYSIOTHERAPY AND MUSCULOSKELETAL ULTRASOUND

Musculoskeletal ultrasound (MSK-US) is a technique in constant evolution and development. It is a tool that is growing in popularity and fast gaining importance in daily clinical practice, both in diagnosis (as an extension of the physical examination) as well as treatment. This technique is used by a range of health professionals, such as radiologists, gynaecologists, sports medicine specialists, emergency medicine physicians, rheumatologists, podiatrists, anaesthetists and physiotherapists, among others.

Depending on the information and objectives sought, the use of ultrasound varies between professionals. From the perspective of physiotherapy, ultrasound is a very useful tool with several advantages.[1] For example, it provides an objective, dynamic, fast, effective, comparative and innocuous study (due to the absence of radiation) of musculoskeletal tissue in real time, which makes it useful from teaching, clinical and research perspectives. However, there are debatable issues, such as the scope of practice and the specific role this new tool can play in clinical physiotherapy practice, as well as its limitations. In spite of this, the primary consideration should be to improve the quality of care provided to the patient in the current economic health situation.

Although MSK-US has been used by the medical collective since 1950, its application in physiotherapy began in the 1980s with the work of Dr Archie Young, a physicist at Oxford University who included physiotherapists within his research team.[2] In 1998 Wayne W Gibbon[3] stated:

> it would appear to be logical that either the ultrasound investigation should be performed by a radiologist with appropriate clinical ... or a clinician/physiotherapist with appropriate ultrasound training and experience ... musculoskeletal ultrasound systems currently being developed are being aimed at the rheumatology, orthopaedic, sports' medicine and, possibly, physiotherapy markets.

Although the use of MSK-US as a tool in physiotherapy dates back several years, its widespread adoption into clinical practice is only beginning to emerge.

The use of MSK-US in the rehabilitation of neuromusculoskeletal disorders has been called rehabilitative ultrasound imaging (RUSI) and was defined by Teyhen in 2006[4] as:

> a procedure used by physical therapists to evaluate muscle and related soft tissue morphology and function during exercise and physical tasks. RUSI is used to assist in the application of therapeutic interventions aimed at improving neuromuscular function. This includes providing feedback to the patient and physical therapist to improve clinical outcomes.

From 2008, physiotherapists have also used MSK-US during invasive techniques, such as percutaneous needle electrolysis techniques which are performed under ultrasound guidance.[5–7]

Thanks to their knowledge of clinical and topographic anatomy and clinical examination, physiotherapists have seized the opportunities available to request and interpret imaging. They have undertaken advanced university and private institutional training courses combined with tutoring in a clinical setting as part of their continuing professional development. In Australia and the UK, there are specific programmes, such as those organized by Sports Medicine Ultrasound Group (courses taught by the physiotherapists Chris Myers and Rob Laus) or by the Dynamic Ultrasound Group Association of Physiotherapists using Ultrasound imaging, promoted by scientific associations (Australian Physiotherapy Association and Chartered Society of Physiotherapy) for their members,

and developed at the universities of Queensland, Sydney and Southampton. In the USA, specialized training is offered in the form of postgraduate programmes offered by private entities. In Spain, the use of MSK-US in the physiotherapy collective is relatively new (since 2008 courses have been taught by the physiotherapists Jacinto Martínez-Payá and Ana de Groot-Ferrando). Currently, the Spanish Association of Physiotherapists, as well as several universities (such as the University of Alcalá de Henares and the CEU San Pablo University in Madrid) and private institutions (such as MVClinic®, Khronos Fisioterapia® or Fisiodocent®), offer different levels of training in MSK-US for physiotherapists. Furthermore, in 2013, the Spanish Society of Ultrasound (a member of the European Federation of Societies for Ultrasound in Medicine and Biology) has specifically expressed its support of the spread of ultrasound training to superior university graduates in all the biomedical sciences.[8] In other European countries, such as Portugal or Italy, physiotherapists are starting to train in MSK-US through private training programmes (for example, those organized by the Master Physical Therapy® company).

4.2 SCOPE OF PRACTICE: MUSCULOSKELETAL ULTRASOUND IN PHYSIOTHERAPY PROCESS

When considering the legal medical liability situation for diagnostic/therapeutic errors based on MSK-US performed by health professionals, the situation is slightly unclear as soon as one goes beyond the traditional radiology department. The scope of practice in physiotherapy is dynamic, evolving together with changes in the evidence base, as well as the policy and the patient's needs. The physiotherapy scope of practice varies from jurisdiction to jurisdiction, and depends on specific licensing guidelines and professional regulations. The World Confederation for Physical Therapy (WCPT) recognizes the diverse social, political and economic environments in which physiotherapy is practised throughout the world. On another front, the European region of the WCPT has adopted a series of European Core Standards of Physiotherapy Practice; however, specific national standards for physiotherapy practice still reflect the unique situation of each country.[9]

In a report from the College of Physical Therapists of British Columbia (Canada), a generic definition regarding the use of MSK-US by physiotherapists has been proposed that encompasses current clinical use. This includes 'applications that result in a physical diagnosis of the structure or movement characteristics of muscles and/or nerves in relation to adjacent structures'.[10]

According to the World Health Organization, physiotherapy is 'the art and science of treatment through therapeutic exercise, heat, cold, light, water, massage and electricity'. Furthermore:

> *physiotherapy includes the performance of electric and manual tests in order to determine the value of the affectation and muscle strength, tests to determine the functional capacities, the range of articular movement and measures of vital capacity, as well as diagnostic aids for the control of evolution.*[11]

The WCPT clearly verifies that the recovery of movement dysfunction and specifically dysfunction of the neuromusculoskeletal system is within the scope of the physiotherapy profession. It also confirms that a physiotherapist is qualified to establish a physiotherapy diagnosis, determine an individual's movement potential and plan and implement programmes, using specialized knowledge, skills and tools, for the prevention or treatment of movement dysfunction.[9] On the other hand, the International Society for Electrophysical Agents in Physical Therapy defines electrophysical agents (EPAs) as the use of electrophysical and biophysical energy for the purposes of evaluation, treatment and prevention of impairments, activity limitations and participation restrictions. Two important points are highlighted in this chapter:

- Evaluation procedures involving EPA include (but are not limited to) ultrasound imaging and electro-neurophysiological testing in order to assist with physiotherapy diagnosis, guide treatment procedures and evaluate treatment outcomes.
- Treatment procedures involving EPA include (but are not limited to) the use of electromagnetic, acoustic and mechanical energies to produce biophysical effects at cellular, tissue, organic and whole-body levels in order to achieve physiological and clinical effects which serve to maintain and optimize health.[12]

In this context, MSK-US is inherent to the process of care in physiotherapy and facilitates the decision making of physiotherapists within their own autonomous practice, for the purposes of assessment, diagnosis, prognosis/planning, intervention and re-examination[9,13–16] (table 4.1).

TABLE 4.1	The use of musculoskeletal ultrasound imaging during physiotherapy procedures gives professionals the opportunity to do the following
Assessment	• Visualize the structure and function of the muscle, tendon, ligament and nerve via static and dynamic tests • Obtain objective soft-tissue measurements
Diagnosis	• Assess and implement the best training and physiotherapy techniques for each individual • Determine the prognosis
Planning	• Establish treatment aims • Provide information on the characteristics of the tissue (i.e. inflammatory or degenerative conditions) • Determine the number of sessions or the type of treatment to be carried out
Intervention	• Give direct, real-time visual feedback to patients during active tasks • Educate patients on their specific muscle dysfunction • Have a tool for guidance during minimally invasive procedures
Reassessment	• Monitor progress in rehabilitation to ensure that any changes to treatment are made at the optimum times • Reconfigure the physiotherapy approach

4.2.1 Assessment

In the examination of individuals with actual or potential impairments, activity limitations, participation restrictions or abilities/disabilities, MSK-US offers the physiotherapist a variety of options. It enables direct visualization of the structure and function of the muscle, tendon, ligament and nerve via static and dynamic tests (real-time images). The static morphological measurements include assessment of the size, shape and structure of the tissue under study (video 4.1) in both healthy and pathological tissues.[17–19] In contrast, the dynamic measures are techniques in real time that offer knowledge regarding changes in muscle length. For example: (1) the sliding capacity of the subscapularis muscle in a patient with limited internal rotation of the glenohumeral joint (video 4.2); (2) muscle activity, for example, activity of the supraspinatus muscle in a patient with difficulty stabilizing the glenohumeral joint, or the extensor carpi radialis brevis muscle in a patient with pain on the lateral epicondyle (video 4.3); and (3) the tendon function, for example distal attachment of the biceps brachii muscle on radial tuberosity (video 4.4).

Another application of MSK-US in physiotherapy is assessment of the morphology and function of the muscle and the remaining soft tissues related to the muscle during exercise and different functional tasks, for example, dynamic assessment of the function of the pelvic floor muscles, both from a transperineal as well as a transabdominal perspective. This provides information regarding the stabilizing function of these muscles, measuring their action of elevation of the neck and base of the bowel via different manoeuvres.[19–23] This also incorporates assessment of the activity of the muscles of the abdominal wall, external oblique, internal oblique, transversus abdominis[22–25] and lumbar multifidus muscles in patients with low-back pain.[26–28]

Moreover, it is possible to carry out ultrasound-guided palpation to correlate with clinical findings, for example, palpation of the Achilles tendon in areas of pain and point tenderness while the tendon is visualized with ultrasound (video 4.5).

As with any form of diagnostic imaging, the idea is not to supersede the physical exam, but to enhance the quality of the physiotherapy diagnosis process in general.

4.2.2 Physiotherapy diagnosis

In physiotherapy, diagnosis[15,16,29] is the result of a process of clinical reasoning that results in identification of existing or potential impairments, activity limitations, participation restrictions, environmental influences or abilities/disabilities of the individual and the analysis of function. This differs from the medical diagnosis, based on the organic and anatomopathological analysis of the illness, the lesion or the trauma. These are, therefore, complementary elements arising from different bodies of knowledge that make it possible to determine the prognosis and improvements together with the most appropriate treatment strategies, depending on the professional (figure 4.1). The purpose of the diagnosis is to guide physiotherapists in determining the prognosis and the most appropriate intervention strategies and to inform patients.[29] Nowadays, it is well known that the medical diagnosis of altered tissue morphology based on the interpretation of imaging studies is

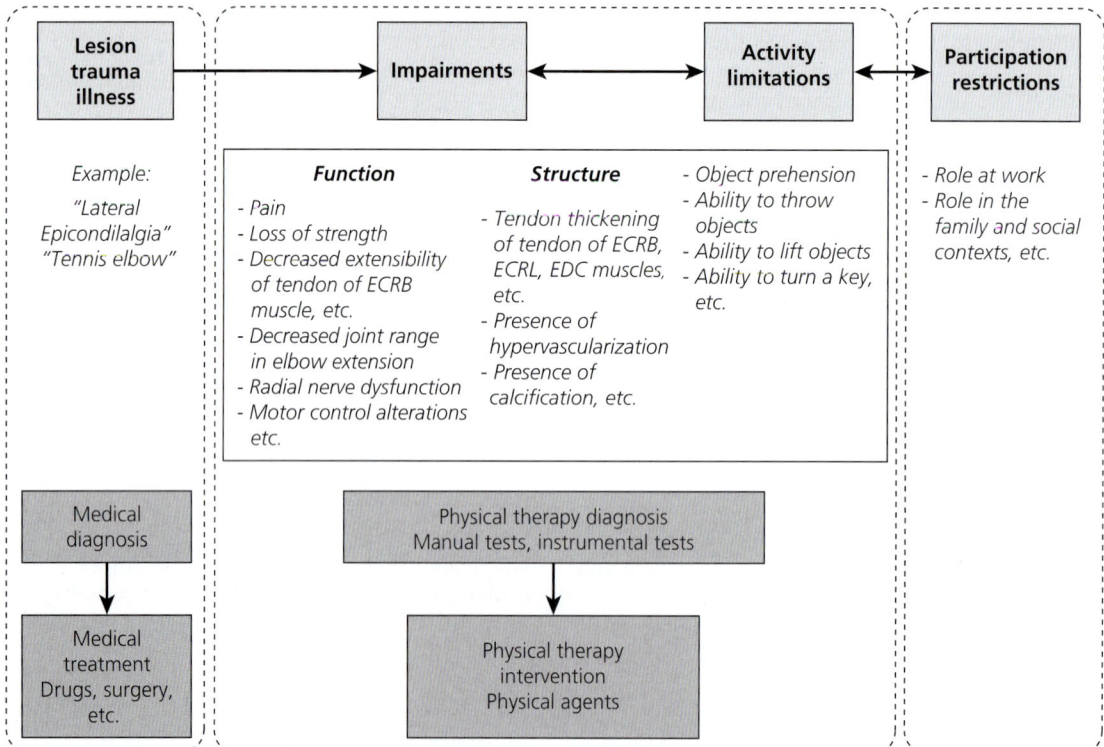

FIGURE 4.1 ■ Conceptual framework – physiotherapy. ECRB, extensor carpi radialis brevis; ECRL, extensor carpi radialis longus; EDC, extensor digitorum communis. (Adapted from the ICF 2001 by Minaya & Valera 2010[30]).

outside the scope of practice available to physiotherapists.

Traditionally, during the process of physiotherapy diagnosis, the physiotherapist has included, within the physical exam, manual and instrumental tests that have enabled the assessment of structure and function of the individual (for example, the Lachmann test provides information regarding stability of the knee). Currently, this information can be complemented with instrumental tests, such as MSK-US or electromyography. So, in the same way that a goniometer is employed differently by different healthcare professionals during their daily clinical practice and, depending on the information sought, their level of training and knowledge, MSK-US is simply an important tool for physiotherapy diagnosis and should be viewed as such.

The Chartered Society of Physiotherapy has developed a series of evidence-based clinical guidelines that highlight the importance of ultrasound in helping to establish a diagnosis for shoulder impingement. MSK-US is a relevant tool in physiotherapy diagnosis owing to its safety, convenience and comparatively low cost in comparison to radiography and magnetic resonance imaging (MRI).[31]

KEY POINTS

The physiotherapist must use all the tools available (manual and instrumental) in order to reach a precise physiotherapy diagnosis that enables improvement of the quality of care and results achieved.

KEY POINTS

Physiotherapy diagnosis is aimed at the analysis of function. Today, the physiotherapy diagnosis is a reality that is necessary for advancement of the profession, recognized by the WCPT, and legally acknowledged by existing legislation.

4.2.3 Treatment planning

Treatment planning, within the process of physiotherapy care, refers to the establishment of aims, including measurable outcome goals negotiated in collaboration with the patient/client, family or caregiver.[29] In this sense MSK-US can help the decision-making process by providing information regarding the characteristics of the tissue (i.e. inflammatory or degenerative conditions) and determining the number of weekly

sessions or the type of treatment to be performed, or, if a red flag is detected, by referring the patient to another healthcare professional. Along these lines, a collaborative study between emergency medicine physicians and physiotherapists indicated that MSK-US may also be valuable in small sports medicine clinics and on match days, when other imaging techniques are not available. In these settings ultrasound has been found to be useful for helping to rule out fractures following ankle or foot sprains.[32]

4.2.4 Intervention

The ultrasound image provides feedback for the patient while working with different active strategies, such as those used to improve motor control of the abdominal muscles and recruitment of the trunk muscles in musculoskeletal dysfunctions where these muscles are involved, for example, patients suffering from chronic lumbopelvic pain.[33,34]

Other applications of MSK-US in physiotherapy, recently developed in the fields of manual therapy and sports physiotherapy, include its use as a guiding tool in minimally invasive procedures, such as the percutaneous needle electrolysis (PNE) techniques for the treatment of tendinopathies (figure 4.2)[5-7] (see chapter 13) or dry needling in myofascial pain syndrome[35] (see chapter 8). In the same way that anaesthetists[36] use MSK-US to guide their interventions and thus achieve safer and more effective anaesthesia, physiotherapists use ultrasound within their scope of competencies in order to treat musculoskeletal tissue (e.g. muscle, tendon,

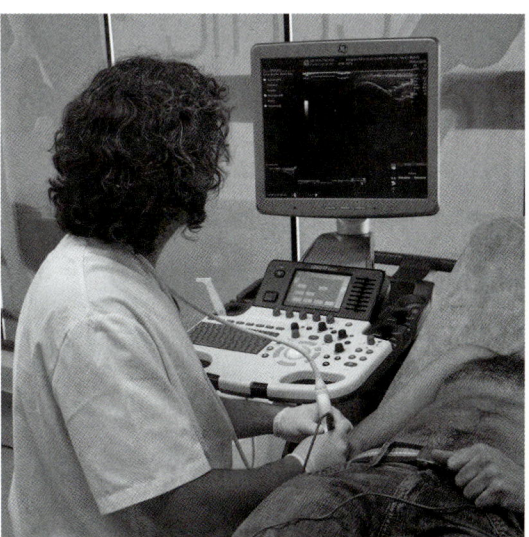

FIGURE 4.2 ■ Application of the ultrasound-guided PNE technique over the epicondyle musculature. (Colour version of figure is available online).

ligament) in a precise, effective and safe manner. This thus improves the results and the cost–benefit relation of the interventions.[6]

It is essential to correlate the information achieved via ultrasound with the clinical findings found in the analysis of function (e.g. pain, alteration of movement pattern, motor control) as, on occasion, the assessment of structure reveals changes that are not clinically relevant. Ultrasound, in a similar manner to other complementary treatments, such as simple radiology (for example, in cervical rectification)[37] or nuclear magnetic resonance (for example, in spinal disc hernias),[38,39] can determine changes in the tissue that are not associated with symptoms.

KEY POINTS

Structural analysis is a necessary practice; however, the information acquired is insufficient on its own to determine the therapeutic procedure.

4.2.5 Reassessment

MSK-US enables the physiotherapist to reassess possible changes in structure and correlate them with improvement in the clinical condition of the patient in the short, medium and long term in an innocuous and rapid manner. This is helpful in order to reconfigure the treatment approach if the desired objectives (aims) are not met, and lead to the patient's discharge if the tissue characteristics have improved as well as quantify the effectiveness of the physiotherapy treatment according to the results obtained.[7,40,41]

4.3 EVIDENCE-BASED PHYSIOTHERAPY MODEL

In recent years, the development of physiotherapy has been primarily motivated by three circumstances:
1. The patient care model, which requires increasing the physiotherapist's responsibility for decision making as a necessary element to improve results.[16]
2. The independent and responsible decision-making process (autonomy), currently considered as one of the characteristics of the profession.[42]
3. The development of the physiotherapy model based on evidence.[43,44]

In the current environment of evidence-based physiotherapy, MSK-US can be a very useful tool. According to this model, it is imperative that physiotherapists be allowed access to the tools that can optimize the effectiveness of their interventions, thus allowing implementation of new knowledge. Likewise, it is important for the professional to stay up to date with any new technological discoveries and the use of new tools that can offer patients more effective and safer care.[6]

In physiotherapy clinical practice (and in medicine) the professional, based on initial information obtained from the patient, generates multiple hypotheses, which are either confirmed or rejected based on the new data found in the assessment and patient diagnosis. The aim of this hypothetical-deductive model[45,46] is to validate the information obtained from the patient via the assessment that must fulfil a dual requirement: be reliable and valid. In contrast to manual clinical tests where the procedure is clearly established, ultrasound tests are in the process of being standardized. As a result, the European Society of Musculoskeletal Radiology has established technical guidelines that are applicable to assessments (*Musculoskeletal Ultrasound Technical Guidelines*).[47]

4.4 ADVANTAGES

The use of MSK-US as a new tool to be applied in the clinical practice of physiotherapy provides many important advantages.

The first to benefit from MSK-US is the user/patient/client, as the person is offered a physiotherapy programme that is more rational as regards the decision-making process. Also, MSK-US enables safer therapeutic strategies, a greater precision in determined techniques (for example, the use of percutaneous needle electrolysis (PNE) for the treatment of tendinopathies) (figure 4.3) and, thus, improvement in effectiveness.

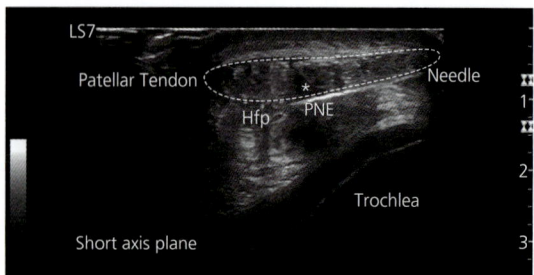

FIGURE 4.3 ■ Visualization of the application technique of ultrasound-guided PNE at the interface between the patellar tendon and Hoffa's fat pad (Hfp) in chronic patellar tendinopathy (*).

Secondly, physiotherapists now have a new, very powerful tool with which to complete the information gathered personally by them, and which can help provide objective information on the changes as well as increase the credibility of the service provided.

Thirdly, the profession itself is benefited – an important aspect worth considering in research studies. The demand and interest in applying evidence and in developing new techniques for physiotherapist practice are constantly growing.

4.5 DIFFICULTIES IN IMPLEMENTATION

There are several circumstances that negatively impact the implementation of MSK-US in physiotherapy:

- Training courses: until recently, physiotherapists have not had access to formal training in MSK-US. At present there are private companies (see section 4.1) that organize training courses for physiotherapists in various countries. There are also universities that have included in their physiotherapy degree course theoretical-practical contents of MSK-US within subjects such as 'Assessment and Diagnosis in Physiotherapy'. This is designed so that future physiotherapists may at least appreciate the possibilities that this tool has to offer. Currently, however, more training programmes in MSK-US, aimed specifically at physiotherapists, are necessary.
- Cost: the current high cost of MSK-US machines makes it necessary for ultrasound imaging in physiotherapy to have a substantial value. This is to improve the decision-making process, the results and cost-effectiveness of the interventions on behalf of the physiotherapist, so that these can be implemented in clinical practice. Otherwise, it will be a tool that can only be found in centres of learning and universities (linked with research and teaching), as well as hospitals and leading clinics. At present, only several commercial brands (General Electric and Sonosite, among others) have increased their activities in the musculoskeletal sector in recognition of the great potential of MSK-US. And, furthermore, they plan specific campaigns targeted towards physiotherapists.
- Capacity of producing three-dimensional (3D) images: together with training in

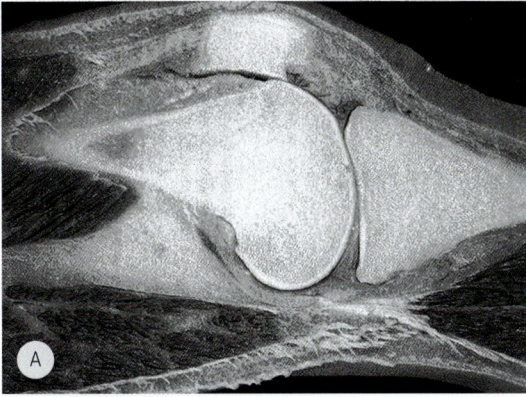

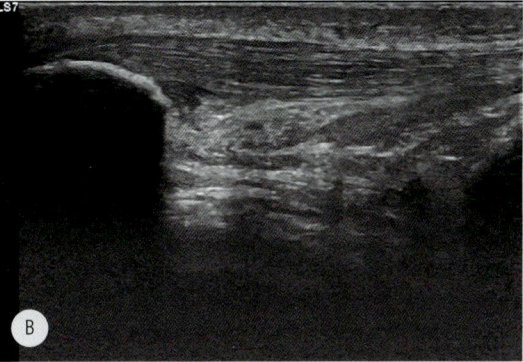

FIGURE 4.4 ■ (A) Longitudinal section of the patellar tendon (cadaver) and (B) its correspondence with the ultrasound image in a live subject. (Colour version of figure is available online).

MSK-US, the professional must be able to 'see the image' in two dimensions, interpret it and mentally transform it into a 3D structure for it to be useful from a clinical point of view (figure 4.4). The technological advances in 3D ultrasound imaging applied to gynaecology will not take long to reach the musculoskeletal field, facilitating visualization of the morphology.

- 'Medical tool': there is some resistance (although this has gradually lessened) from the medical collective to letting physiotherapists have access to and manage MSK-US, mainly because the tool is considered to be diagnostic from a medical point of view. The aims are different, as described at the beginning of this chapter, depending on the type of professional concerned. However, it is necessary to establish practical guides for appropriate and safe use that respects the competencies of the different professionals who use ultrasound. Possibly, in the future, it may be necessary for health boards to define the use of MSK-US for the different professionals involved in the physiotherapy care of the user/patient/client.

4.6 NOVEL APPLICATIONS IN MUSCULOSKELETAL ULTRASOUND

Possibly, it will be a long wait before MSK-US gains recognition as a reference in the clinical physiotherapy practice. This is similar to ultrasound machines being considered a commonplace tool, as an extension of physical exploration and similarly to a goniometer. There is no doubt that MSK-US continues to be developed and there are increasingly more applications for physiotherapy, such as measurement of the joint position,[48,49] measurement of tissue elasticity (sonoelastography)[50–56] (see chapters 6, 13 and 14) or studies in 3D and 4D. All this, together with the development of high-frequency transducers with great resolution and the portability of the machines, makes MSK-US a tool with a great potential and which offers physiotherapists an opportunity to increase the exactness of the physiotherapy diagnosis and interventions.

4.7 CLINICAL CASE

4.7.1 Clinical correlation (figure 4.5)

A 42-year-old male, a policeman, right-handed, comes to the physiotherapy clinic with a medical diagnosis of re-rupture of the left rotator cuff. He had previously undergone surgery 2 years before via arthroscopy with suture of the supraspinatus and subacromial decompression, with a good functional result and no after effects.

At present he suffers from pain in the anterior shoulder which began 5 months previously, and in the absence of any traumatic circumstance. The pain is mechanical, dull and deep, with slight loss of mobility at the end of the range of abduction and both internal and external rotation, with a good motor pattern and without loss of strength. He has undergone conventional

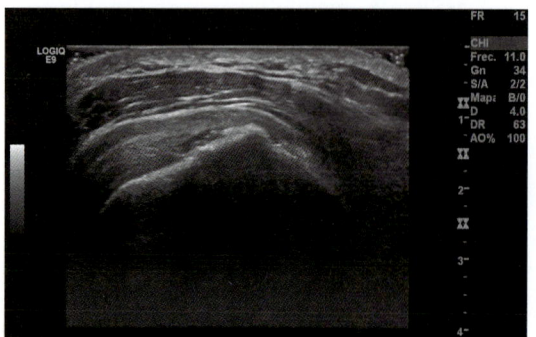

FIGURE 4.5 ■ Longitudinal section of the supraspinatus tendon.

physiotherapy treatment (manual therapy, ultrasound, laser, exercises), with poor results. Due to the results from the MRI ('rupture of the supraspinatus tendon and associated degenerative changes') and failure of more conservative treatment, the orthopaedist proposes a new surgical intervention to repair the rotator cuff and review the acromioplasty via open surgery.

The MSK-US image obtained for the analysis of the structure showed degenerative changes and a loss of continuity in the tissue compatible with the medical diagnosis.

(Clinical case continued on page 489)

4.8 REFERENCES

1. Özçakar L, Tok F, De Muynck M, et al. Musculoskeletal ultrasonography in physical and rehabilitation medicine. J Rehabil Med 2012;44:310–18.
2. Stokes M, Young A. Measurement of quadriceps cross-sectional area by ultrasonography: a description of the technique and its applications in physiotherapy. Physiother Pract 1986;2:31–6.
3. Gibbon WW. Diagnostic ultrasound in sports medicine. Br J Sports Med 1998;32(1):3.
4. Teyhen D. Rehabilitative ultrasound imaging symposium San Antonio, TX. J Orthop Sports Phys Ther 2006;36:A1–3.
5. Valera-Garrido F, Minaya-Muñoz F, Sánchez-Ibáñez JM. Efectividad de la Electrólisis Percutánea Intratisular (EPI®) en las tendinopatías crónicas del tendón rotuliano. Trauma Fund MAPFRE 2010;21:227–36.
6. Minaya-Muñoz F, Valera-Garrido F, Sánchez-Ibáñez JM, et al. Estudio de coste-efectividad de la Electrólisis Percutánea Intratisular (EPI®) en las epicondilalgias. Fisioterapia 2012;34:208–15.
7. Valera-Garrido F, Minaya-Muñoz F, Medina-Mirapeix F. Ultrasound-guided percutaneous needle electrolysis in chronic lateral epicondylitis: short-term and long-term results. Acupunct Med 2014;32(6):446–54. Available at: <http://aim.bmj.com/content/early/2014/08/13/acupmed-2014-010619.full?rss=1>; [Accessed 12 April 2015].
8. Spanish Society of Ultrasound. Statements. Available at: <http://www.seeco.es/index.php/sociedad-espanola-de-ecografia/estatutos>; 2013 [accessed 22 Jan 2014].
9. World Confederation for Physical Therapy. WCPT guideline for the development of a system of legislation/regulation/recognition of physical therapists. London, UK: WCPT; 2011. Available at: <http://www.wcpt.org/guidelines/regulation-legislation>; [accessed 22 Sep 2011].
10. Whittaker JL. Recommendations for the Implementation of Real Time Ultrasound Imaging in Physical Therapy Practice: The Final Report of a College of Physical Therapists of British Columbia, Canada Real Time Ultrasound Imaging Ad Hoc Committee. Vancouver, BC: CPTBC; 2004.
11. World Health Organization. Preamble to the Constitution of the World Health Organization as adopted by the International Health Conference, New York, 19-22 June, 1946; signed on 22 July 1946 by the representatives of 61 States (Official Records of the World Health Organization, no. 2, p. 100) and entered into force on 7 April 1948. Geneva, Switzerland: WHO; 1948.

12. World Confederation for Physical Therapy. International Society for Electrophysical Agents in Physical Therapy (ISEAPT). London, UK: WCPT; 2011. Available at: <http://www.wcpt.org/iseapt>; [accessed 23 Jan 2014].

13. World Confederation for Physical Therapy. Policy Statement: Regulation of the physical therapy profession. London, UK: WCPT; 2011. Available at: <http://www.wcpt.org/policy/ps-regulation>; [accessed 22 Sep 2011].

14. World Confederation for Physical Therapy. Ethical principles. London, UK: WCPT; 2011. Available at: <http://www.wcpt.org/ethical-principles>; [accessed 22 Sep 2011].

15. World Confederation for Physical Therapy. Policy statement: Ethical responsibilities of physical therapists and WCPT members. London, UK: WCPT; 2011. Available at: <http://www.wcpt.org/policy/ps-ethical responsibilities>; [accessed 22 Sep 2011].

16. World Confederation for Physical Therapy. Policy Statement: Direct access and patient/client self-referral to physical therapy. London, UK: WCPT; 2011. Available at: <http://www.wcpt.org/policy/ps-direct-access>; [accessed 22 Sep 2011].

17. Ohberg L, Lorentzon R, Alfredson H. Neovascularisation in Achilles tendons with painful tendinosis but not in normal tendons: an ultrasonographic investigation. Knee Surg Sports Traumatol Arthrosc 2001;9:233–8.

18. Peers KH, Lysens RJ. Patellar tendinopathy in athletes: current diagnostic and therapeutic recommendations. Sports Med 2005;35:71–87.

19. Thompson JA, O'Sullivan PB, Briffa NK, et al. Assessment of voluntary pelvic floor muscle contraction in continent and incontinent women using transperineal ultrasound, manual muscle testing and vaginal squeeze pressure measurements. Int Urogynecol J Pelvic Floor Dysfunct 2006;17:624–30.

20. Thompson JA, O'Sullivan PB, Briffa NK, et al. Altered muscle activation patterns in symptomatic women during pelvic floor muscle contraction and Valsalva manoeuvre. Neurourol Urodyn 2006;25:268–76.

21. Thompson JA, O'Sullivan PB, Briffa NK, et al. Differences in muscle activation patterns during pelvic floor muscle contraction and Valsalva maneuver. Neurourol Urodyn 2006;25:148–55.

22. Hides J, Wilson S, Stanton W, et al. An MRI investigation into the function of the transversus abdominis muscle during 'drawing-in' of the abdominal wall. Spine 2006;31:E175–8.

23. Ainscough-Potts AM, Morrissey MC, Critchley D. The response of the transverse abdominis and internal oblique muscles to different postures. Man Ther 2006; 11:54–60.

24. Richardson CA, Hodges P, Hides JA. Therapeutic Exercise for Spinal Segmental Stabilization in Low Back Pain: Scientific Basis and Clinical Approach. 2nd ed. Edinburgh, UK: Churchill Livingstone; 2004.

25. Teyhen DS, Childs JD, Stokes MJ, et al. Abdominal and lumbar multifidus muscle size and symmetry at rest and during contracted States. Normative reference ranges. J Ultrasound Med 2012;31(7):1099–110.

26. Stokes M, Rankin G, Newham DJ. Ultrasound imaging of lumbar multifidus muscle: normal reference ranges for measurements and practical guidance on the technique. Man Ther 2005;10:116–26.

27. Hodges PW, Pengel LH, Herbert RD, et al. Measurement of muscle contraction with ultrasound imaging. Muscle Nerve 2003;27:682–92.

28. Liu IS, Chai HM, Yang JL, et al. Inter-session reliability of the measurement of the deep and superficial layer of lumbar multifidus in young asymptomatic people and patients with low back pain using ultrasonography. Man Ther 2013;18(6):481–6.

29. World Confederation for Physical Therapy (WCPT). Position Statement. First approved at the 14th General Meeting of WCPT, May 1999. Revised and re-approved at the 16th General Meeting of WCPT, June 2007.

30. Valera-Garrido F, Minaya-Muñoz F, Medina-Mirapeix F, et al. Ecografía musculoesquelética: ¿es una herramienta válida en el razonamiento clínico en fisioterapia? Efisioterapia 2011, [serial on the internet] Available at: <http://www.efisioterapia.net/articulos/ecografia-musculoesqueletica-es-una-herramienta-valida-el-razonamiento-clinico-fisioterapi>; [accessed 12 April 2015].

31. Hanchard NC, Cummins J, Jeffries C. Evidence-based clinical guidelines for the diagnosis, assessment and physiotherapy management of shoulder impingement syndrome. London, UK: Chartered Society of Physiotherapy; 2004.

32. Canagasabey MD, Callaghan MJ, Carley S. The Sonographic Ottawa Foot and Ankle Rules study (the SOFAR study). Emerg Med J 2010;28:838–40.

33. Teyhen DS, Gill NW, Whittaker JL, et al. Rehabilitative ultrasound imaging of the abdominal muscles. J Orthop Sports PhysTher 2007;37:450–66.

34. Henry SM, Teyhen DS. Ultrasound imaging as a feedback tool in the rehabilitation of trunk muscle dysfunction for people with low back pain. J Orthop Sports Phys Ther 2007;37:627–34.

35. Bubnov RV. The use of trigger point 'dry' needling under ultrasound guidance for the treatment of myofascial pain (technological innovation and literature review). LikSprava 2010;5-6:56–64.

36. Hocking G, Mitchell CH. Optimizing the safety and practice of ultrasound-guided regional anesthesia: the role of echogenic technology. Curr Opin Anaesthesiol 2012;25:603–9.

37. Matsumoto M, Fujimura Y, Suzuki N, et al. Cervical curvatura in acute whiplash injuries: prospective comparative study with asymptomatic subject. Injury 1998; 29:775–8.

38. Quiroz-Moreno R, Lezama-Suárez G, Gómez-Jiménez C. Disc alterations of lumbar spine on magnetic resonance images in asymptomatic workers. Rev Med Inst Mex Seguro Soc 2008;46:185–90.

39. Jensen MC, Brant-Zawadzki MN, Obuchowski N, et al. Magnetic resonance imaging of the lumbar spine in people without back pain. N Engl J Med 1994;331: 69–73.

40. Minaya-Muñoz F, Valera-Garrido F, Sánchez-Ibáñez JM, et al. Short- and long-term outcomes of electrolysis percutanous intratisular in lateral epicondylitis. IN: 2nd International Scientific Tendinopathy Symposium, September 27-29, 2012.

41. Sánchez-Ibáñez JM, Alves R, Polidori F, et al. Effectiveness of ultrasound guided percutaneous electrolysis intratendon (EPI®) in the treatment of insertional patellar tendinopathy in soccer player. En: 2nd International Scientific Tendinopathy Symposium, September 27-29, 2012.

42. World Confederation for Physical Therapy. Policy statement: Autonomy. London, UK: WCPT; 2011. Available at: <http://www.wcpt.org/policy/ps-autonomy>; [accessed 22 Sep 2011].

43. Valera-Garrido F, Medina-i-Mirapeix F, Montilla-Herrador J, et al. Fisioterapia basada en la evidencia: un reto para acercar la evidencia científica a la práctica clínica. Fisioterapia 2000;22:158–64.

44. Research Committee (Victorian Branch) of the Australian Physiotherapy Association and Invited Contributors. Evidence-based practice. Aust J Physiother 1999;45: 167–71.

45. Edwards I, Jones M, Carr J, et al. Clinical reasoning strategies in physical therapy. PhysTher 2004;84: 312–30.
46. Rothstein JM, Echternach JL. Hypothesis-oriented algorithm for clinicians: a method for evaluation and treatment planning. Phys Ther 1986;66:1388–94.
47. ESSR Ultrasound Group Protocols. Musculoskeletal Ultrasound Technical Guidelines: Knee. Available at: <http://www.essr.org/html>; [accessed 26 Jul 2010].
48. Kalra N, Seitz AL, Boardman ND, et al. Effect of posture on acromiohumeral distance with arm elevation in subjects with and without rotator cuff disease using ultrasonography. J Orthop Sports PhysTher 2010;40: 633–40.
49. Hing W. The assessment of Mulligan's Shoulder Mobilisation with Movement's by diagnostic ultrasound. 9th Scientific Conference of IFOMT, Rotterdam, Holland; 2008.
50. Langevin HM, Rizzo DM, Fox JR, et al. Dynamic morphometric characterization of local connective tissue network structure in humans using ultrasound. BMC Syst Biol 2007;1:25.
51. Bamber J, Cosgrove D, Dietrich CF, et al. EFSUMB guidelines and recommendations on the clinical use of ultrasound elastography. Part 1: Basic principles and technology. Ultraschall Med 2013;34(2):169–84.
52. Cosgrove D, Piscaglia F, Bamber J, et al. EFSUMB guidelines and recommendations on the clinical use of ultrasound elastography. Part 2: Clinical applications. Ultraschall Med 2013;34(3):238–53.
53. Dewall RJ. Ultrasound elastography: principles, techniques, and clinical applications. Crit Rev Biomed Eng 2013;41(1):1–19.
54. Valera F, Minaya F, Benito A. Cambios estructurales cuantificados con elastografía tras la aplicación de un programa multimodal (EPI® + excéntricos) en las epicondilitis crónicas. En: XIII Congreso Nacional SETLA. Libro de comunicaciones y ponencias. Madrid; 2013.
55. Dewall RJ, Jiang J, Wilson JJ, et al. Visualizing tendon elasticity in an ex vivo partial tear model. Ultrasound Med Biol 2014;40(1):158–67.
56. Chernak Slane L, Thelen DG. The use of 2D ultrasound elastography for measuring tendon motion and strain. J Biomech 2014;47(3):750–4.

CHAPTER 5

SONOANATOMY OF THE MUSCULOSKELETAL SYSTEM

Jacinto J. Martínez Payá • Ana de Groot Ferrando • José Ríos Díaz • Mª Elena del Baño Aledo

First, let me dispose of Socrates because I am sick and tired of this pretense that knowing you know nothing is a mark of wisdom.

ISAAC ASIMOV

KEYWORDS

musculoskeletal ultrasound; Doppler effect; evolution of injury; physical therapy evaluation; therapeutic valuation.

5.1 INTRODUCTION

The thorough knowledge of human anatomy is a decisive factor ensuring correct physiotherapy professional practice. Traditionally, physiotherapists have used their hands as the 'active' element within the care process, together with other tools and instruments. Ultrasound is currently presented as a new tool that offers the possibility of performing assessments and therapeutic validation, as well as being helpful for the purpose of preventing possible complications and the avoidance of unnecessary and inadequate physiotherapy treatments.

Therefore, the aim of this chapter is to describe the ultrasound assessments that are most useful in physiotherapy by correlating human anatomy with the ultrasound image and analysing the artefacts that can distort the image, offering clues to their interpretation.

KEY POINTS

At present, ultrasound has become yet another working tool for the physiotherapist, and an essential element of correct professional practice.

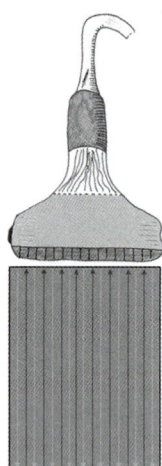

FIGURE 5.1 ■ The ultrasound transducer can both emit ultrasound pulses as well as pick up those that return back to the skin's surface after reflecting in the tissues, which occurs according to the tissue's acoustic impedance. (Colour version of figure is available online).

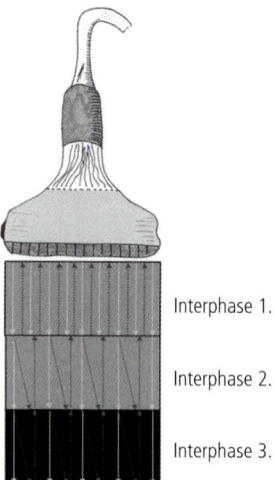

Interphase 1.

Interphase 2.

Interphase 3.

FIGURE 5.2 ■ When an ultrasound beam is projected through a medium it suffers three main types of attenuation. Above, the ultrasound beam is depicted going through three interphases. In the first interphase, some of the pulses are reflected back towards the transducer. In the second interphase, reflection is represented together with refraction, which causes some ultrasound pulses to undergo a change in direction as they change their velocity of transmission. Finally, in the third interphase, reflection, refraction and absorption (shown in black) are represented, as part of the ultrasound beam is transformed into thermal energy. (Colour version of figure is available online).

5.2 ULTRASOUND IN B MODE: ULTRASOUND IS MADE EASIER WITH THE HELP OF PHYSICS AND ANATOMY

The ultrasound transducer has the capacity of emitting and receiving ultrasound beams (thanks to the piezoelectric effect) (figure 5.1). According to the amount of resistance (acoustic impedance) the tissues offer towards the ultrasound beam, the form of the internal structures and the exploratory technique used, these ultrasound beams undergo three types of attenuation concurrently. These are reflection and refraction, which are the two main types (present in all ultrasonographic images), together with another secondary type, absorption (conversion of mechanical energy to heat) and almost unappreciable in diagnostic ultrasound (figure 5.2), in contrast to what occurs in therapeutic ultrasound.[1,2]

The prefix echo- is derived from the effect of the reflection of the ultrasound beam back to the transducer when passing through the tissues and, as such, this leads to an essential attenuation for the obtainment of an ultrasonographic image. It is therefore important to guarantee the greatest reflection possible, as this will enable the best resolution to be obtained. The amount of reflection depends on the angle of tilt of the ultrasound beam. Therefore, when examining the musculoskeletal system, the transducer is placed perpendicular to the direction of the fibres of the structure under study (figure 5.3).

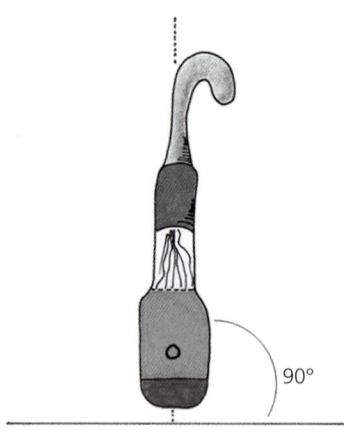

90°

FIGURE 5.3 ■ Lateral view of the transducer highlighting the perpendicularity necessary to perform an ultrasound exploration. (Colour version of figure is available online).

On the other hand, the quantity of reflection is also proportional to the frequency used and the difference in density of the structures under study. This is the reason why, when studying tissues that are both very dense and very superficial (such as the tibia, which entails working with a high frequency), special images appear

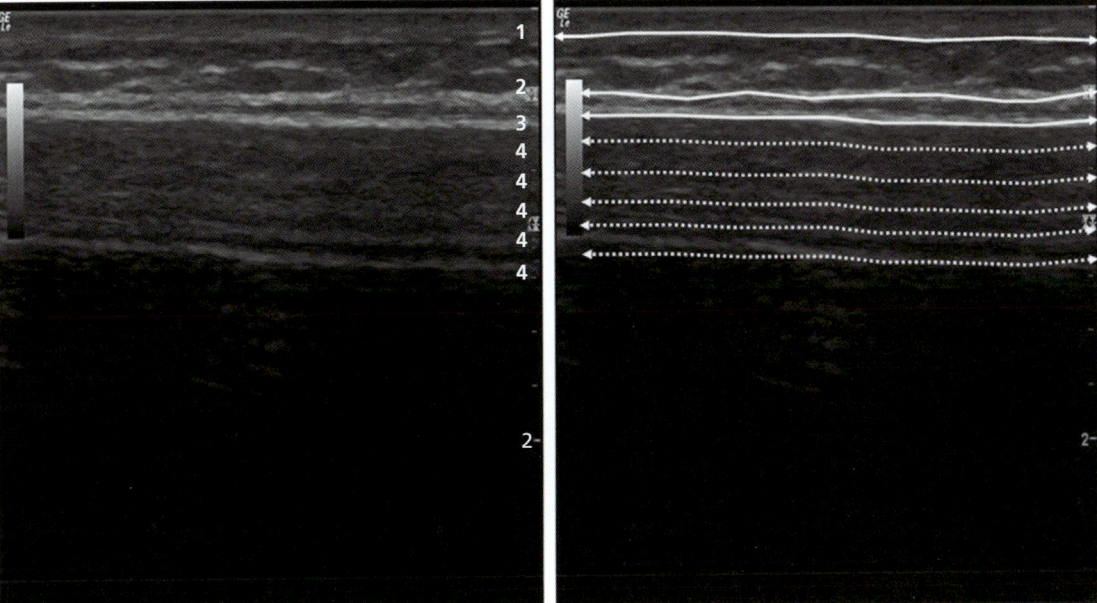

FIGURE 5.4 ■ Longitudinal section of the internal aspect of the tibia. Line 1 indicates the interphase between the skin and the subcutaneous cellular tissue, whereas line 2 signals the interphase between the subcutaneous cellular tissue and the periosteal connective tissue. Line 3 demonstrates the hyperreflective tibial cortex. This hyperechoic structure is repeatedly reflected subjacent to the other structures (line 4).

due to hyperreflection, such as, for example, an image in the mirror (figure 5.4).[3]

Refraction takes place when ultrasound beams change their speed when going through a tissue interphase and therefore alter their wavelength. This causes a change in direction of the ultrasound. This phenomenon is common in transverse explorations of structures with an oval-rounded form, such as the Achilles tendon or the blood vessels, and is also typical for some fibrous strands, such as those of the deltoid muscle. This attenuation is responsible for an artefact called refractile shadowing (figure 5.5), which should not be confused with an acoustic shadow (figure 5.6), related to bone tissue.[4]

Thanks to the reflection phenomenon and its interrelation with the remaining possible attenuations, an ultrasound image is obtained with spots of varying brightness. This is the reason why the normal ultrasound technique is called B mode (or brightness modulation). These bright points are called echogenic points. The tissues that appear brighter (and therefore those that are the most echogenic) are bone and non-specialized connective tissue, which provide support to the remaining musculoskeletal structures. The connective tissue architecture of most of the structures in this system is identical. This explains why the tendon, ligament and nerve are similar in form. The basis for a correct differentiation between these tissues will be revealed

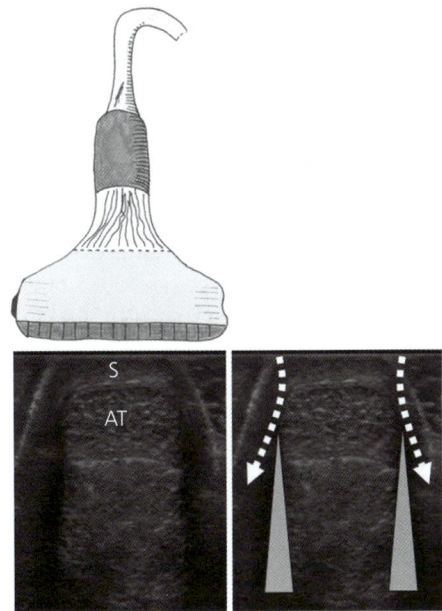

FIGURE 5.5 ■ Transverse view of the Achilles tendon in which the change in direction of the ultrasound beam (discontinuous lines) is visible after changing its velocity at the interphase between the skin (S) and the Achilles tendon (AT), producing a refractile shadow (grey triangles). (Colour version of figure is available online).

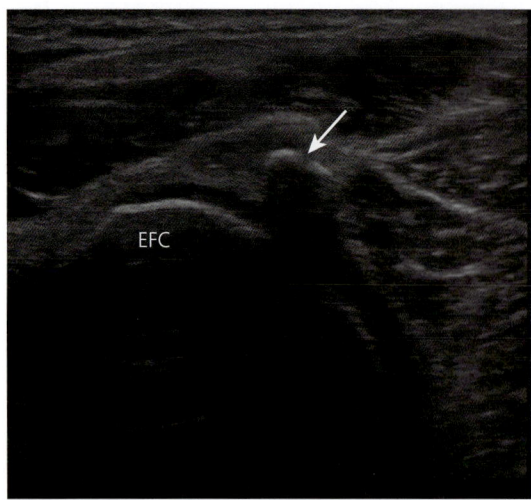

FIGURE 5.6 ■ Longitudinal section of the external femoral condyle (EFC) in which the fabella is visible (white arrow). This is an inconsistent sesamoid bone found in the capsular zone of the external condyle which can lead to confusion with an articular loose body or a degenerative calcifying process. The acoustic shadow is observed both on the condyle as well as on the fabella.

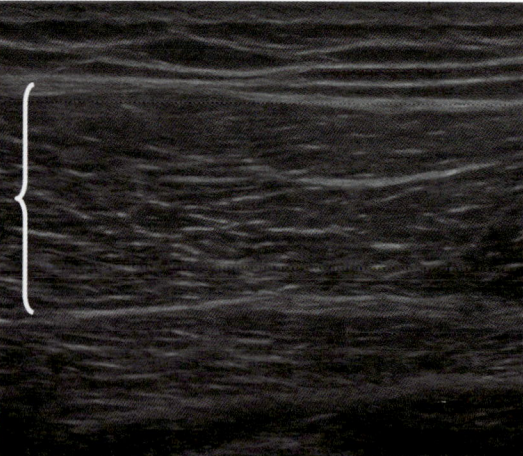

FIGURE 5.7 ■ The bracket highlights a transverse muscular exploration in which the body of the hypoechoic muscle is observed, stabilized within a network of hyperechoic connective tissue.

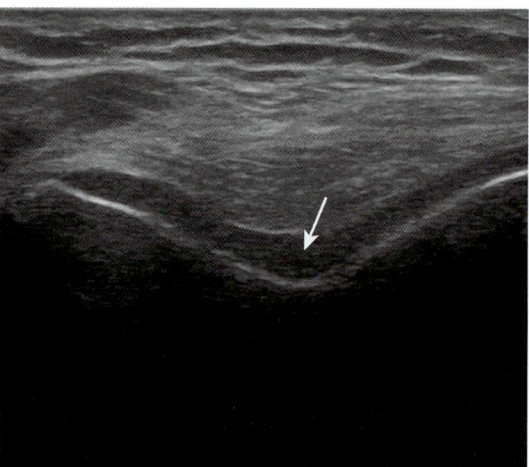

FIGURE 5.8 ■ Ultrasound exploration of the hyaline cartilage of the femoral trochlea (arrow) in maximal knee flexion. An anechoic image is observed covering the articular surface of the femoral trochlea.

subsequently in this chapter. An important aspect to remember here is that the echogenicity of the tissues depends on the speed of reflection which, at the same time, is proportional to tissue density. As previously noted, the bone and non-specialized connective tissue are exceptional; these are very dense tissues that reflect ultrasound waves at a very high speed (in the case of bone, at 4.080 m/s). For the remaining tissues within the musculoskeletal system, the ultrasound waves are reflected at very similar speeds (1.400–1.600 m/s). These considerations, together with the required anatomical knowledge, are the reason why ultrasound is characterized by its difficulty of interpretation and reading. The typical remark made by a person with no formal training who sees an ultrasound image is: 'I don't see anything; it all looks the same'.[5]

In relation to echogenicity, several terms are used:

- Hyperechoic (-genic): very bright interphases associated with very dense or hyper-reflective tissues, such as the bone or the non-specialized connective tissue of the musculoskeletal system (figure 5.7).
- Hypoechoic (-genic): interphases of a weaker brightness, without being altogether anechoic (figure 5.7).
- Anechoic (-genic): interphases with no brightness at all; in other words, they appear black and are neither dense nor reflective. No information is acquired from these structures, e.g. fluid-filled structures or those belonging to the joint cartilage (figure 5.8), due to the absence of echoes.
- Isoechoic (-genic): referring to tissues with similar echogenicities. This is the case of the nerve tendon pairs (figure 5.9), artery–vein, bone–non-specialized connective tissue or articular cartilage–liquid structures.
- Homogeneous image: apart from the particular ultrasound characteristics of each tissue, the homogeneity of its structure and dimensions is what characterizes it as being normal.

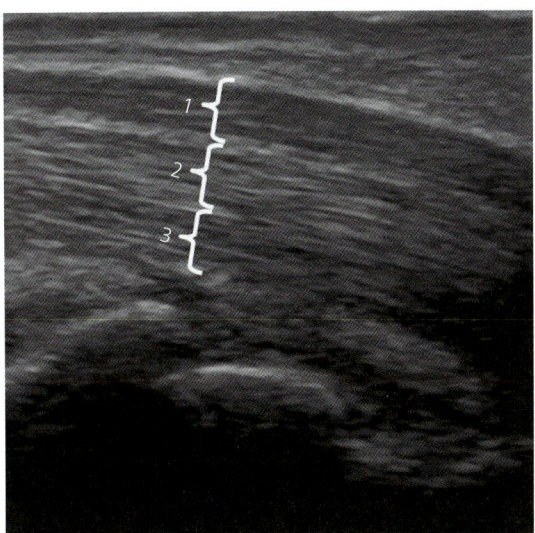

FIGURE 5.9 ■ Longitudinal exploration of the median nerve (bracket 1) as it passes through the carpal tunnel. The nerve is visible passing superficially to the superficial flexor tendon (bracket 2) and the deep flexor tendon (bracket 3) of the index finger. The image demonstrates the similar echogenicity of these structures, which may lead to discrimination difficulties for the operator.

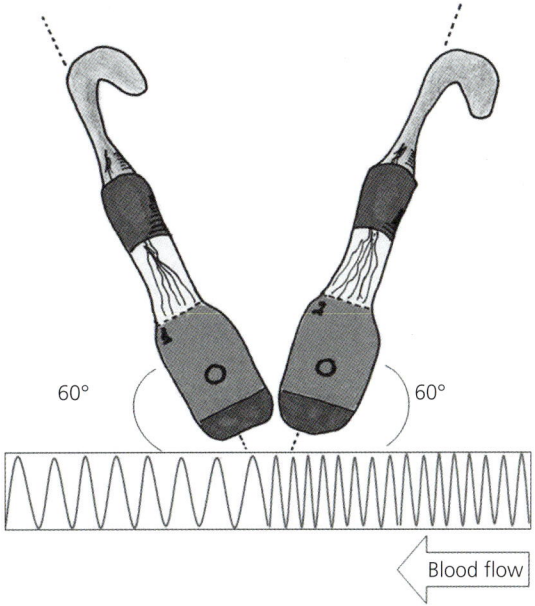

FIGURE 5.10 ■ According to the direction of blood flow, the frequency and length of the wave emitted by the flow will vary depending on whether it is approaching or moving away from the transducer. (Colour version of figure is available online).

- Heterogeneous image: the observation of a heterogeneous ultrasound pattern that notably breaks up the homogeneity when compared to the surrounding structures. When present, this is considered a sign of abnormality. In these circumstances, thorough anamnesis, physical exploration and ultrasonographic knowledge are used to determine the existence or absence of pathology.

KEY POINTS

The first building stone in ultrasound training, regardless of the speciality, begins with a thorough knowledge of its physical principles.

5.3 THE DOPPLER EFFECT AND ITS INDICATIONS IN ULTRASOUND

Haemodynamic studies constitute an important speciality in diagnostic ultrasound within the field of physiotherapy. They enable assessment of the influence that some of the specialized treatment techniques have over the vascular system. The Doppler technique in ultrasound is possible thanks to the discoveries of the Austrian physicist and mathematician, Christian Andreas Doppler (1803–1853). His work, which he named the Doppler effect, was based on the properties of light in movement and has been found to be applicable to all types of waves. Upon this foundation, over 100 years later, the Japanese developed what is known today as the application of the Doppler effect in ultrasound.

A sound wave changes its frequency and wavelength, both when it moves away from an object as well as when it approaches it. If we live opposite a bell tower (a static source of sound), whenever the bells toll and if we are always in the same room, we will hear them at the same intensity, as they produce a sound in a fixed frequency. However, when we are in the same room and we hear an ambulance siren (a moving source of sound) its intensity varies, becoming higher-pitched as it approaches us, and lower-pitched as it moves away. For example, if this ambulance were to emit an original sound of 400 Hz, its frequency would increase and its wavelength would decrease as it approaches, whereas the opposite would be true when it moves away. Blood circulation also produces a sound which can be registered by the ultrasound transducer (figure 5.10). Thanks to the Doppler effect, the blood circulation can be visualized and haemodynamic studies can be performed using ultrasound. Unlike ultrasound in B mode, for the Doppler technique it is necessary to position the transducer with a 60° tilt (Doppler angle) (figure 5.10) in relation to the blood vessel under study. This technique allows for a more precise register of flow within the vessel.

One of the most-used Doppler techniques is colour Doppler (or Doppler colour flow imaging). This shows blood flow represented in two tonalities, with the brightness correlated to the velocity, becoming red if the blood approaches the transducer and blue if the blood flows away from the transducer (figure 5.11). This colouring can actually be inverted by pressing a button, which would then show the artery as blue and the veins red. The advantage of this Doppler technique is not to aid in the differentiation between an artery and a vein, but to be able to assess the possible existence of vascular alterations such as refluxes and turbulences. It is the anatomical and exploratory knowledge that allows us to discern whether the exploration is arterial or venous. The arteries, apart from having thicker walls, maintain a pulse connected with the heart beat and are much less collapsible than veins. On the other hand, in the case of veins, a minimal pressure can provoke a complete collapse (hence the importance of being aware of the exploratory pressure applied). Also, the venous valves are distinguishable and their behaviour worth observing. If we are able to locate major valves, such as those pertaining to the popliteal vein or the great saphenous vein (which ends in the femoral vein), one can appreciate the influence that breathing has on the venous system. During inspiration (inhalation) the valve closes, increasing its diameter significantly, while the opposite occurs during expiration (exhalation). It is interesting to observe that,

during inspiratory apnoea, the valve automatically opens after a few seconds with no need for an expiratory phase (figure 5.12).

On the other hand, we have the colour Doppler energy or power Doppler imaging. The advantage of this technique is that it is less dependent on the angle and more sensitive to the detection of flow in small vessels. For this reason, it is the technique of choice for study of the musculoskeletal system. However, it does not provide information about the direction of flow,

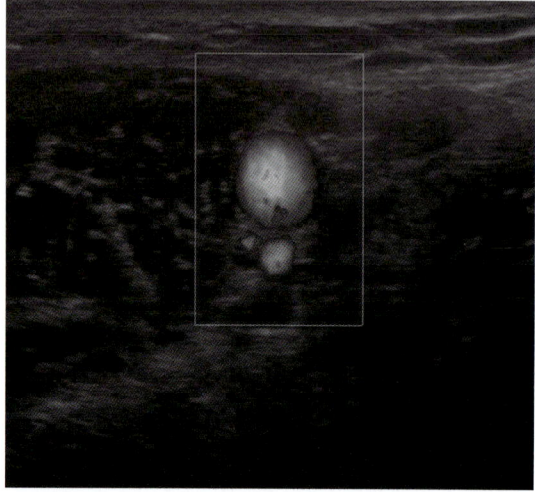

FIGURE 5.11 ■ A haemodynamic study using colour directional Doppler is displayed in which an artery (red) is visible together with its contiguous veins (blue). Differences in brightness and therefore of velocity can be seen between the periphery and the centre of the vessel. (Colour version of figure is available online).

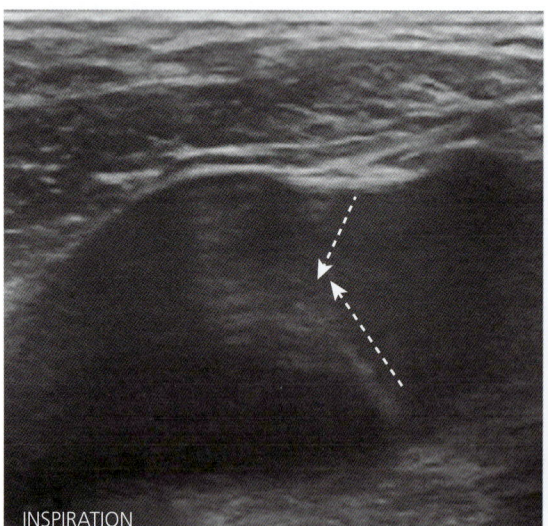
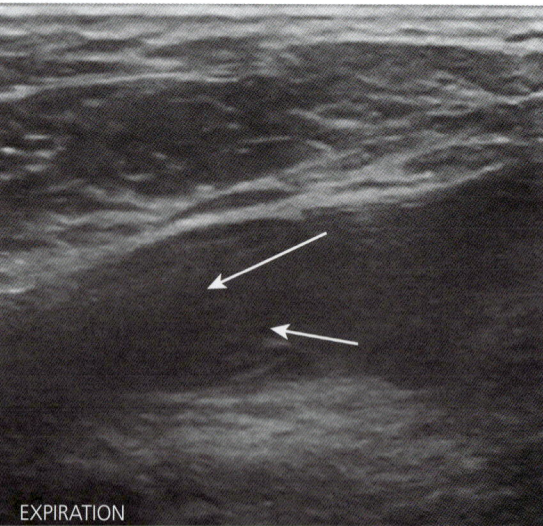

INSPIRATION   EXPIRATION

FIGURE 5.12 ■ Longitudinal exploration of the femoral valve where it passes through the femoral triangle. In the ultrasound image on the left, the valve is visible closing during inspiration (white discontinuous lines), at the same time increasing the diameter of the vessel. Meanwhile, during expiration (right) the valve opens (continuous white lines) and the vein acquires a normal diameter once again.

always showing it in the same orange tone. The brightness of the colour is still correlated with velocity (figure 5.13).[6,7]

KEY POINTS

Because of its greater sensitivity, Colour Doppler Energy is the technique of choice for the study of the musculoskeletal system.

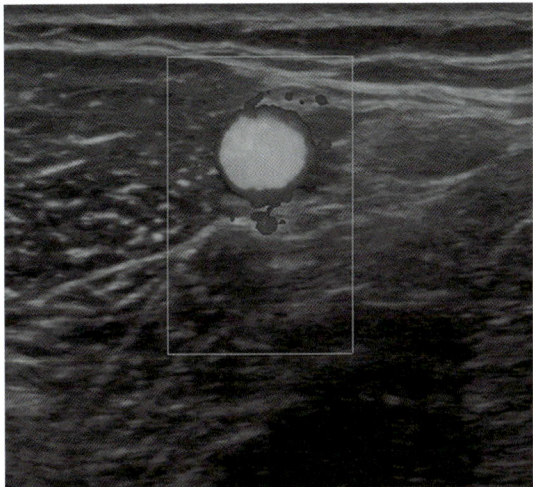

FIGURE 5.13 ■ Haemodynamic study using colour Doppler energy. This Doppler technique is more sensitive to small amounts of fluid, therefore it is the Doppler of choice for the assessment of angiogenesis in the musculoskeletal system. (Colour version of figure is available online).

Both Doppler techniques require a correct optimization, dependent on the exploratory frequency, radiofrequency pulse (RFP) and echogenicity gain. This latter variable will determine whether the Doppler image is clean or full of noise. When the objective is to find small presences of flow, it is recommended to adjust these variables until the possible appearance of noise.

Finally, in general, examinations using Doppler should culminate with a Doppler duplex study as this provides both qualitative and quantitative information regarding the vessel and its blood flow. This technique permits the professional to work simultaneously in B mode, colour Doppler or colour Doppler energy and in pulsed-wave Doppler (PW). PW Doppler displays a histogram where the x-axis corresponds to the velocity (m/s) of flow and the y-axis to time (seconds). The form of the graph depends on whether it involves an artery or a vein. The arterial samples appear with two clear peaks of reference – the systolic and diastolic peaks. However, the venous sample is characterized by presenting a continuous pattern, where the presence of small pulses is curiously related to respiratory frequency and not heart frequency (figure 5.14).

In the study of the arterial system, two types of flow pattern are distinguished: those of high and low resistance. These patterns provide information regarding the tissue they supply, indicating whether the tissue offers more (or

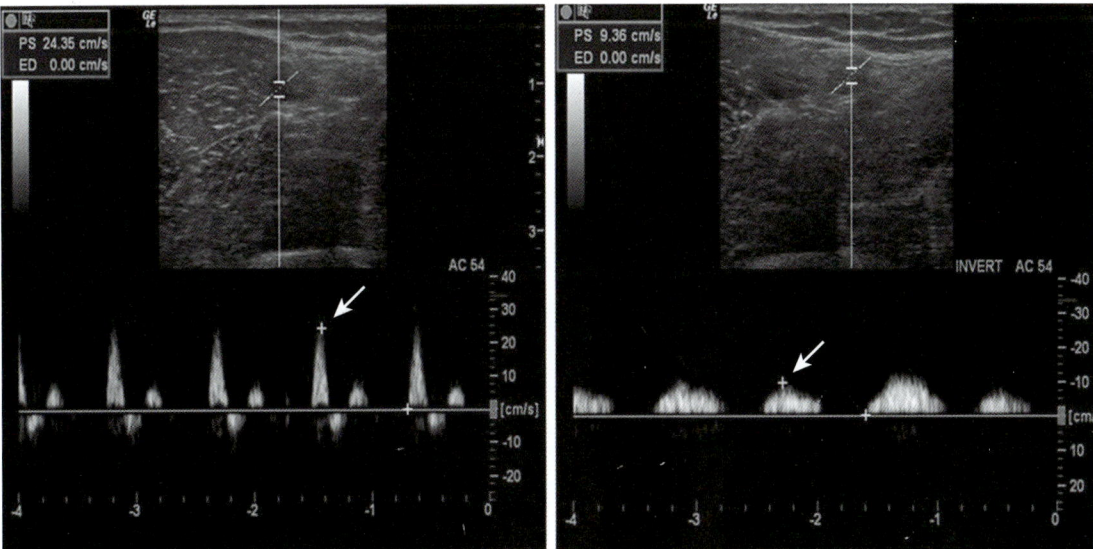

FIGURE 5.14 ■ Comparative haemodynamic arteriovenous study using duplex Doppler (B-mode and pulsed Doppler). Left: a haemodynamic study of the femoral artery; right: haemodynamic study of the femoral vein. Of all the variables, the most important is the systolic peak (white arrow), which corresponds with the maximal fluid velocity.

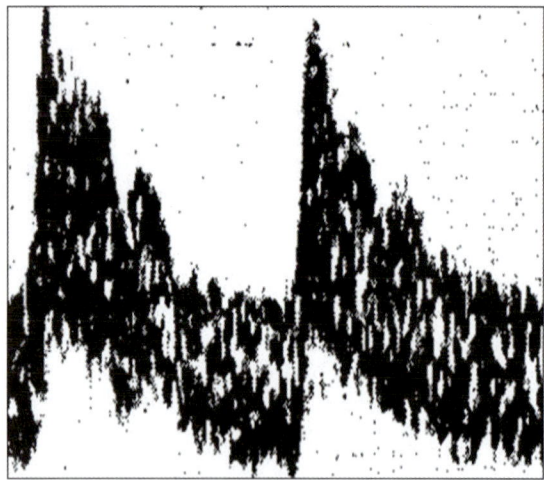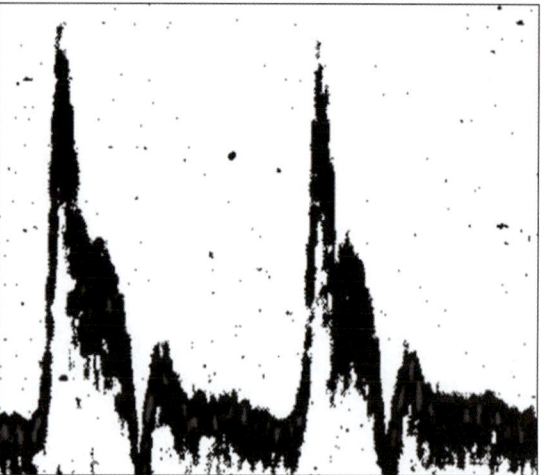

FIGURE 5.15 ■ Comparative haemodynamic study using pulsed Doppler. Left: low-resistance pattern; right: high-resistance pattern. The type of graph is correlated with the resistance that the tissue offers the blood which supplies it and not the resistance of the vessel itself.

less) resistance to the entrance of blood. For example, the pattern of the external carotid artery (which is a vessel that irrigates muscle groups) is of high resistance; however, that of the internal carotid artery (which irrigates the brain) is of low resistance (figure 5.15). The assessment of the arterial pattern is of great interest in the study of angiogenesis by providing indirect information of the state of the tissue, as a result of the repair processes occurring within the musculoskeletal system.

KEY POINTS

'High' or 'low' resistance is related to the resistance the tissue offers to the entrance of blood. For this reason a tissue in repair increases its resistance pattern throughout its recovery process.

Just as occurs in B mode, when PW is performed, a correct image optimization is needed, as the exploration is highly prone to subjectivities. The optimization variables that will be considered are:
- the most reliable Doppler angle
- the centred position of the sample volume of the PW in the interior of the vessel under study
- the RFP most appropriate to the type of flow, and which avoids, as far as possible, potential distortion or aliasing. The RFP is reflected in the histogram as a modification of the speed scale found on the x-axis

- the ascent or descent from the baseline of the graph so that the pattern is framed within the histogram.

5.4 DESCRIPTION AND ANATOMICAL–ULTRASOUND CORRELATIONS WITH THE MUSCULOSKELETAL SYSTEM

Within the musculoskeletal system, it is necessary to make special mention of the non-specialized connective tissue, as it provides a strong and abundant structure for the rest of the tissues forming the locomotor system. It is dense and hyperreflective, which explains why it is observed as a hyperechoic structure. It extends across the musculoskeletal system like the roots of a tree, interrelating some structures with others, whether these are bones, tendons, ligaments, muscles, nerves or even fat itself (figure 5.16).

After a traumatic or degenerative process, an isolated structure will suffer internal changes, provoking more or less pain and incapacity. However, the involvement of its non-specialized connective tissue is responsible for creating a lesional chain during the recovery process and this can ultimately involve other structures found in more or less proximity. For example, there is a clear relation between hoffitis (the degeneration of Hoffa's fat pad) and patellar tendinopathy.

This type of connective tissue, including fascial tissue, also suffers from pathological processes that are more complex to visualize. Notably,

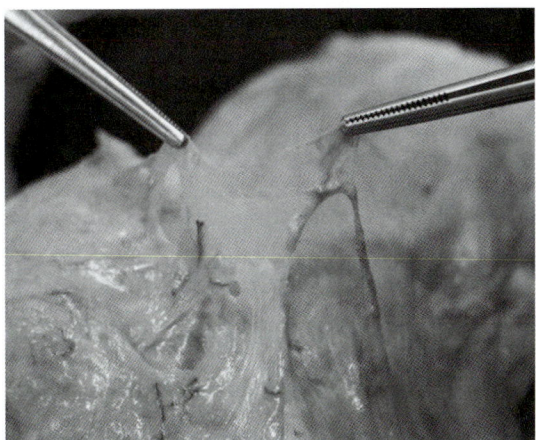

FIGURE 5.16 ■ Image of a knee dissection, in which a fascial network is shown as an example of the connective tissue structure of the musculoskeletal system. (Colour version of figure is available online).

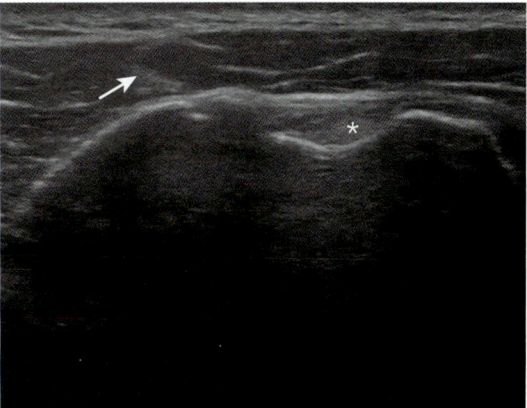

FIGURE 5.17 ■ Transverse section of the long tendon of the biceps brachii (*) in an extracapsular location where it passes by the bicipital groove. White arrow indicates a fibrous strand of connective tissue which separates the anterior and middle fascicles of the deltoid. It is one of the strands which under palpation is often confused with the long tendon of the biceps brachii.

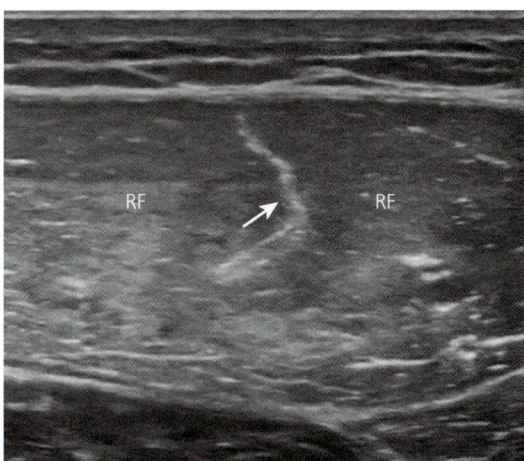

FIGURE 5.18 ■ Transverse section of the rectus femoris (RF). The septum (white arrow) extends intramuscularly in a comma shape from the epimysium, as the projection of the tendon originating in the anterior inferior iliac spine. The shape of the septum depends on the subject, the muscle quality and the injuries the person may have suffered.

an inflammatory infiltration affecting this tissue provokes an increase in width and a loss of echogenicity. This becomes more evident after the comparative study of its contralateral side.

The name itself, 'connective tissue', implies its importance. In other words, it offers structural support and stability. For this reason, after a lesion, and even more so in the case of muscle, restructuring of the connective tissue is one of the most important signs to watch out for in order to confirm correct progression of the injury.

The nerve, tendon, ligament and even fat itself show similar organization. However in the muscle the representation is far more complex. In the muscle, apart from observing the endomysium, perimysium, epimysium and the fascia (all of which are interrelated), one can notice, for example, how, in the case of the deltoid muscle, strands of connective tissue are found following the same trajectory as its muscle fibres (figure 5.17). This finding causes these strands to be confused with other deep tendons that are topographically related, such as the long head of the biceps brachii tendon or the supraspinatus tendon. Therefore, this can be a source of error in the palpation of these structures.[8]

Another element to consider is the presence of intramuscular fibroadipose septa, which continue to the tendon of origin and which are responsible for giving the muscle its characteristic form, together with a point of lesional conflict. This can be observed in muscles such as the rectus femoris (figure 5.18), the hamstrings, adductor longus, tibialis anterior and the deltoid and anconeus muscles, among others. The relation of the muscle fibres with their septa is one

of a true myotendinous junction, and they represent some of the most important points of lesional conflict. For example, in the case of the rectus femoris, its septum is projected to the inferior third of the muscle belly. This anatomical disposition is responsible for the fact that tears in the rectus femoris are commonly located at the point of union with its septum.[9]

On the other hand, the presence of these septa gives the muscle a strand-like texture under palpation, which can cause the clinician to confuse them with simple contractures or inexistent muscle strains. This is typically the case with the adductor longus, rectus femoris or tibialis anterior muscles.

The connective tissue that forms the locomotor system displays a high level of sensitive receptors, which results in the fact that its palpation is always painful, or at least uncomfortable, even in the absence of dysfunction or illness. This challenges the explorations that are normally practised in the assessment of musculoskeletal lesions, as not all that is painful under palpation is due to involvement of the soft tissues. An exhaustive anamnesis, clinical experience, functional testing and the performance of complementary tests, such as ultrasound, are all necessary in order to reach a reliable conclusion, and this requires time.

KEY POINTS

The tissues that form the musculoskeletal system display a similar connective tissue architecture, despite carrying out such diverse functions as, for example, is the case with the nerve and the muscle. As a result, their pathological ultrasound signs follow similar sequences.

5.4.1 Subcutaneous cellular tissue

In normal conditions subcutaneous cellular tissue is displayed as a hypoanechoic area partitioned by walls of hyperechoic connective tissue (figure 5.19). Its quantity depends on the grade of adiposity and the sex of the patient, together with the area under study.

On occasions, an alteration of this characteristic pattern is appreciated. For example, muscle bruising is accompanied by an inflammatory process of the subcutaneous cell tissue adjacent to the bruised area, which is displayed as an increased echogenicity and a loss of its connective architecture. The same scenario can also be accompanied by a break in the subcutaneous lymphatic capillaries, which will result in lymphoedema, found between the subcutaneous cellular tissue and the superficial muscle plane. In assessment of the lymphoedema, it is important to pay special attention to the pressure that one exercises with the transducer, as this can alter the dimensions of the structure.

These ruptures of lymphatic capillaries and of subcutaneous venules are also characteristic in ankle sprains. This would explain why, in just a few minutes, or even sometimes in a few seconds, the volume of the area expands considerably, regardless of the severity of the injury of the external ankle ligament complex.

In varicose processes, an alteration in the image is also observed (thickening, hyperechoicity and loss of the connective pattern) and, furthermore, an increased diameter of the incompetent veins of the superficial venous system can be seen.

The quantity of subcutaneous cellular tissue is a technically determining factor, as it causes considerable limitation in the observation of the subjacent interphases. In these cases the correct manipulation of the frequency, focus and gain is essential in order to correct this technical difficulty.

Accumulations of fat within the joint are found, and these have an important biomechanical role and a similar appearance to the subcutaneous cellular tissue. An example of these are the Hoffa and Kager fat pads, which are very rich in connective tissue (figure 5.20) and which maintain strong adhesions with the patellar tendon and the Achilles tendon, respectively.

5.4.2 Muscle

Intra- and intermuscular stability depends on a network of dense and hyperechoic connective tissue represented by the endomysium, perimysium, epimysium and the fascial tissue itself, all of which are interrelated. The connective tissue represents the compartments within which vessels and nerves relate the internal structure of the muscle with the exterior.

The muscle body is more hyperechoic than the connective tissue that stabilizes it. The most

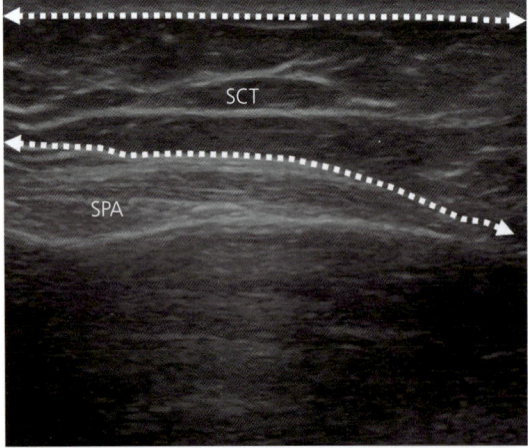

FIGURE 5.19 ■ Longitudinal section of the superficial pes anserinus (SPA) inserting in the internal aspect of the tibia. On its surface, the shape and echogenicity of the subcutaneous cellular tissue (SCT) can be seen, abundant in this area (marked between the two discontinuous lines).

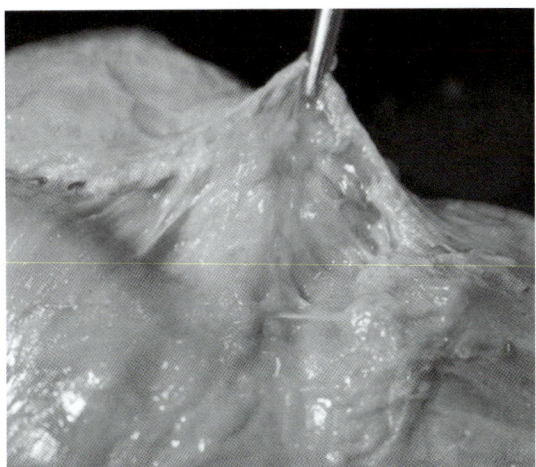

FIGURE 5.20 ■ A knee dissection is shown, demonstrating how traction of the patellar tendon reveals the adipose tissue of Hoffa's fat pad, which is firmly lined by connective tissue which also adheres to the deep aspect of the patellar tendon, implicating it in its biomechanics. (Colour version of figure is available online).

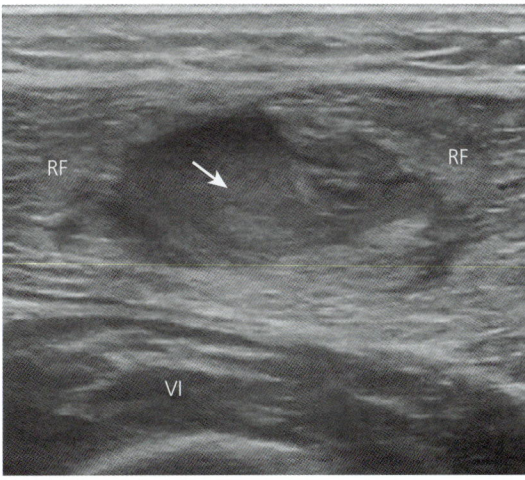

FIGURE 5.21 ■ Transverse exploration of the rectus femoris (RF) and the vastus intermedius (VI). An extremely large partial rupture is observed at the height of its septum. The septum has disappeared and a large haematoma is seen with a hyperechoic solid component, which corresponds to a clot (arrow).

important sign to consider is detection of the correct internal architecture of the connective tissue, for the assessment of a normal state, a macroscopic lesion or return to work or sports after a muscle lesion.

As previously noted, the connective tissue is displayed in a similar manner in all muscles; however certain anatomical variations should be considered. For example, accumulations of connective tissue can be detected. These are called fibroadipose septa and represent intramuscular tendon projections.

The muscle exploration usually begins with transverse views that enable observation of the entire muscle section. These transverse scans can be performed at a medium speed that offers a fast comparison between all portions of the section. Normally the same section of a great muscle belly displays areas with normal reflection and other areas of anisotropy that require correction of the transducer tilt. The anisotropic areas should not be confused with zones susceptible to lesion.

Particular attention must be paid to the amount of pressure applied with the transducer, as excess pressure can potentially modify the dimensions or even hide other pathological signals, such as a haematoma.

Each muscle presents a specific point of conflict where it tends to get damaged. In the case of the rectus femoris (figure 5.21) and the hamstring muscles, this is found in the myotendinous junction between the muscle fibres and their fibroadipose septa. However, in the case of the medial head of the gastrocnemius, a typical lesion is due to a musculoaponeurotic avulsion between the muscle belly and the fascial tissue, corresponding to the origin of the Achilles tendon (figure 5.22). The location of these conflict points also influences the reconstruction period of the connective tissue and, therefore, recovery and return to activity. For this reason, gastrocnemius muscle lesions tend to have a longer recovery process than other muscle bellies.

To date, for a lesion to be visible under ultrasound, it has to be macroscopic and linked to an acute inflammatory reaction, the destruction of its connective architecture and the formation of a haematoma. These signs are subject to the grade of the lesion, together with their location and lesional mechanism (external for contusions or internal due to distension). This means that muscular injuries considered microscopic, for example due to strain, contractures or even trigger points, at present lack clear ultrasound support and therefore the possibility of a precise reading and assessment. In the last few years, tests such as sonoelastography have been introduced as a new way of assessing the musculoskeletal system, and are complementary to basic musculoskeletal ultrasound.[10]

Of all possible signs, the correct reconstruction of the connective network is the most important factor in order both to guarantee correct function and to avoid recurrence. The more serious the injury is, the greater the quantity of muscular and connective tissue to be reconstructed, with the risk of scarring, which

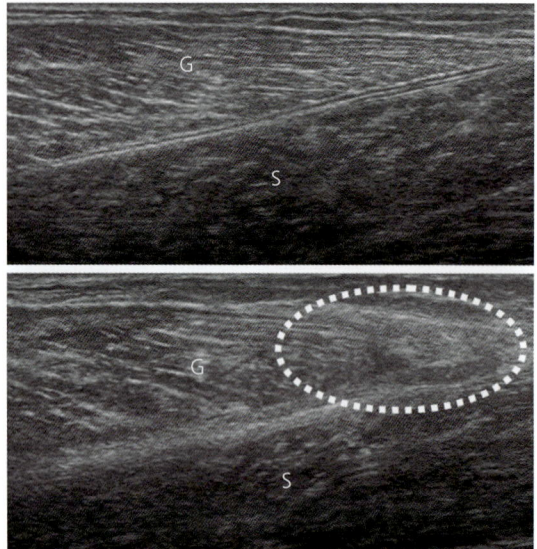

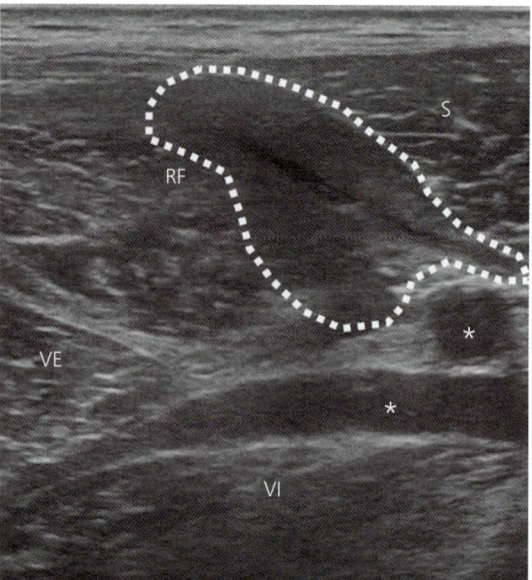

FIGURE 5.22 ■ Comparative contralateral study of a longitudinal exploration of the myotendinous junction of the medial head of gastrocnemius (G) in the Achilles fascia. In the deep muscle plane the soleus muscle (S) is found. In the inferior image, a musculo-aponeurotic avulsion is observed (discontinuous circle) corresponding to signs of an increase in width, a loss of echogenicity and a loss of structure to the connective tissue. It will be very important to monitor progression in this case, in order to avoid the appearance of an ominous interstitial haematoma between the planes of the gastrocnemius and the soleus.

FIGURE 5.23 ■ Ultrasound exam of a professional football player aged 33 years, who attends a consultation in order to monitor his progression after an old tear of the rectus femoris with recurrences. At the time of the ultrasound study, the footballer was not presenting symptoms and was training as normal. A transverse section of the rectus femoris (RF) is shown, topographically related to the vastus externus (VE), vastus intermedius (VI) and sartorius (S) muscles, next to the vascular package (*). The internal aspect of the rectus femoris (discontinuous line) is shown with an increased echogenicity and a loss of its connective tissue architecture, as signs of fibrous scarring of great dimensions with fascial adherences in comparison to other muscle groups. An encapsulated haematoma is also visible on the inside of the scar.

can be quite normal, due to the size of the lesion (figure 5.23). From a functional point of view, an optimal viscoelastic capacity of this fibrous repair tissue is more important than its own dimensions.

It is assumed that, 48–72 hours after the lesion, ultrasound is the technique of choice for the diagnosis of muscle tears. The use of ultrasound in physiotherapy facilitates the performance of repeated studies that enable assessment of a correct progression, as well as avoiding complications related to muscular lesions. These include great muscular fibrosis processes which can cause nervous compression; the formation of large asymptomatic haematomas, which can end up becoming embedded or fibrotic over time; and the development of myositis ossificans related to large muscular contusions, or even compartment syndrome.[11]

KEY POINTS

Of all the ultrasound diagnostic signs related to muscle tissue, the most important is the assessment of the architecture of its connective tissue, as this is directly related to the muscle's performance.

5.4.3 Tendon

Despite the great differences in function and tissue, the tendon presents a similar architecture to the ligament, the nerve and the muscle itself. This is characterized by the disposition of its connective tissue (figure 5.24). The tendon tissue is displayed as a hypoechoic body stabilized by a network of non-specialized hyperechoic connective tissue (endotendon, peritendon, epitendon and paratendon), within which vessels and nerves are found relating the internal and external tendinous structure.

Tendons are minimally vascularized. Therefore, under normal conditions, the Doppler technique will show no flow. Asymptomatic internal flow has only been observed in some patellar tendons of volleyball players, accompanied by thickening and a loss of echogenicity.[12] On the other hand, in some asymptomatic cases, some flow can be observed in the periphery of the tendon.

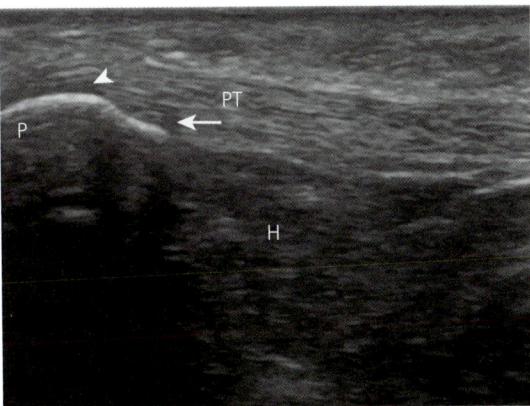

FIGURE 5.24 ■ Longitudinal exploration of the patellar tendon (PT) at its origin on the pole of the patella (P) and topographically located over Hoffa's fat pad (H). In this exploration its deep (arrow) and superficial (arrow head) fibres are seen, connecting to the quadriceps tendon.

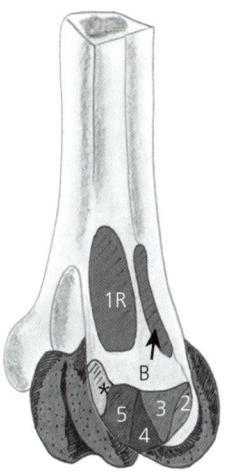

FIGURE 5.25 ■ Lateral posterior view of the distal third of the humerus in which the disposition of the tendons that form the common epicondyle tendon is shown, displacing the brachioradialis (B) and the extensor carpi radialis longus (1R). From anterior to posterior, the following structures are found: the extensor carpi radialis brevis (2), the extensor digitorum (3), the extensor digiti minimi (4) and the extensor carpi ulnaris (5). The anconeus muscle (*) deserves special attention, not only because of its closeness, but also due to its fascial relation with the epicondyle tendon, which therefore ends up implicating it directly in the clinical picture of the epicondylosis. (Colour version of figure is available online).

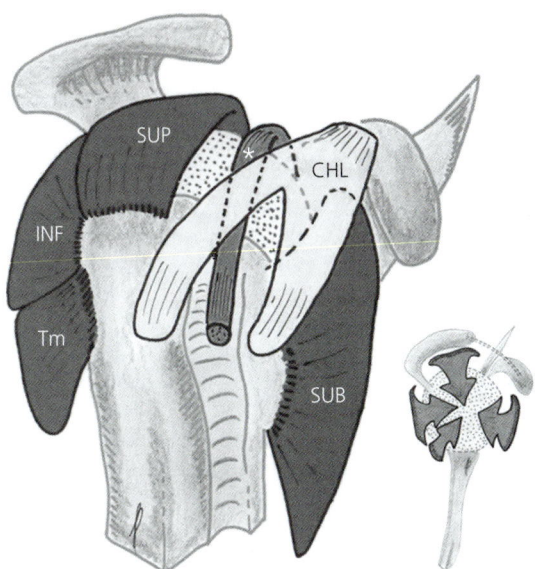

FIGURE 5.26 ■ Location of the rotator cuff and its relation with the long head of the biceps brachii tendon (*) and the coracohumeral ligament (CHL), which constitutes the famous rotator interval, towards which insertion expansions are sent. The integrity of this ligament depends on the stability and behaviour of both the rotator cuff as well as the long head of biceps. The tears in the rotator cuff which cause the most instability are those that affect the rotator interval, which means that the following require mandatory assessment: INF, infraspinatus; SUB, subscapularis; SUP, supraspinatus; Tm, teres minor. (Colour version of figure is available online).

long biceps brachii tendon, the flexors and extensors of the wrist and the ankle, the popliteal, lateral peroneal and tibialis posterior tendons, also show a double sheath which is associated with the synovial membrane.

The ideal ultrasound section will depend on the type of tendon. In general, it is longitudinal in tendons with a single sheath and transverse in those with a double sheath. The acute signs observable in tendinopathies that affect the single sheath tendons are a thickening and loss of echogenicity, and these are easier assessed via a longitudinal section. For tendons with a double sheath, the signs are the increased diameter between the single sheath and the double sheath of more than 2 mm, which justifies a larger quantity of synovial liquid.

Tendons are very anisotropic. At times this can be more of an advantage than an inconvenience, as it aids the discrimination of other tissues found in close proximity, such as the median nerve in the carpal tunnel or the transverse humeral ligament in the long head of the biceps brachii.

Depending on whether a tendon presents a double sheath, the ultrasound assessment of a

There are two types of tendons: those with a single sheath and those with double sheaths. The tendons with a single sheath, such as the patellar, Achilles, epicondylar (figure 5.25), epitrochlear or rotator cuff tendons (figure 5.26), present the paratendon as the last connective tissue layer, whereas those with a double sheath, such as the

TABLE 5.1	Tendons with a single sheath (longitudinal sections). Variables worth considering when monitoring the progression of a simple sheath tendinopathy without loss of continuity
Variable	**Considerations**
Width	The measurement area depends on the site of the tendon lesion
Loss of echogenicity	The number and surface hypoechoic areas are assessed
Calcifications	It is important to consider their diameter and quantity
Angiogenesis	A qualitative and quantitative analysis of flow is performed, considering the number of vessels and the pattern of resistance to flow
Cortical defects	The existence of this defect is noted in the records

TABLE 5.2	Tendons with a double sheath (transverse section). Variables to consider when monitoring the progression in double-sheath tendinopathies without a loss of continuity
Variables	**Considerations**
Single/double-sheath diameter	More than 1.5–2 mm is considered to be pathological. The relation of these tendons with the joint forces one to consider that the excess of fluid could be derived from an articular or tendinous problem
Irregularity of the double sheath	This is a sign of chronicity
Thickening of the double sheath	This receives the name of synovitis and its width is measured
Calcifications	The diameter and quantity of these will be considered
Angiogenesis	A qualitative and quantitative analysis of flow is performed, considering the number of vessels and the pattern of resistance to flow
Tendinosis	If tendinosis is present, the internal structure of the tendon is assessed, following the parameters shown in table 5.1
Detritus within the synovial liquid	If detritus is found within the excess of synovial liquid, this could be due to deposits of cholesterol, uric acid, calcium hydroxyapatite crystals, and also the possible existence of an infectious process accompanied by episodes of fever

tendinopathy must consider specific variables (tables 5.1 and 5.2). It is important to be very precise and thorough while undertaking this assessment, as it enables one to be more objective regarding the evolution the tendinopathy.

In tendons with a simple sheath, the first variable to consider is the width, for which the measurement area will depend on the morphology of the tendon and its area of conflict. Thus, in the case of the patellar tendon, its width is measured 1 cm from the inferior patellar pole (insertion tendiopathies can also be observed in the tibial tuberosity); the Achilles is measured in its belly, at 2–6 cm from its insertion in the calcaneus (as with the patellar tendon, in the calcaneus, insertion tendinopathies are common) (figure 5.27); the epicondylar tendon is measured at the flat bony surface on the lateral aspect of the condyle, paying special attention to its deep fibres, which correspond with the tendon of the extensor carpi radialis brevis. In the case of the epitrochlear tendon, the deformity of its insertion point will require special attention, rather than its

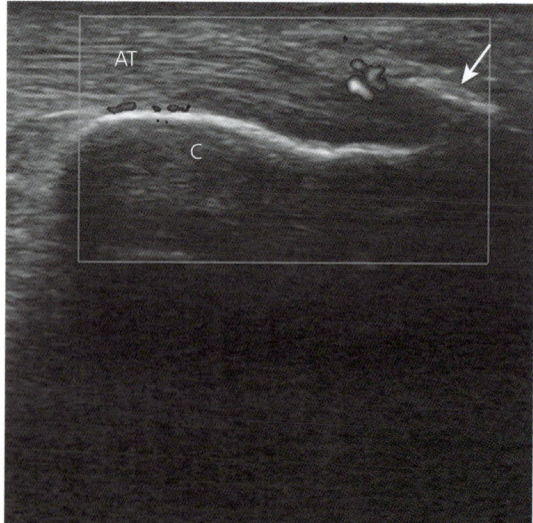

FIGURE 5.27 ■ Longitudinal section of the Achilles tendon (AT) in which an insertion tendinopathy in the calcaneus (C) is displayed with thickening, loss of echogenicity and angiogenesis due to Haglund's deformity (arrow). This situation is usually accompanied by calcaneal bursitis due to the friction. (Colour version of figure is available online).

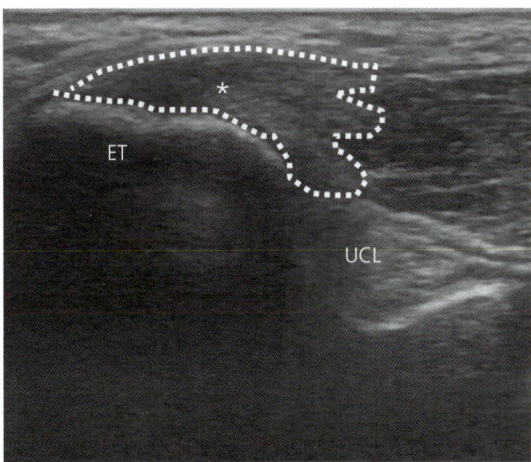

FIGURE 5.28 ■ Longitudinal exploration of the common epitrochlear tendon (*) in its origin on the epitrochlea (ET). The tendon, with a triangular shape, is visibly thickened and displays a loss of echogenicity as signs of a mild tendinopathy. The epitrochlear myotendinous complex must not be confused with the hyperechogenic ulnar collateral ligament (UCL), which is found at its depth.

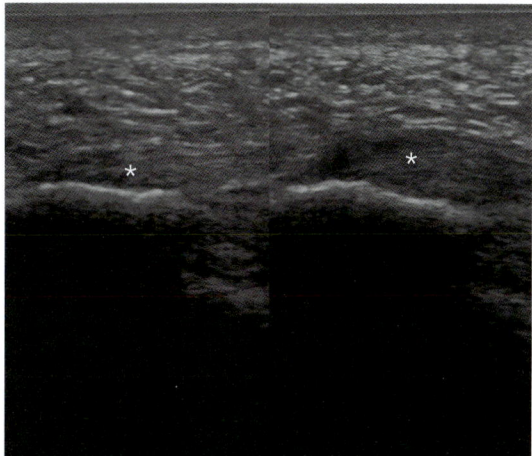

FIGURE 5.30 ■ Comparative contralateral study. Longitudinal exploration of the origin of the plantar fascia (*). Right: the fascia is shown with thickening and a loss of echogenicity, as signs of mild fasciosis.

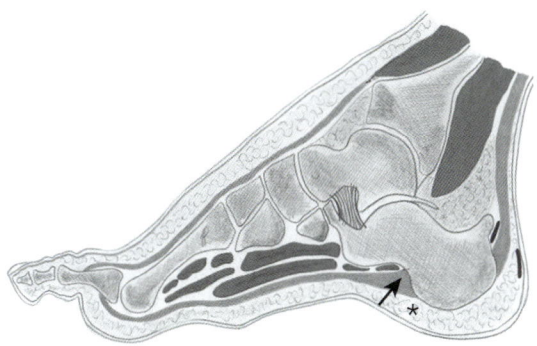

FIGURE 5.29 ■ Sagittal section of the foot and ankle. Observe the origin of the plantar fascia (arrow) on the calcaneus and its relation to the heel fat pad (*). (Colour version of figure is available online).

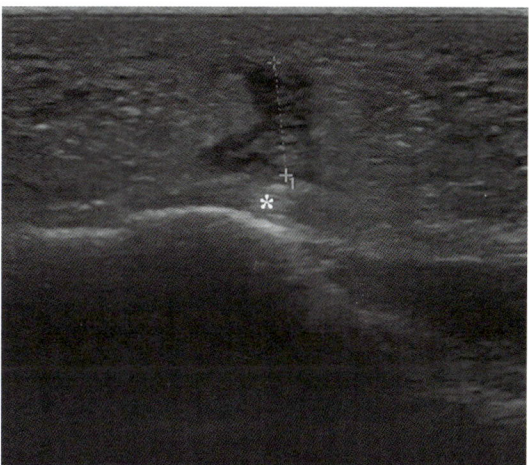

FIGURE 5.31 ■ Longitudinal exploration of the origin of the plantar fascia (*). In the image the fascia is shown with a normal morphoechogenicity, although the heel fat pad shows a hypoanechoic area as a sign of posttraumatic haematoma, simulating a fasciosis symptomatology.

width (figure 5.28) as, due to its triangular morphology, it is impossible to determine an optimal measurement area. For the supraspinatus tendon, measurements are taken 1 cm from the greater tubercle of the humerus.[13]

Among the tendon ultrasound exams, the plantar fascia is also considered (figure 5.29). This structure has a histopathological process that is very similar to that of tendons with a single sheath, and therefore the same ultrasound variables are considered (figure 5.30). The degenerative processes of the plantar fascia usually tend to affect mostly the origin of the fascia in the calcaneus, although this can also be observed within its belly.[7] Similar to what occurs between the patellar tendon at Hoffa's fat pad,[14]

the exams of the plantar fascia are associated with a mandatory study of the heel fat pad which, if found to be affected, would simulate a process of fasciosis (figure 5.31).

KEY POINTS

All ultrasound exams, and even more so when examining a tendon, must be accompanied by a comparative study on the contralateral side. Without this exploratory rule, many minimally degenerative signs could be overlooked.

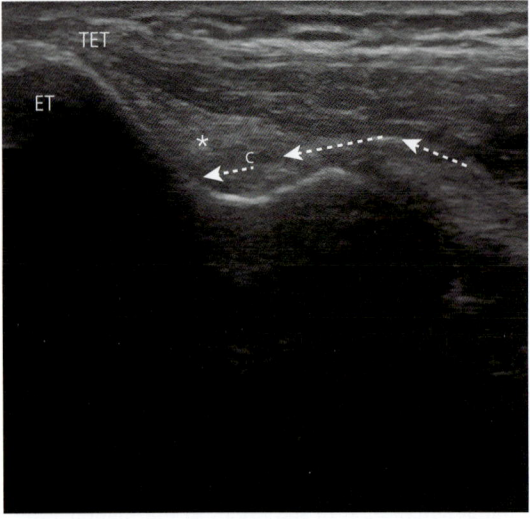

FIGURE 5.32 ■ Longitudinal exploration of a tendon of the epitrochlear muscles (TET). A minimal hypoechoic interphase is observed between the medial compartment of the articular elbow capsule (c) and the medial collateral ligament (*). ET, epitrochlea.

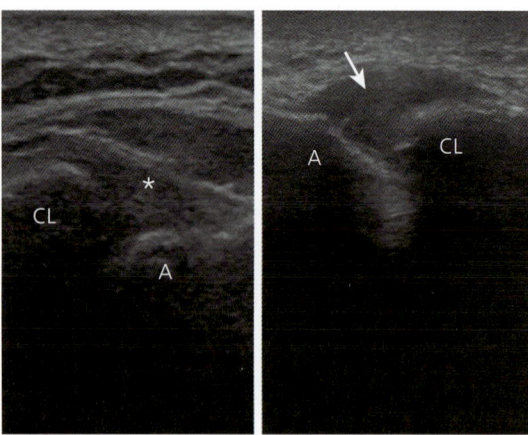

FIGURE 5.33 ■ Comparative contralateral study in an exploration of the acromioclavicular joint. Left: a normal joint is shown in which the articular capsule and the superior acromioclavicular ligament (*) are shown totally joined, ultrasonographically representing the same structure. Right: an unstable joint with excess synovial liquid (arrow) is clearly visible. A, acromion; CL, clavicle.

KEY POINTS

In superficial tendons, such as the epicondyle, it is important to monitor the pressure used for the exploration, as this can alter its width.

5.4.4 The joint and its capsuloligamentous support

The visualization of a normal hyperechoic joint capsule is bound by its dimensions and the amount of support structures it possesses. The study of the femorotibial capsule in an approach to the posterior knee is not at all the same as study of the distal interphalangeal joint. Due to the joint dimensions, the width of the capsule and its proximity to the overlying tissues, in a normal situation it is complicated to discriminate the capsule from the rest of the surrounding tissues (figure 5.32). However, when observing pathological processes, such as posttraumatic arthritis or other articular lesions or capsuloligamentous lesions, the discrimination of this complex is easier, as the contrast between structures is increased, either due to an increase in intra-articular synovial liquid or oedema itself, due to the lesion in the soft tissues (figure 5.33).

As part of the methodological criteria, it is recommended to perform an assessment of the joint during initial explorations. For this purpose, it is important to pay special attention to the possible intra-articular excess of synovial liquid. Once a possible articular lesion is dismissed, the

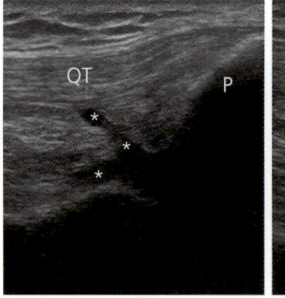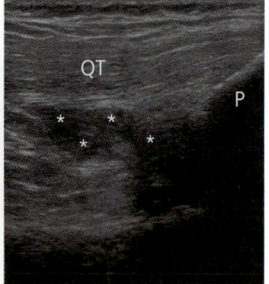

FIGURE 5.34 ■ Comparative contralateral study of a longitudinal exploration of the quadriceps tendon (QT) in its insertion at the base of the patella (P) in order to assess the state of the suprapatellar bursa (*). Right: a bursitis with excess synovial liquid accompanied by pain on weight bearing and joint restriction. The remainder of the soft tissues explored were normal; therefore the treatment was centred on articular stabilization work.

assessment of the soft tissues begins, assessing those that correlate with the symptoms. This is why the exploration of the knee begins with a study of the suprapatellar bursa (figure 5.34), which is usually communicating with the knee joint.

Assessment of the humeroradial and humeroulnar joints in the elbow is further determined by the location of the fat that is found in the radial, coronoid (figure 5.35) and olecranon fossae of the humerus. A situation of articular stress would cause the synovial liquid to project towards the fossae, causing anterior displacement of the previously mentioned fat processes.

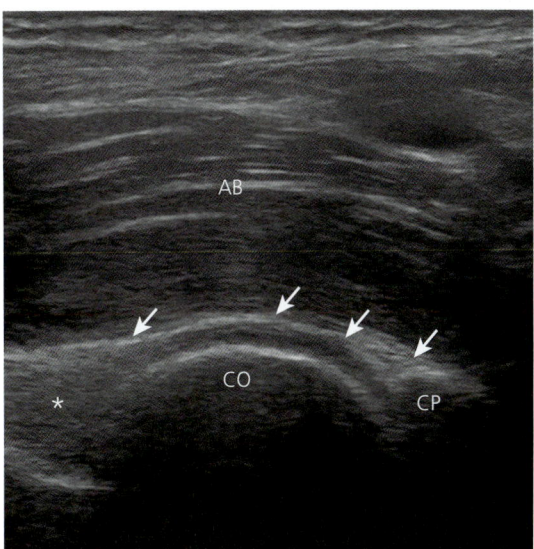

FIGURE 5.35 ■ Longitudinal exploration of the anterior brachialis muscle (AB) where it crosses the humeroulnar joint. This image shows the joint capsule (arrow) and the coronoid fat (*). CP, coronoid process; CO, condyle.

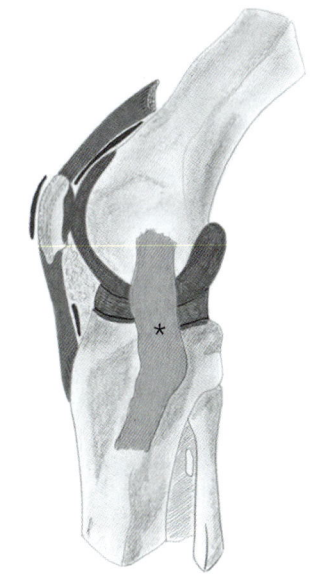

FIGURE 5.36 ■ Lateral view of a knee which shows the superficial fibres of the medial collateral ligament (*) originating in the medial epicondyle of the femur and inserting in the internal and proximal aspect of the tibia. (Colour version of figure is available online).

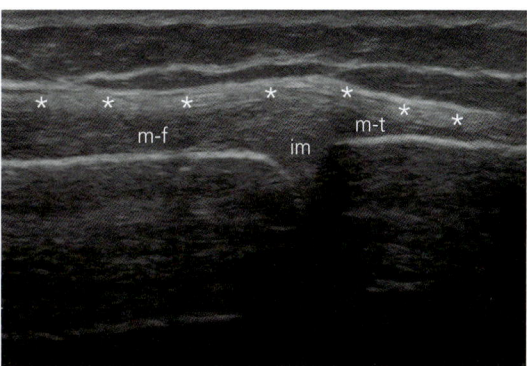

FIGURE 5.37 ■ Longitudinal exploration of the medial collateral ligament where it passes by the articular interline. The superficial and more echogenic fibres (*) are visible passing above the internal meniscus (im), which has a triangular shape and is hyperechogenic. In the second interphase the meniscofemoral (m-f) and meniscotibial (m-t) fibres can be seen.

An excess of articular liquid would cause an increase in articular space, easily verifiable with a comparative study on the contralateral side. If the capsular lesion is large, the joint will lose stability, and therefore it is possible to observe misalignment or even luxation of the articular surfaces. In order to verify the degree of joint stability, dynamic examinations or manual tensioning techniques are advised.

When a capsuloligamentous lesion is assessed, it is advisable to assess the possible cortical defects of the articular surfaces, or the points of capsular insertion that are subject to small bony lesions that are not visible on X-ray.

As with other lesions of the musculoskeletal system, the signs that accompany ligament injuries are thickening and loss of echogenicity (grade I), partial interruption of continuity (grade II) and total rupture (grade III).

In a study of the joint and ligament capsules, the section of choice is longitudinal, as this aids the assessment of signs of normality and of pathology and improves contrast with regard to the periligamentous adipose components. The degeneration and ageing processes imply changes in the ligament which becomes more isoechoic in comparison to the surrounding tissues, and this makes its exploration difficult.[13]

In general, ligaments are narrow, with the exception of the collateral ligaments of the knee or the anterior talofibular ligament, among others. The medial collateral ligament deserves

special mention (figure 5.36), as it displays an evident 2–3 mm width, in which three fascicles are easily differentiated. Thus, a superficial femorotibial fascicle is observed, together with two deep fascicles: the meniscofemoral and meniscotibial fascicles (figure 5.37). As occurs with other soft tissues, the ligaments have conflict areas due to their biomechanical components. The fascicles that are usually affected in the case of sprains of the medial collateral ligament are the femoral origin of the femorotibial (figure

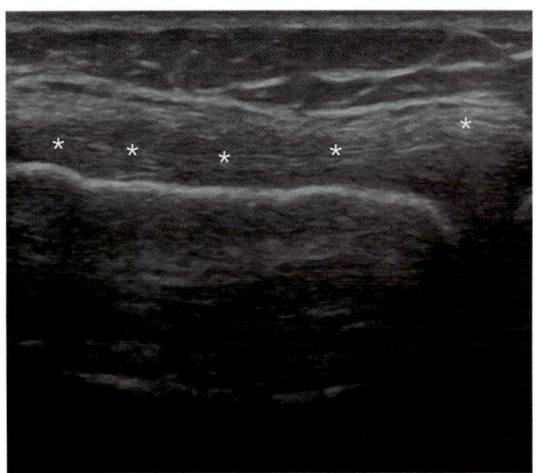

FIGURE 5.38 ■ Longitudinal view of the origin of the medial collateral ligament (*), concretely the femorotibial fibres on the lateral epicondyle.

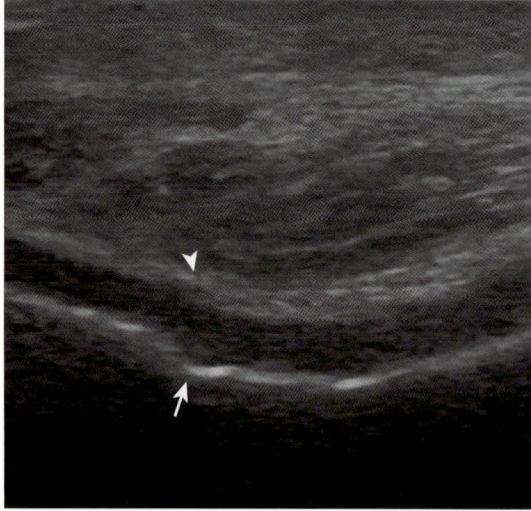

FIGURE 5.39 ■ Ultrasound exploration of the articular cartilage of the femoral trochlea in maximal knee flexion. In the medial portion a small involvement of the subcondral bone is noticeable (arrowhead) related to an irregularity of its overlying cartilage (arrow).

5.38) or the meniscofemoral fascicles, and not the meniscotibial component.

Due to the acoustic shadow caused by the ultrasound beam reflecting on the bone, study of the entire musculoskeletal system is not possible. Some of the structures that are affected by this situation are the anterior and posterior cruciate ligaments of the knee. Only their tibial portion is visible, and this is furthermore made difficult due to the isomorphic echogenicity of the periligamentous fat. However, in the case of disruption in its tibial end, a haematoma may be seen in the proximity of the tibia.

On the other hand, within the joint, it is important to mention the study of the articular cartilage, which is anechoic, and for which a regular width and contour are the easiest signs of appreciable normality (figure 5.39). Its width and exploratory success depend on the joint. For this reason, just as occurs with the cruciate ligaments, the patellar articular cartilage is difficult to assess due to its localization, despite its importance.

Finally, ultrasound is not the best complementary technique for the assessment of hyperechoic fibrocartilage. However, if a lesion exists, it is possible that it can be seen using ultrasound. This is the case with significant meniscal cysts that are characteristic of the external tibial meniscus, and for which their symptomatology and physical exploration simulate degeneration of the iliotibial band (figure 5.40).

5.4.5 Serous synovial bursa

The term bursa comes from the Greek word *prusa*, which means wine skin. This term was adopted due to its characteristic shape, with a maximum width, normally, of around 2 mm.[7,15]

The serous bursae share the same embryonic origin as the joint capsule, and thus can segregate synovial liquid. With regard to their direct or indirect relation with the capsule, two types of bursa may be distinguished: communicating or non-communicating bursae. As previously explained, the exploration of the communicating serous bursae is actually an indirect way of assessing the state of the articulation. On the other hand, the non-communicating bursae can be either superficial or deep. Superficial serous bursae can be due to friction (which explains the existence of bursae named after certain professions), whereas deep bursae are caused by articular degeneration or biomechanical dysfunction.

Non-communicating bursae are treated locally, whereas communicating bursae will also require articular stabilization-type work.

An example of an obvious joint relation is a Baker's cyst, which is considered to be an evagination caused by degeneration of the semimembranosus bursa or of the medial head of gastrocnemius which, in turn, are communicating structures. For this reason, in the interior of the cystic mass, it is common to find loose bodies of a subchondral or meniscal origin. One can also find septa of non-specialized connective tissue. In larger cysts one can observe the duct that communicates the cyst with the bursa, and which opens or closes according to the degree of flexion/extension of the knee (figure 5.41).

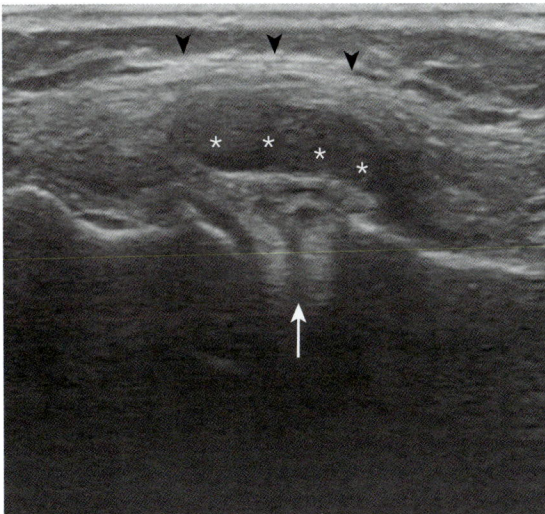
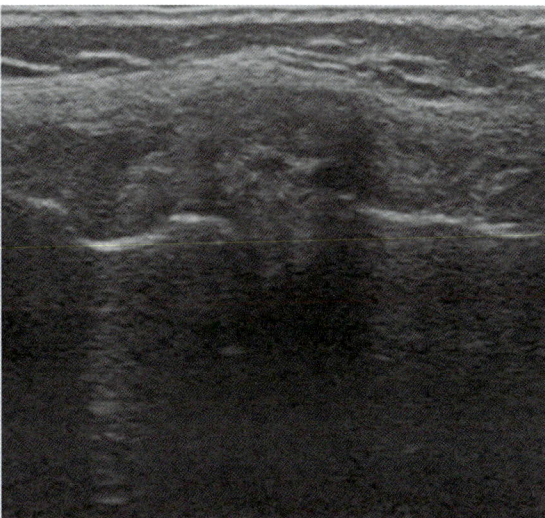

FIGURE 5.40 ■ Comparative follow-up study. An exploration of the external tibial meniscus using the iliotibial band as a window for the approach. Left: the meniscal fissure can be seen (arrow); this communicates the articular space with the water-filled cystic mass (*). The cystic mass is shown projecting towards the surface of the iliotibial band (arrowheads), and palpation in this case would be symptomatic despite the lack of degeneration. Right: the same case after four sessions of percutaneous needle electrolysis, in which the patient was able to return to weight bearing and began gentle continuous jogging with no pain.

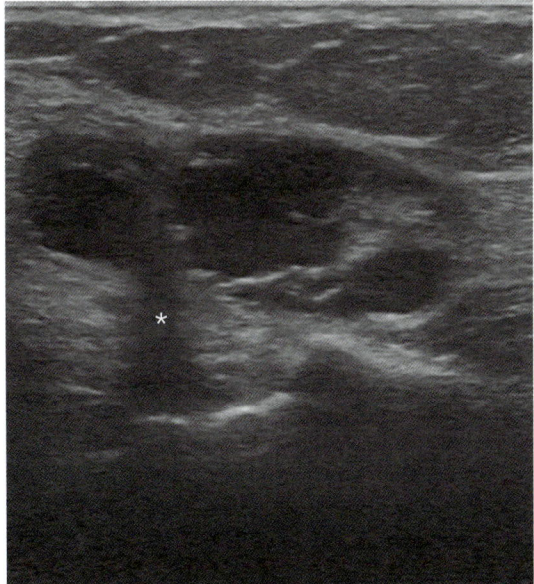

FIGURE 5.41 ■ Posterior approach of the knee in which a multiseptate Baker's cyst is visible communicating with the articular bursa through its characteristic channel (*).

KEY POINTS

The dimensions of a Baker's cyst can invade the interaponeurotic space between the soleus and the medial head of gastrocnemius at the point of its union with the Achilles fascia. This can be confused with a haematoma after muscle aponeurosis avulsion. In this case, the union will be intact and the liquid collection can be followed to the posterior part of the knee.

5.4.6 Bone

Despite the fact that ultrasound is not the best technique for the study of bone lesions, it has been found to be the most sensitive for both assessment of the cortical bone as well as detection of calcifying processes. It is impossible to classify the type of fracture spatially, although it is possible to know of their existence, even when the X-ray has turned out negative.[4]

Thus, it is possible to observe small bony lesions which may have gone unnoticed using radiological techniques, such as the case of hairline fractures of the ribs (figure 5.42), small cortical lesions after ligamentous sprains or even myositis ossificans. Myositis ossificans may be observed under ultrasound 3–4 weeks after the contusion whereas, in order to see this radiologically, an evolution of 3–4 months is the norm.

KEY POINTS

On the other hand, and related to the evolution of soft-tissue lesions, calcifying degenerative processes can be observed far more in advance using ultrasound, in comparison to radiological techniques and, furthermore, they also allow for measurements of increased objectivity.

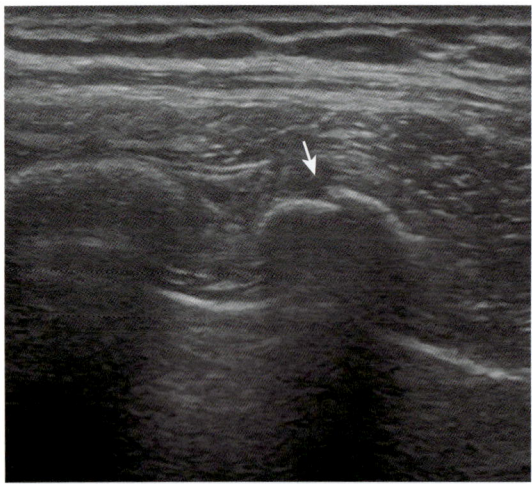

FIGURE 5.42 ■ Transverse costal ultrasound exploration in which a fissure is appreciable (arrow) which did not appear on radiological study.

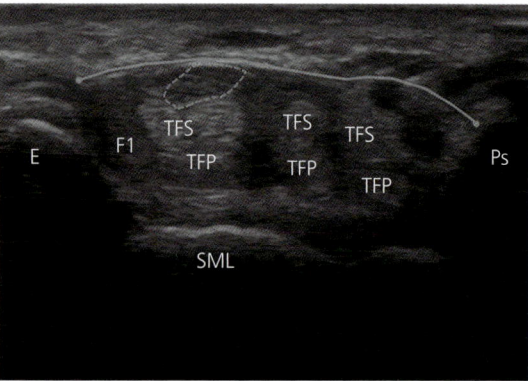

FIGURE 5.43 ■ Transverse view of the median nerve where it passes through the carpal tunnel (concretely, the scaphoid-pisiform section). Topographically we find it related with the following structures: anterior annular ligament (continuous line); TFS, superficial flexor tendons; TFP, deep flexor tendons; F1, flexor hallucis longus tendon; E, scaphoid; Ps, pisiform; SML, semilunar. (Colour version of figure is available online).

5.4.7 Nerve

As explained in previous sections, the nerve has a form and echogenicity similar to that of the tendon and, therefore, it is important to have a thorough anatomical knowledge. Considering how anisotropy-dependent the tendons are, this artefact can be used to discriminate the nerve with more ease.

The echogenicity of the nerve will depend on the structures surrounding it. For this example, the median nerve at the level of the forearm (where it is surrounded by muscle mass) will be viewed as hyperechoic whereas, for example, where it passes through the carpal tunnel and relates with flexor tendons, it can be observed to be hypoechoic.

When one is lacking sufficient experience, it is recommended first to locate the nerves in relation to the muscle masses (where they are discriminated with more ease) and subsequently follow them towards their points of conflict.

The use of ultrasound accompanied by an electrophysiological study has become the technique of choice for the assessment of nerve compressions affecting the peripheral nervous system, displacing magnetic resonance to the second stage. Just like the tendons or muscles, nerves display a hypoechoic matrix related to a network of hyperechoic non-specialized connective tissue (endoneurium, perineurium and epineurium). Perhaps in a transverse section the main differences are apparent with regard to the tendons as, within the nerve, a fascicular axonal disposition is observed (figure 5.43). Unlike the tendons, in a normal situation it is possible to

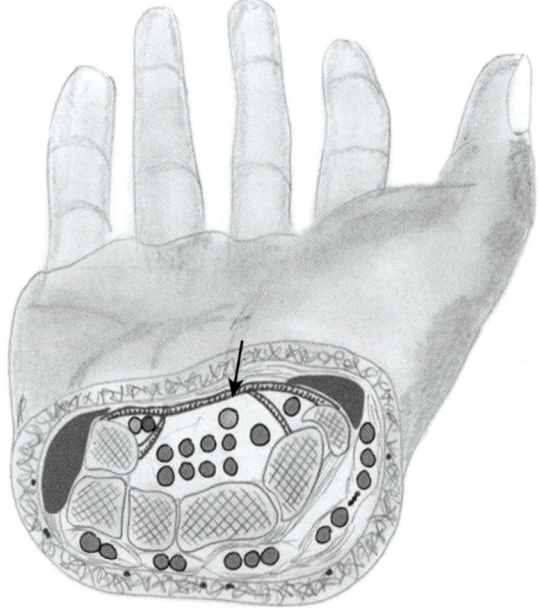

FIGURE 5.44 ■ Transverse section of the wrist in which the median nerve is visible (arrow) passing through the carpal tunnel and its anatomical relation with the flexor tendons. (Colour version of figure is available online).

appreciate a small vascular network accompanying the nerves through the use of colour Doppler.

Nerve compressions are ultrasonographically correlated with three main signs: loss of echogenicity, decrease in width, and increase in surface. Clinically, one of the most frequent nerve compressions encountered is that of the median nerve during its course through the carpal tunnel (figure 5.44). In this case, a longitudinal section is used to assess the difference in width between the compressed section and the healthy proximal portion, prior to the entrance into the carpal tunnel. Some authors consider that this difference in width must not be greater than 3–4 mm. On the other hand, a transverse section is required in order to assess the surface of the nerve, and this is esteemed pathological in cases in which, on account of the oedema, it is more[16] than 9 mm^2.

KEY POINTS

Apart from the static signs (width, echogenicity and surface), the dynamic behaviour of the nerve is considered to be a very important assessment sign, as a compression will entail a movement deficit.

5.5 ARTEFACTS

Topographical knowledge of human anatomy is essential, together with exploratory experience, in order to be successful in a technique as physically complex as ultrasound, in which the appearance of artefacts is frequent. Artefacts are images that do not correspond with real structures and which, during exploration, may be confused with pathological processes. However, the fact of considering them alone can help to distinguish them when they appear. In this sense, according to Van Holsbeeck and Introcaso,[4] there are three major groups of ultrasound artefacts – 'the good, the ugly, and the bad'.

The group of 'good' artefacts includes acoustic shadowing, refractile shadowing, posterior acoustic enhancement and comet tail.

Acoustic shadowing, also known as posterior acoustic shadowing, is exclusively related to the existence of prevailing normal or pathological bone tissue (figure 5.45). The ultrasound waves increase their speed when colliding with the cortical surface, creating a hyperreflection that makes it impossible to observe the echogenicity of the interphases underlying the cortical area. It is possible to appreciate small hyperechogenicity interphases without shadow, which can lead to confusion of a process of fibrous scarring with a calcifying degenerative process. In these cases, the correct position of the focus and the selection of the frequency are key for visualizing the acoustic shadow. Finally, this must not be confused with the dirty shadow (caused by air) in a typical abdominal ultrasound exploration (figure 5.46).

Refractile shadowing, as its name indicates, is linked to the existence of a refraction when

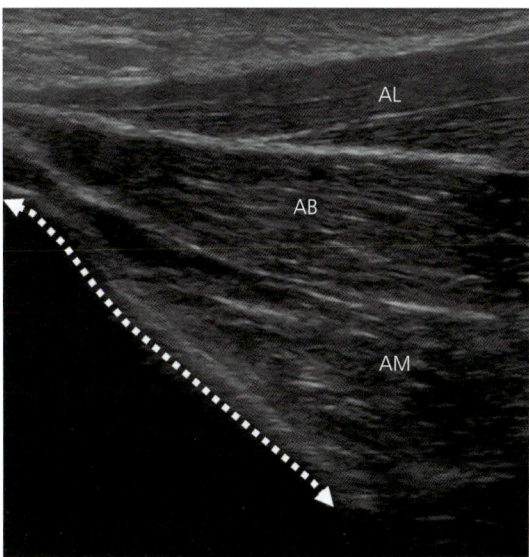

FIGURE 5.45 ■ Longitudinal exploration of the origin of the adductor muscles on the body of the pubis. From superficial to deep, we observe the adductor longus muscle (AL), adductor brevis (AB) and adductor magnus (AM). The discontinuous line shows the hyperechoic image of the cortical bone accompanied by its acoustic shadow.

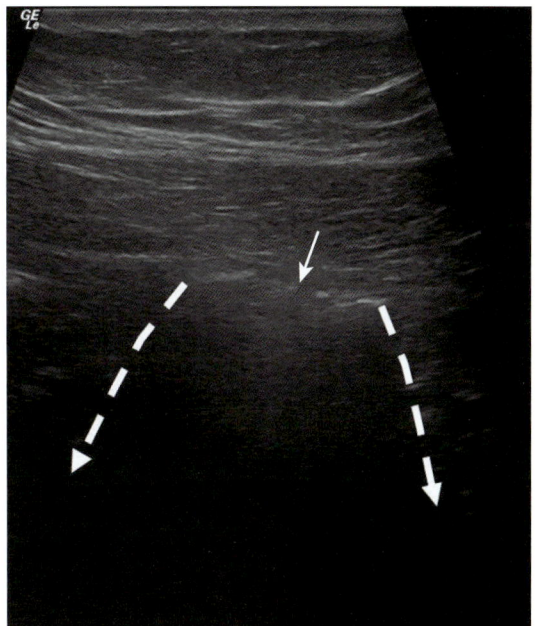

FIGURE 5.46 ■ Abdominal exploration in which the hyperechoic image of air is visible (arrow) accompanied by a dirty shadow (discontinuous arrows).

transversely exploring oval or round structures. This is conditioned by a rapid change in velocity and direction of the ultrasound. It is also common to observe this phenomenon related to fibroadipose muscular strands, where the tissue presents

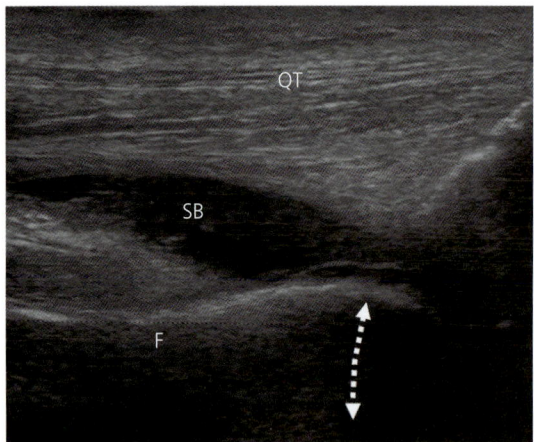

FIGURE 5.47 ■ Longitudinal section of the quadriceps tendon (QT) where the suprapatellar bursa is observed (SB) with an excess of synovial liquid. The posterior acoustic enhancement hides the acoustic shadow of the femur (F).

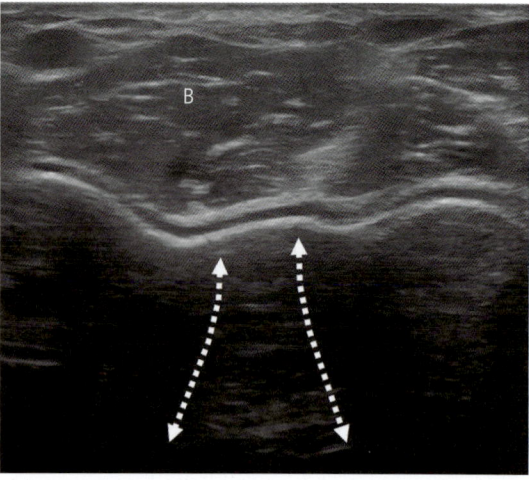

FIGURE 5.48 ■ Transverse view of the brachialis muscle (B). The anterior cortex of the condyle and of the humeral trochlea is very hyperreflectant, and resembles a comet tail (discontinuous arrows).

a fold. This also occurs in total tendon ruptures after the first 'acute' stage.

Posterior acoustic enhancement appears when the ultrasound waves are confronted with liquid anechoic interphases overlying solid reflecting interphases (figure 5.47). When colliding with a liquid surface, these waves increase their propagation velocity, which entails an increase in the echogenicity of the underlying structures. Clinically, this is a sign that helps to distinguish abnormalities of liquid content. On the other hand, it is important to consider that not all fluids will always be related to posterior enhancements, due to the many changes that they may go through and according to their stage of repair. For example, a haematoma changes its behaviour according to its evolution and in relation to the biochemical changes suffered due to the haemoglobin.

Finally, among the so-called 'good' artefacts, the comet tail is found (figure 5.48). This is believed to be a form of reverberation artefact, and appears when the ultrasound waves collide with a strongly reflectant surface (more than the bone itself), such as the case of prosthetic material, crystals or wood splinters. The surface is hyperreflectant enough for the signal to rebound back to the surface of the transducer, and this process is repeated on several occasions. It is also common to observe this as an effect of the bone itself.

This phenomenon entails that the original hyperreflectant interphase is repeated in depth, with its diameter being inversely proportional. This type of artefact aids the detection and localization of osteosynthesis material which may be

suffering from a process of symptomatic fibrotic scarring or small foreign bodies.

Among the 'ugly' artefacts we find electric noise, which is very common and a product of the existence of electromagnetic interferences. This artefact is quickly and easily detected and is not usually confused with abnormalities. It appears frequently, although it is thought that it does not exist close to an electromagnetic source. When it does appear, it is a good time to remind our patients to switch off their mobile phones.

There is a group of artefacts considered 'bad' because they can be confused with pathological processes. Among them we can highlight the mirror image and anisotropy.

In section 5.2, we have already explained the mirror image. It is a typical finding in the exploration of the internal cortex of the tibia and is caused by hyperreflexion due to its density and proximity to the body surface (figure 5.4). In normal conditions, it is just a simple finding, but if it is accompanied by a simple posttrauma-embedded haematoma, this artefact can cause the anechoic interphase to be found over and underlying the cortex, and thus may be confused with more serious bone pathology. In these cases, the knowledge of this phenomenon and the integrity of the cortex are both reassuring signs for the clinician.

Lastly, anisotropy occurs due to refraction caused by a lack of perpendicularity in the exploration. This is a typical finding at the osteotendinous junctions of tendons (and at times inevitable) in longitudinal sections, due to a lack of tension, and which compels examination of the patellar tendon with slight knee flexion or the Achilles tendon in dorsal flexion of the ankle (figure 5.49). This is also evident in transverse sections, due to errors in the angle of the transducer, when one can appreciate virtual disappearance of the tendon. Mainly in the case of transverse sections, it is important to be more vigilant of the tilt angle of the transducer (figure 5.50). Tendons are more anisotropic than nerves, and this knowledge can aid observation, for example, of the median nerve in its passage through the carpal tunnel, by making gentle changes in the angle of the transducer (figure 5.51).

When transverse sections of large muscle masses are performed, anisotropy is also typical in the non-priority areas and those that are distant from the optimal zone. This phenomenon is resolved by simply prioritizing these areas.

Anisotropy is the subject of many frequently asked questions on the subject of ultrasound. This phenomenon, related to the hypoechoic interphase, may at times be confused with a tendinopathy when visualizing a tendon section. In this case, considering the almost inevitable insertion anisotropies that tendons suffer, how can we distinguish an insertion anisotropy from a tendinopathy? The answer is that tendinopathies, during an initial symptomatic phase, apart from their decreased echogenicity, are correlated with an increased width and lack of internal

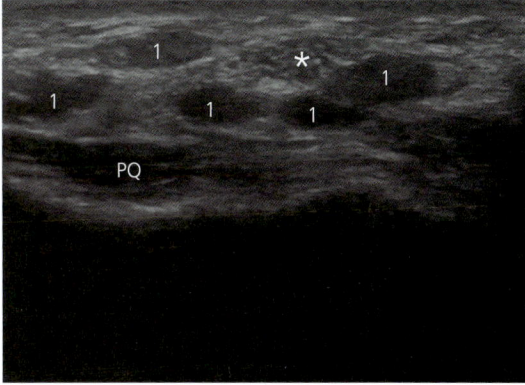

FIGURE 5.51 ■ Transverse exploration of the anterior compartment of the distal third of the forearm. At the centre of the image, the median nerve is observed (*) accompanied by the flexor tendons (1). In depth, the pronator quadratus muscle (PQ) is visible. The flexor tendons appear with a loss of echogenicity due to anisotropy, which improves the ability to discriminate the nerve.

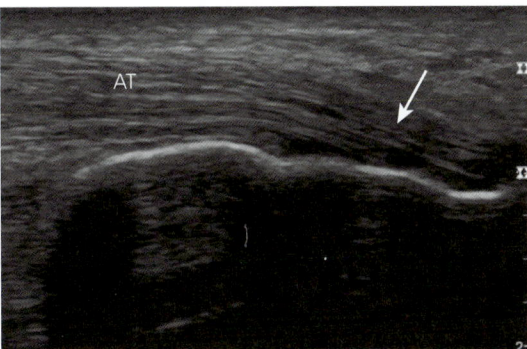

FIGURE 5.49 ■ Longitudinal exploration of the insertion of the Achilles tendon (AT). Despite pre-tensioning the structure, a loss of echogenicity is observed (white arrow) as a sign of insertion anisotropy.

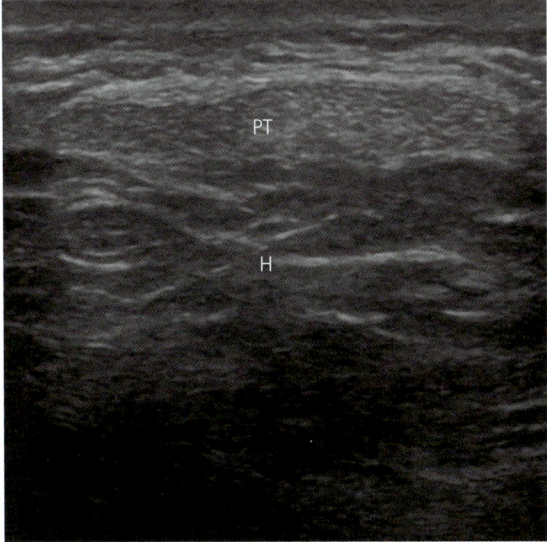 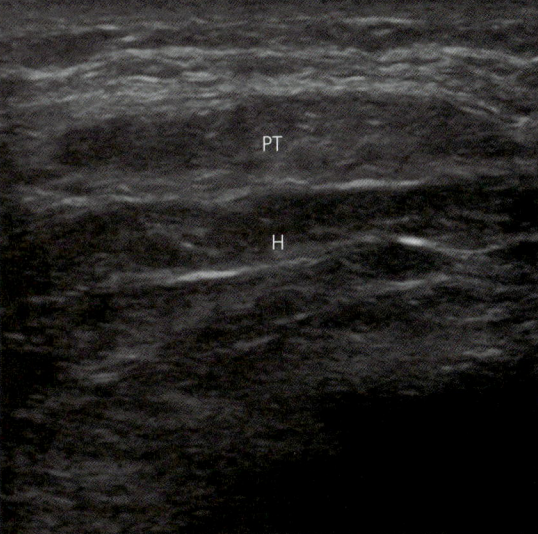

FIGURE 5.50 ■ Transverse exploration of the patellar tendon (PT) at 1 cm from the inferior pole of the patella, in which Hoffa's fat pad (H) is observed in depth. The image on the left has been taken correctly, whereas on the right, the transducer has been incorrectly angled, and this causes the tendon to be shown with a great loss of echogenicity as a sign of anisotropy.

structure. On the other hand, in the case of anisotropy, the findings are restricted to an isolated loss of echogenicity that can be corrected by rectifying the angle of the transducer.

5.6 REFERENCES

1. Mc-Nally E. Ecografía musculoesquelética. Madrid: Marbán; 2008.
2. Jiménez JF. ECO musculoesquelética. Madrid: Marbán; 2010.
3. Ríos V. Manual de ecografía musculoesquelética. Madrid: Editorial Médica Panamericana; 2010.
4. Van Holsbeeck MT, Introcaso JH. Ecografía musculoesquelética. Madrid: Marbán; 2008.
5. Bueno A. Ecografía musculoesquelética esencial. Madrid: Editorial Médica Panamericana; 2011.
6. Bianchi S, Martinoli C. Ecografía musculoesquelética. Madrid: Marbán; 2011.
7. Jiménez JF. Ecografía del aparato locomotor. Madrid: Marbán; 2007.
8. De Groot A, Martínez-Payá JJ, Ríos-Díaz J, et al. Error en la palpación del tendón largo del bíceps braquial. Estudio guiado mediante ecografía. XI Jornadas Nacionales I Congreso Internacional de Fisioterapia de la Actividad Física y el Deporte. Madrid; 2009. p. 174.
9. Balius R. Ecografía musculoesquelética. Badalona: Editorial Paidotribo; 2007.
10. Sikdar S, Shah JP, Gebreab T, et al. Novel applications of ultrasound technology to visualize and characterize myofascial trigger points and surrounding soft tissue. Arch Phys Med Rehabil 2009;90:1829–38.
11. Balius R. Patología muscular en el deporte. Barcelona: Elsevier (Masson); 2005.
12. De Groot A, Ríos-Díaz J, Martínez-Payá JJ, et al. Comportamiento morfo-ecogénico y textural del tendón rotuliano frente a estímulos de estrés. XI Jornadas Nacionales I Congreso Internacional de Fisioterapia de la Actividad Física y el Deporte. Madrid; 2009. p. 201.
13. Martínez-Payá JJ. Anatomía ecográfica del hombro. Herramienta de prevención, diagnóstico, investigación y validación de técnicas terapéuticas. Madrid: Editorial Médica Panamericana; 2008.
14. Ly JQ, Bui-Mansfield LT. Anatomy of and abnormalities associated with Kager's fat Pad. AJR 2004;182: 147–54.
15. Brasseur JL, Tardieu M. Ecografía del sistema locomotor. Barcelona: Masson; 1999.
16. Altinok T, Baysal O, Karakas HM, et al. Ultrasonographic assessment of mild and moderate idiopathic carpal tunel syndrome. Clin Radiol 2004;59:916–25.

CHAPTER 6

ULTRASOUND APPLICATIONS TO VISUALIZE AND CHARACTERIZE MYOFASCIAL TRIGGER POINTS AND SURROUNDING SOFT TISSUE

Jay P. Shah • Juliana Heimur

Doctors pour drugs of which they know little, to cure diseases of which they know less, into human beings of which they know nothing.

VOLTAIRE

CHAPTER OUTLINE

KEYWORDS

Doppler; blood flow; nodule; local twitch response; myofascial pain syndrome (MPS); sonoelastography; ultrasound.

6.1 INTRODUCTION

Myofascial pain syndrome (MPS) describes a chronic pain condition that arises from muscle and its connective tissue. MPS is a specific non-inflammatory condition, characterized by regional pain that often presents in select quadrants of the body. A prominent characteristic of MPS is the presence of one or more myofascial trigger points (MTrPs) – discrete, hyper-irritable nodules found within taut bands of skeletal muscle. MPS arises from active MTrPs which cause pain in local and/or distant tissue in particular referral patterns. The prevalence of MPS is high, affecting up to 85% of patients in pain management cases,[1,2] and similar levels in general medicine[3] and dental clinics.[4] MTrPs are often an unidentified source of pain and muscle dysfunction and diagnosis depends exclusively on subjective measures. Ultrasound has been explored as an objective, reliable and repeatable diagnostic test for evaluation of MTrPs. This chapter discusses the use of two-dimensional (2D) grey-scale, Doppler and vibration sonoelastography to visualize and characterize MTrPs and surrounding soft tissue better.

6.2 MYOFASCIAL PAIN SYNDROME

6.2.1 Current diagnostic criteria

MTrPs arise from clusters of contraction knots in adjacent muscle fibres (figure 6.1). They may present in active or latent states. Spontaneous pain is indicative of an active MTrP, and this pain can be reproduced and exacerbated by pressure

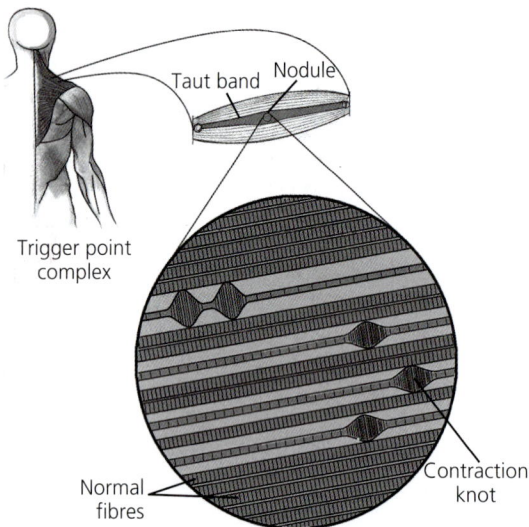

FIGURE 6.1 ■ Schematic of a trigger point complex. A trigger point complex in a taut band of muscle is composed of multiple contraction knots. (Adapted from Simons DG, Travell JG. Myofascial Pain and Dysfunction: The Trigger Point Manual. Vol. 1 Upper Half of Body. 2nd ed. Baltimore, MD: Williams & Wilkins; 1999, and original figure by sv: Användare: Chrizz.) (Colour version of figure is available online).

on the nodule. Latent MTrPs do not cause spontaneous pain but have the similar physical findings of palpable nodules within a taut band of skeletal muscle. When firm digital pressure is applied, latent MTrPs may elicit pain. In fact, the pain pressure threshold has been shown to be significantly different in active and latent MTrPs when compared to normal sites.[5] Both types of MTrP may cause referral pain to distant and seemingly unrelated areas, muscle dysfunction, weakness and a limited range of motion.

Patient history and physical examination are critical in identifying MTrPs. The patient's reported pain patterns can help to suggest which muscles are involved. A clinician trained in muscle examination techniques must palpate the muscle to identify a taut band. The nodule along the taut band which elicits the maximum tenderness is the MTrP. *Myofascial Pain and Dysfunction: The Trigger Point Manual* contains detailed instructions for examination.[6]

A characteristic finding of an MTrP is the presence of a local twitch response (LTR). This is an involuntary, localized contraction of muscle fibres that is both rapid and transient. It can be elicited with mechanical palpation, particularly with the dry needling technique. Muscle shortening is not evident through imaging, therefore needle insertion is a valuable tool to confirm the presence of an MTrP.[7] However, eliciting an LTR requires a high degree of skill and is thus considered an unreliable method of evaluation.

MTrP diagnosis depends upon examiner experience and training, which raises concerns of its validity. Some studies found low interrater reliability among examiners in their attempts to identify MTrPs.[8,9] Low interrater reliability may be due in part to the lack of an official list of diagnostic criteria. To adjust for the inconsistency, Gerwin et al.[10] outlined essential criteria for an MTrP: (1) an exquisitely tender spot found in a taut band of muscle; (2) an LTR and/or referred pain to distant sites upon manual palpation or needling of the tender spot; (3) restricted range of motion; (4) reproduction of the patient's pain complaint through pressure on the MTrP; (5) regional muscle weakness; and (6) autonomic symptoms. The fourth criterion is only applicable to active MTrPs since latent MTrPs do not cause spontaneous pain.

6.2.2 New lines of assessment

MTrPs are often an unidentified source of pain and muscle dysfunction and diagnosis depends exclusively on subjective measures. Therefore, there is a need for an objective, reliable and repeatable diagnostic test for evaluation of MTrPs. Promising lines of research have emerged using existing forms of technology. In the 1950s, surface electrodes were used to identify low-resistance points on the skin.[11] Thermography was later used to image MTrPs[12,13] and differentiate active from latent sites.[14] Shock-wave technology was even considered in MTrP identification.[15] Chen et al.[16] succeeded in using magnetic resonance elastography for this purpose.

Our group explored the use of ultrasound to visualize MTrPs, surrounding soft tissue and vasculature. This technology provides non-invasive, real-time imaging and is suitable for use in a clinical office. Ultrasound is readily available and has the potential to characterize viscoelastic properties of myofascial tissue,[17] quantify haemodynamic changes, provide measures of tissue performance and demonstrate structure and function correlations.[18–20] It provides a method to obtain descriptive information of tissue, such as the presence of fat, fibre and fluid, in addition to its mechanical properties.[21,22]

6.2.3 Methods of investigation

To investigate myofascial pain, healthy volunteers and individuals suffering from neck pain enrolled in our protocols. Participants underwent physical examination by a physiatrist to determine the presence or absence of MTrPs in the upper trapezius muscle, according to standard clinical criteria.[6] Four sites were marked on each participant as active MTrPs, latent MTrPs or normal tissue. Pain pressure threshold was measured at each site using pressure algometry. Following the physical examination, sonography was performed by examiners who were blinded to the site classifications and clinical status of the participant. The upper trapezius was visualized in three stages: 2D grey-scale imaging, Doppler and vibration sonoelastography.[5,17,23–26]

Physical examination

Physical examinations revealed certain trends. Medially located MTrPs had a higher prevalence than those in the lateral upper trapezius muscle. Furthermore, one study[23] showed that 83% of active MTrPs had symmetrical active or latent MTrPs bilaterally. Active MTrPs had lower pain pressure thresholds than latent MTrPs, and these latent MTrP sites had significantly lower pain pressure thresholds than normal control sites. It was determined that pain pressure threshold is a fair classifier of active versus normal sites but a poor classifier between other site types. However, the visual analogue scale separated active from latent MTrPs well.[23]

Diagnostic ultrasound technology

Diagnostic ultrasound is extensively used for non-invasive real-time imaging of soft tissue, such as muscle, tendon, fascia and blood vessels.[17] Further, it is a low-risk method to obtain descriptive information of tissue and assess its properties.[21,22] Our group investigated the feasibility of ultrasound imaging in visualizing MTrPs and surrounding muscle. Throughout each study, we used the Philips iU22 clinical ultrasound system with a 12.5 MHz linear array L12-5 transducer.[5,23,26] Sonoelastography was performed using an external vibrational tool of approximately 92 Hz.[23–25] SonixRP ultrasound system (Ultrasonix, Vancouver, BC) and a 5–14 MHz linear array transducer were used for later investigation of vibration sonoelastography.[24,25] To examine shear waves through the upper trapezius, we used a vibrational tool with a variable power supply, allowing us to vibrate the muscle at different frequencies.[24]

Grey-scale imaging

Participants were seated upright in a comfortable position. The upper trapezius was visualized using longitudinal and transverse views on B-mode 2D grey-scale imaging. Normal sites appeared to have uniform fibre orientation throughout the tissue (figure 6.2A). MTrPs appeared as focal hypoechoic regions (darker than the surrounding area), elliptical or band-like in shape, and with increased fibre alignment heterogeneity[5,17,24] (figure 6.2B). These sites corresponded with the location of the palpable nodule from the physical examination. Under ultrasound imaging, a single MTrP often appeared as multiple, smaller nodules in close proximity to one another. Hypoechoic areas from active and latent MTrPs were significantly larger than those sites marked as normal; however there was no significant difference in size between active and latent MTrPs.[5]

Blood flow

Using Doppler ultrasound, we investigated the vasculature and circulation of the marked sites and their surrounding tissue, specifically the ascending branch of the transverse cervical artery and any other arteries or enlarged arterioles in the neighbourhood region. Our group measured peak systolic velocity (PSV) and minimum diastolic velocity (MDV) near marked sites. Two calculations were used to assess blood flow. The resistive index (RI) is commonly used in vascular diagnosis, as it indicates the resistance of the end-organ vascular bed. The RI is the ratio of the difference in peak systolic and minimum diastolic velocities to the peak systolic velocity, shown in the equation $RI = ([PSV - MDV]/PSV)$. An $RI = 1$ in muscle indicates normal, non-diastolic flow. However, $RI < 1$ indicates elevated diastolic flow and decreased vascular bed resistance, while $RI > 1$ indicates negative diastolic flow and increased vascular bed resistance. The pulsatility index (PI) was also examined, as this quantifies the level of flow oscillation between systole and diastole, as seen in the equation $PI = ([PSV - MDV]/mean\ velocity)$.[5]

Blood vessels were visualized using colour Doppler imaging in the immediate vicinity of the MTrPs, occasionally very close to the MTrP itself. Studies showed that active MTrPs have significantly higher peak systolic velocities and negative diastolic velocities, along with significantly lower minimum diastolic, when compared to latent MTrPs and normal muscle[5,26] (figure 6.3). RI was used to identify negative diastolic flow. Our first study revealed differences between active and latent MTrPs, as 69% of active MTrPs showed unique Doppler flow waveforms with retrograde diastolic flow compared to only 16.7% of latent MTrPs.[5] A later study confirmed that the occurrence of retrograde diastolic flow was significantly higher in active and latent sites when compared to normal muscle tissue.[23]

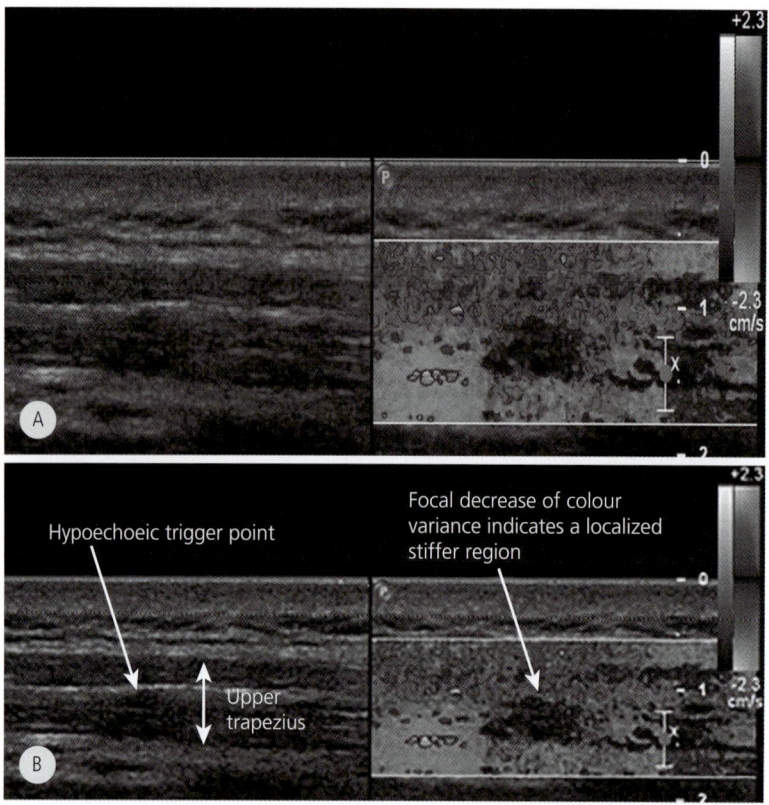

FIGURE 6.2 ■ (A) Normal upper trapezius muscle. A myofascial trigger point is not palpable and the normal muscle appears isoechoic and has uniform colour variance. (B) Upper trapezius muscle with a palpable myofascial trigger point. A hypoechoic region and a well-defined focal decrease of colour variance indicating a localized stiffer region are visible. (Colour version of figure is available online).

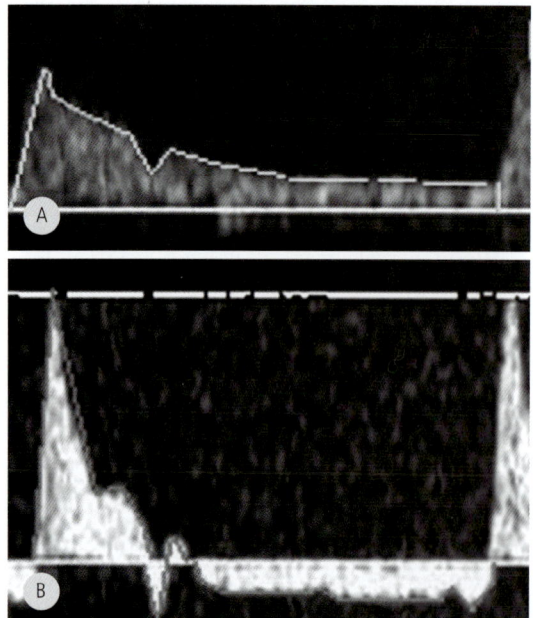

FIGURE 6.3 ■ (A) Doppler velocity spectrum near a latent myofascial trigger point (MTrP). (B) Doppler velocity spectrum near an active MTrP. (Colour version of figure is available online).

The PI is indicative of flow oscillation within the vasculature. Using spectral Doppler imaging, our group found that active and latent MTrPs had highly pulsatile flow more often than normal muscle tissue, though there were no significant differences between active and latent MTrPs.[5,23,26] PI therefore has the ability to distinguish MTrPs from normal sites. Thus, we are able to conclude that MTrPs are associated with blood flow abnormalities.[23]

Vibration sonoelastography

Vibration sonoelastography utilizes an external vibration source of less than 1000 Hz. Used in conjunction with Doppler, our group performed sonoelastography in two stages. The first implemented the Philips iU22 clinical ultrasound system with an external hand-held vibrating massager with a modified flat-head attachment head. Colour Doppler variance imaging was performed while inducing vibrations of ~92 Hz. The hand-held vibrational tool was placed 2–3 cm from each marked site. Colour variance mode was used to image wave propagation from the vibrational tool through selected muscle tissue. Accordingly, MTrPs appeared as focal areas of reduced vibration amplitude, indicating a region of increased tissue stiffness. Further, these areas of reduced vibration amplitude corresponded with the localized hypoechoic regions observed in 2D grey-scale imaging for all subjects.[5]

The 92 Hz tool was also used to analyse the cross-section area of marked sites. On sonoelastography, sites of active MTrPs were significantly larger than latent MTrPs and palpably normal tissue. Further, latent MTrPs were significantly larger than normal muscle tissue. Thus, it was concluded that area measurements are excellent classifiers of site type and could robustly distinguish among active MTrPs, latent MTrPs, and palpably normal sites. However, when compared to sensitivity of pain, there was no linear correlation between pain pressure threshold and hypoechoic area of the MTrP. In this study, it was concluded that vibration sonoelastography was an effective method for measuring the cross-section area of MTrPs and the size was excellent in determining the site type.[23]

Later studies implemented varying frequencies in sonoelastography. A hand-held vibrational tool with a variable power supply was fabricated[24,25] in conjunction with the previously mentioned modified flat-head attachment.[5] This tool allowed the muscle tissue to be externally vibrated at selected frequencies of 60 Hz, 110 Hz, 160 Hz and 200 Hz. Using the SonixRP US system, raw data were acquired from both symptomatic and asymptomatic patients. Upon analysis, active MTrPs in the upper trapezius muscle had significantly higher shear modulus than palpably normal tissue, indicating stiffer tissue. This method was therefore capable of quantitatively measuring region-specific shear properties in both muscle tissue harbouring active MTrPs and normal tissue.[24] When high-frequency excitations (>100 Hz) were used, shear wave speeds were significantly higher in active MTrPs and their surrounding tissue in comparison to palpably normal tissue.[25]

6.3 DISCUSSION AND CONCLUSION

The pathogenesis of myofascial pain is not yet fully understood. A few postulations on MTrP formation exist, including Simons' integrated hypothesis. This hypothesis proposes that a lack of adenosine triphosphate leads to an 'energy crisis' which perpetuates an initial sustained sarcomere contracture, or an MTrP. Muscle fibre contraction can cause capillary constriction, compromising circulation and thus increasing local metabolic demands. Ischaemia and hypoxia sensitize peripheral nociceptors and thereby cause more pain and tenderness at the MTrP.[15,27–29] Findings from our group support Simons' integrated hypothesis.[5,17,23–26,30]

Our studies used ultrasound to characterize the soft-tissue environment of the upper trapezius muscle. Results of 2D grey-scale imaging confirm that significant tissue abnormalities and morphological changes are associated with MTrPs. Active and latent MTrPs appear as one or more focal hypoechoic regions on grey-scale and colour variance ultrasound imaging. These hypoechoic areas are absent in palpably normal myofascial tissue. Differences in echogenicity of MTrPs compared to normal tissue suggest a disruption of normal muscle fibre structure and local tissue characteristics. The hypoechoic regions may be indicative of contraction knots resulting from increased muscle fibre recruitment and contraction, local injury, localized regions of ischaemia[5] and/or low-level muscle contractions accompanying stereotypical movement patterns.[31,32] It should be noted, however, that some hypoechoic regions were observed when nodules were not palpable on physical examination.[5] Echotexture and echogenicity of muscle under ultrasound may depend on additional factors that lead to this observation, such as density, spacing between fibres, orientation of fibres, fat or fluid content or tissue heterogeneity.

Ultrasound imaging enables clinicians to investigate the vasculature and blood flow characteristics of myofascial tissue. Results from our investigation associate distinct blood flow disturbances with the pathophysiology of MTrPs. The Doppler blood flow waveforms near active MTrPs showed increased systolic velocities and flow reversal with negative diastolic velocities – results that were significantly different from latent MTrPs and normal, uninvolved muscle. These findings are indicative of a highly resistive vascular bed. An increase in vascular resistance at sites containing active MTrPs is consistent with blood vessel compression, caused either by sustained contracture at the MTrP or constriction caused by oxidative stress or hypoxia. Blood vessel compression may be sufficient to induce local hypoperfusion, hypoxia and other pathophysiological developments, leading to the pain, tenderness and nodularity of an active MTrP. Previous studies have shown that high intramuscular pressure significantly impedes local blood flow. This suggests that pain secondary to active MTrPs may be caused indirectly by decreased blood flow to the nodule, further supporting Simons' integrated hypothesis.[15,29] Hypoperfusion may lead to the observed low partial pressure of oxygen (PO_2) and contractures, as low PO_2 is probably associated with a lack of adenosine triphosphate.[5] A study of tissue oxygenation indicated a focal region of hypoxia at the centre of the MTrP and a surrounding region of hyperoxia.[33] In fact, low oxygen levels are potent factors to release bradykinin, a sensitizing agent for muscle nociceptors.[5,23,26] Furthermore, inflammation, haemodynamic stress, hypoxia and tissue distress at the MTrP may lead to vascular remodelling[33] at the site of the nodule.

Beyond the resistivity of blood vessels, arteries in the neighbourhood of both active and latent MTrPs had highly pulsatile blood flow more often than palpably normal muscle tissue. Two explanations could account for the difference in pulsatility: an increase in outflow resistance and/or an increase in the compliance and volume of the vascular compartment. Increased outflow resistance could be due to a number of factors, including muscle contracture at the MTrP that compresses the capillary/venous bed, anatomical influences related to the geometry of the apex of the upper trapezius muscle that apply external compression, local vasoconstriction due to inflammation or externally applied pressure by the ultrasound transducer. An increased vascular volume acts as a reservoir into which the blood flows during systole and flows out during diastole. The significance of an increased vascular volume is not yet fully understood but it may help to elucidate the pathophysiological mechanisms of MTrPs and myofascial pain. We have observed that active MTrPs predominantly present in the apex of the upper trapezius and therefore the anatomy could, indeed, contribute to their formation.[5,23,26] Previous studies revealed elevated levels of proinflammatory mediators and other neuropeptides associated with vasodilatory and angiogenic effects in the vicinity of active MTrPs.[30,34] These biochemicals may play a role in the observed blood flow waveforms.

Our group used vibration sonoelastography to investigate MTrPs and normal muscle quantitatively. MTrPs appeared as focal regions of reduced vibration amplitude, indicative of increased stiffness compared to surrounding tissue. It is believed that these stiffer nodules are a result of muscle fibre contractures. We found vibration sonoelastography to be an effective method for measuring MTrP size and excellent in distinguishing among active MTrPs, latent MTrPs and palpably normal tissue. However, there was no correlation between MTrP size and pain pressure threshold, suggesting that other

mechanisms may contribute independently to MTrP size and sensitivity.[23] The presence of sensitizing biochemicals such as neuropeptides and catecholamines may influence the pain sensitivity of myofascial tissue, as elevated levels were previously found in active MTrPs.[34] By vibrating the upper trapezius at high frequencies, we observed that shear wave speeds were higher in symptomatic tissue than normal muscle tissue. Thus, it may be concluded that increased tissue heterogeneity exists at active MTrPs and their surrounding tissue.

Our team sought to investigate a novel application of ultrasound to identify and characterize abnormalities associated with MTrPs and their surrounding soft-tissue environment. Findings from our sonographic studies may help to elucidate the pathophysiological mechanisms underlying the development and natural history of myofascial dysfunction, as we have shown differences between active MTrPs, latent MTrPs and palpably normal tissue. We have been able to understand better the complex environment surrounding MTrPs by studying objective measurements such as blood flow, MTrP size and mechanical shear properties of the region. Ultrasound was selected since the technology is safe, non-invasive, cost-effective and readily available in the clinical setting. It is our aim to help establish objective diagnostic criteria for the identification and classification of MTrPs through a method that is more reliable, sensitive and specific than physical examination alone. These qualities enable it to be used in longitudinal monitoring of MTrPs. By examining changes in size, appearance, stiffness and/or blood flow, clinicians may objectively measure treatment outcomes.

6.4 LIMITATIONS

While we believe that ultrasound technology has applicability in the field of myofascial pain, there are several limitations to our studies that should be acknowledged. The ultrasound transducer used in our studies created 2D images. However, the MTrP is a three-dimensional nodule. To assess the MTrP more accurately, a three-dimensional ultrasound transducer should be used in future studies. Though the sonographer attempts consistency among participants, the operator technique is difficult to control and is determined subjectively. The amount of pressure and the angle at which the transducer is applied to the skin are not quantitatively assessed.[5,26] Additionally, vibration sonoelastography is very sensitive to the position of the hand-held vibrational tool. The shear wave can be missed if the tool and ultrasound transducer are not properly positioned. To address this issue and ensure shear wave propagation, we used real-time visualization of the phase image to allow the user to adjust the positions of the transducer and vibrational tool on to the skin.[24] Concerning blood flow waveforms, we did not measure reproducibility, nor did we analyse systemic changes.[26] Though some painfree control participants were studied, most 'normal' sites were marked at least 5 cm from MTrP sites on symptomatic individuals.[23] Finally, a single physiatrist and sonographer performed all examinations and we did not assess intraobserver and interobserver variabilities.[5,26] A definitive model for the aetiology of myofascial pain and MTrPs is premature; however, we believe that our application of ultrasound expands upon current knowledge and brings us closer to developing a model of the pathophysiology of MTrPs and their objective treatment measures.[5,23]

6.5 Acknowledgements

We would like to acknowledge all members of our research team: Katherine Armstrong, Tadesse Gebreab, Lynn H Gerber, Paul Otto, Diego Turo and Siddhartha Sikdar.

6.6 REFERENCES

1. Gerwin RD. Classification, epidemiology, and natural history of myofascial pain syndrome. Curr Pain Headache Rep 2001;5:412–20.
2. Fishbain DA, Goldberg M, Meagher BR, et al. Male and female chronic pain patients categorized by DSM-III psychiatric diagnostic criteria. Pain 1986;2: 181–97.
3. Skootsky SA, Jaeger B, Oye RK. Prevalence of myofascial pain in general internal medicine practice. West J Med 1989;151:157–60.
4. Graff-Radford B. Myofascial trigger points: Their importance and diagnosis in the dental office. J Dent Assoc S Afr 1984;39:249–53.
5. Sikdar S, Shah JP, Gebreab T, et al. Novel applications of ultrasound technology to visualize and characterize myofascial trigger points (MTrPs) and surrounding soft tissue. Arch Phys Med Rehabil 2009;90:1829–38.
6. Travell JG, Simons DG. Myofascial pain and dysfunction: the trigger point manual. VI and VII ed. Baltimore: Williams & Wilkins; 1999.
7. Travell JG, Rinzler SH. The myofascial genesis of pain. Postgrad Med 1952;11:434–52.
8. Njoo KH, Van der Does E. The occurrence and interrater reliability of myofascial trigger points in the quadratus lumborum and gluteus medius: a prospective study in non-specific low back pain patients and controls in general practice. Pain 1994;58(3):317–23.
9. Wolfe F, Simons DG, Friction JR, et al. The fibromyalgia and myofascial pain syndromes: a preliminary study of tender points and trigger points in persons with fibromyalgia, myofascial pain syndrome and no disease. J Rheumatol 1992;19:944–51.
10. Gerwin RD, Shannon S, Hong CZ, et al. Interrater reliability in myofascial trigger point examination. Pain 1997;69(1–2):65–73.
11. Sola AE, Williams RL. Myofascial pain syndromes. Neurology 1956;6(2):91–5.
12. Diakow PR. Thermographic imaging of myofascial trigger points. J Manipulative Physiol Ther 1988;11(2): 114–17.
13. Kruse RAJ, Christiansen JA. Thermographic imaging of myofascial trigger points: a follow-up study. Arch Phys Med Rehabil 1992;73(9):819–23.
14. Diakow PR. Differentiation of active and latent trigger points by thermography. J Manipulative Physiol Ther 1992;15(7):439–41.
15. Simons DG. Review of enigmatic MTrPs as a common cause of enigmatic musculoskeletal pain and dysfunction. J Electromyogr Kinesiol 2004;14(1):95–107.
16. Chen Q, Bensamoun S, Basford JR, et al. Identification and quantification of myofascial taut bands with magnetic resonance elastography. Arch Phys Med Rehabil 2007;88(12):1658–61.
17. Sikdar S, Shah JP, Gilliams E, et al. Assessment of myofascial trigger points (MTrPs): a new application of ultrasound imaging and vibration sonoelastography. In: 30th Annual International Conference of the IEEE, Engineering in Medicine and Biology Society. Vancouver, BC; 2008.
18. Chi-Fishman G, Hicks JE, Cintas HM, et al. Ultrasound imaging distinguishes between normal and weak muscle. Arch Phys Med Rehabil 2004;85:980–6.
19. Hicks JE, Hawker TH, Jones BL, et al. Diagnostic ultrasound: its use in the evaluation of muscle. Arch Phys Med Rehabil 1984;65:129–31.
20. Saltzstein RJ, Anoff JV, Shawker TH, et al. Ultrasound sector scanning used to define changes in muscle configuration. Scand J Rehabil Med 1989;21:209–12.
21. Sikdar S, Beach KW, Vaezy S, et al. Ultrasonic technique for imaging tissue vibrations: preliminary results. Ultrasound Med Biol 2005;31:221–32.
22. Shamdasani V, Bae U, Sikdar S, et al. Research interface on a programmable ultrasound scanner. Ultrasonics 2000;48:159–68.
23. Ballyns JJ, Shah JP, Hammond J, et al. Objective sonographic measures for characterizing myofascial trigger points associated with cervical pain. J Ultrasound Med 2011;30:1331–40.
24. Ballyns JJ, Otto P, Shah JP, et al. Evaluation of shear properties in muscle via novel superficial elastography technique. In: IEEE Ultrasonics Symposium. 2011.
25. Ballyns JJ, Turo D, Otto P, et al. Office-based elastography technique for quantifying mechanical properties of skeletal muscle. J Ultrasound Med 2012;1209–19.
26. Sikdar S, Ortiz R, Gebreab T, et al. Understanding the vascular environment of myofascial trigger points using ultrasonic imaging and computational modeling. In: 32nd Annual International Conference of the IEEE EMBS. Buenos Aires, Argentina; 2010.
27. Jarvholm U, Styf J, Suurkula M, et al. Intramuscular pressure and muscle blood flow in supraspinatus. Eur J Appl Physiol Occup Physiol 1988;58:219–24.
28. Otten E. Concepts and models of functional architecture in skeletal muscle. Exerc Sport Sci Rev 1988;16: 89–137.
29. Gerwin RD, Dommerholt J, Shah JP. An expansion of Simons' integrated hypothesis of trigger point formation. Curr Pain Headache Rep 2004;8(6):468–75.
30. Shah JP, Gilliams EA. Uncovering the biochemical milieu of myofascial trigger points using in-vivo microdialysis: An application of muscle pain concepts to myofascial pain syndrome. J Bodyw Mov Ther 2008;12(4): 371–84.

31. Chen Q, Basford J, An KN. Ability of magnetic resonance elastography to assess taut bands. Clin Biomech 2008;23(5):623–9.

32. Treaster D, Marras WS, Burr D, et al. Myofascial trigger point development from visual and postural stressors during computer work. J Electromyogr Kinesiol 2006;16(2):115–24.

33. Pierce SM, Skalak TC. Microvascular remodeling: a complex continuum spanning angiogenesis to arteriogenesis. Microcirculation 2003;10(1):99–111.

34. Shah JP, Danoff JV, Desai M, et al. Biochemicals associated with pain and inflammation are elevated in sites near to and remote from active myofascial trigger points. Arch Phys Med Rehabil 2008;89:16–23.

CHAPTER 7

INVASIVE ULTRASOUND-GUIDED TECHNIQUES IN PHYSIOTHERAPY

Fermín Valera Garrido • Francisco Minaya Muñoz

If you really believe in yourself, nothing will be beyond your possibilities.
WAYNE DYER

CHAPTER OUTLINE

KEYWORDS

probe; transducer; needle tip; needle shaft; focus; gain; depth; target; ultrasonographic guidance; safety; needle visibility; in-plane approach; out-of-plane approach.

7.1 PHYSIOTHERAPY AND INVASIVE ULTRASOUND-GUIDED TECHNIQUES

Ultrasound is an excellent tool available to physiotherapists for the purpose of visualizing and assessing the musculoskeletal system.[1–4] Furthermore, the performance of invasive techniques under direct visualization of musculoskeletal ultrasound has an increasing number of applications,[5–7] as it enables a clearer localization of the target structure. This not only increases the precision of the intervention,[8–15] but also improves the safety of the technique,[16–21] produces improved results[22,23] and has an overall cost benefit.[24]

KEY POINTS

The application of invasive musculoskeletal techniques under the guidance or direction of ultrasound imaging has shown improved results and a reduction in the overall cost of interventions.

A range of studies have demonstrated that the localization of the target structure based on palpation methods alone is prone to error. Several studies have compared infiltrations guided by palpation compared to contrast radiology or fluoroscopy. The results have shown that the needle is incorrectly placed inside the target tissue between 10% and 70% of the time.[8–13]

Ultrasound allows for the procedure to be performed in real time with continuous control of the needle position, and monitoring of the application of a therapeutic agent on behalf of the professional. In accordance, several studies have demonstrated the effectiveness of ultrasound-guided procedures in the musculoskeletal system, resulting in positive results in comparison to conventional systems.[14,15] The current generation of systems and high-frequency probes provides an excellent description of the musculoskeletal tissues, and offers a detailed view of the different structures (e.g. tendon, muscle, ligament).

KEY POINTS

The present-day technology allows one to 'see' rather than 'imagine' the structures.

A range of professionals (such as anaesthetists, cardiologists, gynaecologists, rheumatologists and physiotherapists) rely on ultrasound images in order to improve the effectiveness and safety of their procedures. In all the aforementioned cases, the visualization of the anatomical structures, such as the vessels, nerves and organs found in areas close to the target tissue, guarantee the safety of the application.[16–21] Furthermore, ultrasound is useful for detecting anatomical variations (such as an unusual location of a nerve or the presence of additional nerves or vessels) which are not usually detected with conventional types of assessment tools such as palpation.

The use of ultrasound guidance during minimally invasive techniques in physiotherapy is relatively recent and has been associated with the development of percutaneous needle electrolysis techniques, such as the EPI® technique[25,26] and dry needling.[27] The ultrasound image provides the physiotherapist with key information in order to establish therapeutic targets for the use of physical agents. Examples of procedures that benefit from ultrasound guidance are the destruction of neovascularized areas associated with chronic tendinopathies via the use of electric currents[28] or the vaporization of the haematic contents in the case of a muscle rupture.[29] This is similar to the use of ultrasound guidance by orthopaedic surgeons while performing infiltrations with sclerosing substances[30] or aspirations.[31] The great advantage is that the clinical result of the treatment is seen in real time.

KEY POINTS

When combined with invasive physiotherapy techniques, ultrasound enables a precise and safe approach of the target structure in real time.

In recent years, a growing number of physiotherapists have introduced ultrasound devices into their clinical practice in order to improve patient care. This process has been facilitated by the numerous technological advances, the portability of the devices and a reduction in their costs, together with the emergence of specialized training opportunities.

The safety and effectiveness of ultrasound-guided techniques in physiotherapy depend on various factors: correct image optimization and visualization of the target area, improvement in the technique of needle visualization and the establishment of safety measures. Our primary aim with this chapter is to provide readers with the opportunity to gain the knowledge and develop the skills to perform invasive ultrasound-guided techniques in daily clinical practice.

7.2 PROCEDURES FOR IMPROVING IMAGE VISUALIZATION

Despite the differences between the different machines and brands available on the market with regard to appearance and options, all machines have the same basic functions that the physiotherapist can manipulate in order to optimize the image. These are frequency and probe selection, depth, focus, gain, colour Doppler (CD) and power Doppler. The goal is to improve the axial and lateral resolution of the image surrounding the target area to be treated.

7.2.1 Frequency and probe selection

The ultrasound wave is characterized by a frequency (f), a wavelength (delta) and a constant speed of propagation within the soft tissue (1540 m/s). Selection of the appropriate fre-

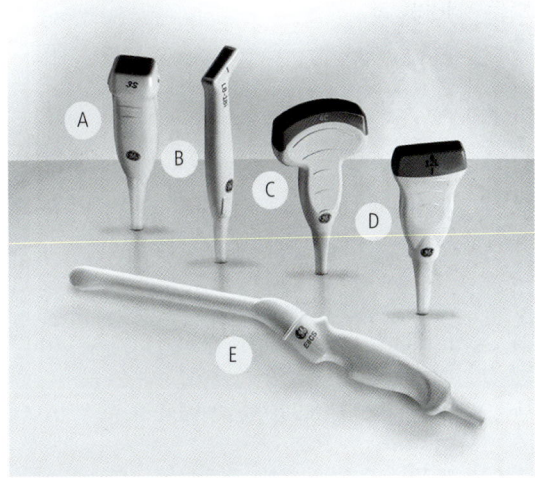

FIGURE 7.1 ■ Probe or transducer. (A) Linear probe for cardiology. (B) Linear 'hockey stick'-type probe. (C) Curvilinear probe. (D) Linear conventional probe (E) Vaginal probe. (Courtesy of General Electric®.) (Colour version of figure is available online).

quency is probably the most decisive element for the purpose of image optimization. The most common frequency range in musculoskeletal ultrasound lies between 5 and 13 MHz. In this way, the high frequencies provide superior axial resolution (for example, at 5 MHz axial resolution is 0.6 mm while, at 12 MHz, it is 0.25 mm), but they have less penetration strength.

↑ Frequency = ↑ Resolution

↓ Frequency = ↑ Penetration

The probe (transducer) most commonly used in musculoskeletal ultrasound is lineal (figure 7.1B and D), as it is the best way for an ultrasound beam to fall perpendicularly over the straight structures of the musculoskeletal system (e.g. tendon, ligament). Far less frequently, the curvilinear probe is used (figure 7.1C), in this case for deeper structures (for example, the piriformis muscle). Some ultrasound machines provide the option of increasing the field of view and simulating that a curved probe is being used. This is called 'virtual convex imaging', given that these devices electronically increase the field of view from rectangular to trapezoidal. This is especially useful for visualizing muscle tissue (figure 7.2).

The use of frequency transducers (10–15 MHz) is best suited for visualizing superficial structures (2–4 cm), whereas the middle frequency transducers (5–10 MHz) are preferably used in areas found at a depth of 5–6 cm. Most of the probes used are multifrequency (for example, 7–12 MHz). The ultrasound machines predeterminally establish a central frequency that they deem to be optimal, according to the type of study (for example, musculoskeletal,

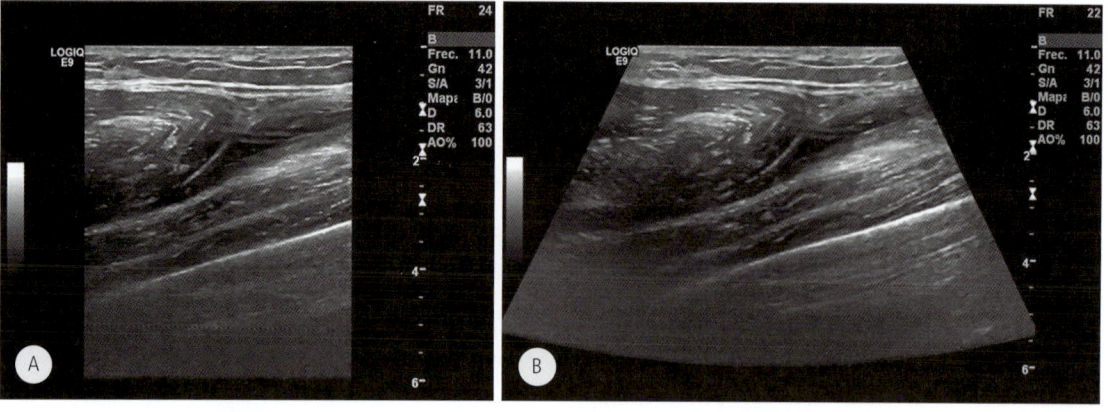

FIGURE 7.2 ■ Field of view. (A) Linear image. (B) Virtual convex image.

small areas) and the anatomical area (for example, knee, shoulder). However, the professional should modify the ultrasound wave frequency emitted by the transducer. As a recommendation, the highest possible frequency is selected (i.e. with the highest resolution) whenever the required depth is met for visualization of the target structure.

Another important factor in relation to the probe is its size. Different-shaped models are available according to the area to be studied (figure 7.1). For instance, linear probes with a smaller contact surface (i.e. 'hockey stick') are better suited to small and irregular areas, as they provide a better-suited approach for anatomical areas such as the foot or the hand.[9]

7.2.2 Depth

Depth refers to the possibility of increasing or decreasing the field of view and must be adjusted according to the target structure in order to ensure correct visualization. On the right-hand side of the screen the depth is shown in centimetres (figure 7.3).

At first, it is recommended to increase the field of view (i.e. increase depth) (figure 7.3A) as this will permit identification of areas of anatomical landmarks and those that are clinically relevant; after this, the field of view is decreased (less depth) (figure 7.3B) and the image is centred over the target area (figure 7.3C).

If an important structure, such as a vessel or a nerve, is found close to the target, the depth should be adjusted accordingly in order to achieve a more complete view and to improve safety.

In more superficial structures (for example, the carpal tunnel) the image can be improved by applying more gel between the probe and the skin.

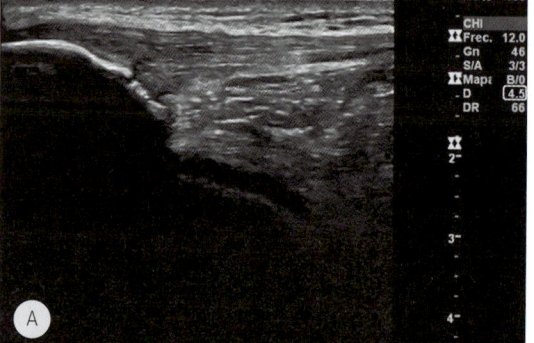

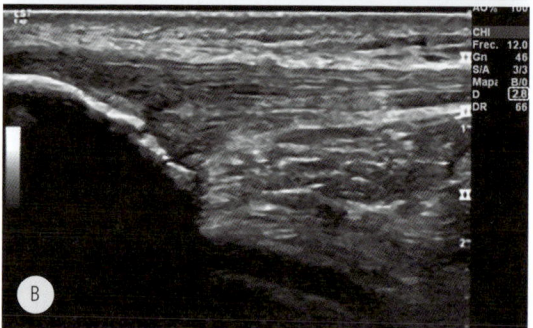

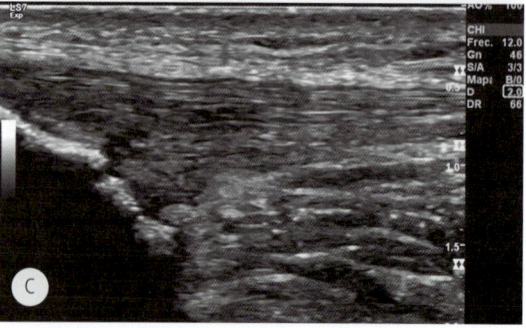

FIGURE 7.3 ■ Depth. Longitudinal section on the patellar tendon at different depths (A–C). (A) Wide field of view in order to identify areas of anatomical references. (B) and (C) Appropriate depth for centring the image on the target area. The depth (D) appears on the right-hand side of the image, marked within a rectangle.

The depth must be adjusted in order to improve the image and increase the safety of the procedure.

7.2.3 Focus

The focus or focal zone is the limit in which ultrasound waves converge and begin to diverge. It is a site with improved lateral resolution.

The present ultrasound machines allow the possibility of (1) adjusting the focal zone to different depths within the field of view (figure 7.4A–C) and (2) establishing multiple focal zones, thus managing to centre the projection of the ultrasound beam upon the structure to be assessed or treated (figure 7.4D). However, the increase in the number of focal zones can degrade temporal resolution, as the machine will need more time to read the ultrasound wave and process each image. The position of the focus is generally represented with a small arrow at the right or left of the image (figure 7.4). It is recommended that the focus is positioned slightly deeper (1 cm) to the area of interest.

Image optimization is achieved by positioning the focus or the focal zones over the target tissue.

7.2.4 Gain

The gain establishes how white or bright (hyperechoic) or how dark (hypoechoic) the image on the screen appears (figure 7.5A). By increasing the gain, the amount of white (brightness) increases. In contrast, by decreasing the gain, the image appears altogether darker. By adjusting the gain of the image, the goal is that the professional should be able to recognize the structures under study more easily; for this reason, the adjustments of the gain depend on the professional's preferences. With most machines it is possible to adjust the gain automatically, and this is the option most commonly used.

It is important to bear in mind that, by increasing the gain, the lateral resolution decreases and that by making the image darker, real information regarding the target area may be lost (figure 7.5B and C). For example, in a pathological patellar tendon, an excessive increase of gain will brighten the image to the point of obscuring the visible areas of involvement, creating a false

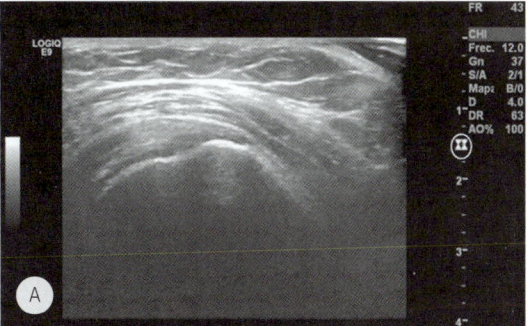
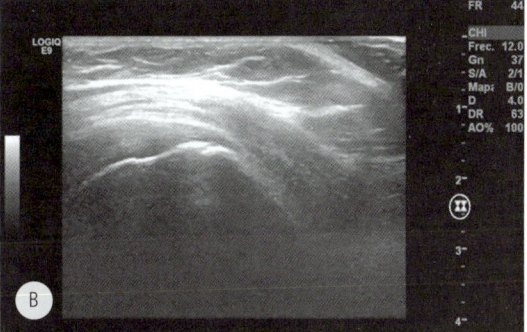
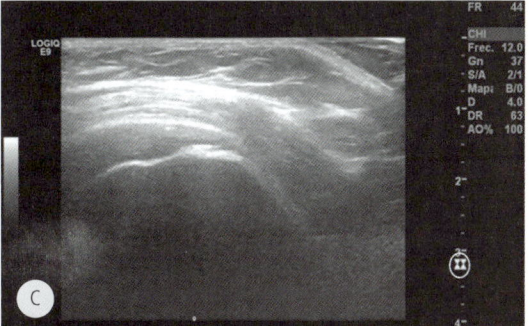
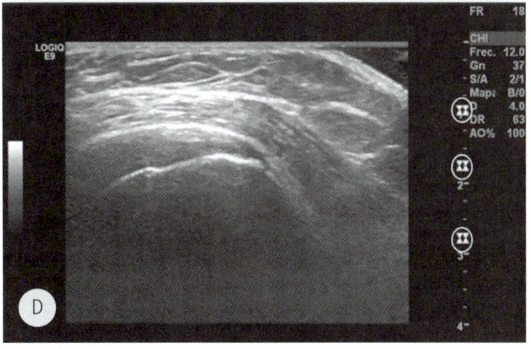

FIGURE 7.4 ■ Focus. Adjusting the focus to different depths over the supraspinatus tendon in a longitudinal ultrasound section. (A) Optimal focus. (B) and (C) Examples of focus with error. (D) Adjustment using different focuses. The focus appears on the right-hand side of the image marked within a circle.

negative, whereas, by decreasing the gain, it is possible to 'lose' the hyperechoic relevant focal zone, by darkening the image, creating a greater area involved and leading to an incorrect diagnosis.

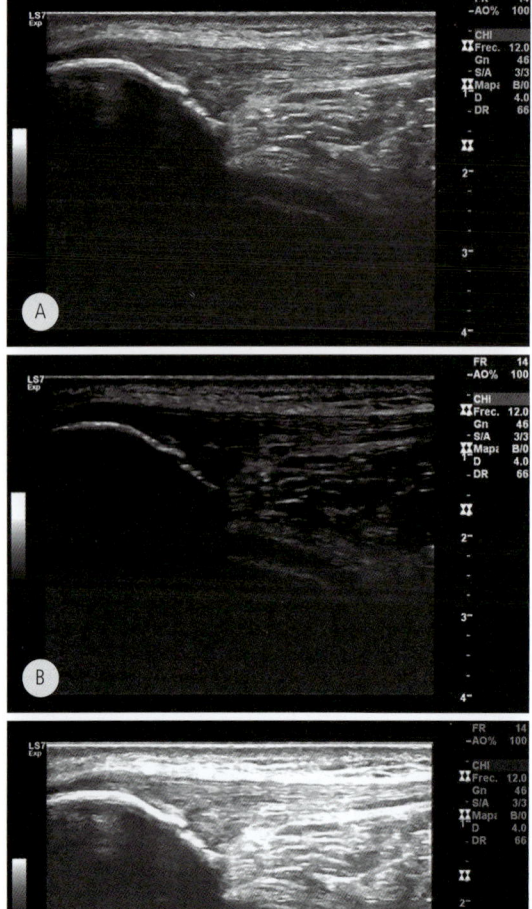

FIGURE 7.5 ■ Gain. (A) Optimal gain. (B) Not enough gain. (C) Excessive gain.

7.2.5 Time gain compensation (TGC)

The TGC function, similar to the gain, enables adjustment of brightness. Unlike the gain, which increases or decreases overall brightness, the TGC allows the operator to adjust the brightness independently at different depths within the field. Most machines have a TGC control with a set of small sliders that allow for adjustment of less to more gain at specific levels of depth. In this way, the TGC is normally used to increase the gain of the deeper structures. In the remaining situations, the control of TGC is usually positioned in the central area.

7.2.6 Grey maps

The machines normally offer maps with both different colour tones and degrees of contrast (figure 7.6). Professionals must determine the concrete settings with which they are most comfortable and those that offer the greatest image detail.

7.2.7 Compound and harmonic imaging

Compound imaging technology enables acquisition of multiple images of the same object taken from different angles within the same plane (spatial compound imaging) or acquired at different frequencies (frequency compound imaging) and combining them into a single image. The ultrasound systems by GE Healthcare offer a compound function (CrossXBeam™) designed to improve the image.[32] The images thus obtained show less granulation and increased definition of the borders and subsequently produce a cleaner image (with less noise) (figure 7.7).

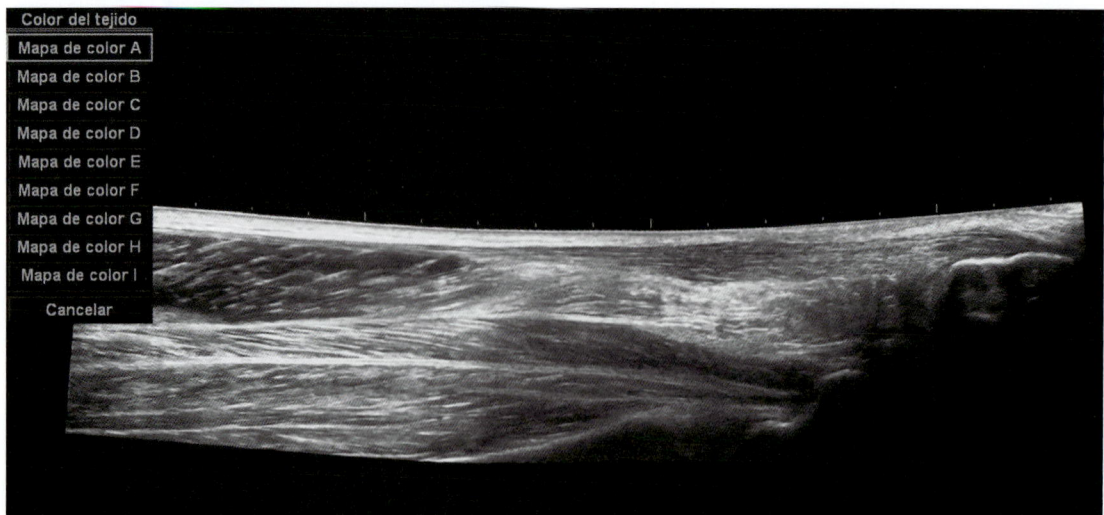

FIGURE 7.6 ■ Colour map of the Achilles tendon in a panoramic image. (Colour version of figure is available online).

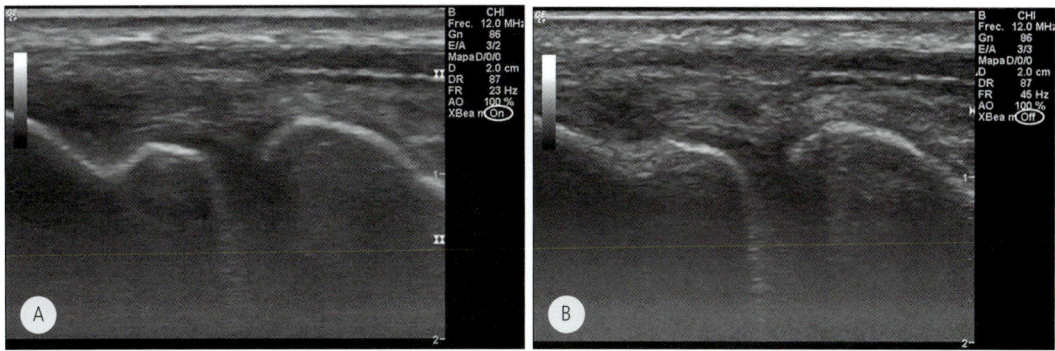

FIGURE 7.7 ■ (A) CrossXBeam™ on. (B) CrossXBeam™ off. Views of a longitudinal ultrasound section over the epicondylar tendon. (A) appears less grainy and has better image definition than (B).

Tissue harmonic imaging creates an image using echoes at twice the emitted frequency; this higher-frequency harmonic signal is spontaneously generated by propagation through tissues.[33]

7.2.8 Probe manipulation

When manipulating the probe, there are several elements worth noting in order to optimize the image. PART is an acronym for pressure, alignment, rotation and tilt.

Pressure

Correct pressure application can considerably improve image quality. The increase in pressure affects the echogenicity of the tissue (it appears more anechoic) and shortens the distance to the structure of interest (target zone), which can introduce error into the calculation of distance from the skin to the target area, as well as an error in quantification of the width of a structure (for example, when quantifying the width of a tendon).

On occasion more pressure is applied intentionally. For instance, firm pressure upon the probe is used for the purpose of differentiating a vein (which collapses with pressure) and an artery (which does not collapse), during an ultrasound-guided procedure and in order to reach a greater depth with the needle, thus reducing the distance to the target, and in order to direct the ultrasound beam to an area of interest. In this case, more pressure is applied to one side of the probe and this causes it to angle.

Alignment

It is important for the probe to be positioned on the appropriate plane, due to the narrow width of the ultrasound beam (as little as 1 mm at the focal zone of high-frequency transducers) and slight movements can move the target structure and the needle outside the field of view.

Likewise, the transducer in B-mode can be placed perpendicular to the target zone in order to increase the quality of the image. If the angle of the probe is perpendicular, or close to perpendicular, more ultrasound waves will be reflected back to the transducer, which will result in a better image. If the ultrasound waves are parallel to the surface of the target area (an angle of incidence of more than 45°), the image will appear more blurred.

KEY POINTS

The transducer must be placed in the correct plane and perpendicular (in B mode) to the target structure.

Rotation and tilt

The image can be improved by tilting or rotating the probe, thus adjusting the angle of the ultrasound beam. By manipulating the probe, the direction of the ultrasound beam is modified and different images are obtained of the same structure until the ideal image is obtained. In the soft tissues, especially tendons and nerves, the phenomenon of anisotropy is an important consideration (see chapter 5).

7.2.9 Dominant eye

The dominant eye is the one with the most visual acuteness or acuity and with superior visual depth, whereas the other eye mainly dominates peripheral and spatial vision. Based on the combined information from both eyes, a three-dimensional image is formed in our brain.

The fact of having a dominant eye can affect what we see and how we see; therefore the professional must find out if the vision in one eye predominates. It may be vital to use that eye in order to improve the quality of observations. Thus, if the professional's dominant eye is the right one, the target tissue will be placed on the right-hand side of the ultrasound screen during an in-plane approach (see section 7.6.4).

Eye dominance can be tested in many ways. A straightforward way to find out which eye is dominant is as follows:

1. Completely extend both arms and place them at the level of the eyes.
2. Form a triangle between the thumbs and the index fingers, leaving a small hole through which one can see.
3. Through the hole, pick out an object to observe which does not surpass the size of the hole.
4. Close the left eye. If the image changes (the angle of view changes), the left eye is dominant.
5. If the image remains unaltered, the right eye is dominant.

Another important aspect to consider is the dominant hand, as right-handed operators prefer a right-hand screen bias so that they can see their hands and the display during the procedure.

KEY POINTS

The professional must be aware of which eye is dominant and align it with the dominant hand during ultrasound-guided invasive techniques.

7.3 PROCEDURES FOR IMPROVING IDENTIFICATION OF THE TARGET ZONE

Once the image has been optimized and before beginning treatment on the target tissue, it is important to ensure that it is the clinically relevant tissue. It is not about 'pricking' a faulty image with a needle, but of approaching the actual injured tissue. For this purpose, different strategies can be established in order to improve identification of the truly affected (target) area.

7.3.1 Clinical correlation

In the process of physiotherapy evaluation and diagnosis, a physiotherapist usually combines manual testing (e.g. orthopaedic tests, palpation) with instrumental tests (for example, musculoskeletal ultrasound) for the purpose of identifying any alterations (at the level of function and structure) and limitations experienced during activity. With regard to the order of these procedures, the anamnesis and manual physical exploration take place before the instrumental assessment with ultrasound. Ultrasound serves to confirm previous hypotheses and to set the therapeutic goal (which must occur after all the information has been correlated). In other words, the ultrasound finding (for example, a focal hypoechoic region over the inferior pole of the patella) must correlate with the patient's clinical condition and previous tests (e.g. selective pain on palpation of the inferior pole of the patella, difficulty going down stairs).

KEY POINTS

A "target structure" must not be approached without a confirmed clinical correlation.

Sonopalpation (edge technique)

The edge of the transducer may be used as a palpation tool and to elicit feedback from the patient regarding pain-sensitive structures.

7.3.2 Systematizing the ultrasound assessment

It is important to systematize the exploration of the different anatomical regions with assessment protocols.[34] An ultrasound study must include at least the examination of the longitudinal and transverse plane in order to obtain valid and precise information regarding the structure under study and to approach the whole anatomical area (see section 7.3.3). The evaluation in both longitudinal and transverse planes enables an orthogonal image of the target structure to be attained and decreases the error associated with a possible anisotropy.

Whenever possible, the static study must be complemented with a dynamic analysis of the tissue (for example, by asking the patient to abduct the shoulder in order to assess the dynamic behaviour of the supraspinatus and the subacromial impingement).

7.3.3 Scanning

Together with the study in the transverse and longitudinal plane, it is recommended that a scan be performed in order to assess the anatomical region of interest thoroughly and thus avoid errors.[35] It is important to consider that the image obtained by ultrasound represents a two-dimensional section of a structure that has three dimensions. Therefore, it is recommended that

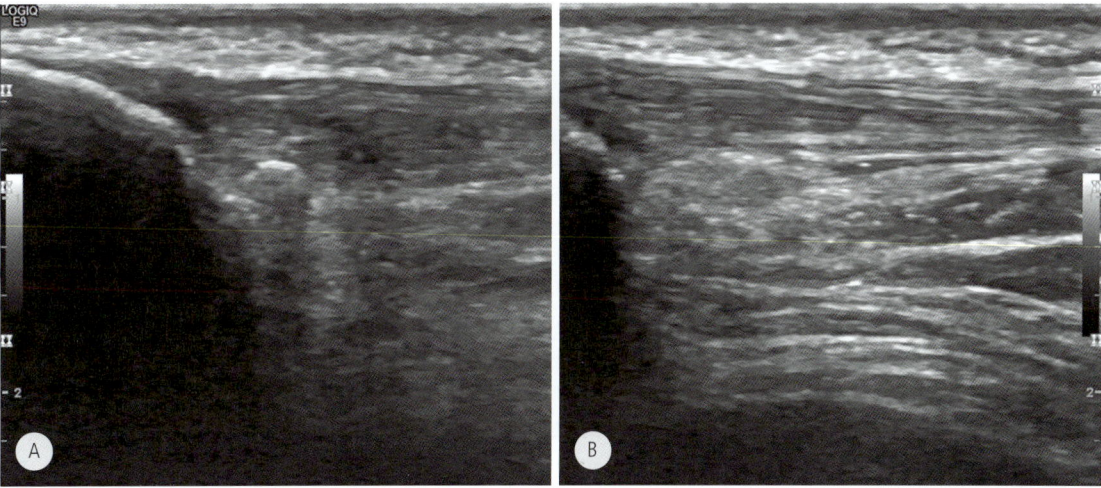

FIGURE 7.8 ■ Contralateral study. Longitudinal ultrasound section showing degenerative changes in both patellar tendons. (A) Asymptomatic. (B) Symptomatic.

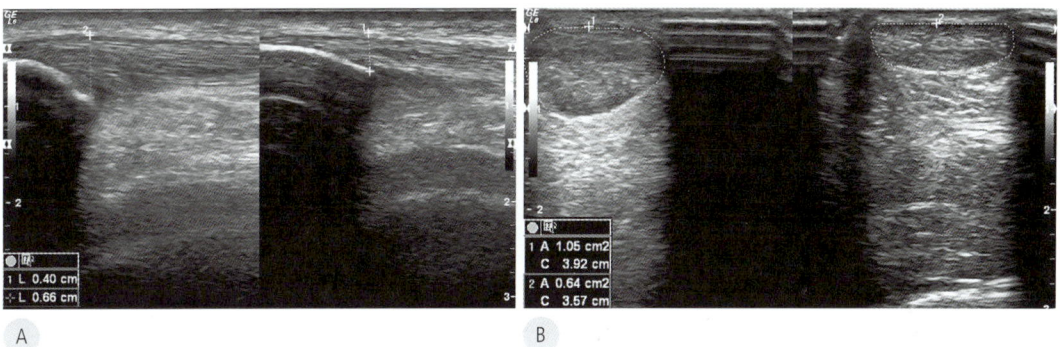

FIGURE 7.9 ■ Contralateral study. Measurement. Dual image of the patellar tendon. (A) Longitudinal section. (B) Transverse section.

multiple sections are viewed, as this will allow the professional to reconstruct the target structure mentally in the three dimensions. This process requires the professional to have a thorough knowledge of the anatomical region.

7.3.4 Contralateral study

A comparative study of the contralateral (supposedly healthy) side is usually recommended (right-to-left comparison), or at least a study of the asymptomatic portion of the structure under study. This is in order to be able to compare and highlight the normal structures from the presumably pathological ones, as well as to have a clearer idea of the differences or similarities between them.

In the case of tendinopathies, bilateral involvement is frequent, as well as the presence of degenerative changes that affect the individual bilaterally (for example, in runners); sometimes these are accompanied by clinical symptoms, at other times not at all[36–38] (figure 7.8). To date, there is a lack of studies focusing on patterns of normality of the soft tissue.

Many devices allow for the screen to be divided, with the benefit of displaying the images one beside the other (dual option), thus facilitating comparative measures between structures (figure 7.9).

7.3.5 Panoramic study

The newer ultrasound devices include the option of conducting a panoramic study of the anatomical structure (for example, the LogiqView® by GE®). This option is particularly useful for study of the structure as a whole (figure 7.10) and allows for easier identification of the area of interest.

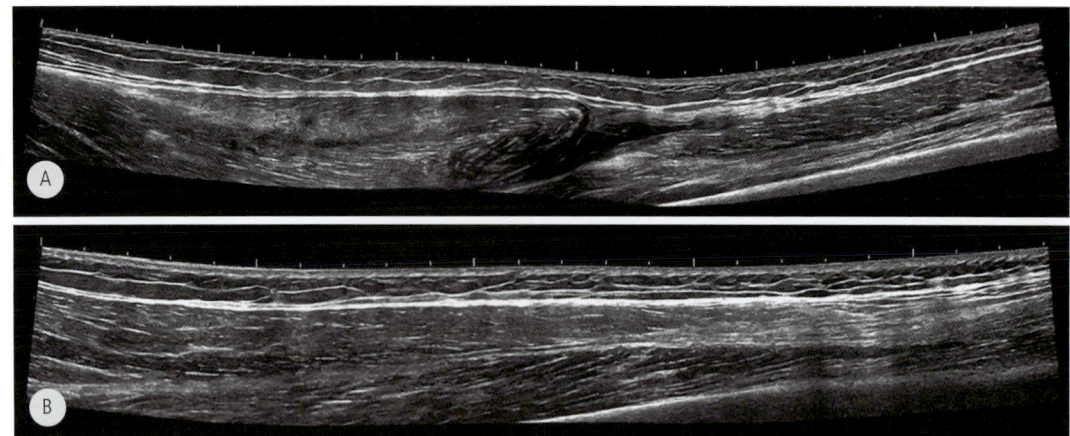

FIGURE 7.10 ■ Panoramic image. (A) Loss of continuity in the myotendinous junction of the rectus femoris. (B) Healthy muscle.

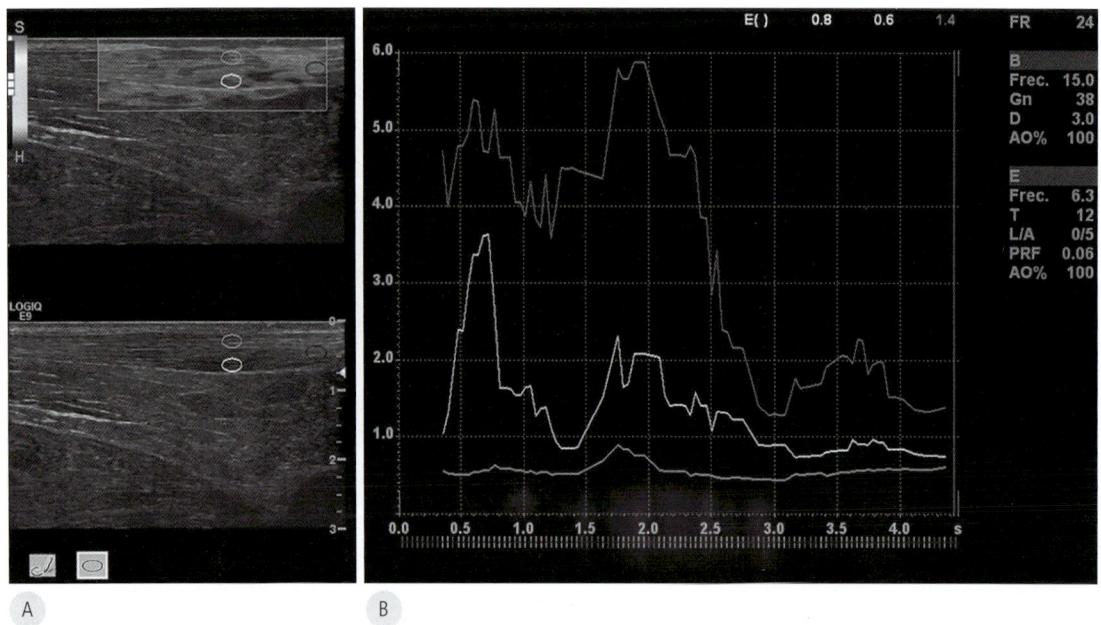

FIGURE 7.11 ■ Elastography. (A) Top: an elastography image, with its correspondence in B-mode (bottom). (B) Elastographic image analysis. Quantitative display of elasticity of the tissue in the different areas selected. (Colour version of figure is available online).

7.3.6 Elastographic study

Sonoelastography is a new technique that has been incorporated into ultrasound devices for analysing the elasticity of tissues. In this manner, the changes in tissue elasticity are represented on the screen, similar to a map of colours, from blue (more rigid tissue) to red (more elastic tissue). The use of sonoelastography associated with B-mode offers extra information for the professional, therefore enabling a more precise analysis of the structure, with identification of the areas of interest and their quantification[39,40] (figure 7.11).

7.4 SAFETY MEASURES IN INVASIVE ULTRASOUND-GUIDED TECHNIQUES

Before beginning the ultrasound-guided approach, a series of safety procedures must be performed.

7.4.1 Positioning

There are three factors associated with adequate positioning in the application of invasive echo-guided procedures: the ultrasound device, the patient and the professional or operator.

Ultrasound device

- This must be placed at a comfortable distance.
- The screen must be placed directly in front of the operator.
- The angle of the device and the screen must be adjusted in order to reduce reflections to a minimum.
- It is recommended that the screen on the device be placed at the level of or slightly below the operator's eyes. This will avoid the operator adopting a forced position and/or a maintained flexion plus protraction of the cervical spine.

Patient

- It is important that the patient feels comfortable and safe.
- If the patient is apprehensive, the screen on the device must be placed outside the patient's visual field.

Operator

- The operator must be positioned as close to the patient as possible.
- The operator's back must be supported. Thus, it is recommended to use a chair or a stool that offers support in the lumbar region, and which allows for height adjustment.
- Avoid a position of dorsal kyphosis.
- Reduce cervical and ocular tension.
- The operator must look straight ahead and avoid having to turn the head or the body.

All of these elements will increase the comfort and safety of the procedure, as well as reduce the risk of complications.

7.4.2 Material

The material needed in ultrasound-guided invasive physiotherapy techniques must be sterile and be placed on a cart or a table so that it is easily accessible.

- Antiseptic spray for healthy skin. These are products (such as Cutasept® or Skin-Des®) that have a wide-spectrum disinfectant action, with bactericidal, fungicidal, tuberculocidal, microbactericidal and virus inactivation (hepatitis B, human immuno-deficiency virus) effects. The skin must be sprayed prior to the procedure and left to dry for around 1 minute.
- Sterile gel. The gel has a double function: to contribute to the formation of an echographic image, by decreasing the difference of impedance between the air and the skin, and as a lubricant, as it allows for easier manipulation of the transducer. The gel used in invasive ultrasound-guided invasive physiotherapy procedures must be sterile (for example, Aquasonic®). It is important to make sure of this because the gel that is usually used in physiotherapy services is not sterile. Monodose presentations of product are also available (20 grams).
- Probe covers or protective devices. The transducer must not be sterilized in an autoclave and the use of disinfectant liquids for cleaning it can damage it. For this reason, and to guarantee the sterility of the transducer, different strategies can be used: (1) a sterile glove; (2) a latex condom-type cover; (3) adhesive transparent lamina such as Opsite® Flexigrid® (Smith & Nephew) or Tegaderm® (3M). In any case, it is important to ensure that air does not become trapped between these and the probe in order to avoid distorting the image. For this reason it is recommended to place the gel on the transducer before covering it.
- The use of probe covers is no substitute for cleaning and disinfection between procedures (see chapter 1).
- Non-sterile gloves. It is important to select a correct glove size, so that the glove fits snugly on to the professional's hand.
- Sterile needles. The puncture needles must be sterile.
- Sterile gauze. This is used after removing the needle, for the purpose of applying pressure to the treatment area. Normally the puncture needle used in invasive physiotherapy techniques (see chapter 2) does not provoke bleeding after extraction, as the soft tissue itself collapses the access path after the needle is removed. If a capillary is perforated, pressure placed upon the sterile gauze for approximately 30 seconds is usually enough to cut the blood effusion.
- 70% Alcohol. 70% alcohol has a superior disinfectant strength in comparison to 95% alcohol.
- Medical waste disposal or sharps container: see chapter 1.

KEY POINTS

A disinfection process combined with the use of a sterile gel and a probe cover is an accepted method of infection control for ultrasound transducers.

KEY POINTS

It is always useful to confirm which side of the transducer corresponds with which side of the screen, in order to identify the correct orientation of the image.

7.4.3 Probe orientation and the image on the screen

Before beginning the invasive approach and advancing the needle, it is important to be sure of the position of the probe in relation to the tissue and the representation of the image on the screen. It is important to remember that the transducers present a marker on one of the sides that coincides with the left-hand side of the screen (figure 7.12) and which will help with image orientation.

On the contralateral side, when a transducer is positioned transverse to the longitudinal axis, the right side of the patient corresponds with the left side of the ultrasound image and the left side corresponds with the right side of the image.

If we position the transducer longitudinally to the axis, the left side of the ultrasound image will correspond with the superior part of the transducer and the right side of the ultrasound image will correspond with the inferior aspect of the transducer.

7.4.4 Doppler

Doppler technology (see chapter 5) is based on the change of frequency of the ultrasound beam when it encounters a moving object (such as the blood cells in a vessel), which causes the beam to be reflected back towards the source that originated it at a different frequency. The frequency increases if the object (blood cells) moves towards the source that originated the beam (transducer) and decreases if the object moves away from it. In contrast with B-mode, Doppler registers the image better when the ultrasound beam is more parallel to the direction of the flow. In other words, when the incidence angle is close to 90° there is less flow, and colour may not appear on the screen, which can give a false-negative indicative of 'no flow'.

Both CD and power Doppler imaging (PDI) technologies are useful adjuncts to invasive physiotherapy procedures for two reasons: (1) they allow for the identification of vessels close to the target area or in the path of the needle (figure 7.13); and (2) because determined structures, such as the tendon, present a neovascularization process in the case of degeneration (figure 7.14), which is one of the therapeutic objectives.[37,38]

CD expresses the data of change in frequency in a colour spectrum (red–blue). The colour scale has a directional character, so that the red spectrum corresponds to the flow that moves

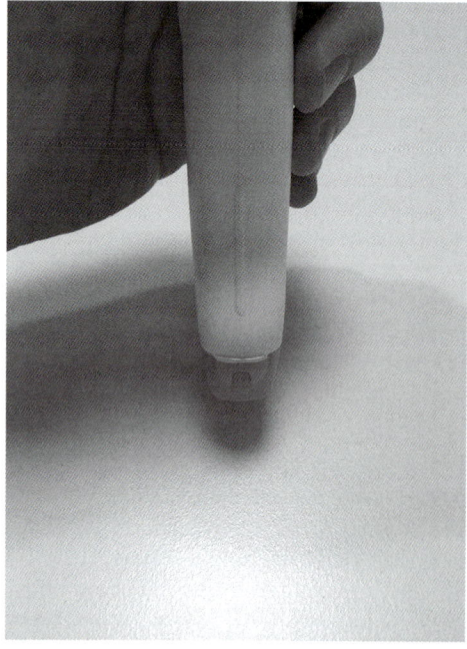

FIGURE 7.12 ■ Marker on the lateral side of the transducer – useful for establishing the correct orientation of the image on the ultrasound screen. (Colour version of figure is available online).

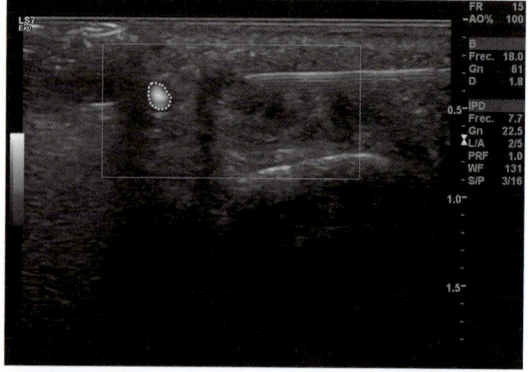

FIGURE 7.13 ■ Power Doppler colour. Identification of vascular structures close to the target tissue and in the path of the needle. The vascular element shows up as marked with discontinuous lines. (Colour version of figure is available online).

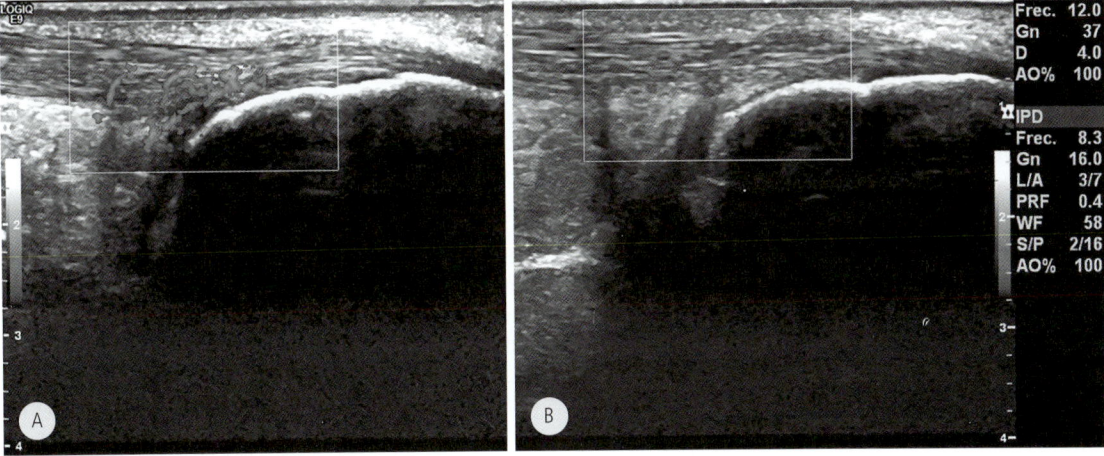

FIGURE 7.14 ■ Power Doppler colour. (A) Neovascularization displayed in the Achilles tendon in a longitudinal ultrasound section. (B) Contralateral Achilles tendon without hypervascularization. (Colour version of figure is available online).

towards the transducer and the blue spectrum is the one that moves away. PDI is different from CD in that it represents the width of the Doppler signal and not the frequency, in orange.

PDI is more sensitive to slow flow in smaller vessels than CD (and therefore it is very useful in processes such as tendinopathies) and is not affected by an unfavourable tilt angle.

KEY POINTS

Before initiating any treatment approach, it is important to analyse the presence of vessels close to the target area or in the pathway of the needle.

KEY POINTS

PDI is less angle-dependent and more sensitive to slow flow, allowing for the visualization of smaller vessels.

7.4.5 Measurement and needle selection

Once the target area is identified it is important to measure the distance from the skin to the target in order to select the most appropriate needle (i.e. one that guarantees safety in the application of the technique). Note that 0.5–1 cm must be left outside the skin (see chapters 1 and 2). For example, if the target is located at 21.4 mm, a needle measuring 30 mm long will be used rather than one of 25 mm.

7.4.6 Needle tip visualization

Correct needle tip visualization that is maintained throughout the duration of a treatment approach on a target structure is of special importance in order to minimize complications. It has been demonstrated that this is one of the most frequent errors[41] made among novice practitioners.

KEY POINTS

Do not continue advancing the needle if you lose sight of the needle tip on the ultrasound screen.

7.5 PROCEDURES FOR IMPROVING NEEDLE VISUALIZATION

Needle visualization depends on a range of factors, such as the characteristics of the needle used, the type of tissue that it goes through (the more fluid a tissue is, the more echogenic the needle becomes),[42] the technology of the transducer and the ultrasound equipment,[43] as well as the professional's knowledge regarding potential artefacts and experience regarding image interpretation.[41]

Therefore, the elements that can improve the process of needle visualization can be classified into:

- improvements in echogenicity of the needle, such as the type of needle, the diameter, length, place and angle of insertion or orientation with regard to the probe
- technical improvements related to the transducer resolution (dependent on the

density and type of piezoelectric crystals) and ultrasound equipment, as well as the processor on the device, and the presence of the Doppler or the B-Steer system, which improves ultrasound beam reflection

- improvements in the abilities of the professional, such as the use of phantoms and simulated application on cadavers.

KEY POINTS

Correct needle visualization is essential in order to ensure the safety and efficacy of ultrasound-guided invasive techniques in physical therapy.

7.5.1 Type of needle

The needles used in ultrasound-guided physiotherapy techniques are conventional (see chapter 2), in contrast with the new echogenic improvements that are used, for instance, in the field of anaesthesia.[44,45] Echogenic needles are engineered to increase the reflection of ultrasound waves back towards the transducer. The materials and type of needle used determine the increase in echogenicity. Future avenues of research for improving visualization include the development of more echogenic needles in musculoskeletal ultrasound intervention.

7.5.2 Needle gauge

A larger-calibre needle is more easily visualized for two reasons: firstly, because it causes a greater change in acoustic impedance and secondly, because the needle can intercept the ultrasound beams better and therefore there is a greater probability of the beam being reflected again to the transducer and provoking a brighter signal. Nonetheless, it is important to consider that a larger-calibre needle causes more discomfort for the patient during both insertion and advancement of the needle within the tissue.

The needles commonly used in invasive physiotherapy techniques, such as dry needling or percutaneous needle electrolysis, have a diameter of 0.30 mm, 0.32 mm or 0.35 mm. During injection techniques, the most commonly used needle has a diameter of 0.80 mm (21G) or 1.3 mm (18G).

7.5.3 Needle length

In general terms, longer needles are easier to visualize than smaller needles as they generate a greater ultrasound reflection.[46] However, this can generate more discomfort for the patient, as more tissue has to be penetrated in order to reach the target.

7.5.4 Insertion angle, insertion site and echogenicity

The angle and site of the needle insertion, in relation to the transducer, play a critical role in optimizing needle visualization (figure 7.15).[47–49] By following these recommendations an optimum and reliable needle approach is obtained.

In theory, the best image is obtained when the ultrasound beam emitted by the probe and the needle are situated at 90° from each other. If the needle is inserted too close to the probe or the angle is excessively perpendicular (acute) to the skin, the ultrasound beams will not contact properly with the needle and visibility will be reduced. Shaft visibility decreases more sharply than tip visibility. Identification of the needle tip is more difficult when a more oblique trajectory is used to reach targets found at a deeper level.

A series of recommendations can be established for approaching the structures of the musculoskeletal system susceptible for treatment with invasive physiotherapy techniques (see sections 7.6.4 and 7.6.5).

KEY POINTS

Needle tip and shaft visibility decrease gradually with steeper angles.

7.5.5 Needle bevel orientation

Certain techniques call for the use of bevelled needles (for example, during infiltrations); in these cases, needle bevel orientation is an important consideration for enhancing needle tip visibility. Needle tip visibility is better when the bevel opening is oriented either directly facing the ultrasound beam (0°) or facing 180° away from the beam.[46,50]

7.5.6 Hydrolocation

Hydrolocation involves injection of a small amount of fluid (0.5–1 mL) in order to confirm needle tip position via the production of both tissue movement and the appearance of a small anechoic 'pocket'.[51] The needle tip (which appears as a bright echogenic structure) is highlighted by the contrast between it and the anechoic pocket of fluid. For this purpose, sterile water can be used as well as normal saline, an

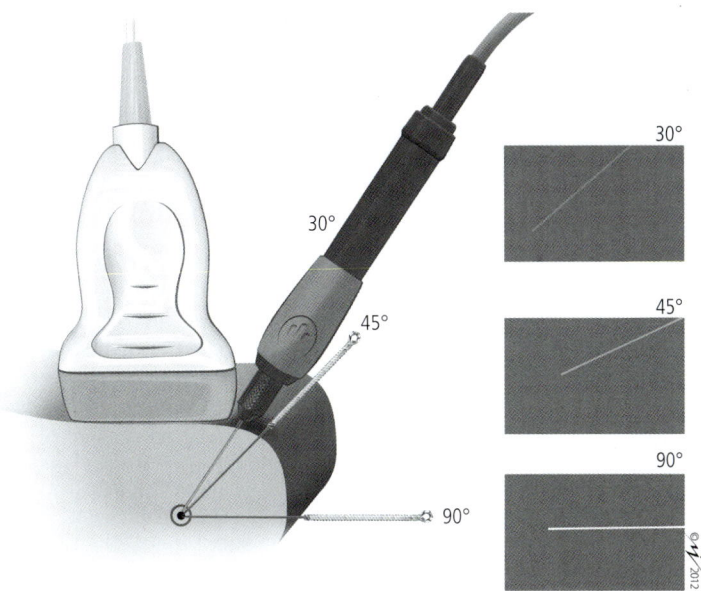

FIGURE 7.15 ■ Insertion angle of the needle. The definition of the image obtained on the ultrasound (rectangles on the right) varies according to the insertion angle. The more perpendicular the angle between the needle (90°) and the ultrasound beam (probe), the better the visualization of the needle. (Colour version of figure is available online).

injection of local anaesthetic or 5% dextrose. Further injection of fluid also aids in opening up the space between anatomical structures (hydrodissection), thus creating an obstacle-free path for further needle repositioning.

7.5.7 Needle–beam alignment

The approach or orientation of the needle relative to the transducer can be longitudinal or transverse (see sections 7.6.4 and 7.6.5). In both cases it is important to align the needle adequately in relation to the transducer so that the ultrasound beam can 'find' the needle and properly reflect the image on to the screen (figure 7.16). If the needle is not correctly visible after insertion, it may be helpful to perform slight tilting or rotation movements in order to 'find' the needle.

7.5.8 Doppler ultrasound

Movement of an object within an ultrasound beam produces a Doppler shift in the frequency of the reflected echoes. The Doppler function available on most modern ultrasound machines modulates this frequency shift into a colour signal, and is commonly used to detect blood flow. It may also be used to locate a moving needle tip against a stationary background as small advances and withdrawals ('chicken-pecking' technique) will cause the needle to appear highlighted in colour (figure 7.17).[52–54]

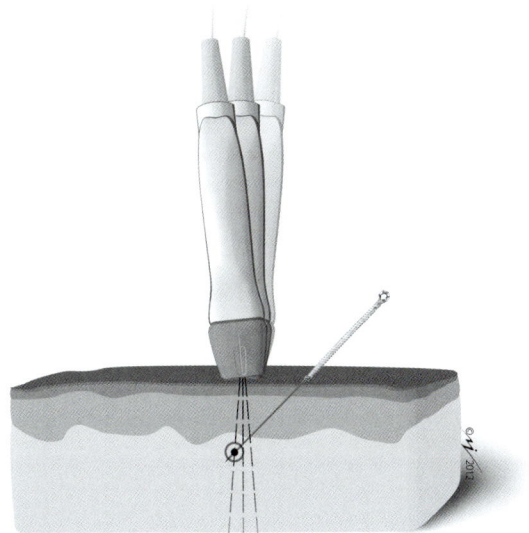

FIGURE 7.16 ■ Probe needle alignment. Small movements of the probe enable correct alignment of the ultrasound beam in relation to the needle. (Colour version of figure is available online).

7.5.9 Electronic beam steering

The needles that penetrate the tissues with excessive tilt angles produce reflections in the more distal part that escape from the probe, thus not contributing to the formation of the image. Electronic beam steering is a technology that allows the ultrasound beam to be tilted relative to the

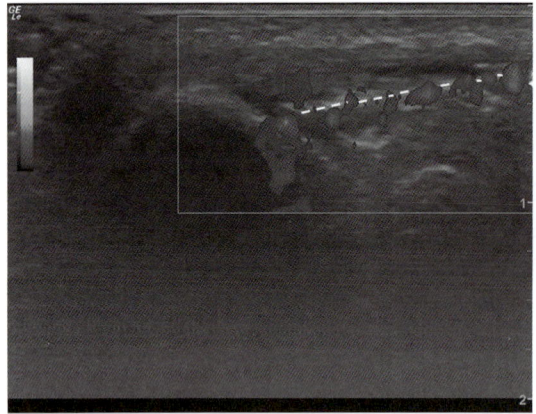

FIGURE 7.17 ■ Doppler. The Doppler mode helps to distinguish the needle (represented by the discontinuous line), detecting its movement. (Colour version of figure is available online).

transducer, therefore increasing the needle beam angle of incidence towards 90°, for example. The ultrasound systems by GE Healthcare offer a beam-steering function (B-Steer) designed to improve needle visibility[55] (figure 7.18).

7.5.10 Phantom training

In ultrasound, phantoms are models that simulate a body part or structure and that are used to improve the factors affecting the approach and visibility of a needle during ultrasound-guided interventions. Phantom training enables the practice of simulated interventions so that they do not have to be performed for the first time on the patient. It also serves to improve the confidence of the professional, as well as to develop

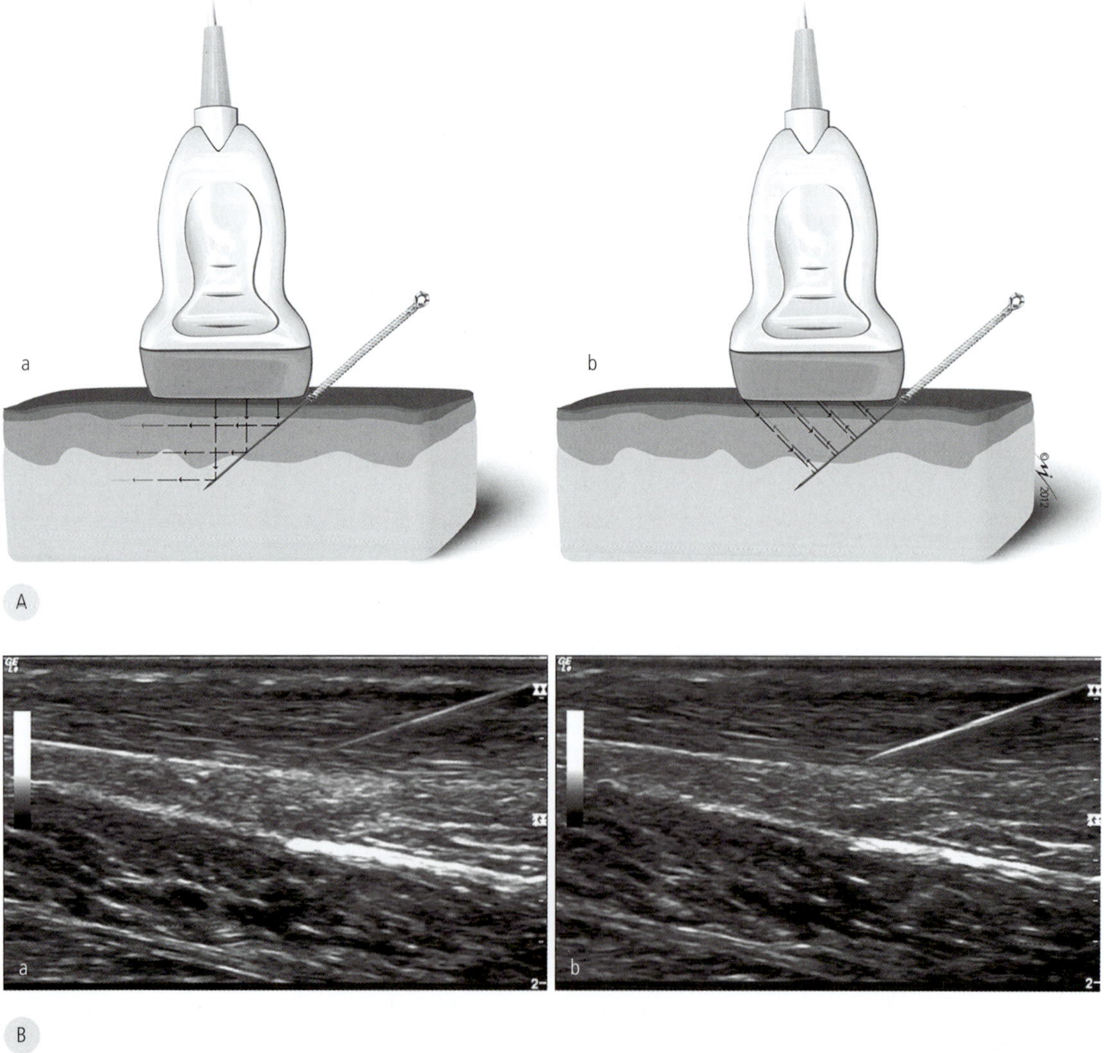

FIGURE 7.18 ■ B-Steer. (A) (a) Conventional orientation of the ultrasound beam. (b) Lateralization of the ultrasound beam 30° towards the needle. (B) (a) B-Steer deactivated in a longitudinal approach over the Achilles tendon. (b) B-Steer activated. (Colour version of figure is available online).

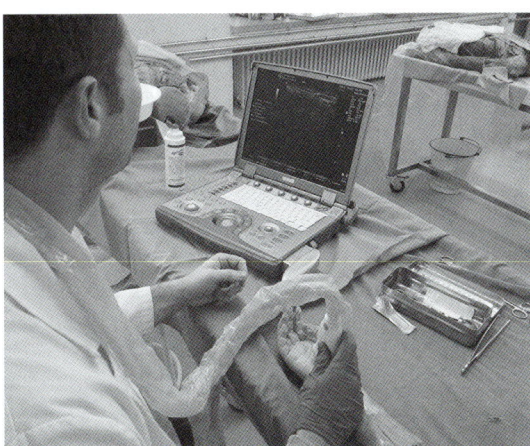

FIGURE 7.19 ■ Simulated application on a cadaver. (Colour version of figure is available online).

eye–hand coordination during application of the technique.[56]

Different types of phantom exist: homemade built models,[57] blue phantoms or anatomical models (for example, a lumbar spine). For training purposes it is also possible to use turkey legs or pig feet.

7.5.11 Cadaver training

Apart from the phantoms, there are other options available to help professionals improve their dexterity and interventional skill, such as cadaver training[58,59] (see chapter 3) (figure 7.19). For this purpose, unembalmed cadavers are preferred – the 'fresher' the cadaver, the better. This type of training has great value, as inferred by the study by Peuker and Grönemeyer,[60] which concludes that all the traumatic lesions described in the review could have been avoided if the professionals had a better knowledge of theoretical and applied anatomy. This knowledge constitutes an important factor of the ongoing quest of providing efficient and safe treatment.

7.6 NEEDLE APPROACH TECHNIQUES

Before describing the procedure and the different types of needle approach techniques available, it is necessary to establish the terminology and a series of general considerations:

7.6.1 Terminology

- Probe position relative to the anatomic structure:
  - longitudinal
  - transverse

- Needle position relative to the probe:
  - in-plane (long axis): needle parallel to the probe's long axis
  - out-of plane (short axis): needle parallel to the probe's short axis.

7.6.2 General considerations

- Before beginning treatment, the professional and patient must be positioned properly, comfortably and safely.
- The ultrasound device must be placed directly facing the professional (whether on the same side as the approach area or on the contralateral side). The aim is to avoid the operator having to turn his or her trunk or head in order to see the screen.
- The professional must be situated on the same side as the area of the needle approach.
- Soft lighting is preferable in order to facilitate visualization of the image on the screen.
- The probe is usually managed with the non-dominant hand and with the needle held in the dominant hand.
- The probe must be held firmly and as close as possible to the contact surface. The professional's transducer hand and fingers should be resting on the patient to prevent unintentional slipping of the transducer, and reduce fatigue as well as unintentional transducer movement.
- The target structure must be clearly visible and must correlate with the clinical history and physical exam of the patient. Sonopalpation is recommended.
- If the patient presents diffuse pain over the region, invasive approaches are not advised.
- It is important to establish the position of the probe once the desired image of the target structure is obtained.
- Place the target area in the centre of the screen, or as close as possible to the theoretical path of the needle.
- Measure the distance between the skin and the target in order to select the appropriate needle (see clinical case, chapter 4).
- In general, the path of the needle must be the shortest distance between the skin and the target area in order to minimize risks.
- The transducer must always be moved in order to 'find' the needle, and not the other way around. It is not recommended to move the probe and the needle at the same time.
- The visualization of the shaft and the needle tip decreases gradually with the

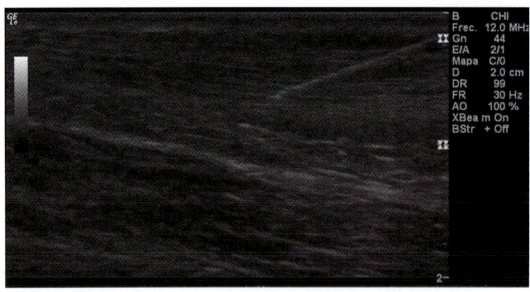

FIGURE 7.20 ■ Echo-localization of the needle with the help of electrolysis. Observe the hyperechoic image of the needle after application of a minimal dosage and its comparison regarding the conventional image and with B-Steer activated (figure 7.18).

angle of the needle tip, with the shaft less visible than the tip.

- The needle must not be advanced unless the tip is identified or visualized.
- It is usually difficult to maintain visualization of the exact location of the needle during the entire process of advancing the needle and, in most cases, its localization is determined by a series of indirect signs, such as:
  - movement of the tissues produced by the needle advancing
  - visualization of a posterior acoustic shadow or a comet tail (artefacts) coinciding with the tip at the same time as the needle advances.
- It is important to develop a 'feel of depth' with the needle.
- Percutaneous needle electrolysis techniques, such as EPI®, allow the professional to confirm the location of the needle tip by applying minimal doses of electric current,[61] which causes the needle to become more hyperechoic (figure 7.20).
- Save the images and/or videos with the information relating to the patient, the anatomical area, the side (right/left) and the date of the procedure.

7.6.3 Description of the invasive ultrasound-guided technique

In order to perform an invasive technique correctly with ultrasound guidance, professionals are obliged to switch their attention methodically (on–off) between two elements throughout the procedure. These are the needle–probe ensemble and the ultrasound screen. The following sequence of steps is recommended:

1. Visualize the image in the target area of the screen (screen 'on').
2. Maintain the probe in that plane (do not move the transducer), hold the needle (or needle holder) and pay attention to the correct alignment of the needle with the probe (needle–probe: 'on'). Do not focus attention on the screen (screen: 'off').
3. Insert and perform a slight advancement of the needle over the skin (screen: 'off').
4. Visualize the tip of the needle on the screen (screen 'on'). Needle–probe: 'off'.
5. Begin advancing the needle towards the target. Small changes in the pathway can be performed based on feedback from the screen (screen: 'on'), paying special attention to the position of the needle and the probe (needle–probe: 'on'). In this procedure, eye–hand coordination is essential. Maintain the needle aligned with the probe in order not to lose the needle from the plane of the ultrasound beam.
   - If the needle tip disappears during the procedure, the needle must not be advanced any further. It is recommended to: (1) withdraw the needle partially and slightly change the trajectory or (2) redirect the probe (see section 7.2.8) until the needle is once more identified. As a general rule, do not move the needle in order to find the probe. The professional must advance towards the target structure only when the needle 'appears' on the screen.
   - If the whole needle is lost, withdraw the needle in order to find the best possible approach and to realign the needle with the plane of the ultrasound wave. In the case of a novice practitioner, different linear array transducers may negatively influence the performance of ultrasound-guided needle advancement.[62] In these cases a standard 38-mm transducer is preferred to a 25-mm hockey stick transducer.
6. Apply the invasive physiotherapy technique to the target tissue.

Box 7.1 lists the tasks that are helpful for performing invasive ultrasound-guided physiotherapy techniques.

7.6.4 In-plane approach

The in-plane approach is also named the longitudinal or long-axis approach.

Characteristics

- The needle passes below the transducer following its longitudinal axis (long axis) (figure 7.21A and B).

- The entire needle and the tip are visualized (figure 7.21B) (video 7.1).
- The longitudinal approach requires the needle to be perfectly aligned with the transducer and the structure (figure 7.22A). If the needle alignment with the transducer is not correct, it is possible that what is identified as the tip is actually a part of the needle shaft (figure 7.22B) or that it has been left outside the plane of the ultrasound (figure 7.22C).
- In general, the needle shaft and its tip are more visible when inserted at an angle of less than 30° (figure 7.23).
- If the structure is superficial (e.g. patellar tendon, Achilles tendon, rotator cuff), it is recommended to insert the needle close to the probe (approximately 1 cm apart) in the most parallel angle as possible that allows for an approach on the target structure (figure 7.24A). In this manner, the distance to the target structure decreases, and therefore the potential risks decrease and the discomfort is lessened.
- If the structure is deep (e.g. rectus femoris, joint hamstrings tendon), it is recommended that the point of introduction of the needle into the skin is not too close to the probe so that the insertion angle is not too acute. It is suggested that the insertion point be at a distance from the probe equal to the depth of the target (figure 7.24A): i.e. if the target is found at 2 cm depth, the needle will be inserted at 2 cm from the probe.

- The optimal position of the target structure on the ultrasound screen is on the opposite side of the needle insertion and must coincide with the dominant eye.

7.6.5 Out-of-plane approach

The out-of-plane approach is also called the transverse or short-axis approach.

Characteristics

- The needle passes beneath the probe following its transverse axis (short axis) (figure 7.25).
- The tip is only observed as a bright point (hyperechoic) (figure 7.25) (video 7.2). The needle shaft is not visible.
- In general, the needle tip is better visualized when the angle of insertion is greater than 60° (figure 7.26).
- Whether the structure is superficial or deep, move the needle as close as possible to the transducer, seeking the most perpendicular insertion angle possible to facilitate visibility of the needle tip (figure 7.24B).
- It is important to develop the perception of the depth of the needle. Otherwise it is possible that what is identified as the needle tip is, in reality, part of the needle shaft, with the associated risk of puncturing a neighbouring structure (figure 7.27).
- A 'walk-down' technique has been suggested to aid out-of-plane needle tip visualization during the transverse needle approach (figure 7.28). This consists of inserting the needle at a distance from the transducer equivalent to the depth of the target, so that the tip will eventually intersect the ultrasound beam and target at a trajectory angle of approximately 45°. The initial insertion angle should, however, be shallow so as to facilitate detection of the needle tip. The needle is then incrementally angled and 'walked down', with the tip visualized at progressively greater depths until the target is reached.[63] Potential disadvantages of this technique include the need for multiple needle passes and a long needle track to reach deeper targets, both of which may increase patient discomfort.
- The optimal position of the target structure on the ultrasound screen is at its middle. It is advisable to keep the region of interest at the centre of the screen and puncture the skin at the centre of the probe to improve needle localization during the procedure. The needle is identified via the

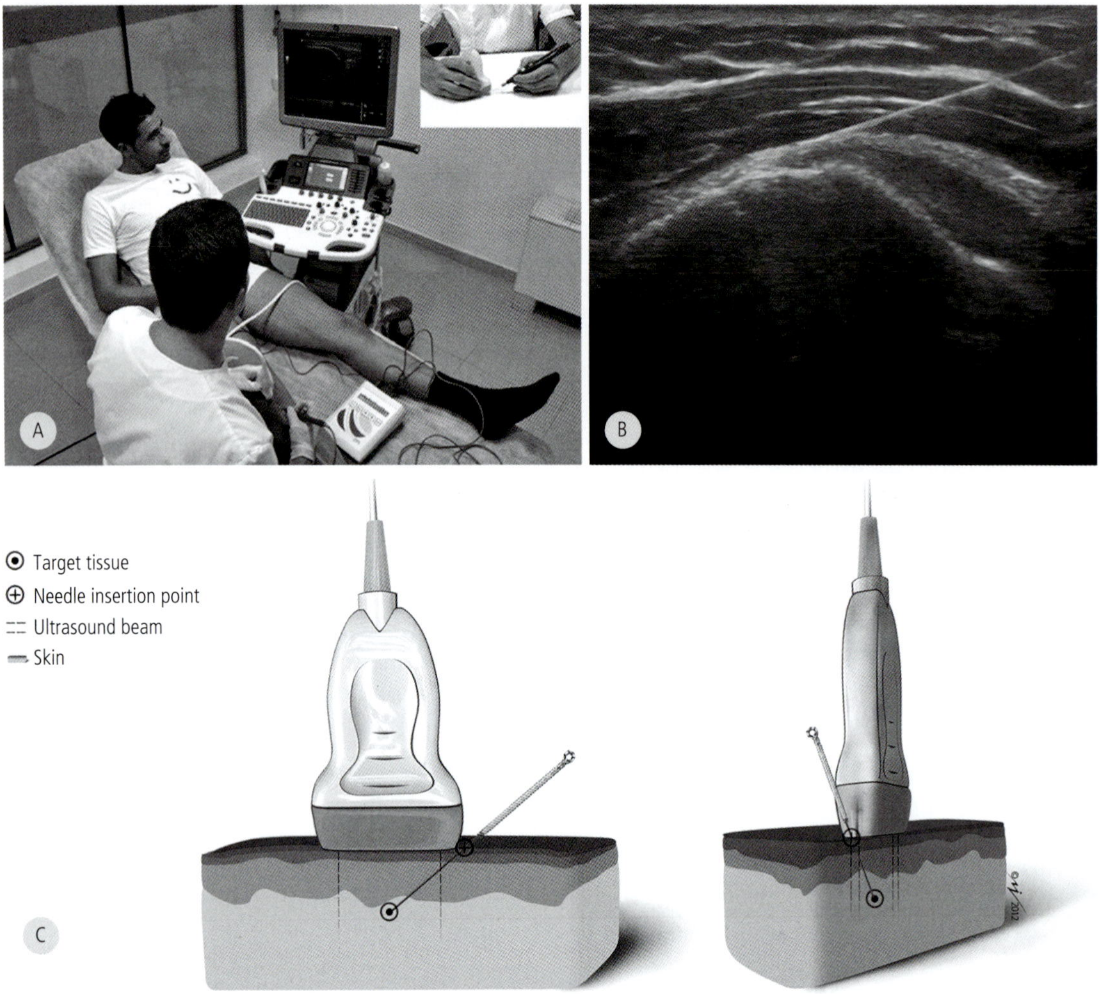

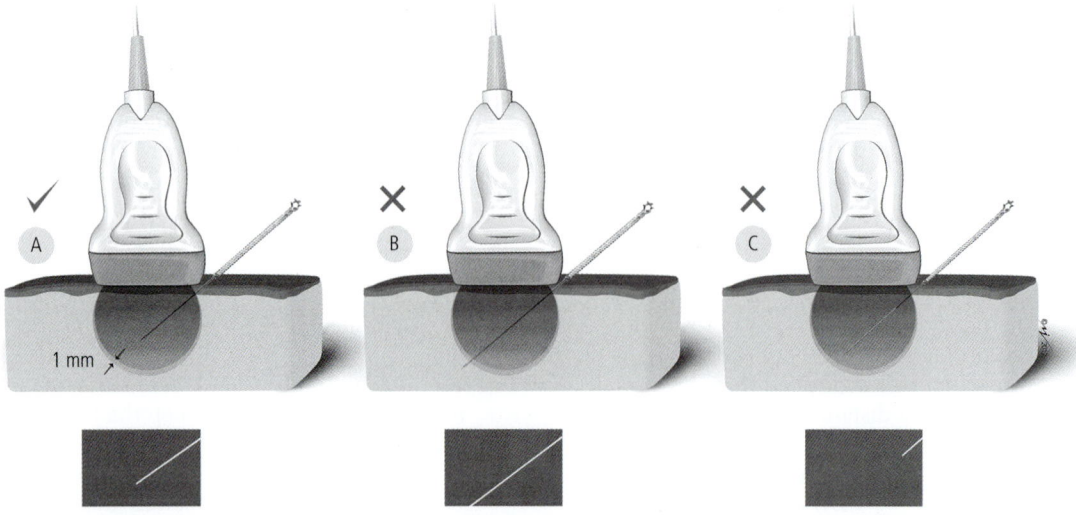

FIGURE 7.21 ■ (A) Longitudinal approach or long axis. Application on the patellar tendon. The top right image displays the direction of the needle and how it passes beneath the probe. (B) Longitudinal approach or approach on the long axis over the supraspinatus tendon. (C) Longitudinal approach or long-axis approach in (left) frontal view and (right) lateral view. (Colour version of figure is available online).

⊙ Target tissue
⊕ Needle insertion point
⚌ Ultrasound beam
⬗ Skin

FIGURE 7.22 ■ Alignment of the needle with the probe in a longitudinal approach. (A) Correct alignment and tip of the needle over the target tissue. (B) Correct alignment and tip of the needle situated just outside the target tissue. (C) Incorrect alignment. Tip of the needle outside the plane. (Colour version of figure is available online).

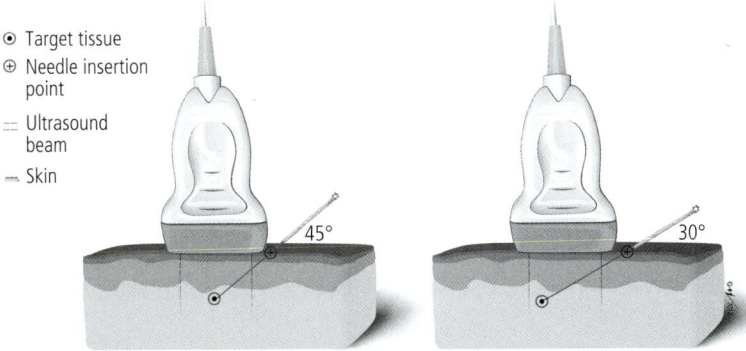

FIGURE 7.23 ■ Insertion angle of the needle in a longitudinal approach. The visualization of the needle improves the more parallel it is to the skin (30° compared to 45°), but this requires going through more tissue. (Colour version of figure is available online).

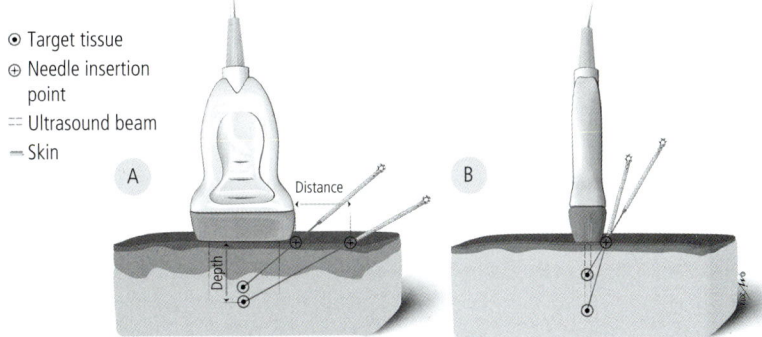

FIGURE 7.24 ■ Insertion angle in (A) longitudinal approach and (B) transverse approach. Superficial and deep structures. (Colour version of figure is available online).

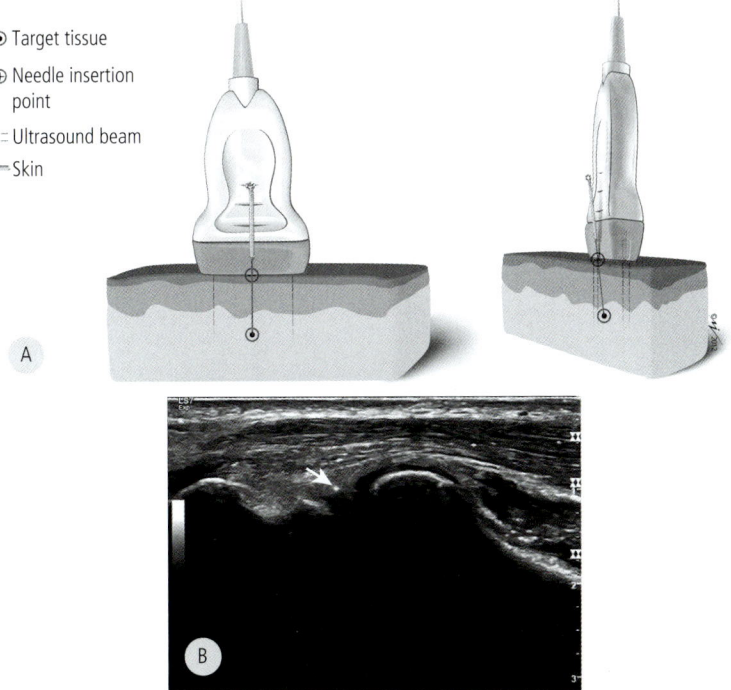

FIGURE 7.25 ■ (A) Transverse or short-axis approach seen from a frontal view (left) and a lateral view (right). (B) Transverse or short-axis approach on the extensor carpi radialis brevis tendon and the humeroradial capsule. The white arrow marks the hyperechoic point that identifies the tip of the needle. (Colour version of figure is available online).

⊙ Target tissue
⊕ Needle insertion
   point
== Ultrasound beam
— Skin

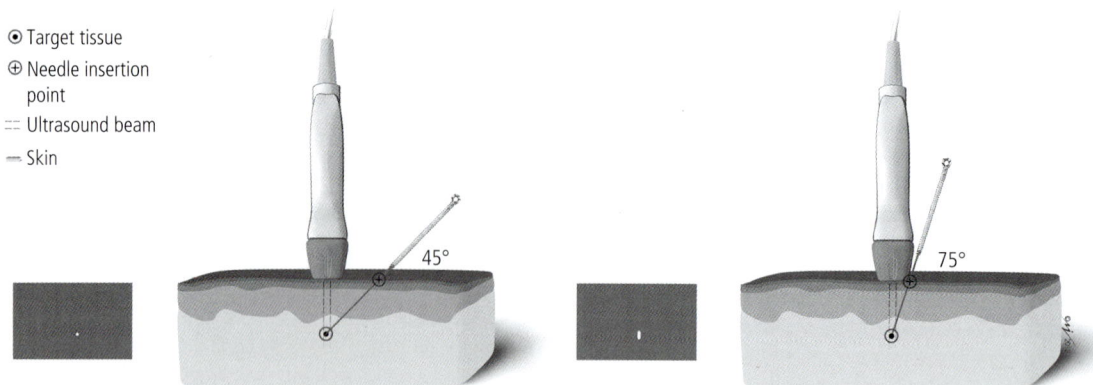

FIGURE 7.26 ■ Insertion angle of the needle in a transverse approach. The area of needle visualization (rectangle) is greater the more perpendicular the insertion is on the skin. (Colour version of figure is available online).

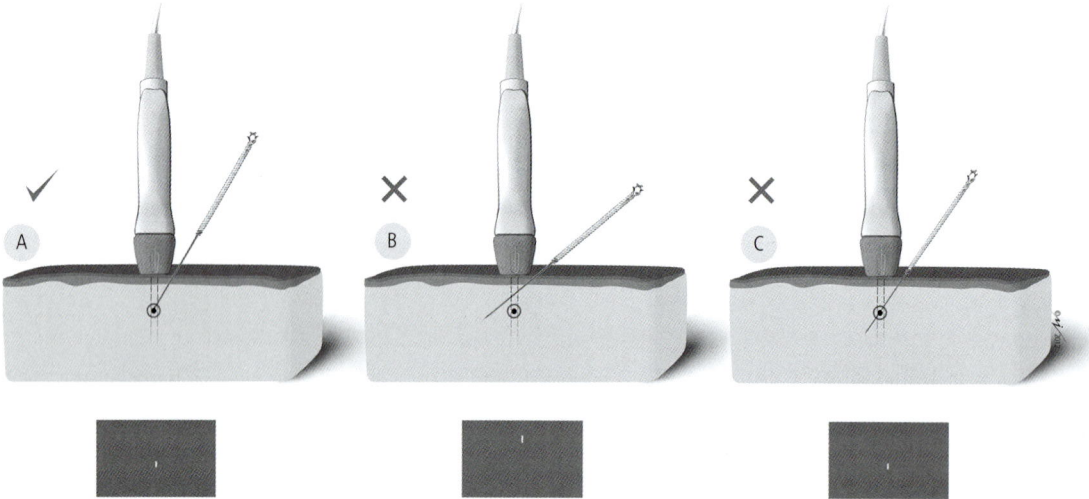

FIGURE 7.27 ■ Alignment of the needle with the probe in a transverse approach. (A) Correct alignment and tip of the needle over the target tissue. (B) Correct alignment and tip of the needle outside the plane. (C) Correct alignment and tip of the needle situated just outside the target tissue. (Colour version of figure is available online).

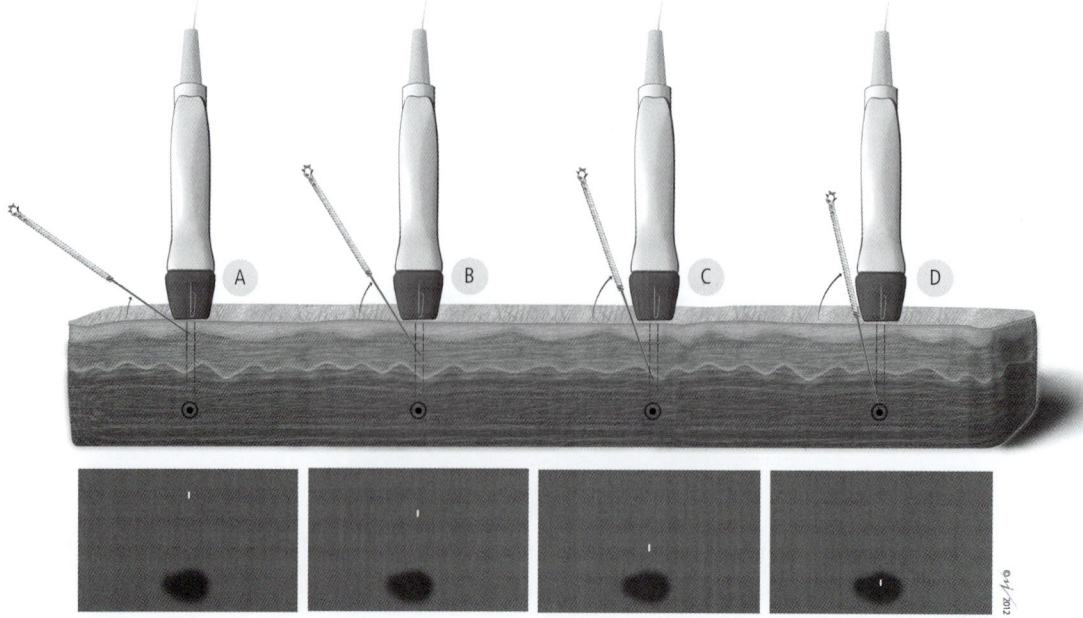

FIGURE 7.28 ■ (A–D) The 'walk-down' technique. (Colour version of figure is available online).

ring-down artefact, shadowing or by jiggling the needle. Sliding or fanning the probe may also help.

7.6.6 In-plane versus out-of-plane approach (table 7.1)

When should the transverse or longitudinal approaches be used?

Within the techniques of invasive physiotherapy, the selection of one or other approach will depend on the professional's choice, considering that:

- The superiority of one approach over the other has not been demonstrated.
- The longitudinal approach allows for complete visualization of the shaft and the needle tip and is the usual approach selected by physiotherapists, although the transverse approach enables a more three-dimensional image.
- The longitudinal approach is usually easier to perform than the transverse approach.
- The longitudinal approach comes with the inconvenience that the muscle planes that are crossed are greater than with a transverse approach, which could lead to greater patient discomfort.
- The transverse approach is commonly used in small joints such as the acromioclavicular joint or the interphalangeal joints.
- Nerve stimulation may be especially suited to the out-of-plane approach.
- A small footprint of the probe ('hockey stick') (figure 7.1B) is occasionally more advantageous for in-plane needle advancement, allowing professionals to place the needle entry closer to the target and thus also shortening the distance to the target.

- There are structures for which, due to their characteristics, one is almost 'obligated' to use a certain type of approach, such as the longitudinal approach of tendons during percutaneous needle electrolysis, in order to ensure that the tissue repair occurs in the correct direction or, for instance, the use of the transverse approach for interventions on the pubic symphysis.

7.6.7 Anterograde–retrograde linear threading approach

The anterograde or retrograde linear threading approach establishes a needle direction in relation to the target structure; this can be either in front of the target (anterograde approach) (figure 7.29) or from the target backwards (retrograde approach). In this case, once the needle is inserted into the target location, the tissue is stimulated in a retrograde fashion (e.g. deep fascia/paratenon of the Achilles tendon and Kager's fat pad) (video 7.3). These techniques are performed on their own or in combination depending on the location to be treated.

7.6.8 Grid approach

This approach is, in fact, a strategy that the professional may establish in order to optimize application of the invasive technique upon the target tissue. It consists of imagining the target structure being divided into a grid in order to select one area (or several areas) for treatment (figure 7.30).

7.6.9 Indirect approach

The indirect approach or indirect technique can be used for superficial structures, such as the

---

TABLE 7.1   Comparison of in-plane and out-of-plane approaches

Approach	Advantages	Disadvantages
In-plane	Most direct visualization. It allows visualization of the entire needle, including its tip The amount of unimaged needle path is typically small Better in tendons	Partial line-ups (creating a false sense of security when the needle tip is not correctly identified) Requires more space for probe and needle placement Longer paths and therefore the needle passes through more structures
Out-of-plane	Shorter needle path than with in-plane approaches Simultaneous anterior–posterior and lateral–medial perspective of the structure Most similar to other approaches (palpation) Useful in limited spaces at region of interest Better in small joints and nerve stimulation	Unimaged needle path, crossing the plane of imaging without recognition Requires more eye–hand coordination

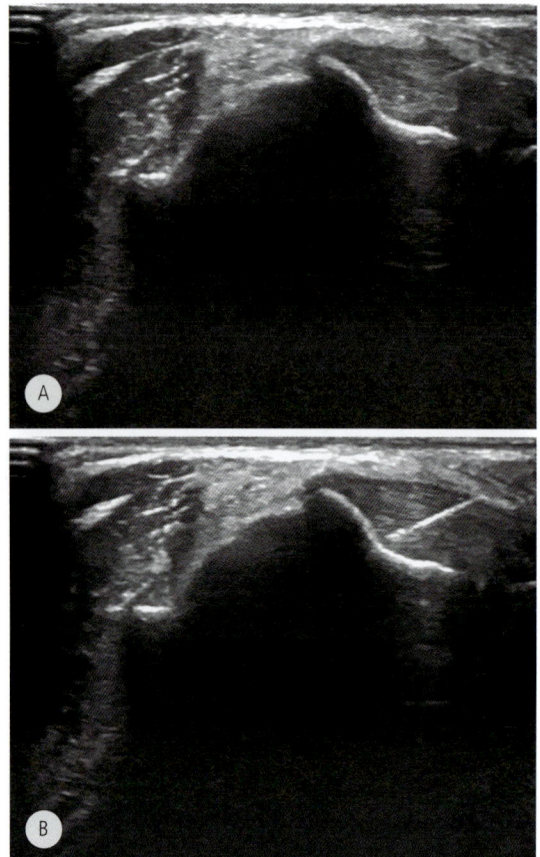

FIGURE 7.29 ■ Longitudinal approach in anterior tracing over the extensor carpi radialis brevis tendon. (A) The tip of the needle is visible. (B) It is advanced towards the target tissue.

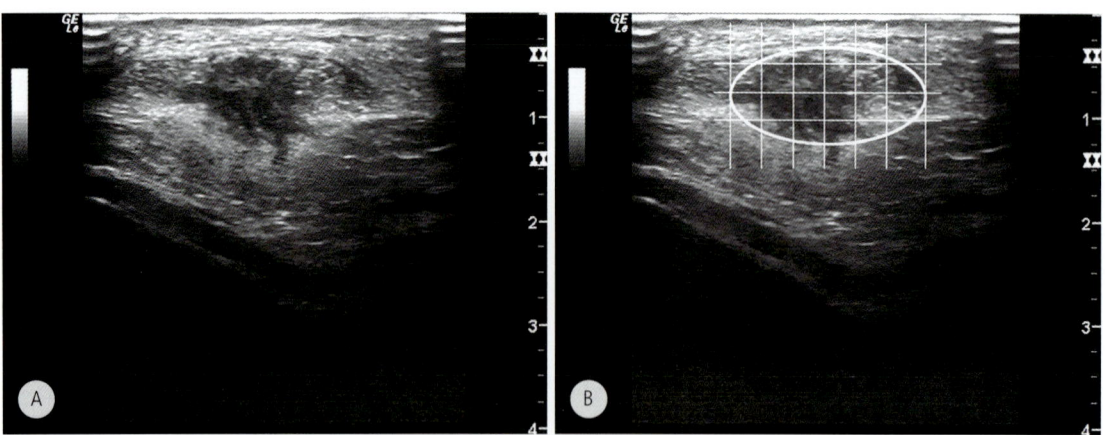

FIGURE 7.30 ■ (A, B) Grid approach on the patellar tendon.

acromioclavicular joint, or in those areas where the use of the probe and the needle is not viable.

This consists of:
- evaluating and identifying the target structure with the help of the ultrasound machine
- marking the limits of the target using a skin marker
- inserting the needle between the limits without the help of the ultrasound
- applying invasive physiotherapy treatment without ultrasound guidance.

The indirect approach cannot be considered ultrasound-guided or ultrasound-directed.

7.6.10 The freehand approach or the use of a support system on the probe

The techniques of invasive physiotherapy are usually applied bimanually. In other words, the probe is handled with one hand (non-dominant hand) and the needle with the other (the dominant hand). This is what is commonly known as the 'freehand technique' although, paradoxically, it is a procedure that does not leave the professional with any free hand for manipulating the ultrasound. It is necessary to set down the transducer in order to manipulate the machine, or, ideally, it requires two people in order to apply the ultrasound-guided procedure.[64–66]

The other system that can be used is that in which the needle is attached to the probe through a guide. This method has been developed mainly in anaesthesia and allows the professional to keep one hand free and achieve a better alignment with the needle and the ultrasound beam. The inconvenience is that this requires a longer needle and as a result, this may affect the professional's kinaesthetic sense during needle insertion (see wand effect, chapter 2, section 2.1).

7.7 ARTEFACTS

The puncture needle usually presents a posterior acoustic shadow or comet tail (artefacts) (see chapter 5) which coincides with the tip (figure 7.13), at the same time as it advances within the tissue.

7.8 ADVANTAGES AND DISADVANTAGES OF ULTRASOUND-GUIDED PROCEDURES

Despite the great advantages related to ultrasound-guided procedures, there are a number of related difficulties.

7.8.1 Advantages

In relation to the patient:
- It is a safe and effective procedure.
- It is a procedure without ionizing radiation.

In relation to the professional:
- It allows for real-time visualization of the needle position and application of the technique.
- It provides improved results.

In relation to the administration:
- There is a good quality/cost relation.

7.8.2 Disadvantages

In relation to the professional:
- It is operator-dependent. Ultrasound imaging examinations require operators to possess extensive knowledge regarding normal anatomy so that abnormal conditions can be easily recognized. For example, if the professional fails to perform examinations correctly, this may put patients at risk of having further unnecessary techniques. Reliability studies are necessary to determine the various pitfalls and the strategies available to improve examinations.
- The learning curve is slow.
- Invasive ultrasound-guided techniques require extensive hands-on experience in order to handle the ultrasound probe and the needle (or the needle holder) simultaneously.

In relation to the technique, there is:
- Limited field of view.
- Incomplete assessment of the bone and the joints.
- Limited penetration.
- Difficulty performing the ultrasound-guided application in certain small areas with the conventional probes, as there is a lack of available space. In these cases, the use of small linear probes (hockey stick type) (figure 7.1B) or the indirect approach (see section 7.6.9) are options worth considering.

In relation to the devices:
- Devices have variable quality and cost.

KEY POINTS

Due to the enormous advantages of ultrasound-guided procedures, they should be the methods of choice for the variety of invasive techniques of the musculoskeletal system.

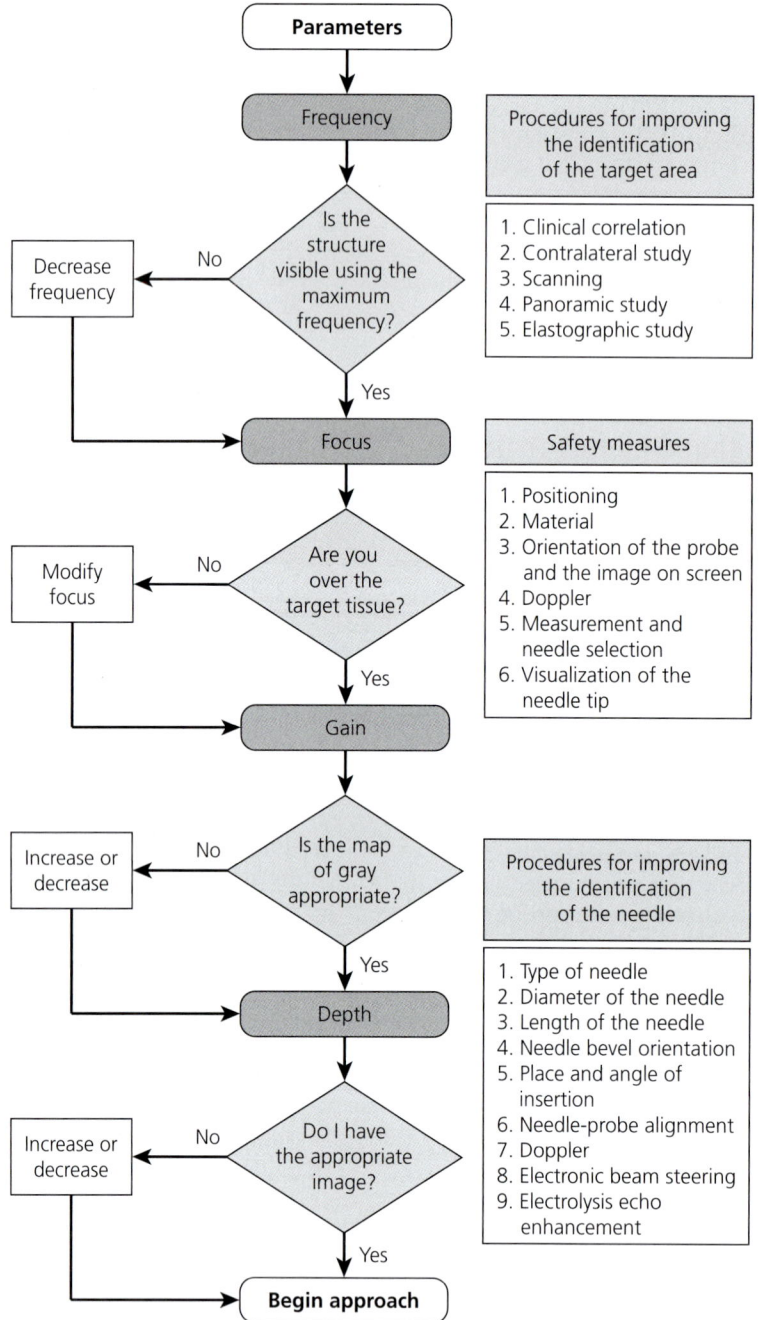

FIGURE 7.31 ■ Algorithm: procedures for improving image visualization and summary tables of the procedures for improving needle identification, target area and the safety of the application.

7.9 ALGORITHM

The most relevant characteristics of the ultrasound-guided procedures in physiotherapy are shown in an algorithm[67] in order to facilitate the decision-making process for the physiotherapist with regard to the process of improving the image, together with a summary table for the remaining considerations (figure 7.31).

Conflict of interest declaration

The authors declare that they have no conflicts of interest.

7.10 REFERENCES

1. Lento PH, Strakowski JA. The use of ultrasound in guiding musculoskeletal interventional procedures. Phys Med Rehabil Clin N Am 2010;21(3):559–83.

2. Valera F, Minaya F, Sánchez JM, et al. Ecografía musculoesquelética: ¿es una herramienta válida en el razonamiento clínico en fisioterapia? 2011. Available at: <http://www.efisioterapia.net/articulos/ecografia -musculoesqueletica-es-una-herramienta-valida-el -razonamiento-clinico-fisioterapi> [Accessed 1 Sept. 2012].

3. Valera F, Minaya F, Sánchez JM, et al. Mitos y realidades en fisioterapia: tendinitis versus tendinosis. I Congreso Internacional de Electrólisis Percutánea Intratisular (EPI®). Libro de comunicaciones y ponencias. Madrid: 2011.

4. Valera F, Minaya F, Sánchez J, et al. Correlación clínica e instrumental en el síndrome de dolor miofascial, ¿es posible identificar con ecografía musculoesquelética un punto gatillo miofascial? En: XI Congreso Nacional SETLA: Ponencias y Comunicaciones. Gijón, 2011; p. 145-6.

5. Smith J, Finnoff JT. Diagnostic and interventional musculoskeletal ultrasound: part 2. Clinical applications. PM R 2009;1(2):162–77.

6. Louis LJ. Musculoskeletal ultrasound intervention: principles and advances. Radiol Clin North Am 2008;46: 5–533.

7. Adler RS, Sofka CM. Percutaneous ultrasound-guided injections in the musculoskeletal system. Ultrasound Q 2003;19(1):3–12.

8. Jones A, Regan M, Ledingham J, et al. Importance of placement of intra-articular steroid injections. BMJ 1993;307(6915):1329–30.

9. Raza K, Lee CY, Pilling D, et al. Ultrasound guidance allows accurate needle placement and aspiration from small joints in patients with early inflammatory arthritis. Rheumatology (Oxford) 2003;42(8):976–9.

10. Eustace JA, Brophy DP, Gibney RP, et al. Comparison of the accuracy of steroid placement with clinical outcome in patients with shoulder symptoms. Ann Rheum Dis 1997;56:59–63.

11. Zingas C, Failla JM, van Holsbeeck M. Injection accuracy and clinical relief of de Quervain's tendonitis. J Hand Surg Am 1998;23:89–96.

12. Helm AT, Higgins G, Rajkumar P, et al. Accuracy of intra-articular injections for osteoarthritis of the trapeziometacarpal joint. Int J Clin Pract 2003;57(4):265–6.

13. Jo CH, Shin YH, Shin JS. Accuracy of intra-articular injection of the glenohumeral joint: a modified anterior approach. Arthroscopy 2011;27(10):1329–34.

14. Balint PV, Kane D, Hunter J, et al. Ultrasound guided versus conventional joint and soft tissue fluid aspiration in rheumatology practice: a pilot study. J Rheumatol 2002;29(10):2209–13.

15. Kane D, Balint PV, Sturrock RD. Ultrasonography is superior to clinical examination in the detection and localization of knee joint effusion in rheumatoid arthritis. J Rheumatol 2003;30(5):966–71.

16. Grassi W, Farina A, Filippucci E, et al. Sonographically guided procedures in rheumatology. Semin Arthritis Rheum 2001;30:347–53.

17. Sofka CM, Collins AJ, Adler RS. Use of ultrasonographic guidance in interventional musculoskeletal procedures: a review from a single institution. J Ultrasound Med 2001;20:21–6.

18. Sofka CM, Adler RS. Ultrasound guided interventions in the foot and ankle. Semin Musculoskelet Radiol 2002;6:163–8.

19. Kapral S, Greher M, Huber G, et al. Ultrasonographic guidance improves the success rate of interscalene brachial plexus blockade. Reg Anesth Pain Med 2008;33(3): 253–8.

20. Perlas A, Brull R, Chan VW, et al. Ultrasound guidance improves the success of sciatic nerve block at the popliteal fossa. Reg Anesth Pain Med 2008;33:259–65.

21. Redborg KE, Antonakakis JG, Beach ML, et al. Ultrasound improves the success rate of a tibial nerve block at the ankle. Reg Anesth Pain Med 2009;34:256–60.

22. Sibbitt WL Jr, Peisajovich A, Michael AA, et al. Does sonographic needle guidance affect the clinical outcome of intraarticular injections? J Rheumatol 2009;36(9): 1892–902.

23. Hall S, Buchbinder R. Do imaging methods that guide needle placement improve outcome? Ann Rheum Dis 2004;63(9):1007–8.

24. Sibbitt WL Jr, Band PA, Chavez-Chiang NR, et al. A randomized controlled trial of the cost-effectiveness of ultrasound-guided intraarticular injection of inflammatory arthritis. J Rheumatol 2011;38(2):252–63.

25. Valera-Garrido F, Minaya-Muñoz F, Sánchez-Ibáñez JM. Efectividad de la Electrólisis Percutánea Intratisular (EPI®) en las tendinopatías crónicas del tendón rotuliano. Trauma Fund Mapfre 2010;21(4):227–36.

26. Valera-Garrido F, Minaya-Muñoz F, Medina-Mirapeix F. Ultrasound-guided percutaneous needle electrolysis in chronic lateral epicondylitis: short- and long-term results. Acupunct Med 2014. In press.

27. Bubnov RV. The use of trigger point 'dry' needling under ultrasound guidance for the treatment of myofascial pain (technological innovation and literature review). Lik Sprava 2010;(5–6):56–64.

28. Minaya-Muñoz F, Valera-Garrido F, Sánchez-Ibáñez JM, et al. Estudio de coste-efectividad de la Electrólisis Percutánea Intratisular (EPI®) en las epicondilalgias. Fisioterapia 2012;34(5):208–15.

29. Valera-Garrido F, Minaya-Muñoz F, Sánchez-Ibáñez JM Efecto de la Electrólisis Percutánea Intratisular (EPI®) en las roturas musculares agudas. Caso clínico de la lesión de 'tennis leg'. Comunicación. II Congreso Regional de Fisioterapia de la Universidad de Murcia, Murcia, 2012.

30. Hoksrud A, Ohberg L, Alfredson H, et al. Ultrasound-guided sclerosis of neovessels in painful chronic patellar tendinopathy: a randomized controlled trial. Am J Sports Med 2006;34(11):1738–46.

31. Fessell DP, Jacobson JA, Craig J, et al. Using sonography to reveal and aspirate joint effusions. AJR Am J Roentgenol 2000;174(5):1353–62.

32. Sarmiento-Gomez J, Owen CA, Washburn MJ Advantages of using SRI-HD and CrossXBeam imaging technology in an aortic occlusion patient: Case report. Madrid: General Electric Healthcare; 2006.

33. Mesurolle B, Bining HJ, El Khoury M, et al. Contribution of tissue harmonic imaging and frequency compound imaging in interventional breast sonography. J Ultrasound Med 2006;25:845–55.

34. Beggs I, Bianchi S, Bueno A, et al. ESSR Ultrasound Group Protocols. Musculoskeletal Ultrasound Technical Guidelines: Knee. <http://www.essr.org/html/img/pool/ knee.pdf>; [Accessed: 1 Sept. 2012].

35. Jamadar DA, Jacobson JA, Caoili EM, et al. Musculoskeletal sonography technique: focused versus comprehensive evaluation. AJR Am J Roentgenol 2008; 190(1):5–9.

36. Cook JL, Khan KM, Kiss ZS, et al. Asymptomatic hypoechoic regions on patellar tendon ultrasound: a 4-year clinical and ultrasound follow-up of 46 tendons. Scand J Med Sci Sports 2001;11:321–7.

37. Cook JL, Malliaras P, De Luca J, et al. Neovascularization and pain in abnormal patellar tendons of active jumping athletes. Clin J Sport Med 2004;14(5):296–9.

38. Malliaras P, Purdam C, Maffulli N, et al. Temporal sequence of greyscale ultrasound changes and their relationship with neovascularity and pain in the patellar tendon. Br J Sports Med 2010;44(13):944–7.

39. Munirama S, Satapathy AR, Schwab A, et al. Translation of sonoelastography from Thiel cadaver to patients for peripheral nerve blocks. Anaesthesia 2012;67(7):721–8.

40. Jiménez JF, Martínez F, Ramos DJ, et al. La sonoelastografía en el diagnóstico de una rotura del tendón supraespinoso. Archivos de Medicina del Deporte 2012; XXIX(148):632–6.

41. Sites BD, Gallagher JD, Cravero J, et al. The learning curve associated with a simulated ultrasound-guided interventional task by inexperienced anesthesia residents. Reg Anesth Pain Med 2004;29(6):544–8.

42. Wiesmann T, Bornträger A, Neff M, et al. Needle visibility in different tissue models for ultrasound-guided regional anaesthesia. Acta Anaesthesiol Scand 2012;56: 1152–5.

43. Hebard S, Hocking G. Echogenic technology can improve needle visibility during ultrasound-guided regional anesthesia. Reg Anesth Pain Med 2011;36(2): 185–9.

44. Hocking G, Mitchell CH. Optimizing the safety and practice of ultrasound-guided regional anesthesia: the role of echogenic technology. Curr Opin Anaesthesiol 2012;205:603–9.

45. Guo S, Schwab A, McLeod G, et al. Echogenic regional anaesthesia needles: a comparison study in Thiel cadavers. Ultrasound Med Biol 2012;38(4):702–7.

46. Bondestam S, Kreula J. Needle tip echogenicity. A study with real time ultrasound. Invest Radiol 1989;24: 555–60.

47. Nichols K, Wright LB, Spencer T, et al. Changes in ultrasonographic echogenicity and visibility of needles with changes in angles of insonation. J Vasc Interv Radiol 2003;14:1553–7.

48. Schafhalter-Zoppoth I, McCulloch CE, Gray AT. Ultrasound visibility of needles used for regional nerve block: an in vitro study. Reg Anesth Pain Med 2004;29:480–8.

49. Chapman GA, Johnson D, Bodenham AR. Visualisation of needle position using ultrasonography. Anaesthesia 2006;61:148–58.

50. Hopkins RE, Bradley M. In-vitro visualisation of biopsy needles with ultrasound: A comparative study of standard and echogenic needles using an ultrasound phantom. Clin Radiol 2001;56:499–502.

51. Reisig F. Büttner J. Ultrasound-guided thoracic paravertebral block for acute thoracic trauma: continuous analgesia after high speed injury. Anaesthesist 2013;62(6): 460–3.

52. Feld R, Needleman L, Goldberg BB. Use of needle vibrating device and color Doppler imaging for sonographically guided invasive procedures. AJR Am J Roentgenol 1997;168:255–6.

53. Armstrong G, Cardon L, Vilkomerson D, et al. Localization of needle tip with color Doppler during pericardiocentesis: In vitro validation and initial clinical application. J Am Soc Echocardiogr 2001;14:29–37.

54. Jones CD, McGahan JP, Clark KJ. Color Doppler ultrasonographic detection of a vibrating needle system. J Ultrasound Med 1997;16:269–74.

55. Cheung S, Rohling R. Enhancement of needle visibility in ultrasound-guided percutaneous procedures. Ultrasound Med Biol 2004;30(5):617–24.

56. Hocking G, Hebard S, Mitchell CH. A review of the benefits and pitfalls of phantoms in ultrasound-guided regional anesthesia. Reg Anesth Pain Med 2011;36(2): 162–70.

57. Wilkin R, Hamm R. How to make a cheap and simple prostate phantom. J Ultrasound Med 2010;29(7): 1151–2.

58. Edgcombe H, Hocking G. Sonographic identification of needle tip by specialists and novices: a blinded comparison of 5 regional block needles in fresh human cadavers. Reg Anesth Pain Med 2010;35:207–11.

59. Partington PF, Broome GH. Diagnostic injection around the shoulder: hit and miss? A cadaveric study of injection accuracy. J Shoulder Elbow Surg 1998;7(2): 147–50.

60. Peuker E, Grönemeyer D. Rare but serious complications of acupuncture: traumatic lesions. Acupunct Med 2001;19(2):103–8.

61. Cockburn JF, Khosh SK. Electrolytic echo enhancement: a novel method to make needles more reflective to ultrasound. J Med Imaging Radiat Oncol 2014;58(2): 203–7.

62. Davies T, Townsley P, Jlala H, et al. Novice performance of ultrasound-guided needle advancement: standard 38-mm transducer vs 25-mm hockey stick transducer. Anaesthesia 2012;67(8):855–61.

63. Tsui BC, Dillane D. Needle puncture site and a 'walkdown' approach for short-axis alignment during ultrasound-guided blocks. Reg Anesth Pain Med 2006; 31:586–7.

64. Bradley MJ. An in-vitro study to understand successful freehand ultrasound guided intervention. Clin Radiol 2001;56:495–8.

65. Phal PM, Brooks DM, Wolfe R. Sonographically guided biopsy of focal lesions: A comparison of freehand and probe-guided techniques using a phantom. AJR Am J Roentgenol 2005;184:1652–6.

66. Hatada T, Ishii H, Ichii S, et al. Ultrasound-guided fine-needle aspiration biopsy for breast tumors: Needle guide versus freehand technique. Tumori 1999;85: 12–14.

67. Medina F, Meseguer AB, Montilla J, et al. Los algoritmos clínicos: una herramienta necesaria en fisioterapia. Fisioterapia Actual 2000;33–41.

PART **IV**

DRY NEEDLING

CHAPTER 8

DRY NEEDLING OF MYOFASCIAL TRIGGER POINTS

Orlando Mayoral del Moral • Isabel Salvat Salvat

We hit each trigger area with a hypodermic needle attached to an empty syringe; we used a rapid peppering motion in the same manner as when injecting a solution. That dry-needling worked too.

JANET G. TRAVELL (*OFFICE HOURS: DAY AND NIGHT. THE AUTOBIOGRAPHY OF JANET TRAVELL, M.D.,* P. 258)

KEYWORDS

dry needling; myofascial pain syndrome (MPS); myofascial trigger points (MTrPs); local twitch response.

8.1 INTRODUCTION

Dry needling (DN) is a treatment technique consisting of the introduction of different types of needles through the skin and into the body, without injection or extraction of substance or fluid. In other words, the mechanical stimulus of the needle alone is used, and this causes a series of effects on the subject, with the goal of treating different pathologies.[1-4] Although an increasing number of treatment indications are being discovered for this technique,[2,5] until now, the major developments in the use of DN have come with the treatment of myofascial pain syndrome (MPS), which represents the main field of action.[6]

MPS is defined as the ensemble of symptoms and signs caused by myofascial trigger points (MTrPs).[6] When a patient is diagnosed with MPS, it is important to specify the muscle, muscle group and anatomical region where the MTrPs considered responsible for the MPS are to be found.

An MTrP is clearly defined as an hyperirritable focal point found on a taut band of muscle

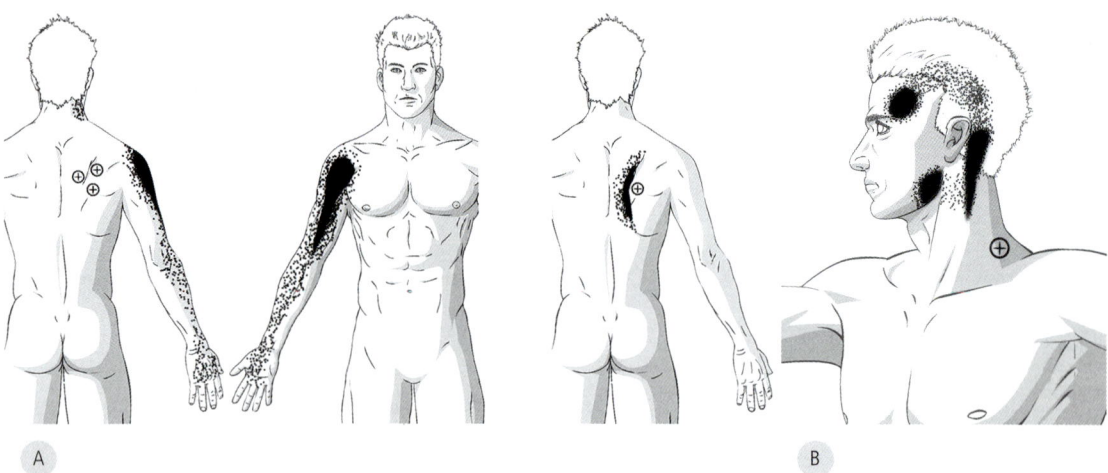

FIGURE 8.1 ■ Patterns of referred pain pertaining to (A) the infraspinatus muscle and (B) the trapezius muscle. The '+' marks represent the most common locations of the myofascial trigger points (MTrPs). The area shaded in black represents the region where the patient feels the pain when the MTrP is active. (Adapted from: Simons et al.[6]). (Colour version of figure is available online).

fibres[6] and which produces signs of hyperalgesia and, frequently, of allodynia, when it is mechanically deformed with stimuli such as compression. It may even provoke other symptoms or signs, such as referred pain (figure 8.1), motor disorders (e.g. inhibition, weakness, movement restriction,[6] disorder in patterns of motor activation[7,8]) and autonomic alterations.[6]

Currently, the most accepted aetiopathogenic theory on the development of MTrPs is known as the integrated hypothesis, formulated by David Simons in 1996,[9] and thereafter extended.[6,10–13] According to this hypothesis, MTrPs are small contractures caused by dysfunctions in the motor end-plates, capable of generating tension in the band where they are located. These dysfunctions are characterized by an excessive activity of acetylcholine, which could be due to different problems at presynaptic, synaptic and postsynaptic levels.[13] The tension created by the contractures of the sarcomeres causes hypoxia and localized deterioration of the tissues, which is accompanied by pH acidity and liberation and accumulation of multiple sensitizing and nociceptive substances,[14] causing peripheral sensitization. These processes are responsible, firstly, for the exquisite local pain of MTrPs and, secondly (after inducing central sensitization), for the referred pain which is characteristic of MTrPs.[15–17]

According to this hypothesis, MTrPs constitute a clear example of a self-perpetuating phenomenon,[10,13,18] independently of the fact that their original causes may have disappeared.[6] This complicates the task of their inactivation and elimination, and explains why DN techniques can be more effective than conservative treatments.[19–21] This tendency for self-perpetuation also supports the idea that the treatment of MPS must consist of two phases[2,3,22]: a first stage, in which there is an attempt to control the pain via treatment of the relevant MTrPs for that MPS, and a second stage, in which all the aetiological and perpetuating factors of the MTrPs are attempted to be both controlled and eliminated.[6,23]

As will be revealed, DN has proven to be effective in the treatment of MTrPs, which, as has been explained, only represents the first phase of treatment for MPS.[2,3] This first phase is essential, but frequently insufficient, particularly in the management of chronic cases.

8.2 CLASSIFICATION OF DRY NEEDLING AND ITS MODALITIES

There are various DN modalities known for the treatment of MTrPs, and these can be classified in different ways, according to the various classification criteria.[2,5] The most commonly used classification criterion is the depth of needle insertion, or, more exactly, the distinction of whether the needle reaches the MTrP or whether it stays on the tissues lying directly above it.[2] According to this, the different DN modalities can be classified into two categories[2,5]:

- superficial DN (SDN) techniques, in which the needle does not reach the MTrP and stays in the tissues immediately overlying it
- deep DN (DDN) techniques, in which the needle reaches the MTrP and passes through it.

Examples of SDN are Peter Baldry's technique,[24,25] and Fu's subcutaneous needling technique.[26,27] Examples of DDN are Hong's fast-in and fast-out technique,[28,29] Gunn's intramuscular stimulation technique[30] and the miniscalpel-needle release technique.[31,32]

8.2.1 Baldry's superficial dry needling technique

In the early 1980s, the acupuncturist Peter Baldry was treating a patient with arm pain due to MPS in the anterior scalene muscle. Fear of producing a pneumothorax led Dr Baldry to avoid introducing the needle as far as the muscle. Instead, he decided to place it only as far as the superficial tissues overlying the MTrP, leaving it in for a short period of time. As a result, on removing the needle, he found that both the hyperalgesia of the MTrP and the arm pain had disappeared.[33,34] After this success, he decided to try it on other parts of the body, where it proved to be just as successful in deep muscles, not only for decrease in pain, but also, according to his subsequent reports, for disappearance of any taut band existing prior to treatment.[25,33,34]

The application of the technique differentiates between patients who are more or less sensitive to it, known as so-called weak, medium and strong responders (see chapter 2). Strong responders are very sensitive to the technique and can experience a negative response if the stimulation is too intense. As it is impossible to predict the category of specific patients, Baldry recommends that, in the first session, a stimulation that sequentially increases in intensity be used, according to the patient's response, followed by a treatment of the different MTrPs one by one (of the indicated MTrPs), using the so-called 'jump sign'[6] and the amplitude of mobility as selection criteria to assess its effectiveness.[25] Therefore, one begins by introducing the needle 5–10 mm deep into the tissues overlying the MTrP, and leaving it in place for 30 seconds before removal. If, upon removal, the jump sign persists, the needle is reintroduced, leaving it for 2–3 minutes, after which the persistence or disappearance of the jump sign is assessed. In the few cases where this sign may be found to persist (i.e. with weak respondents) the needle is reintroduced into the same place and left for longer, applying intermittent turns as a form of manual stimulation.[25] Although Baldry does not specify the duration of the application of the technique in weak responders, the recommendation, from our experience, would be 10–15 minutes.

Once the patient's category has been determined, the adapted technique is applied in subsequent sessions taking into consideration both the time and type of stimulation at this sensitivity, bearing in mind that various MTrPs can be treated at the same time (according to Baldry, this refers to all the active MTrPs found in the patient).

Baldry recommends performing one session per week, except in cases of very severe pain, where treatments on alternate days are recommended. Normally, the duration of the effects from each session is progressively longer each time, allowing for either patient discharge or decrease in the frequency of treatments after the third session. This regime is also useful in cases of long-standing chronic pain, and it is possible for the treatment to be repeated every 4–8 weeks for an indefinite period. In the event that the treatment fails to achieve satisfactory results in the first three sessions, a review of both the diagnosis as well as the therapeutic method used is recommended.

In our opinion, one of the great advantages of Baldry's SDN is the immediate rise in the pain threshold,[19] which allows for application of manual techniques which are better tolerated and, therefore, have a higher likelihood of success. In other words, SDN is an excellent and convenient complement to manual treatments.[8,20]

8.2.2 Fu's subcutaneous needling technique

Fu's subcutaneous needling technique, also known as the technique of floating acupuncture or floating puncture, dates back to 1996. However, few studies have proven the usefulness of the technique for the treatment of MTrPs, except for two small studies by its developer. In these, the technique is described, with somewhat contradictory explanations as to its usefulness for the immediate relief of pain and function in patients with low-back pain[26] and neck pain.[35] The technique is performed with special needles of 1 mm diameter and 31 mm length, solid and with a bevelled tip (figure 8.2). The entire needle, except for the tip (3 mm), is covered by a plastic tube similar to an intravenous catheter. In fact, Dr Fu has surmised that, if special needles are not available, common needles with intravenous catheters can be used instead.[27] The needle is inserted, approximately 7–8 cm from the MTrP that it seeks to treat,[35] until it makes contact with the muscle layer. Immediately after this, it is removed several millimetres to avoid the needle touching the muscle or its fascia for the rest of the procedure. Subsequently, the needle is oriented completely into the horizontal plane and fully inserted into the subcutaneous tissue in the

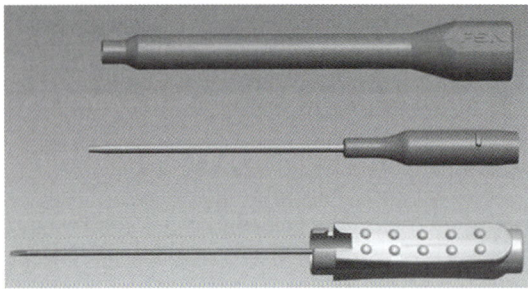

FIGURE 8.2 ■ Needle with catheter used in Fu's subcutaneous dry needling technique. (Colour version of figure is available online).

direction of the MTrP. In order to avoid the possible scenario of the needle manipulations eventually sectioning the tissue and causing bleeding, it is recommended to remove the needle slightly in relation to the catheter, so that the tip of the needle is covered by it. Then the clinician begins manipulating the needle by moving the handle from one side to another in parallel to the skin of the patient, which will generate a 'windscreen wiper' movement of 25–35° amplitude. This movement is repeated 200 times for 2 minutes, after which the needle is removed, leaving the catheter inserted and fixed with surgical tape to avoid it falling out. The catheter is left in the subcutaneous tissue for a variable amount of time, 2–8 hours in acute cases, and 24 hours in chronic cases. According to Fu and Xu, in acute cases a single treatment may be sufficient, while in chronic cases, several treatments may need to be repeated on alternate days.[27]

The manipulation applied to the needle must be completely painfree and it must be able to produce a decrease in the patient's pain. If movement of the needle causes pain, the needle should be repositioned, as it is possible that the needle is inserted either too superficially or too deeply.[27] In our opinion one must be extremely careful with asepsis when using this technique, both before inserting the needle as well as afterwards, together with leaving the catheter in the subcutaneous tissue. More precisely, it is recommended to use the cap usually administered with these types of needles in order to close the handle of the catheter and cover everything with sterile dressing (preferably made of polyurethane), so as to minimize the risk of infection.

8.2.3 Hong's fast-in and fast-out DDN technique

Chan-Zern Hong's DDN technique, known as the 'fast-in and fast-out technique', is probably one of the techniques that is most often used in the treatment of MTrPs. This technique was initially conceptualized as an infiltration technique for MTrPs.[6,28] Dr Hong himself considers that it should be performed using intramuscular or monopolar electromyographic needles, seeing as, in his opinion, the acupuncture needles are too fine and flexible for reliable execution of the technique (C-Z Hong personal communication). Nevertheless, correct training in the use of acupuncture or DN needles enables correct use in the application of this technique.

Once the MTrP is located and established as precisely as possible, the technique consists of inserting the needle until it passes through it, with the intention of provoking local twitch responses (LTRs) (video 8.1). Clinically, it is observed that speed is critical to obtain these LTRs, in that they are more easily obtained if the needle enters faster rather than slower.[28] The needle has to be inserted quickly in order to provoke the LTR, and immediately after, a fast exit is recommended in order to try as far as possible to remove the needle from the taut band by the time the LTR occurs. If one wishes to change the direction of the puncture, the needle is removed from the taut band and the muscle, but not from the patient, leaving the tip of the needle in the subcutaneous tissue. The fast-ins and fast-outs of the needle are performed repeatedly until either the LTRs are exhausted, or the patient's tolerance threshold is met. Some studies have demonstrated that the puncture or infiltration of MTrPs is more effective if LTRs are provoked.[36,37]

KEY POINTS

The LTR is one of the most striking characteristics of MTrPs. It consists of provocation of an involuntary brief, transitory and isolated contraction of the fibres that form the taut band when the MTrP is stimulated via determined manual explorations or rapid insertion of the needle.

8.2.4 Gunn's intramuscular stimulation technique

This is not a simple needle manipulation technique, but an entire diagnostic and therapeutic concept focused mainly on the treatment of chronic pain. According to Chan Gunn, MTrPs are always secondary to radiculopathy,[30] or, more extensively, to alteration of the nervous system.[38] Although conceptually very different, the Gunn technique is very similar to the spinal segmental sensitization technique of Andrew Fischer,[39–41]

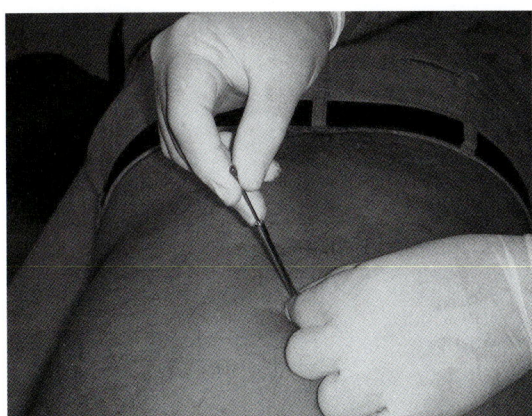

FIGURE 8.3 ■ Plunger recommended by Chan Gunn for inserting and manipulating needles, in the intramuscular stimulation technique by said author. (Colour version of figure is available online).

from the point of view of the diagnostic and therapeutic protocol.[42]

With regard to the technique of needling, Chan Gunn recommends the use of acupuncture needles that are inserted and manipulated using a plunger (figure 8.3), enabling fast ins and outs, in a manner similar to those recommended by Hong, but also adding twists to the needle in both directions once the needle has entered the MTrP (or 'muscle knot', according to Gunn's own terminology) or even percutaneous electrostimulation through the plunger using a dermometer.

8.2.5 DDN miniscalpel-needle release technique

A recent study[31]analysed the effectiveness of a taut band release technique using a needle which was introduced in the year 2007[32] and which is known as the miniscalpel needle. This study compared this technique with DDN in the treatment of MTrPs of the upper trapezius. The miniscalpel needle has a width of 1 mm (as opposed to the 0.30 mm of the acupuncture needle used in the study) and its tip is flat and sharp, similar to a scalpel blade. The results from the miniscalpel needle group were significantly superior to those of the DDN group at 3-month follow-up, and both were better than those of the control group, who performed self-stretching exercises for the upper trapezius (the self-stretching exercises were also performed by the subjects from both puncture groups). A previous study was unable to demonstrate the superiority of the results depending on the width of the needle used in the infiltration of MTrPs,[43] and therefore it is recommended that more studies

are undertaken to support the results of using the miniscalpel needle before considering more widespread use of the technique. In any case, nowadays, because of its greater aggressiveness, its use could be proposed in cases that are unresponsive to acupuncture needles or DN.

8.3 DIAGNOSTIC IMPORTANCE OF DRY NEEDLING

There are several reasons why DN and, more specifically, DDN are of interest in diagnostics. The most obvious is its demonstrated capacity to provoke referred pain more effectively than other types of manual stimulation of the MTrP, such as compression,[44] contraction or stretching. Although the referred pain provocation is not considered to be an essential diagnostic criterion,[1,6] clinically, it is tremendously useful as it establishes the greater or lesser relevance of the MTrPs, according to whether the provoked referred pain is or is not recognized by the patient as his or her habitual pain. The superiority of DDN for the provoking referred pain from MTrPs is especially noticeable in deep muscles such as the multifidus or the supraspinatus, in which manual stimulation rarely achieves this, and it thus becomes an invaluable diagnostic tool.[1]

On the other hand, thanks to the well-known 'wand' phenomenon,[1,45] the needle becomes a palpation tool which allows the physiotherapist to 'feel' differences in the stiffness of the tissues which are explored[1,4] (once one acquires experience in its use). This could entail several advantages: from avoiding inserting the needle into the peritoneum, to treating the rectus abdominis (as one can 'feel' the posterior wall of the rectus abdominis sheath[1]), to avoiding touching the spinal dura mater by using contact with the vertebral lamina as a reference, among other examples.

KEY POINTS

According to the 'wand' phenomenon, described by Daniel Dennett,[45] when an object is touched through a wand or stick which is held in one hand, the complex kinaesthetic and tactile mechanisms that are triggered allow one to feel through the wand, experimenting the (false) feeling of having nerve endings at the tip of the wand.

Although LTRs are not considered to be essential criteria for the diagnosis of MTrPs, due to the low interexaminer reliability achieved in published studies[46,47] and the difficulty or impossibility of manually achieving them in deep muscles, they constitute a first-order finding of the presence of an MTrP, which some consider to be pathognomonic.[6] Apart from therapeutic interest in DDN,[36,37] the finding of an LTR with a needle (and its visualization, whether it be direct in superficial muscles, or through ultrasound in deeper ones) constitutes one of the main indicators of having performed the puncture of an MTrP, which implies an important support for diagnostics.

8.4 THERAPEUTIC EFFECTIVENESS AND INDICATIONS OF DRY NEEDLING

One cannot emphasize enough the importance of the exact and precise diagnosis of MTrPs[3,5] and of the MPS[5] in order to achieve effective DN. Without a good diagnosis, DN turns into an imprecise intervention with unpredictable results.

Usually, Steinbrocker[48] is cited as the first to have described the effectiveness of punctures without infiltration for the treatment of pain: 'The mere insertion of a needle somewhere in the region of pain, without introducing analgesic solutions, also has been reported to give frequent lasting relief'. Since then, a number of works have been published in which the effectiveness of DN has been exposed. Some have demonstrated an effectiveness of DDN similar to that of infiltrations of different substances for the treatment of MTrPs.[36,49–52] This allows for extrapolation of the documented results of infiltrations to DDN.

However, the reviews available on the effectiveness of DN always reach the same conclusions. Cummings and White, in their systematic review,[53] conclude that direct puncture of MTrPs seems to be an effective technique, although it has not proved to be superior in effectiveness to placebo in clinical trials. These authors conclude that 'controlled clinical trials are needed in order to investigate whether puncture has a greater effect than placebo on pain in MTrPs'. More recent systematic reviews on DN have come to similar conclusions.[54,55] Due to the invasive nature of DN, it is complicated to design double-blind controlled studies against placebo.[2,4,16] The different models of placebo needles and the simulated puncture methods are called into question, as it is considered that all of them entail some kind of physiological stimulus which, therefore, disqualifies them from being authentic placebo.[56] With this in mind, and in order to avoid this problem, our team carried out a randomized controlled trial, as opposed to a double-blind placebo on the effectiveness of DDN of MTrPs in the prevention of myofascial pain after total arthroplasty of the knee.[57]

In our study, an expert examiner explored 40 patients in search of MTrPs in the muscles of the lower extremity several hours before surgery for joint replacement. The patients were then assigned either to a group of real DDN or to a group of simulated DDN. Immediately after the anaesthesia and before commencing the surgical intervention, DDN was performed on all of the previously diagnosed MTrPs in patients belonging to the group of real DDN, whereas the patients from the group of simulated DDN were not provided with any treatment, although the physiotherapist who applied the DDN was in the surgery room throughout the anaesthesia process and simulated DDN immediately afterwards. Given that the patients could not feel a thing, they were completely blind regarding the assigned group, just as the examiner of the MTrPs was also blind throughout the presurgical explorations and during the follow-up at the first, third and sixth month after the intervention. The patients from the group of real DDN experienced less pain after surgery, with statistically significant differences in the postsurgical request for analgesics ($p = 0.02$) and in the rate of change for the scores measured using the visual analogue scale (VAS) 1 month after surgery (VAS > 4; $p = 0.03$; entry–attribute–value = 0; $p = 0.04$). The results from this study show the superiority of the DDN as opposed to placebo, resulting in an innovative and very interesting placebo methodology for DDN.[2]

Although much more research is certainly needed, until now, different studies have demonstrated the effectiveness of DN in myofascial shoulder pain,[58] hemiparetic shoulder pain,[59] chronic subacromial impingement syndrome,[21] arm pain caused by MTrPs in the infraspinatus muscle,[60] alterations of the motor activation patterns of the shoulder,[8] low-back pain,[50,54,61–65] cervical and lumbar radiculopathies,[66–68] chronic cervical pain[69] caused by whiplash syndrome,[38] cervical pain concurrent with a sensation of respiratory difficulty,[70] chronic thoracic myofascial postsurgical pain,[71] chronic myofascial pain of the knee,[72] anterior idiopathic pain of the knee,[73] chronic pain in patients with foot arthrodesis,[74] myofascial pain and temporomandibular dysfunction,[75,76] chronic myofascial pain in different locations,[77] postherpes pain,[78,79] migraine,[80] tension headache,[81] chronic headache,[52,82] pain from total postarthroplasty of the knee,[57] spasticity in incomplete tetraplegias[83] and in infantile cerebral palsy.[84]

Electromyographic studies have found that the technique is able to inhibit end-plate noise in the treated areas.[37] The presence of end-plate noise and its prevalence are considered to be objective data for the existence of MTrPs[85] and the grade of irritability,[86] respectively.

Using microanalysis techniques, Shah et al.[14] have demonstrated that the LTR provoked by DDN causes an immediate decrease in the concentration of existing nociceptive and sensitizing substances located in the area of the MTrP. This could explain why DDN frequently causes an immediate reduction in pain.[14]

Recently, Ballyns et al.[87] have shown using objective ultrasound measurement that DDN can alleviate cervical pain, while at the same time decreasing the size of the MTrP.

Based on the pain typically involved in treatment with DDN techniques, these types of puncture have been attributed to be a cause of central sensitization.[41] Nevertheless, as we have previously explained, the referred pain from the MTrPs is a clear manifestation of the existence of a central sensitization.[15,17] Thus, it is possible to affirm that DDN is, in fact, a technique that consists of reverting this sensitization, due to its demonstrated effectiveness for the elimination of existing pain. A recent study elegantly demonstrated the aforementioned capacity of DDN to decrease or eliminate the central sensitization related to MTrPs, inducing clear segmentally mediated antinociceptive effects.[88]

With regard to the clinical indications of DN, apart from its use in MTrPs (already described), new empirical evidence is suggesting its value in other pathologies such as for the treatment of enthesopathies and tendinopathies (insertional MTrPs),[89–91] for non-MTrPs such as those found within the ligaments,[92] the joints or in scar tissue (C-Z Hong personal communication) or for spasticity.[84] Further studies are needed to explore the usefulness of DN in these cases.

8.5 MECHANISMS OF ACTION OF DRY NEEDLING IN MYOFASCIAL TRIGGER POINTS

It is reasonable to assume that the mechanisms of action, which are used to explain the beneficial effects of DN in the treatment of MTrPs, should be different in the case of SDN as opposed to DDN. Some of the mechanisms that are detailed below have clearly been identified, whereas others are eminently hypothetical and evolve according to the progress of new knowledge regarding the aethiopathogenesis of the MTrPs.

8.5.1 Mechanisms of action of superficial dry needling

Given that, in SDN, the needle does not go through the MTrP, its possible effects cannot, in principle, be justified with regard to mechanical effects; rather, the invoked mechanisms are to be found fundamentally in the field of neurophysiology. A first approach to this matter could be made using the concept of 'analgesia by hyperstimulation', as described by Melzack, and referring to the application of a harmful stimulus in the nervous system to alleviate pain by inducing the activation of complex endogenous pain-modulating mechanisms.[33] The most likely mechanisms of action of superficial needling are:

- the stimulation of A-δ nerve fibres performed by inserting a needle into the skin overlying the MTrP. This can suppress the pain mediated by the muscular nociceptors of the C fibres (involved in myofascial pain proceeding from MTrPs) by different means[93]:
  - via direct action over the inhibitory enkephalinergic inhibitory interneurons situated on the border of lamina I and II of the dorsal horn of the spinal cord
  - via indirect action over the enkephalinergic interneurons through the descending inhibitory serotoninergic system
  - via a stimulating effect on the descending noradrenergic system
  - via activation of the diffuse inhibitory controls of nociception,[94,95] which can also be activated by the peripheral C fibres,[96] via collaterals that connect the neospinothalamic tract with the dorsal reticular subnucleus of the spinal cord
- the well-known capacity for stimulation using needles to induce secretion of endogenous opioid peptides (e.g. enkephalins, dynorphins)[33,97]
- the gate-control theory. The stimulation of A-β nerve fibers tends to 'close' the gate and inhibit the transmission of pain to the superior centres[98]
- hypothetical action over the autonomous nervous system,[99] which is known to modulate the activity of MTrPs.[11,100–102]

Currently, several important aspects concerning the SDN technique are unknown, such as whether its effectiveness is superior to placebo; the optimal application time; the duration of its effects and the relation between these parameters; as well as the suitability of combining it with other treatments. No studies have researched whether insertion of the needle over the MTrP (as dictated by Baldry) is more effective than needling over the dermatome corresponding to the myotome of the muscle with the MTrP. In this way it guarantees a segmental correspondence between cutaneous A-δ and/or A-β fibres and the muscular nociceptors that allow blockage of the muscle's nociceptors.

8.5.2 Mechanisms of action of deep dry needling

In principle, all the mechanisms invoked for SDN can also be applied to DDN, including the induction mechanism for the secretion of endogenous opioid peptides.[103]

As has been explained previously, there seems to be a clear correlation between obtaining an LTR and the therapeutic effectiveness of DDN.[36,37,66,67] With this in mind, a series of possible mechanisms of action are exclusive to DDN regarding their effect on MTrPs:

- Cleansing of nociceptive sensitizing substances produced by the LTR[14]: the works by Shah et al. have demonstrated that active MTrPs have a significantly high concentration of bradykinin, substance P, calcitonin gene-related peptide (CGRP), tumour necrosis factor, interleukin-1β, serotonin and noradrenaline, among others. It has also been demonstrated that the concentration of these substances immediately decreases the provocation of an LTR. It is important to highlight that, in these studies, the LTR is obtained using the same microdialysis needle with which the biochemical medium of the MTrPs is analysed in vivo, which only serves to increase the reliability of the study. We have already briefly commented on the importance of these substances with regard to the pain caused by MTrPs and their perpetuation. The decrease in concentration caused by the LTR is understood to be something that is extraordinarily useful for the reduction of the related peripheral and central sensitizations.
- pH elevation: the same study[14] demonstrates how the LTR is able to elevate the pH of the MTrP zone significantly. In the introduction it was also stated that the acidity existing in the MTrPs directly affects their worsening and perpetuation. It is considered that acid pH causes peripheral sensitization, decreases acetylcholinesterase expression, increases acetylcholine activity and promotes the liberation of sensitizing substances such as CGRP, all of which contribute to accentuating the dysfunction of the motor end-plate causing the MTrPs.[11,12]

- Mechanical rupture of the fibres and/or the affected motor end-plates[4,6,28,104,105]: the limited magnitude of the lesions caused in the muscle fibres and/or in their innervation would allow for their repair and restitution ad integrum of the injured myocytes and a new synaptogenesis over a period of 1–2 weeks[104,105].
- Local stretch of the shortened cytoskeletal structures[106,107] of the fibres close to the needle which have not been destroyed by the needle. This stretch can contribute to normalization of the length of the shortened sarcomeres. Additionally, this stretch could normalize the titin which, due to the maintained contracture, hypothetically has derived in titin gel and maintains the myosin adhered to the Z band.[22,107–109] Assuming that the needle can locally stretch the muscle fibres, it may be appropriate to twist the needle during the puncture procedure. The twist causes a rolling of the connective tissue around the needle, and demonstrates that insertion of the needle accompanied by rotation causes an orientation that is more parallel to the collagen fibres.[110]

8.6 CLINICAL CASE

8.6.1 Dry needling in a case of temporomandibular pain

A patient attended the clinic suffering from severe restriction of the mandibular opening which began the previous week after a visit to the dentist when she was required to keep her mouth wide open (maximum width) for about an hour. The patient had an interincisal opening of 9 mm, with a hard end-feel and spontaneous pain in the upper right maxillary molars and in the right mandibular region (VAS 48/100) which was aggravated when opening of her mouth was forced (63/100). The dentist dismissed a dental cause for the restriction of mobility and pain, and told the patient that the cause was musculoarticular. He prescribed passive exercises with a clothes peg in order to try and gain mobility. After a week of performing the exercises with no more result than an increase in pain, the patient decided to consult the physiotherapist, seeing as the limitation of mobility was starting to interfere in her quality of life and she could not eat (she was only allowed liquids and purées) or speak normally.

Given the activator mechanism, consisting of maintained overstretching of the jaw elevator muscles, and the well-known capacity for these muscles, especially the masseter muscle, to limit mandibular opening when they present MTrPs, the muscular exploration of the patient was centred on the jaw elevator muscles (both masseters, both temporals and both medial pterygoid muscles). The manual exam revealed the presence of an important tension in both masseters, especially the right one, in which an MTrP was also found with allodynia, located in a specially taut band of this muscle. There were no striking findings in any of the temporal muscles. Due to the limited mandibular opening, manual intraoral exam of the medial pterygoid muscles was impossible. Extraoral palpation of the inferior insertion of both muscles in the inner side of the angle of the mandible did not show any hypersensitivity of the area. The manual exam of both temporomandibular joints also failed to reveal any anomaly beyond restriction of mobility.

In the first session, the treatment consisted of the application of manual release (compression and massage) of the MTrPs of the left masseter and DDN of the MTrP of the right masseter with a needle of 0.16×25 mm, followed by spraying and stretching both muscles. After treatment, the opening increased to 2.1 cm. The patient was asked to apply local heat to both masseters three times a day, followed by active self-stretching exercises (yawning) and was given an appointment for 2 days later.

After 48 hours, examination revealed that the mobility that was gained had been virtually completely lost once again. The existence of a perpetuating factor hampering the complete and long-lasting inactivation of the MTrPs of the masseter muscles was consequently considered. One of the most frequent causes is the existence of MTrPs in the upper trapezius, whose zone of referred pain includes the zone of the masseter muscle (figure 8.1B). Examination of this muscle showed the existence of an active MTrP in the clavicular fibres of the right trapezius. The patient described the pain that she felt when the therapist was pressing the MTrP seemed familiar and that previously, she had suffered neck pain for which she had received physiotherapy treatment, something that she had not admitted to in the initial anamnesis. After the invasive treatment was applied using DN in this MTrP, the mobility of the interincisal opening reached 3.2 cm, without any treatment to the masseter.

In the manual treatment of both masseters, which was applied afterwards, the patient restored her normal mobility with a completely free mandibular opening (4.3 cm).

The 1-week posttreatment check-up revealed that the mobility gained in the second session was maintained and that the pain decreased. The patient was discharged, and given gentle home exercises of postisometric relaxation of both trapezius muscles and for both masseters.

(Clinical case continued on page 489)

8.7 REFERENCES

1. Mayoral O. Fisioterapia invasiva del síndrome de dolor miofascial. Fisioterapia 2005;27:69–75.
2. Mayoral Del Moral O. Dry needling treatments for myofascial trigger points. J Musculoskelet Pain 2010; 18(4):411–16.
3. Mayoral-del-Moral O, Torres-Lacomba M. Fisioterapia invasiva y punción seca. Informe sobre la eficacia de la punción seca en el tratamiento del síndrome de dolor miofascial y sobre su uso en fisioterapia. Cuest Fisioter 2009;38(3):206–17.
4. Dommerholt J, Mayoral del Moral O, Gröbli C. Trigger point dry needling. J Man Manip Ther 2006; 14(4):E70–87.
5. Mayoral del Moral O. Fisioterapia invasiva en el síndrome de dolor miofascial: Avances y formación. In: Gómez-Conesa A, Rodríguez R, Alcocer MA, editors. XIV Congreso Nacional de Fisioterapia. El Fisioterapeuta 2.0. Nuevos estudios, nuevos métodos. Madrid: Asociación Española de Fisioterapeutas; 2012. p. 55–61.
6. Simons DG, Travell JG, Simons LS. Dolor y disfunción miofascial. El manual de los puntos gatillo. Mitad superior del cuerpo. 2nd ed. Madrid: Editorial Médica Panamericana; 2002.
7. Ibarra JM, Ge HY, Wang C, et al. Latent myofascial trigger points are associated with an increased antagonistic muscle activity during agonist muscle contraction. J Pain 2011;12(12):1282–8.
8. Lucas KR, Polus BI, Rich PA. Latent myofascial trigger points: their effects on muscle activation and movement efficiency. J Bodyw Mov Ther 2004;8(3):160–6.
9. Simons DG. Clinical and etiological update of myofascial pain from trigger points. J Musculoske Pain 1996; 4(1/2):93–121.
10. Simons DG. Review of enigmatic MTrPs as a common cause of enigmatic musculoskeletal pain and dysfunction. J Electromyogr Kinesiol 2004;14(1):95–107.
11. Gerwin RD, Dommerholt J, Shah JP. An expansion of Simons' integrated hypothesis of trigger point formation. Curr Pain Headache Rep 2004;8(6):468–75.
12. Bron C, Dommerholt JD. Etiology of myofascial trigger points. Curr Pain Headache Rep 2012;16(5):439–44.
13. McPartland JM, Simons DG. Myofascial trigger points: translating molecular theory into manual therapy. J Man Manip Ther 2006;14(4):232–9.
14. Shah JP, Phillips TM, Danoff JV, et al. An in vivo microanalytical technique for measuring the local biochemical milieu of human skeletal muscle. J Appl Physiol 2005;99(5):1977–84.
15. Mense S, Simons DG, Russell IJ. Muscle Pain. Understanding its nature, diagnosis, and treatment. Baltimore: Lippincott Williams & Wilkins; 2001.

16. Dommerholt J. Dry needling-peripheral and central considerations. J Man Manip Ther 2011;19(4):223–7.

17. Hoheisel U, Mense S, Simons DG, et al. Appearance of new receptive fields in rat dorsal horn neurons following noxious stimulation of skeletal muscle: a model for referral of muscle pain? Neurosci Lett 1993;153(1): 9–12.

18. Mayoral O. Mecanismos analgésicos de la punción seca en el síndrome de dolor miofascial. In: Fisioterapia y dolor; 2005. Madrid: Escuela Universitaria de Fisioterapia ONCE; 2005. p. 95–101.

19. Martínez JM, Mayoral O, Torres M, et al. Randomized pilot study on the immediate effectiveness of the treatment of latent myofascial trigger points in infraspinatus muscle: ischemic compression versus superficial dry needling. In: MYOPAIN 2010. VIII World congress on myofascial pain and fibromyalgia. 2010 3–7 October; Toledo (Spain): International Myopain Society; 2010. p. 17 <http://c.ymcdn.com/sites/www.myopain.org/resource/resmgr/docs/abstracts-book-myopain-2010-.pdf>; [Accessed 8-10-2012].

20. Edwards J, Knowles N. Superficial dry needling and active stretching in the treatment of myofascial pain – a randomised controlled trial. Acupunct Med 2003;21(3): 80–6.

21. Ingber RS. Shoulder impingement in tennis/racquetball players treated with subscapularis myofascial treatments. Arch Phys Med Rehabil 2000;81(5):679–82.

22. Mayoral O, Torres R. Tratamiento conservador y fisioterápico invasivo de los puntos gatillo miofasciales. In: Patología de partes blandas en el hombro. Madrid: Fundación MAPFRE Medicina; 2003.

23. Gerwin RD. Factores que promueven la persistencia de mialgia en el síndrome de dolor miofascial y en la fibromialgia. Fisioterapia 2005;27(2):76–86.

24. Baldry P. Superficial versus deep dry needling. Acupunct Med 2002;20(2–3):78–81.

25. Baldry PE. Acupuncture, trigger points and musculoskeletal pain. 3rd ed. London: Elsevier-Churchill Livingstone; 2005.

26. Fu ZH, Chen XY, Lu LJ, et al. Immediate effect of Fu's subcutaneous needling for low back pain. Chin Med J (Engl) 2006;119(11):953–6.

27. Fu Z-H, Xu J-G. A brief introduction to Fu's subcutaneous needling. Pain Clinic 2005;17(3):343–8.

28. Hong C-Z. Considerations and recommendations of myofascial trigger points injection. J Musculoskelet Pain 1994;2(1):29–59.

29. Hong C-Z. New trends in myofascial pain syndrome. Zhonghua Yi Xue Za Zhi (Taipei) 2002;65(11):501–12.

30. Gunn CC. The gunn approach to the treatment of chronic pain, intramuscular stimulation for myofascial pain of radiculopathic origin. 2nd ed. New York: Churchill Livingstone; 1996.

31. Ma C, Wu S, Li G, et al. Comparison of miniscalpel-needle release, acupuncture needling, and stretching exercise to trigger point in myofascial pain syndrome. Clin J Pain 2010;26(3):251–7.

32. Wang C, Xiong Z, Deng C, et al. Miniscalpel-needle versus triggerpoint injection for cervical myofascial pain syndrome: a randomized comparative trial. J Altern Complement Med 2007;13(1):14–16.

33. Baldry PE. Acupuncture, trigger points and musculoskeletal pain. 2nd ed. London: Churchill Livingstone; 1993.

34. Baldry PE. Myofascial pain and fibromyalgia syndromes. Edinburgh: Churchill Livingstone; 2001.

35. Fu ZH, Wang JH, Sun JH, et al. Fu's subcutaneous needling: possible clinical evidence of the subcutaneous connective tissue in acupuncture. J Altern Complement Med 2007;13(1):47–51.

36. Hong C-Z. Lidocaine injection versus dry needling to myofascial trigger point. The importance of the local twitch response. Am J Phys Med Rehabil 1994;73(4): 256–63.

37. Chen JT, Chung KC, Hou CR, et al. Inhibitory effect of dry needling on the spontaneous electrical activity recorded from myofascial trigger spots of rabbit skeletal muscle. Am J Phys Med Rehabil 2001;80(10): 729–35.

38. Gunn CC, Byrne D, Goldberger M, et al. Treating whiplash-associated disorders with intramuscular stimulation: a retrospective review of 43 patients with long-term follow-up. J Musculoskelet Pain 2001;9(2): 69–89.

39. Imamura M, Kaziyama HHS, Hsing WT, et al. Efficacy of a segmental neuromyotherapy approach to improve pain pressure threshold in patients with severe osteoarthritis of the knee. J Musculoske Pain 2007;15(Suppl. 13):25.

40. Ga H, Choi JH, Park CH, et al. Dry needling of trigger points with and without paraspinal needling in myofascial pain syndromes in elderly patients. J Altern Complement Med 2007;13(6):617–24.

41. Fischer AA. Treatment of myofascial pain. J Musculoskelet Pain 1999;7(1/2):131–42.

42. Fischer AA. New injection techniques for treatment of musculoskeletal pain. In: Rachlin ES, Rachlin IS, editors. Myofascial pain and fibromyalgia: trigger point management. Mosby; 2002. p. 403–19.

43. Yoon SH, Rah UW, Sheen SS, et al. Comparison of 3 needle sizes for trigger point injection in myofascial pain syndrome of upper- and middle-trapezius muscle: a randomized controlled trial. Arch Phys Med Rehabil 2009;90(8):1332–9.

44. Hong C-Z, Kuan TS, Chen JT, et al. Referred pain elicited by palpation and by needling of myofascial trigger points: a comparison. Arch Phys Med Rehabil 1997;78(9):957–60.

45. Dennett D. La conciencia explicada. Una teoría interdisciplinar. 1st ed. Barcelona: Paidós Ibérica S.A.; 1995.

46. Gerwin RD, Shannon S, Hong CZ, et al. Interrater reliability in myofascial trigger point examination. Pain 1997;69(1–2):65–73.

47. Bron C, Franssen J, Wensing M, et al. Interrater reliability of palpation of myofascial trigger points in three shoulder muscles. J Man Manip Ther 2007;15(4): 203–15.

48. Steinbrocker O. Therapeutic injections in painful musculoskeletal disorders. J Am Med Assoc 1944;125: 397–401.

49. Jaeger B, Skootsky SA. Double blind, controlled study of different myofascial trigger point injection techniques. Pain 1987;4(Supl):S292.

50. Garvey TA, Marks MR, Wiesel SW. A prospective, randomized, double-blind evaluation of trigger-point injection therapy for low-back pain. Spine 1989;14(9): 962–4.

51. Ga H, Choi JH, Park CH, et al. Acupuncture needling versus lidocaine injection of trigger points in myofascial pain syndrome in elderly patients – a randomised trial. Acupunct Med 2007;25(4):130–6.

52. Venancio Rde A, Alencar FG, Zamperini C. Different substances and dry-needling injections in patients with myofascial pain and headaches. Cranio 2008;26(2): 96–103.

53. Cummings TM, White AR. Needling therapies in the management of myofascial trigger point pain: a systematic review. Arch Phys Med Rehabil 2001;82(7): 986–92.

54. Furlan AD, van Tulder M, Cherkin D, et al. Acupuncture and dry-needling for low back pain: an updated

systematic review within the framework of the Cochrane Collaboration. Spine 2005;30(8):944–63.

55. Tough EA, White AR, Cummings TM, et al. Acupuncture and dry needling in the management of myofascial trigger point pain: a systematic review and meta-analysis of randomised controlled trials. Eur J Pain 2009;13(1):3–10.

56. Lund I, Lundeberg T. Are minimal, superficial or sham acupuncture procedures acceptable as inert placebo controls? Acupunct Med 2006;24(1):13–15.

57. Mayoral O, Martín MT, Martín S, et al. Randomized, double blind, placebo-controlled clinical trial about the effectiveness of myofascial trigger points dry needling in the prevention of myofascial pain after total knee arthroplasty. In: MYOPAIN 2010. VIII World congress on myofascial pain and fibromyalgia. 2010 3–7 october; Toledo (Spain): International Myopain Society; 2010. p. 19 <http://c.ymcdn.com/sites/www.myopain.org/resource/resmgr/docs/abstracts-book-myopain-2010-.pdf>; [Accessed 8-10-2012].

58. Ceccheerelli F, Bordin M, Gagliardi G, et al. Comparison between superficial and deep acupuncture in the treatment of the shoulder's myofascial pain: a randomized and controlled study. Acupunct Electrother Res 2001;26(4):229–38.

59. DiLorenzo L, Traballesi M, Morelli D, et al. Hemiparetic shoulder pain syndrome treated with deep dry needling during early rehabilitation: a prospective, open-label, randomized investigation. J Musculoske Pain 2004;12(2):25–34.

60. Hsieh YL, Kao MJ, Kuan TS, et al. Dry needling to a key myofascial trigger point may reduce the irritability of satellite MTrPs. Am J Phys Med Rehabil 2007; 86(5):397–403.

61. Ceccherelli F, Rigoni MT, Gagliardi G, et al. Comparison of superficial and deep acupuncture in the treatment of lumbar myofascial pain: a double-blind randomized controlled study. Clin J Pain 2002;18(3): 149–53.

62. Pérez-Palomares S, Oliván-Blázquez B, Magallón-Botaya R, et al. Percutaneous electrical nerve stimulation versus dry needling: effectiveness in the treatment of chronic low back pain. J Musculoske Pain 2010;18(1): 23–30.

63. Gunn CC, Milbrandt WE, Little AS, et al. Dry needling of muscle motor points for chronic low-back pain: a randomized clinical trial with long-term follow-up. Spine 1980;5(3):279–91.

64. Itoh K, Katsumi Y, Kitakoji H. Trigger point acupuncture treatment of chronic low back pain in elderly patients – a blinded RCT. Acupunct Med 2004;22(4): 170–7.

65. Macdonald AJR, Macrae KD, Master BR, et al. Superficial acupuncture in the relief of chronic low-back pain. Ann R Coll Surg Engl 1983;65:44–6.

66. Chu J. Twitch-obtaining intramuscular stimulation. Observations in the management of radiculopathic chronic low back pain. J Musculoskelet Pain 1999;7(4): 131–46.

67. Chu J. Twitch-obtaining intramuscular stimulation (TOIMS): long term observations in the management of chronic partial cervical radiculopathy. Electromyogr Clin Neurophysiol 2000;40(8):503–10.

68. Chu J. Early observations in radiculopathic pain control using electrodiagnostically derived new treatment techniques: automated twitch-obtaining intramuscular stimulation (ATOIMS) and electrical twitch-obtaining intramuscular stimulation (ETOIMS). Electromyogr Clin Neurophysiol 2000;40(4):195–204.

69. Itoh K, Katsumi Y, Hirota S, et al. Randomised trial of trigger point acupuncture compared with other acupuncture for treatment of chronic neck pain. Complement Ther Med 2007;15(3):172–9.

70. Aun NC. Treating subjective shortness of breath by inactivating trigger points of the levator scapulae muscles with acupuncture needles. J Musculoske Pain 1996;4(3):81–5.

71. Cummings M. Myofascial pain from pectoralis major following trans-axillary surgery. Acupunct Med 2003; 21(3):105–7.

72. Cummings M. Referred knee pain treated with electroacupuncture to iliopsoas. Acupunct Med 2003; 21(1–2):32–5.

73. Naslund J, Naslund UB, Odenbring S, et al. Sensory stimulation (acupuncture) for the treatment of idiopathic anterior knee pain. J Rehabil Med 2002;34(5): 231–8.

74. Tateishi M, Imamura M, Hsing WT, et al. Study of the effectiveness of dry needling in the treatment of chronic pain in people with foot arthrodesis. J Musculoske Pain 2007;15(Suppl. 13):39.

75. McMillan AS, Nolan A, Kelly PJ. The efficacy of dry needling and procaine in the treatment of myofascial pain in the jaw muscles. J Orofac Pain 1997;11(4): 307–14.

76. Gonzalez-Perez LM, Infante-Cossio P, Granados-Nunez M, et al. Treatment of temporomandibular myofascial pain with deep dry needling. Med Oral Patol Oral Cir Bucal 2012;17(5):e781–5.

77. Lewit K. The needle effect in the relief of myofascial pain. Pain 1979;6(1979):83–90.

78. Okada M, Stump P, Lin TY, et al. The occurrence of latent and active myofascial trigger points in patients with post-herpetic neuralgia. J Musculoske Pain 1998; 6(Suppl. 2):29.

79. Weiner DK, Schmader KE. Postherpetic pain: more than sensory neuralgia? Pain Med 2006;7(3):243–9, discussion 250.

80. Hesse J, Mogelvang B, Simonsen H. Acupuncture versus metoprolol in migraine prophylaxis: a randomized trial of trigger point inactivation. J Intern Med 1994;235(5):451–6.

81. Karakurum B, Karaalin O, Coskun O, et al. The 'dry-needle technique': intramuscular stimulation in tension-type headache. Cephalalgia 2001;21(8):813–17.

82. Issa TS, Huijbregts PA. Physical therapy diagnosis and management of a patient with chronic daily headache: a case report. J Man Manip Ther 2006;14(4): E88–123.

83. Fresno MJ, Mediavilla P, Mayoral O. Dry needling of myofascial trigger points for hypertonia spastica in incomplete spinal cord injuries. Report of two cases. J Musculoske Pain 2004;12(Suppl. 9):75.

84. Herrero P, Mayoral O. A case study looking at the effectiveness of deep dry needling for the management of hypertonia. J Musculoske Pain 2007;15(2):55–60.

85. Couppé C, Midttun A, Hilden J, et al. Spontaneous needle electromyographic activity in myofascial trigger points in the infraspinatus muscle: a blinded assessment. J Musculoskelet Pain 2001;9(3):7–16.

86. Kuan TS, Hsieh YL, Chen SM, et al. The myofascial trigger point region: correlation between the degree of irritability and the prevalence of endplate noise. Am J Phys Med Rehabil 2007;86(3):183–9.

87. Ballyns JJ, Shah JP, Hammond J, et al. Objective sonographic measures for characterizing myofascial trigger points associated with cervical pain. J Ultrasound Med 2011;30(10):1331–40.

88. Srbely JZ, Dickey JP, Lee D, et al. Dry needle stimulation of myofascial trigger points evokes segmental anti-nociceptive effects. J Rehabil Med 2010;42(5): 463–8.

89. Connell DA, Ali KE, Ahmad M, et al. Ultrasound-guided autologous blood injection for tennis elbow. Skeletal Radiol 2006;35(6):371–7.

90. James SL, Ali K, Pocock C, et al. Ultrasound guided dry needling and autologous blood injection for patellar tendinosis. Br J Sports Med 2007;41(8):518–21, discussion 522.

91. Suresh SP, Ali KE, Jones H, et al. Medial epicondylitis: is ultrasound guided autologous blood injection an effective treatment? Br J Sports Med 2006;40(11):935–9, discussion 939.

92. Travell J. Office hours: day and night. The autobiography of Janet Travell, M.D. Cleveland: The New American Library; 1968.

93. Bowsher D. The physiology of stimulation-produced analgesia. Acupunct Med 1991;9(2):58–62.

94. Le Bars D, Dickenson AH, Besson JM. Diffuse noxious inhibitory controls (DNIC). II. Lack of effect on non-convergent neurones, supraspinal involvement and theoretical implications. Pain 1979;6(3):305–27.

95. Le Bars D, Dickenson AH, Besson JM. Diffuse noxious inhibitory controls (DNIC). I. Effects on dorsal horn convergent neurones in the rat. Pain 1979;6(3):283–304.

96. Le Bars D, Villanueva L, Bouhassira D, et al. Diffuse noxious inhibitory controls (DNIC) in animals and in man. Patol Fiziol Eksp Ter 1992;4:55–65.

97. Baldry P. Management of myofascial trigger point pain. Acupunct Med 2002;20(1):2–10.

98. Melzack R. Folk medicine and the sensory modulation of pain. In: Wall PD, Melzack R, editors. Textbook of pain. 3rd ed. Edinburgh: Churchill Livingstone; 1994. p. 1209–17.

99. Simons DG. Literature reviews. Myofascial pain syndromes-MTrPs. J Musculoskelet Pain 2002;10(4):71–86.

100. Hubbard DR. Chronic and recurrent muscle pain: pathophysiology and treatment, and review of pharmacologic studies. J Musculoske Pain 1996;4(1/2):124–43.

101. Dommerholt J. Muscle pain syndromes. In: Cantu RI, Grodin AJ, editors. Myofascial manipulation. theory and clinical application. 2nd ed. Gaithersburg: Aspen Publishers, Inc.; 2001. p. 93–140.

102. Chen JT, Chen SM, Kuan TS, et al. Phentolamine effect on the spontaneous electrical activity of active loci in a myofascial trigger spot of rabbit skeletal muscle. Arch Phys Med Rehabil 1998;79(7):790–4.

103. Fine PG, Milano R, Hare BD. The effects of myofascial trigger point injections are naloxone reversible. Pain 1988;32(1):15–20.

104. Mayoral O, Santafé M, Salvat I, et al. Cell implications of dry needling injury to muscle tissue. a pilot study. In: MYOPAIN 2010. VIII World congress on myofascial pain and fibromyalgia. 2010 3-7 octubre; Toledo (Spain): International Myopain Society; 2010. p. 48 <http://c.ymcdn.com/sites/www.myopain.org/resource/resmgr/docs/abstracts-book-myopain-2010-.pdf>; [Consultado 8-10-2012].

105. Mayoral del Moral O, Santafé Martínez M. Lesión muscular por punción seca: Regeneración vs. Reparación. In: Fernández Chinchilla JA, editor. Fisioterapia y deporte. Actualizaciones en regeneración muscular y tendinosa. Madrid: Escuela Universitaria de Fisioterapia ONCE; 2011. p. 192–200.

106. Chu J. The local mechanism of acupuncture. Zhonghua Yi Xue Za Zhi (Taipei) 2002;65(7):299–302.

107. Dommerholt J. Dry needling in orthopaedic physical therapy practice. Orthopaedic Practice 2004;16(3):11–16.

108. Wang K. Titin/connectin and nebulin: giant protein rulers of muscle structure and function. Adv Biophys 1996;33:123–34.

109. Simons DG. Understanding effective treatments of myofascial trigger points. J Bodyw Mov Ther 2002;6(2):81–8.

110. Langevin HM, Churchill DL, Cipolla MJ. Mechanical signaling through connective tissue: a mechanism for the therapeutic effect of acupuncture. FASEB J 2001;15(12):2275–82.

DRY NEEDLING FOR HYPERTONIA AND SPASTICITY (DNHS®)

Pablo Herrero Gallego • Sandra Calvo Carrión • María Ortiz Lucas

Never walk on the travelled path because it only leads where others have been.
ALEXANDER GRAHAM BELL

KEYWORDS

DNHS®; dry needling; spasticity; hypertonia; plasticity; Botulinum toxin; upper motor neuron syndrome.

9.1 INTRODUCTION

Many studies to date have investigated the effectiveness of dry needling of myofascial trigger points (MTrPs) for the treatment of myofascial pain.[1] While this is becoming a widely accepted treatment option for many patients, it is not commonly used in patients with neurological conditions. In this field of research, a study was performed showing that hemiparetic patients receiving a programme of dry needling and rehabilitation exercises may benefit from a significant reduction in the frequency and intensity of pain.[2]

Although some of the pain that a hemiplegic patient may experience may have at least a partial myofascial origin, there are no published data on the prevalence of MTrPs for this type of patient. Therefore, with the knowledge available, we cannot know for certain if the prevalence is higher or lower than in patients without a central nervous system (CNS) lesion. In theory, one would expect the prevalence to be higher, as the lesion to the CNS theoretically constitutes an activation and perpetuation mechanism for MTrPs[3] and, furthermore, the lesion, apart from being of a great magnitude, never completely disappears.

Apart from their relation with pain, it is a well-known fact that MTrPs are able to provoke other types of sensory, motor and vegetative dysfunctions (such as weakness and proprioceptive dysfunctions). If MTrPs were to develop following a CNS lesion then it is possible that they could partially contribute to the movement dysfunction that some patients with CNS damage may experience.

Physiotherapists have carried out research on the use of dry needling to treat hypertonia and/or spasticity.[4–6] To date there have been several conference presentations[4,5] and an article published by Herrero and Mayoral,[6] which was the first manuscript to describe the use of dry needling to improve hypertonia and spasticity. This paper provided detailed information regarding the diagnostic criteria and application protocol, as well as providing several hypotheses to explain why changes in spasticity or hypertonia may occur. This new application of dry needling for the purpose of treating hypertonia and spasticity was named the DNHS® technique (Dry Needling for Hypertonia and Spasticity). Since then, research has evolved and many things have changed; for example, the DNHS® technique is no longer focused solely on the treatment of spasticity and hypertonia but is also used to treat other movement dysfunctions.

As a result of the latest research and based on extensive clinical experience, this chapter provides new updates to this technique, advancing new essential and diagnostic criteria, changes in the protocol and a thorough analysis of some aspects that could not have been explained or hypothesized in 2007.

Although these series of published clinical experiences[4–6] are lacking the evidence to permit establishment of a clear cause-and-effect relationship, they are a starting point when considering that there is a certain relationship between the MTrPs and phenomena such as hypertonia and spasticity, and that dry needling can be used in the treatment of these problems.

Furthermore, there are additional arguments related to this connection, such as the use of botulinum toxin type A (BTX A), both for the treatment of pain provoked by MTrPs[7–10] as well as for hypertonia and spasticity,[11–17] which demonstrates that the target structure on which BTX A acts is the same as in dry needling (although BTX A often spreads beyond the motor end-plate zone, whereas DNHS® is thought to be more local). There is a distinct difference in the mechanism of action of dry needling, which is mechanical (rupture of motor end-plates), whereas that of BTX A is chemical (inhibition of the liberation of acetylcholine [ACh]); however, the target structure is still the motor end-plate. Another difference is that there is no limit to the number of muscles that may be treated with dry needling, whereas the infiltration of BTX A comes with a clear limit in dosage, due to its neurotoxicity.[18–20] A further argument in support of this technique is the fact that dry needling has been shown to be as effective as infiltration of substances such as lidocaine or BTX A in the deactivation of MTrPs, especially when accompanied by a local twitch response (LTR).[21–25] Based on the data presented, dry needling is a therapeutic tool that could be just as effective as BTX A in the treatment of hypertonia and spasticity.

The technique of DNHS® presents many similarities with dry needling of MTrPs in myofascial pain syndrome (MPS), although it uses different diagnostic criteria and the application procedure is also different. Furthermore, as the name implies, the goal is not the treatment of myofascial pain, but rather the reduction of hypertonia and spasticity and an improvement in function for the patient with damage to the CNS.

9.2 PHYSIOPATHOLOGY OF SPASTICITY

The upper motor neuron syndrome (UMNS), which can seem a vague concept, is, in fact, very useful for defining the characteristics and symptoms that a person who has suffered damage to the CNS may experience. These symptoms (or characteristics) can be divided into two large groups: positive or negative (figure 9.1). The positive signs, such as spasticity, are characterized by a certain type of muscular hyperactivity, whether this be concerning an excessive muscular contraction or some sort of inappropriate muscle contraction. The negative signs, such as weakness or loss of skill, are characterized by a reduction in motor activity.[26]

Regarding the positive characteristics, the term spasticity is inconsistently defined and this inconsistency needs to be addressed and resolved.[27] Spasticity is just one of the positive characteristics of the UMNS, although at times the term is used incorrectly to refer to other positive UMNS characteristics or even the ensemble of them. Another term that often gets confused with spasticity is hypertonia. Part of this confusion lies in the fact that some of the

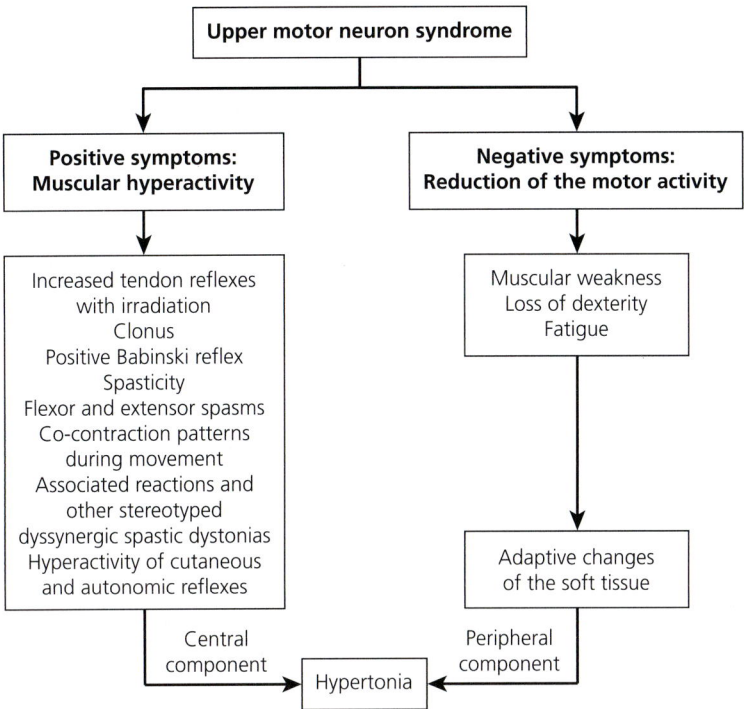

FIGURE 9.1 ■ Characteristics (positive and negative symptoms) of upper motor neuron syndrome and how these influence the development of the central and peripheral component of hypertonia.[26,38]

clinical scales that are used to measure spasticity are actually measuring stiffness.[28]

In the case of the term hypertonia, the most commonly accepted definition is 'increased resistance to passive movement', although it has also been defined as an 'increased response to stimuli'. However, clinically, when hypertonia is found accompanying a movement dysfunction, it is difficult to determine the main factors influencing the aetiology of the movement dysfunction and of the hypertonia itself.

In general terms, hypertonia is usually divided into two large components,[29] one of which is categorized as 'neural' or 'central', while the other is considered 'biomechanical' or 'peripheral' (figure 9.1). Although in theory the difference appears clear, in reality it is not, as at times not only are they overlapping, but they also influence one another. Clinically, it is also very difficult to establish a clear distinction between both these components, aggravated by the fact that there are no scales to allow us to differentiate between them. Frequently, it is the 'velocity-dependent' characteristic that is used to differentiate the central component from the peripheral component, although this is not altogether correct, as muscles, just like any viscoelastic tissue, also show velocity-dependent behaviour when stretched. Furthermore, for the

measurement of hypertonia, it is important to consider the influence of both the velocity and length dependency. For this reason, it is thought that the development of contractures (i.e. peripheral component) could be one of the phenomena contributing to the worsening of the myotatic reflex,[6] which would be further evidence of the overlap between the central and peripheral components of hypertonia.[30]

In order to understand the peripheral components of hypertonia it is important to recognize the contribution of the viscoelastic behaviour of the muscle and tendons. On the one hand, we can find thixotropy-like changes in the viscoelastic properties of the muscle. Thixotropy is a form of resistance to muscle stretch due to an intrinsic stiffness of the muscle fibres resulting from cross-linking of actin and myosin filaments, which is dependent on the history of limb movement.[31] In the case of muscles, it is easy to see how, in the morning, as soon as one wakes up, there is a certain rigidity, which decreases with movement. According to some authors, the thixotropic component does not seem to be relevant in the case of patients with CNS damage.[32] Notwithstanding this debate, it is important to consider this factor when performing research studies, as carrying out comparisons between different measurements taken at different times

---

BOX 9.1 **Descending tracts for movement control involved in spasticity**

1. **Direct tracts**. These participate in the voluntary control of movement. They are differentiated into two tracts:
   - *Corticospinal tracts*. The first motor neuron originates in the cerebral cortex and descends to the spinal cord. There, it synapses with the second motor neuron, which innervates the skeletal muscles of the trunk and extremities via the corresponding spinal motor nerves. The fibres decussate, either at the level of the medulla oblongata (roughly 85%) or at the spinal cord (approximately 15%), and therefore one side of the brain controls most of the movement of the opposite side of the body
   - *Corticobulbar tracts*. The first motor neuron also originates in the cerebral cortex, and descends to the motor nuclei of the cranial nerves. There, it synapses with the second motor neuron, which goes on to innervate the skeletal muscles of the head and neck according to the pair of cranial motor nerves with which they synapse. In a similar fashion to the corticospinal tract, the fibres are crossed; therefore one side of the brain controls most of the movement of the opposite side of the body
2. **Indirect tracts** (tracts originating in the brainstem). These participate in the involuntary control of movement, i.e. automatisms, motor control, balance and regulation of muscle tone.

There are several indirect tracts, two of which are:
- *Reticulospinal tract:* the lesion of this tract leads to spasticity. Originating from the reticular nuclei of the brainstem, it descends to the spinal cord, where it synapses with the motor neurons of the axial muscles and the muscles close to the extremities. There are two separate fascicles: an anterior or medial one (*activator* of the spinal reflexes) and a dorsal or lateral one (*inhibitor* of spinal reflexes).[26] This tract also receives afferents from the cerebral cortex, which *activates* this tract[26,38,72]
- *Vestibulospinal tract*: originating from the lateral vestibular nucleus and connecting to the spinal cord, where it synapses with interneurons and also directly with motor neurons. This tract is involved in the *activation* of the spinal reflexes but it seems to have a lesser role in the production of spasticity[26,37]

The reticulospinal tract contributes to gross movements such as locomotion, posture and control of balance. In contrast, the corticospinal tract is more involved with the fine control of movement.[73] In this sense, lesions of the corticospinal tract are likely to affect the control of precise, voluntary movements in the distal extremities, while lesions of the reticulospinal tract cause a greater dysfunction of global motor control.[74]

---

and with different previous experiences to movement may be a source of important bias.

Besides thixotropy, soft tissues demonstrate creep and hysteresis properties when subjected to load, whether this is in the form of repeated stretch cycles or previous movement experience.[31,33] These phenomena explain the molecular rearrangements that cause tissues to deform when load is applied. When the viscoelastic soft tissues remain immobile, the increase in stiffness can be rapid if the central components of muscle activation coexist. This can lead to the formation of fixed contractures, which, unlike thixotropy, seem to contribute significantly to peripheral components of hypertonia.[32]

Spasticity represents the central or neural component of hypertonia. In the scientific literature different definitions are found under this term, to the point that the definition of spasticity is still evolving while the afferent component is gaining in relevance. Some definitions found in the literature are:
- A velocity-dependent increase in the tonic stretch reflex with exaggerated tendinous reflexes, as a result of hyperexcitability of the stretch reflex, with an UMNS[34] component.

- A velocity-dependent increase in hypertonia with a catch when a threshold is exceeded.[35]
- Disordered sensorimotor control, resulting from an upper motor neuron lesion, presenting an intermittent or sustained involuntary activation of muscles.[36]

In order to understand the concept of spasticity, it is necessary first to understand the different types of descending pathways for movement control that may be involved (box 9.1).

Regarding the physiopathology of spasticity, it is said that an isolated injury of the corticospinal tract does not cause spasticity, but rather it is caused by a lesion of the dorsal or lateral reticulospinal tract,[26] as it is involved in the inhibition of spinal reflexes. In this latter circumstance, an imbalance occurs between the excitatory control mechanisms and the inhibitors of the spinal reflexes, which could then cause the clinical picture of spasticity. This imbalance seems to be caused mainly by a loss of supraspinal inhibition of these reflexes.[26] Also, the degree of spasticity depends on the type of CNS lesion (figure 9.2). If the lesion affects the cortical information that activates the dorsal or lateral reticulospinal tract (i.e. a lesion at the level of the cerebral cortex or

— Corticonuclear tract
··· Anterior or medial reticulospinal tract
-- Dorsal or lateral reticulospinal tract
〰 Damage

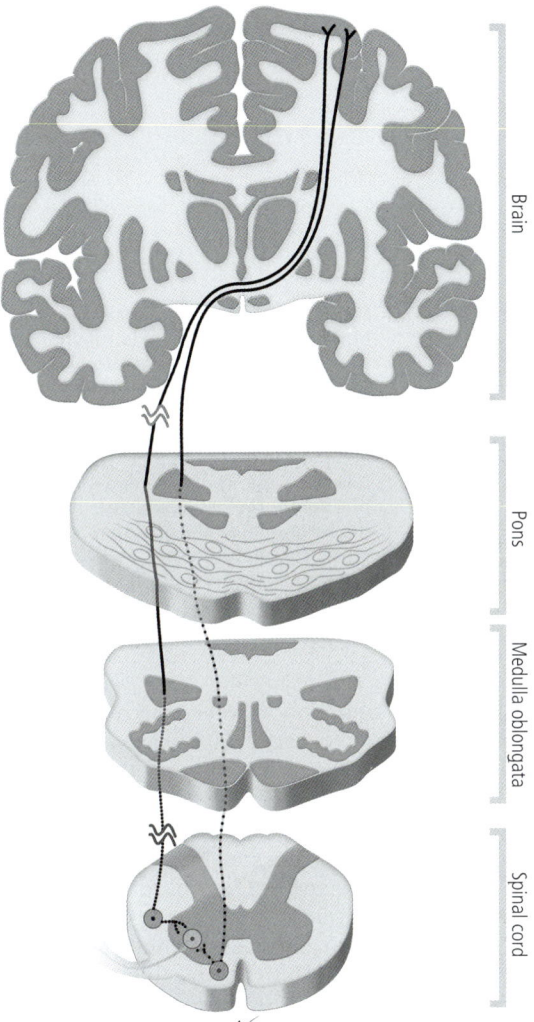

Brain

Pons

Medulla oblongata

Spinal cord

FIGURE 9.2 ■ Influence of a lesion of the reticulospinal tract in the development of spasticity. The interruption of the information from the dorsal or lateral reticulospinal tract is related to the appearance of spasticity, due to the lack of inhibition affecting spinal reflexes. This can be the result of a lesion in the tracts that transmit the cortical information that activate this tract or due to a lesion at some point along the pathway. This would lead to a clinical picture of mild or severe spasticity, respectively. (Colour version of figure is available online).

the internal capsule), a loss of activation would occur in this tract, as it would no longer have such a potent inhibitory effect on the spinal reflexes and this would produce a clinical picture of mild spasticity. If the lesion occurs through the pathway of the dorsal or lateral reticulospinal tract (caused by a lesion at the brainstem or spinal cord), there would be a complete loss of

inhibition of the spinal reflexes that regulate this pathway, and therefore the clinical picture would be of a more severe spasticity.[26,37]

In these types of lesion it is important to consider the potential involvement of other spinal tracts,[26,37,38] in which case:

- A partial lesion of the spinal cord that only affects the dorsal or lateral reticulospinal tract but not the excitatory reflex tracts (anterior or medial reticulospinal tract and the vestibulospinal tract) would lead to a more severe clinical picture.
- If there is a complete lesion affecting the spinal cord, both the inhibitory tracts and the tracts subserving the reflexes, all control over reflexes would be lost and hyperactivation of reflexes would be observed.

However, it seems that the mechanisms contributing to an imbalance between the activation/inhibition of reflexes is rather complex. Frequently, the appearance of hyperreflexia occurs after a period of decreased reflexes. In such a case, adaptive changes in the neural pathways may have caused the onset of spasticity mediated by the following possible mechanisms[26,30,37]:

- The axonal sprouting phenomenon: the afferent fibres create new collateral branches (sprouts) which connect to synapses that previously were inhibitory, changing them to excitatory.[26]
- The excitotoxic mechanism (figure 9.3): this occurs when acute pain is transformed into chronic pain. In this case, a strong or prolonged nociceptive stimulus provokes the liberation of substance P and glutamate, which produce the opening of calcium channels into the cell. The presence of maintained levels of calcium in the cell's interior will produce cell death by apoptosis. It seems that the inhibitory interneurons that synapse with nociceptive central neurons are especially sensitive to this excitotoxic phenomenon. This phenomenon could occur in spasticity over time, if lack of inhibition of the reticulospinal tract leads to an excessive liberation of neurotransmitters at a medullary level. However, for death by apoptosis to occur as well, it would be necessary for the inhibitory interneurons that synapse with the motor neurons of the skeletal muscles also to be sensitive to this excitotoxicity phenomenon.
- Changes in the sensitivity of the receptors (denervation supersensitivity).[39,40] This phenomenon consists of an increase in the ACh receptors that are distributed over the whole surface of the muscle fibre.

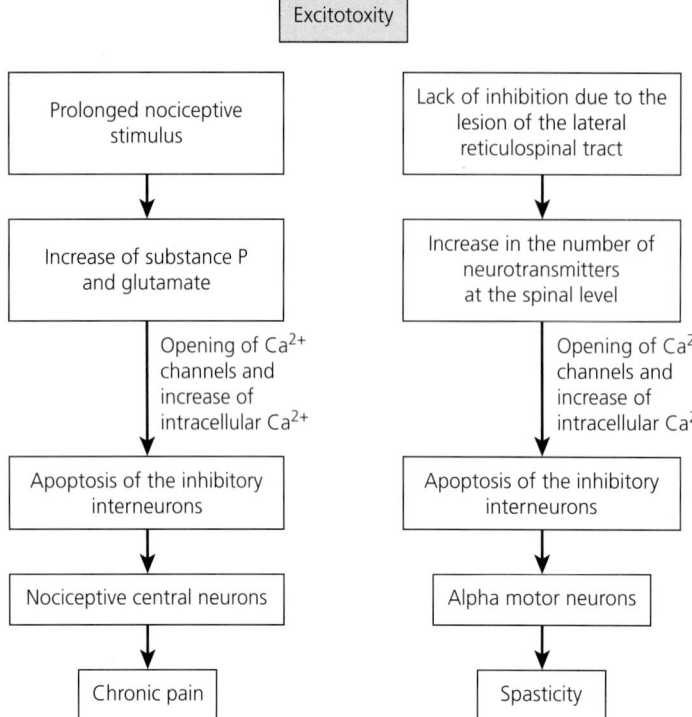

FIGURE 9.3 ■ Hypothesis on the functioning of the excitotoxic mechanism in spasticity, using an analogy of this phenomenon applied in development of chronic pain. In the case of nociception, the inhibitory interneurons that synapse with the central nociceptive neurons are more sensitive to this phenomenon. In spasticity, it is the inhibitory interneurons that synapse with the alpha motor neurons that are more sensitive to the effects of excitotoxicity.

Based on the physiopathology of spasticity, another element that enters into the equation is the possible hyperexcitability of the myotatic reflex (or stretch reflex). According to some authors, this reflex is elicited when the muscle is stretched quickly and dynamically and the type Ia afferent fibres from the neuromuscular spindle are activated. In the spinal cord, these fibres synapse with the motor neurons that innervate that muscle, activating them, which in turn produces a muscle contraction. This reflex also has a static component: when the muscle is subjected to a slow and static stretch, the type II fibres of the muscle spindle are activated. These fibres synapse with excitatory interneurons, which in turn, synapse with the motor neurons of the muscle that is contracting. In patients with spasticity, an alteration in the latency of the stretch reflex has been described in the form of a reduction or delay of this reflex.[41] In relation to this, there are opposing opinions on whether spasticity is indeed an alteration of the myotatic reflex (an increase in excitability or a decrease in the activation threshold) or other reflexes, or whether it is a pathological reflex in itself.[38]

Various spinal mechanisms have been thought to intervene in the alteration of reflexes and research suggests that, rather than producing an alteration in a single spinal tract, a chain of alterations is produced in different spinal tracts as a consequence of the poor processing of the afferent information together with a lack of inhibition of the motor neurons.[30,37]

The phenomenon, thought to intervene in the physiopathology of spasticity at the level of the spinal cord level, includes:

- Reduced reciprocal inhibition, which is produced by activation of the type Ia fibres of the neuromuscular spindle. During reciprocal inhibition, the fibres synapse with inhibitory interneurons which, in turn, produce relaxation of the antagonistic muscles by inhibiting the motor neurons that they innervate. Furthermore, these inhibitory interneurons are activated by the stimulus originating from the descending motor pathways. A lesion of these descending fibres would be responsible for reduction of the reciprocal inhibition of spasticity and would provoke the appearance of pathological muscular co-contraction of the antagonists. Additionally, the appearance of an excessive reciprocal inhibition has also been reported, which would produce muscular weakening.[26,30,42]

- Reduced postactivation depression (homosynaptic depression) of the type Ia fibres of the neuromuscular spindle. During this phenomenon, a decrease in the liberation of the neurotransmitters of the type Ia fibres occurs immediately after their activation, with resulting decrease in activation of the motor neurons that they innervate. This lasts for 10–15 seconds and only affects the fibres Ia that are activated. It seems that this mechanism could play a more causal role in the development of spasticity than presynaptic inhibition (presented below).[30,43,44]

- Reduced presynaptic inhibition of the type Ia fibres of the neuromuscular spindle. This is a closed-loop feedback system due to activation of the type Ia fibres that activate the inhibitory interneurons in order to inhibit these sensitive fibres. It lasts 300–400 ms and affects the Ia fibres, whether these are activated or not. This phenomenon has been observed to occur in some, but not all, patients with spasticity.[30,37,41,42,45]
- Alteration of the autogenic inhibition mechanism of the type Ib fibres of the Golgi tendon organ. The muscle contraction causes a stretch to the tendon, which, in turn, activates the Ib fibres of the Golgi tendon organ that triggers the tendon reflex. The activation of inhibitory interneurons then occurs, which inhibits the motor neurons of the muscle. Both an excitation and an inhibition of this mechanism have been described in patients with spasticity.[30,37,41]
- A decreased activation threshold of the spinal motor neurons due to creation of plateau potentials in the membrane. These potentials are produced, either by a reduction in the repolarizing output currents, or by the opening of voltage-dependent calcium channels by serotoninergic or noradrenergic innervation of the motor neurons. Additionally, this can occur without the mediation of these neurotransmitters. This phenomenon could also take place within the interneurons; however, this has not been demonstrated in humans due to the associated difficulties. These plateau potentials can affect the motor neurons responsible for reciprocal innervation and could explain the partial or total loss of the reciprocal inhibition which is observed in spasticity.[30,46]

In contrast, the link between the following phenomena and their role in the presence of spasticity has been refuted:

- Increased neuromuscular spindle afferents, which produce a larger discharge of impulses in the motor neurons.[30,37,46]
- Modifications in the recurrent inhibition of the Renshaw cells which block inhibition of the motor neurons. In this process, when a motor neuron is activated, a collateral branch of its axon activates inhibitory Renshaw neurons which, in turn, deactivate the motor neuron that initiated the impulse and the synergistic motor neurons. It also inhibits the gamma motor neurons and the Ia inhibitory interneurons (which participate in reciprocal inhibition).[30,37,41]

Today, it is well accepted that spasticity is only partially responsible for hypertonia, and that other positive characteristics of UMNS (the main component for hypertonia) and alterations in the viscoelastic properties of the muscle (the peripheral component of hypertonia) contribute to the increased resistance to passive movement.[26,47–51]

9.3 HYPOTHESIS OF THE DNHS® TECHNIQUE

We shall analyse the different levels that may be altered in a patient with a CNS lesion and relate these to the technique of DNHS®, in order to hypothesize about the possible mechanisms of action of the DNHS® technique.

9.3.1 At the level of the muscle fibre and motor end-plate

A review of studies has summarized the alterations affecting the musculature of patients with spasticity at the level of the muscle fibre and motor end-plate. The following phenomena have been described[52]:

- Increased fibre size variability. The muscle fibres lose their polygonal and juxtaposed forms, which are replaced by rounded and 'moth-eaten' forms.
- Increased extracellular space in some cases. A large amount of poorly organized extracellular material is observed in spastic muscle bundles compared with normal bundles and the mechanical properties are of inferior quality compared to those of a normal muscle.
- Increased collagen concentration.
- There is no consensus regarding the predominance of type I or type II fibres.
- Increased active muscle stiffness may be due to an increase in the number of cross-bridges attached during contraction or to an increase in stiffness per cross-bridge.
- The only direct measurement of fibre length that has ever been performed in

children with spastic diplegia has shown the fibre length to be normal. There is no evidence of fibre length changes due to spasticity.

- A shortened muscle–tendon unit has been found while the sarcomeres within the fibres are actually lengthened.

In a more recent study an increase in passive stiffness was observed in children with cerebral palsy, accompanied by an increase in collagen tissue and a decrease in the diameter of the muscle fibre in the hamstring muscles.[53] An increased *in vivo* sarcomere length was also found. In this study, differences in the mechanical properties of the muscle fibre or in the size of the titin were not observed; the authors concluded that the increase in passive tension is due to the change in stiffness of the extracellular matrix and the increase in length of the sarcomere *in vivo* and therefore not due to any intracellular modification.

In these patients the sarcomere was longer than the optimal length of a sarcomere, which supports the idea that the sarcomeres are overstretched. The muscles would be supporting larger tensions due to changes in the properties of the extracellular material and change in the length of the sarcomeres. The increased length of the sarcomeres would indicate the impossibility of the muscle adding sarcomeres in series. The alteration of the extracellular matrix could inhibit the activation or proliferation of the satellite cells and even induce its proliferation towards extracellular tissue. Fibrosis and lack of growth would create a vicious circle, leading to muscle contracture.

In the cited publications[52,53] there are no apparent references to MTrPs or possible dysfunctions of the motor end-plate as being responsible for increased rigidity. However, it seems possible that these types of motor end-plate dysfunctions occur frequently in patients with spasticity, as one of the most common mechanisms for the formation of MTrPs is repeated contraction in shortened positions, which occurs frequently in these patients. Considering the integrated hypothesis described by Simons et al.,[3] the maintained contraction of the sarcomeres that form the MTrPs is the result of a dysfunction of the motor end-plates associated with those muscle fibres. This dysfunction is provided by an increased concentration of ACh in these dysfunctional motor end-plates (due to excess liberation or decrease in acetylcholinesterase), and is worsened by the acidic medium[54] of the MTrPs, which blocks the action of the acetylcholinesterase. Also, as previously indicated, in spastic patients it is thought that there is a greater sensitivity to ACh, which is reflected by an increase in the number of ACh receptors over the entire surface of the muscle fibre. Therefore, all these factors – the increase in concentration of ACh, the acidic medium and the increase in number of ACh receptors – could contribute to the structural changes that are produced in spastic muscles, and this could end up producing the development of MTrPs in the soft tissue. However this has not been studied in patients with spasticity.

Domingo et al.[55] describe the destruction of the neuromuscular junction and its posterior regeneration after dry needling in the healthy muscle tissue of mice. Considering that the average size of human myocytes is 40–45 μm and that the calibre of the needles used in dry needling is 160–450 μm, the mechanism of action would entail the rupture of myocytes.[55] After the puncture there is an inflammatory reaction that is clearly observable 24 hours after the lesion. The regeneration phase is initiated 3 days after the puncture, which is when cleaning of the necrotic remains is observed in the injured area, with the non-injured parts of the muscle fibres being preserved. The satellite cells are activated and transformed into myoblasts and these initiate the mitotic proliferation. The myoblasts fuse with themselves and with the healthy areas of the muscle fibres, forming myotubes, which begin the synthesis of actin and myosin. This occurs between days 3 and 5 postpuncture. On the fifth day after the lesion, most of the cytoplasm contains neoformed contractile organ. Not all myoblasts are fused, and the remains are transformed into satellite cells. A week after the lesion, recovery is complete.

According to the same study, at the level of the nerve, axonal destruction of the injured zone takes place posttreatment and degenerative changes occur distal to the injured section (Wallerian degeneration), with consequent disappearance of the synapsis. The ACh receptors are dispersed over the surface of the muscle fibre, the myelin disappears and the Schwann cells surround the axons to phagocytose the injured areas. Three days after the puncture, the appearance of neural growth cones and the reinnervation of the end-plates by very fine axons covering a large area of the muscle fibre are observed. Afterwards, the receptors are concentrated around the cones and the axons, forming functional neuromuscular synapses. The reinnervation is a faster process compared to muscular regeneration as, in 3 days, the neuromuscular connections are re-established.

Consequently, the following factors could explain the clinical improvements in motor response that are observed after the application of a DNHS®:

- The ACh is synthesized in the synaptic bouton via choline acetyl transferase. One of the substrates, choline, is obtained from the extracellular medium via transporters.[56] The mechanical destruction of the axon and the synaptic bouton could lead to a reduction in ACh levels, as synthesis of ACh would be prevented due to a lack of choline transporters.
- The effect of dry needling when it achieves an LTR would be cleansing sensitizing substances,[54] which would also allow an improved function of acetylcholinesterase.
- The normalization of the characteristics of the muscle fibres will cause a reprogramming and/or modification of the afferent information that goes from the skeletal muscle to the spinal cord and this would allow a transitory normalization of information processing at a central level and therefore improve the motor response.

9.3.2 Spinal reflexes

After the application of DNHS® on MTrPs in patients with spasticity, the emergence of an LTR has been found, as well as the so-called global increase in spasticity.[6] The difference between these is that the LTR is defined as a 'transient contraction of a group of tense muscle fibres (taut band) of the trigger point'. The contraction of the fibres occurs in response to the stimulation (or in general because of sudden palpation or puncture) of the same trigger point, or sometimes, of a trigger point close by.[3] In contrast, the global increase in spasticity, or global twitch response (GTR), (which is the preferred term due to the inconsistencies related to the term 'spasticity') is defined as a 'contraction of a muscle or muscle group on a global level, at times accompanied by an increase in axial tone'.[6] These two responses are observed in the case of patients with a CNS lesion, whether or not they feel pain.[6]

If we relate the LTR to spinal reflexes, the LTR could be a polysynaptic spinal reflex with a reduced influence from the supraspinal component.[57] A possible hypothesis could be that both the LTR and the myotatic reflex are spinal polysynaptic reflexes that share at least a large part of the afferent, spinal and efferent pathways. Therefore, activation of this reflex while applying the DNHS® technique could cause a neuromodulator effect on the myotatic reflex (or other reflexes), causing an improvement in spasticity.[6] Furthermore, this neuromodulation

could produce the phenomenon of neuronal plasticity via the modification of a threshold of neuronal activation which, in the case of a patient with damage to the nervous system, could favour an improvement in function by activating the compensatory pathways (opening the silent or ineffective synapses) or by creating new collaterals.[58,59]

In contrast, with regard to the GTR, it has been observed that on occasion this is found to be associated with an LTR while, other times, it occurs in an isolated manner. It is necessary to bear in mind that sometimes the LTR is not perceivable visually nor through the use of tactile palpation. In these circumstances, the only way to be aware of the existence of an LTR is with information transmission through the needle or by visualization under ultrasound.

With the application of the DNHS® technique, it is observed that the GTR is not limited solely to the treated side but, in the case of bilateral involvement, it can be manifested also on the opposite side. In these cases, the therapeutic effects observed after achieving a GTR are observed on the contralateral side.[6] Although no research to date has studied this phenomenon and neither are there enough data available to enable a comparison of both responses, in animal models, a remote effect has been described when an MTrP is punctured over other MTrPs of other muscles, both ipsilateral and contralateral.[60] For this reason, our hypothesis is based on the fact that the GTR could, in fact, be a polysynaptic spinal reflex of greater complexity than the LTR. It is known that a sensitized nervous system can show alterations, such as a decrease in the activation threshold to external stimuli or the activation of neighbouring neurons which, under a normal physiological situation, would not be activated.[61] Interestingly, certain studies have shown that the puncture of MTrPs in a sensitized nervous system (due to active MTrPs) can cause electromyographic activity in the MTrPs of the contralateral side.[62] In a similar manner, in the case of a patient with a lesion of the CNS, our hypothesis is that the presence of MTrPs could cause activation of synergists (agonists and antagonists) on both homolateral and contralateral sides, based on the current knowledge base.[60,62]

The information entering the spinal cord from the posterior horns is received by the convergent neurons that receive information from various body areas, such as the joints, fascia and skin. However, not all inputs will cause an action potential.[63] Each spinal neuron will have multiple synapses that could be excitatory or inhibitory, or active or silent. The activation or non-activation of an action potential depends on the combination of all the inputs that the neuron receives.[64] When the puncture is applied, the spinal cord receives a new input which would then be integrated together with the rest of the inputs previously described, and which would act by normalizing the effector muscle response.

9.3.3 Neural CNS pathways

The effect of dry needling on skeletal muscle could possibly be reflected at the level of the brain in a transitory modulation of the neural pathways implicated in the development of spasticity. In a recent study[65] using electroencephalography (EEG) to assess the effects of the application of the DNHS® technique in two patients who had suffered from a cerebrovascular accident, an improvement in cortical processing was described; this could possibly explain different functional changes found in patients with the application of dry needling alone. Within the results obtained using the EEG, changes are observed in the correspondence between the frontal/prefrontal regions as well as a decrease in discordance. This shows that, in specific regions, there is an increased phase coherence for the different frequencies. Hypothetically, this could be a positive indicator of the information processing associated with the neuronal activity, which may facilitate the functional changes experienced by patients. These findings reveal a new line of research requiring further investigation to understand the effect of DNHS® in patients with a CNS lesion.

Apart from the already cited effects described in the treatment of MTrPs for myofascial pain, in the case of neurological patients, the effect of the DNHS® technique could lie not only in peripheral improvements, but also in the indirect effects that these changes could have on the CNS. In relation to these indirect effects, it could be hypothesized that the local decrease in ACh concentration should have positive effects over the CNS, by decreasing the potentially irritating effect that ACh has on the CNS, either because it could be transported in a retrograde manner to the neuronal body (which seems unlikely), or because it was somehow sending sensitizing afferents to the CNS. Together with these indirect and local effects, the phenomenon of denervation supersensitivity[39] could be added. This phenomenon proposes the existence of a greater sensitivity to ACh, as reflected by an increase in the number of ACh receptors on the entire surface of the muscle fibre.[26,30,37]

However, these effects are temporary and therefore correspond with what is observed clinically, as the lesion at the level of the CNS still remains and acts as a perpetuating factor. The duration of part of these effects could be related to the time it takes to re-establish the neuromuscular junction, which, as detailed previously, has been shown to take 3 days,[55] while others may last longer, or indeed, indefinitely.

9.3.4 Summary of the working hypotheses to explain the changes that occur with the DNHS® technique

- Changes at the level of the motor end-plate and the muscle fibre:
  - A decrease in the levels of ACh, due to breakage of the motor end-plate.
  - Cleansing of sensitizing substances via the LTR or GTR.
  - Normalization of the muscle fibre and, therefore, of the afferents.
- Changes at the spinal level:
  - Neuromodulation of the myotatic reflex, and possibly other reflexes.
  - Neuronal plasticity phenomena.
- Changes at the level of the superior CNS centres:
  - Improvement in sensorimotor processing.

9.4 THERAPEUTIC EFFECTS OF THE DNHS® TECHNIQUE

In relation to the peripheral component of hypertonia, it is known that the maintenance of shortened positions for a long time (as is the case for these patients) produces changes in the biomechanical properties of the muscle fibres due to immobilization and lack of contractility. This, in turn, entails a loss of functional motor units, atrophy of muscle cells, physiological and metabolic changes in the fibres (transformation of the type of fibre) and an increase in rigidity (e.g. proliferation of connective tissues together with mechanical changes in the fibres).[66,67] This component can be improved by treating MTrPs with dry needling so as, on the one hand, to destroy the dysfunctional motor end-plates and, on the other, to lavage the nociceptive and sensitizing substances which are responsible, in part, for the persistence of localized contracture.[54]

The central component is related to the changes in the membrane properties of the alpha motor neurons and the decrease of their activation threshold, as well as to an altered inhibition of the efferent pathways.[30] The MTrPs which, by definition, present a sensorimotor alteration, could be partially influencing this anomalous information processing within the CNS, analogous to what occurs in the central sensitization phenomenon. Moreover, it has been observed that the deactivation of MTrPs achieves improvements in sensorimotor information processing in patients with a CNS lesion.[6] It is probable that the LTRs or GTRs obtained could somehow have improved the central information processing, at least on the medullar levels where these were produced.[60,65]

At the time of writing, the application of DNHS® in patients with movement alterations of a central origin (concretely, in spastic and ataxic patients) has been related to clinically observed improvements in the global execution of movement. Based on clinical experience, improved motor control is often seen immediately after puncture and is generally maintained for an average of 2–4 weeks. The greater effects, lasting 3–7 days, may be related to the time it takes to re-establish the neuromuscular junction; however, this has not been demonstrated. For instance, considering that this longer-lasting change could hypothetically be due to the opening of determined neuronal connection pathways at a medullary level (analogous to the concept of segmentary spinal sensitization) and the interrelations with the agonist–antagonist muscles (segmentally mediated and influenced by modification of reflex responses, such as the LTR), there are determined clinical changes in some patients which may only be due to changes of sensorimotor information processing at a higher level, i.e. in the CNS.[6]

The MTrPs are related to both components of hypertonia: they can influence the peripheral component due to their effect on the viscoelastic properties of the muscle, and the central component by modifying sensorimotor information.

9.5 APPLICATION METHODS OF THE DNHS® TECHNIQUE

Although originally the technique of DNHS®[6] was conceived for the treatment of hypertonia and spasticity and was registered with this acronym as the objective was the treatment of these problems, at present it is more involved with finding functional changes. In fact, the studies upon which it is based currently use movement analysis and diagnostic tests such as EEG.[65]

In order to ensure the most effective application of the DNHS® technique, we have established a series of guidelines for therapists. These are based on MPS guidelines, however, adapted to neurological patients and comprehend a series of essential and confirmatory diagnostic criteria, together with a guide to the procedure, an appli-

---

BOX 9.2	Essential diagnostic criteria used in DNHS®

1. Within the ensemble of taut bands, the one that displays the highest degree of tension (in muscles that are accessible)
2. The nodular zone within the band or the more sensitive area, if this exists
3. Assessment of the movement and function of the patient
4. Restriction of the range of movement, an increase in the resistance to passive movement or the triggering of a myotatic reflex, or other reflexes

---

cation guideline and a series of indications and contraindications.

9.5.1 Essential and confirmatory diagnostic criteria

The essential diagnostic criteria used in DNHS® have been defined based on those established for the identification and diagnosis of MTrPs[3] (box 9.2).

With regard to the first criterion, this is based on the 'palpable taut band (in accessible muscles)' used in trigger point treatments. The DNHS® technique has modified this, as generally there are many taut bands that are palpable in a patient with a CNS lesion, and the palpation is therefore directed at determining which of these displays the highest degree of tension.

The criterion 'exquisite spot tenderness by pressure applied upon a nodule in the taut band' used in MPS is not valid for most neurological patients, as generally these present with some type of sensory alteration, whether this be superficial or deep, which prevents them from determining which is the most sensitive point. It is also important to consider that many patients have cognitive disorders that do not allow them to assess or adequately express which is the most sensitive spot among various possibilities. In these cases, the DNHS® technique seeks to determine which area shows a larger thickening in the tissue, as active MTrPs have been associated with greater lesional areas.[68]

Regarding the criterion 'patient's recognition of current pain complaint by pressure on the tender nodule' used in MPS, this is modified, considering that the pain is not usually the reason for consultation. Instead, the criterion 'assessment of movement and function of the patient' is preferred, whether this consists of visual or laboratory tests of movement analysis. Furthermore, referred pain is not considered, as this is not a common occurrence with puncture in patients with CNS lesions.

BOX 9.3	Confirmatory diagnostic criteria used in the DNHS® technique

1. Visual or tactile identification of a global or local twitch response
2. 'Neural release' (release from a contraction or maintained relaxation)
3. Electromyographic demonstration of the spontaneous electric activity, a typical sign of active loci in the tender nodule of a taut band

BOX 9.4	Application procedure for the DNHS® technique

1. Place the muscle to be treated in a position of submaximal stretch
2. Perform explorations of myofascial trigger points using the needle, while controlling the stability of the segment until there is significant cessation in excessive muscular activity (which generally takes place immediately after a local or global twitch response); this is known as 'neural release', as it implies structures such as the neuromuscular junction
3. Maintain the position for a brief period until the neural release appears or contraction ceases
4. Remove the needle to the skin layer and then move the treated muscle into a position of submaximal stretch before proceeding with further needle explorations

The criterion 'painfully restricted stretch range of motion' used in MPS is substituted by 'restriction of the range of motion, increase of resistance to passive movements or triggering of the myotatic reflex' seeing as, as revealed by the previous criterion, pain is not the main characteristic for consideration.

The confirmatory diagnostic criteria used in the DNHS® technique have been defined based on those established for the identification and diagnosis of MTrPs[3] (box 9.3).

The confirmatory diagnostic criteria used in the DNHS® technique (box 9.3) are also defined based on those used in MPS. In this case, the first criterion is the 'visual or tactile identification of a GTR[6] or LTR induced by needle penetration of the nodule'. It is common to see or identify an LTR via palpation after inserting a needle, but on occasions there are patients in whom a GTR can be found.

Regarding the criterion 'referred pain or altered sensation with pressure of tender nodule', this is no longer used, due to the reasons already stated. In its place, the criterion of 'neural' or 'neuromuscular release' is used, understood as a relaxation response or a decrease/cessation of abnormal contractile activity, perceived as a decrease in the stretch resistance that the muscle presents, and which is generally achieved after the appearance of an LTR or GTR due to mechanical denervation of the end-plate. This relaxation allows for repositioning of the muscle in an increased degree of stretch until a new increased resistance to stretch is perceived by the physiotherapist. The term 'neural release' is used, as this abnormal and excessive muscular activity is considered mainly to have a central origin, although, as explained previously, it may also be considered to be partially provoked due to the spontaneous electric activity in the dysfunctional motor end-plates.

The third confirmatory finding coincides exactly with the one employed in MPS as it considers spontaneous electric activity to be partially responsible for the increased resistance to passive movement.

9.5.2 Application procedure for the DNHS® technique

As opposed to dry needling in MPS, where the muscle is needled under slight stretch, the application procedure for the DNHS technique (described in box 9.4) requires the muscle to be positioned in submaximal stretch (understood as the stretch that takes the muscle close to the end range but without applying maximal force). The exception for this is in the case of a muscle that does not show a great increase in activity, in which case it is not necessary to insist so much on attaining a position of submaximal stretch. The reason is twofold: on the one hand, it aids in palpation as, in general, these muscles tend to be very shortened and therefore, the submaximal stretch allows for a more precise differentiation of the taut bands, and especially of the nodular zones, considered to be the essential diagnostic criteria. On the other hand, and most importantly, submaximal stretch is used for reasons that are in agreement with the neurophysiology of 'neural release', previously described as a confirmatory diagnostic criterion.

From the point of view of the muscular contraction, the more elongated the muscle, the more difficult it is for the cross-bridges between actin and myosin to be established.[69] For this reason, the muscle is positioned in submaximal stretch so that the 'neural release' can occur more easily and this will facilitate the repositioning of the muscle into a new position of submaximal stretch. This criterion is only applied when treating muscles with an important excess of muscular activity and whenever palpation of the MTrPs is optimal within that degree of stretch. If this is not possible, a mid-range position can also be used, if this enables palpation of the MTrPs, especially when practising a pincer palpation.

After placing the muscle in a position of submaximal stretch, the area is explored with the needle in search of the 'neural release', which usually occurs right after the LTR or the GTR, although at times these are not easily perceived, especially in deep muscles, in which case release alone is perceived. Note that it is important to appropriately immobilize the segment that is being needled, as, at times, the intensity of the LTR or the GTR is quite high.

The LTR or GTR that occurs prior to the neural release can occasionally generate an increase in contractile activity for a brief period of time (1–3 seconds on average). Therefore, the immobilization during this period should be maintained until the neural release is perceived, which will then allow for the muscle to be placed into a new position of submaximal stretch.

After this, the muscle is repositioned to a new position of submaximal stretch. If the needle remains within the muscle while the limb is repositioned into submaximal stretch, the needle will bend. For this purpose, it is recommended to remove the needle to the skin layer (without completely taking it out), to move the muscle to a new position of submaximal stretch and from there proceed with a new insertion.

Regarding the patient's position, this is usually ascertained according to the person's own functional limitations or by the position which the person finds most comfortable, although in any case, the patient should be lying down, as in any dry needling technique.

9.5.3 Application guidelines

A 7–10-day break period between sessions is recommended in order to respect the repair stages of a neuromuscular lesion.[70,71]

The clinical experiences and studies that have taken place to date indicate that an improvement in the patient occurs in the first three to four treatment sessions.[6] On average, the first and second sessions are those that demonstrate the greatest change, whereas after three or four sessions, the beginning of the plateau phase begins in which the changes are difficult to perceive and treatment is less effective. For this reason, the application guideline for the DNHS® technique consists of different treatment series, each made up of three to four sessions[6] separated by an interval of 7–10 days.

The number of MTrPs and/or muscles to treat (there are muscles which may contain various MTrPs) can vary according to different aspects although, when possible, it is recommended to treat all MTrPs that are located in muscles which exhibit hyperreactivity, excessive muscular contractions or those that are partially responsible for associated reactions or movement dysfunctions which are intended to be improved. Therefore, the recommendation is that, once a patient is assessed and the muscles that most contribute to the movement dysfunction are identified (due to an excess of activity), the physiotherapist is the one who, according to the time available, the layout of the physiotherapy session or the knowledge of the tolerance of the patient (in those cases in which dry needling is painful) must determine the number of MTrPs to treat. Once the physiotherapist has decided the number of MTrPs to treat after examining the patient, it is recommended that, as a basic rule, the needling be performed in a proximal to distal order, as, according to the patterns of pain reference areas and dysfunction published,[3] 85% of muscles have a pattern which is at least partially peripheral and therefore their ability to influence other muscles will be greater when this sequence is followed. However, this aspect still requires further research, and it seems that at least in some muscles the currently published patterns for pain and dysfunction are not applicable to neurological patients in terms of spasm or referred inhibition. An example of this are the adductor pollicis and the first dorsal interosseous muscles. Despite being defined as following a local-type pattern, these muscles generate important inhibition effects, both in the hand as well as in the rest of the upper extremity.

While one of the criteria used in the treatment of myofascial pain is the performance of dry needling until no further LTRs in the MTrPs are obtained, in the case of a neurological patient this is not so. This is because of the large amount of LTRs or GTRs which can be obtained that limit the compliance for this criterion. On many occasions, it is observed that, although the amount of LTRs and GTRs considerably decreases, they continue to appear. This would mean prolonging treatment in a large number or, in the worst case, when needling is painful, sensitizing the patient. For this reason, when LTRs or GTRs continue to occur after a variable number of in-and-out motions with the needle, the physiotherapist's own judgement is necessary to move on to treat other points. In any case, it is the physiotherapist who decides the number of punctures to perform, based on clinical reasoning, clinical experience and the knowledge of the patient at hand.

In dry needling, needles are used of a length that adapts to the area treated, while exercising precaution so that the needle is not inserted up to the handle. The minimum length is 25 mm as the technique is based on deep dry needling. With regard to calibre, needles with a minimum of 0.25 mm width are preferred in the case of needles measuring 25 mm in length, and a calibre of 0.30 or 0.32 mm for those of 40 mm in length and greater, as the hypertonia and changes in the properties of the tissue described previously impede the entrance and management of small-calibre (0.16 mm) needles.

Considering that the factors of activation and perpetuation persist indefinitely in a patient with a CNS lesion, the treatment after the first round of punctures is centred on carrying out a global re-education programme which will allow for activation of the muscles treated with the DNHS® technique. The performance of a new series then continues once the improvements obtained begin to display a certain regression or, rather, if there is no regression, when a prudent period of time has passed according to the physiotherapist's judgement (it has been confirmed that the effects can last from several weeks to several months, depending on the severity of the perpetuation factors and the initial state of the patient).

9.5.4 Indications

DNHS® is indicated at present for muscles that display an increased passive resistance (analytically assessed), or for those which, prior to the performance of a functional assessment, show that they are impeding a determined motor function for the patient. In order to facilitate this analysis, the MTrPs themselves are considered to be activators and/or perpetuators of other MTrPs. In this case, special attention is given to the muscles that are synergists of the affected muscle, either as agonists or antagonists of a certain movement, as the presence of MTrPs in the affected muscle can cause overuse or excitation/inhibition of the MTrPs of the related muscles, analogous to what has been shown for MPS.

Furthermore, the relation between muscles that segmentally share the same innervation or that are related to the same spinal segments is assessed, as, according to the hypothesis proposed by the DNHS® technique, a neuromodulatory effect may occur.[65] We consider that this neuromodulatory effect may be increased during dry needling, not just via needling of the muscle under study, but also via the needling of the multifidus muscles of the spinal segment related to the spastic muscle, although, at present, there are no studies available that demonstrate this clinical perception.

DNHS® is applied to the muscles that are functionally altered, together with their agonists and antagonists and those that share the same innervation, seeking to facilitate an effect of neuromodulation.

As a concept, DNHS® does not use terminology to differentiate active and latent MTrPs, as pain is neither the reason for consultation nor the treatment goal. Preferably, as explained in the application guidelines section (section 9.5.3), an order or hierarchy for needling the MTrPs is established, so that, after the patient assessment, all the muscles are treated according to the established order of importance, within the limiting circumstances of time or, eventually, of pain provoked by the needling. In order to establish this hierarchy, the reference to bear in mind is that 85% of referred pain patterns are peripheral.[3] Although, in the case of neurological patients, it has not yet been demonstrated that the increase in activity is transmitted in a predominantly distal manner, we consider this reference as a general rule.

In some concrete cases, clinical experience has shown exceptions to this rule, finding muscles which exercise a strong inhibitory effect in a proximal direction, which is the case for the adductor pollicis and the first dorsal interosseous (video 9.1). However, the fact that each patient generally has a large number of muscles affected means that all the effort is directed towards performing deep dry needling on muscles that show an increased resistance to passive movement. Nonetheless, perhaps future studies will show effectiveness in treating muscles that do not display this characteristic. For example, our clinical experience is that the needling of certain MTrPs produces increased recruitment of inhibited muscles, or muscles with lack of strength.

With regard to the type of muscles that display the best response to the application of the DNHS® technique, those that commonly show a high abnormal muscle activity and an exacerbated myotatic reflex are highlighted. In contrast, those in which assessment indicates that the increased resistance to passive stretch is due to a consolidation in the soft tissue offer a worse prognosis, as this is not an indication for the application of DNHS®. Although it is generally common to find some typical patterns, patients with CNS lesions present a wide clinical variability, even with very similar lesions, which also depends on the posture. For this reason, it is not possible to provide a list of muscles to treat, although we can share our experience of those that have demonstrated better results since we started using this technique in 2005, both in the clinic as well as in research projects. One of the criteria considered is the prioritization of biarticular or polyarticular muscles over monoarticular muscles, although there are exceptions to this, such as the soleus.

In the case of the upper limb, according to our experience, it is common to find excessive activity in the upper trapezius, pectoralis major, teres major, lattisimus dorsi, biceps brachii, brachialis anterior, brachioradialis, pronator teres, flexor digitorum superficialis and flexor digitorum profundus, adductor pollicis and the first dorsal interosseous muscles.

In the case of the lower limb, the rectus femoris, hamstrings, gastrocnemius, soleus, flexor digitorum longus, flexor hallucis longus and tibialis posterior muscles are highlighted.

9.5.5 Prognosis

With regard to resistance to passive movement, the effects are usually greater and of increased duration in the upper limbs rather than the lower limbs, possibly because of the activation factor represented by the person's weight placed on the lower limbs. However, with regard to functional changes, the largest improvements are found in the lower limbs and, in general, in those patients who have a more active mobility and functionality. The fact that it is easier to achieve functional improvements in the lower limbs we believe is due to the high representation that the upper limbs have in the brain, especially with regard to the hand.[72]

9.5.6 Contraindications

The contraindications and dangers of DNHS® are the same as those with dry needling of MTrPs. Because this treatment modality is directed at patients with neurological involvement, other relative contraindications must be considered, such as sensory alterations and the use of anticoagulants and epilepsy.[65] In these cases, usually a trial treatment is first carried out which is not very aggressive (two to three insertions into each MTrP), followed by a rest period to assess whether the patient shows a positive response. Furthermore, it is recommended to speak to the medical specialists attending the patient in order to discuss whether the contraindication is valid or not. However, in daily clinical practice this is quite straightforward and the only patients for whom treatment is contraindicated are those who are considered at risk. The criteria to consider a patient at risk are not clear as all the existing references are for infiltrations with botulinum toxin, and the lesion produced by this type of needle, which is of a larger calibre and bevelled, cannot be compared to the lesion made by a filiform needle used for dry needling.

Therefore, in the case of patients with anticoagulant medication, if dry needling is agreed on, very deep punctures should be avoided in the first sessions (to avoid uncontrolled bleeding) or in places that are especially dangerous (e.g. compartment syndrome).

On a more practical level, seeing as the topic of how to apply dry needling in patients who are on anticoagulants usually creates lots of doubt for physiotherapists, this can be possibly resolved by asking the patient if, when he or she goes for blood tests, the doctor recommends interruption of the anticoagulant medication. In comparison, the needles used to draw blood are of a much greater calibre, and are bevelled, and therefore if these types of procedures do not entail a risk, dry needling should not either. An important consideration here is that, in the case of dry needling, several punctures are performed, whereas blood tests and infiltration with botulinum toxin tend to use a single puncture. However, regardless of this factor, we consider that, in the case of dry needling, the area of the lesion and the risk of bleeding are notably lower than that of infiltration with botulinum toxin.

9.6 CLINICAL CASE

9.6.1 Hypertonia of the upper limb poststroke

A 55-year-old woman, who had suffered an ischaemic cerebrovascular accident 6 months previously, attends a physiotherapy consultation complaining of difficulty in performing isolated functional movements with her affected hand.

An assessment of the mobility and hypertonia of the affected upper limb is conducted, which reveals the following findings:

- Grade 1+ hypertonia in the modified Ashworth scale affecting the thumb abduction movement
- Grade 2 hypertonia affecting extension of the elbow, wrist and fingers as well as forearm supination. No hypertonia is found when passive elbow extension is performed with a closed fist (wrist and fingers in flexion), but this increases gradually when performed with an open hand (wrist and fingers in extension)
- Normal range of movement in all the joints.

If we were to apply the DNHS® technique, what muscles would you select for treatment? In which order would you treat them? Why?

(Clinical case continued on page 489)

9.7 Acknowledgements

The authors would like to thank Professor Dr. Anand D. Pandyan and Isabel Quintero for their assistance and advice in the scientific review of this chapter.

9.8 REFERENCES

1. Kietrys DM, Palombaro KM, Azzaretto E, et al. Effectiveness of dry needling for upper-quarter myofascial pain: a systematic review and meta-analysis. J Orthop Sports Phys Ther 2013;43(9):620–34.

2. DiLorenzo L, Traballesi M, Morelli D, et al. Hemiparetic shoulder pain syndrome treated with deep dry needling during early rehabilitation: A prospective, open-label, randomized investigation. J Musculoske Pain 2004;12(2):25–34.

3. Simons DG, Travell JG, Simons LS. Dolor y disfunción miofascial. El manual de los puntos gatillo. Vol 1. Mitad superior del cuerpo. 2nd ed. Madrid: Editorial Médica Panamericana; 2002. p. 735–7.

4. Fresno MJ, Mediavilla P, Mayoral O. Dry needling of myofascial trigger points for hypertonia spastica in incomplete spinal cord injuries. Report of two cases. J Musculoske Pain [Abstract] 2004;12(9):75.

5. Trenado J, Herrero P, Ventura AL, et al. Tratamiento de puntos gatillo miofasciales en el paciente con daño cerebral adquirido: un ensayo clínico. Toledo, Spain: I Jornadas Nacionales de Dolor Miofascial; 2009.

6. Herrero P, Mayoral O. A case study looking at the effectiveness of deep dry needling for the management of hypertonia. J Musculoske Pain 2007;15(2):55–60.

7. Ernberg M, Hedenberg-Magnusson B, List T, et al. Efficacy of botulinum toxin type A for treatment of persistent myofascial TMD pain: a randomized, controlled, double-blind multicenter study. Pain 2011;152(9):1988–96.

8. Qerama E, Fuglsang-Frederiksen A, Kasch H, et al. A double-blind, controlled study of botulinum toxin A in chronic myofascial pain. Neurology 2006;67(2):241–5.

9. Behmand RA, Tucker T, Guyuron B. Single-site botulinum toxin type a injection for elimination of migraine trigger points. Headache 2003;43(10):1085–9.

10. Safarpour D, Jabbari B. Botulinum toxin A (Botox) for treatment of proximal myofascial pain in complex regional pain syndrome: two cases. Pain Med 2010;11(9):1415–18.

11. Ozcakir S, Sivrioglu K. Botulinum toxin in poststroke spasticity. Clin Med Res 2007;5(2):132–8.

12. Francisco GE. Botulinum toxin for post-stroke spastic hypertonia: a review of its efficacy and application in clinical practice. Ann Acad Med Singapore 2007;36(1):22–30.

13. Bakheit AM, Fedorova NV, Skoromets AA, et al. The beneficial antispasticity effect of botulinum toxin type A is maintained after repeated treatment cycles. J Neurol Neurosurg Psychiatry 2004;75(11):1558–61.

14. Gugala B, Snela S. Effectiveness of botulinum toxin in diminishing lower limbs spasticity in children with diplegic form of cerebral palsy. Chir Narzadow Ruchu Ortop Pol 2011;76(2):91–5.

15. Tomásová Z, Hlustík P, Král M, et al. Cortical activation changes in patients suffering from post-stroke arm spasticity and treated with botulinum toxin a. J Neuroimaging 2013;23(3):337–44.

16. Béseler MR, Grao CM, Gil A, et al. Walking assessment with instrumented insoles in patients with lower limb spasticity after botulinum toxin infiltration. Neurologia 2012;27(9):519–30.

17. Molenaers G, Van Campenhout A, Fagard K, et al. The use of botulinum toxin A in children with cerebral palsy, with a focus on the lower limb. J Child Orthop 2010;4(3):183–95.

18. Cobb DB, Watson WA, Fernández MC. Botulism-like syndrome after injections of botulinum toxin. Vet Hum Toxicol 2000;42(3):163.

19. Partikian A, Mitchell WG. Iatrogenic botulism in a child with spastic quadriparesis. J Child Neurol 2007;22(10):1235–7.

20. Tilton AH. Injectable neuromuscular blockade in the treatment of spasticity and movement disorders. J Child Neurol 2003;18(Suppl. 1):S50–66.

21. Hong CZ. Lidocaine injection versus dry needling to myofascial trigger point. The importance of the local twitch response. Am J Phys Med Rehabil 1994;73(4):256–63.

22. Ay S, Evcik D, Tur BS. Comparison of injection methods in myofascial pain syndrome: a randomized controlled trial. Clin Rheumatol 2010;29(1):19–23.

23. Ga H, Choi JH, Park CH, et al. Acupuncture needling versus lidocaine injection of trigger points in myofascial pain syndrome in elderly patients – a randomised trial. Acupunct Med 2007;25(4):130–6.

24. de Venâncio RA, Alencar FG, Zamperini C. Different substances and dry-needling injections in patients with myofascial pain and headaches. Cranio 2008;26(2):96–103.

25. de Venâncio RA, Alencar FG, Zamperini C. Botulinum toxin, lidocaine, and dry-needling injections in patients with myofascial pain and headaches. Cranio 2009;27(1):46–53.

26. Sheean G. The pathophysiology of spasticity. Eur J Neurol 2002;9(Suppl. 1):3–9, discussion 53–61.

27. Malhotra S, Pandyan AD, Day CR, et al. Spasticity, an impairment that is poorly defined and poorly measured. Clin Rehabil 2009;23(7):651–8.

28. Pandyan AD, Johnson GR, Price CI, et al. A review of the properties and limitations of the Ashworth and modified Ashworth Scales as measures of spasticity. Clin Rehabil 1999;13(5):373–83.

29. Katz RT, Rymer WZ. Spastic hypertonia: mechanisms and measurement. Arch Phys Med and Rehabil 1989;70(2):144–55.

30. Nielsen JB, Crone C, Hultborn H. The spinal pathophysiology of spasticity – from a basic science point of view. Acta Physiol 2007;189(2):171–80.

31. Hagbarth KE, Hägglund JV, Nordin M, et al. Thixotropic behavior of human finger flexor muscles with accompanying changes in spindle and reflex responses to stretch. J Physiol 1985;368:323–42.

32. Vattanasilp W, Ada L, Crosbie J. Contribution of thixotropy, spasticity, and contracture to ankle stiffness after stroke. J Neurol Neurosurg Psychiatry 2000;69(1):34–9.

33. Pandyan AD, Granat MH, Stott DJ. Effects of electrical stimulation on flexion contractures in the hemiplegic wrist. Clin Rehabil 1997;11(2):123–30.

34. Lance JW. Pathophysiology of spasticity and clinical experience with baclofen. In: Feldman RG, Koella WP, editors. Spasticity: disordered motor control. London: Year Book Medical; 1980. p. 185–204.

35. Sanger TD, Delgado MR, Gaebler-Spira D, et al. Classification and definition of disorders causing hypertonia in childhood. Pediatrics 2003;111(1):e89–97.

36. Pandyan AD, Gregoric M, Barnes MP, et al. Spasticity: clinical perceptions, neurological realities and meaningful measurement. Disabil Rehabil 2005;27(1–2):2–6.

37. Mukherjee A, Chakravarty A. Spasticity mechanisms – for the clinician. Front Neurol 2010;1:149.

38. Barnes MP, Johnson GR. Upper motor neurone syndrome and spasticity. Clinical management and

neurophysiology. 2nd ed. New York: Cambridge Medicine; 2008.

39. Merlie JP, Isenberg KE, Russell SD, et al. Denervation supersensitivity in skeletal muscle: analysis with a cloned cDNA probe. J Cell Biol 1984;99(1 Pt 1):332–5.

40. Streichert LC, Sargent PB. The role of acetylcholinesterase in denervation supersensitivity in the frog cardiac ganglion. J Physiol 1992;445:249–60.

41. Voerman GE, Gregoric M, Hermens HJ. Neurophysiological methods for the assessment of spasticity: the Hoffmann reflex, the tendon reflex, and the stretch reflex. Disabil Rehabil 2005;27(1–2):33–68.

42. Katz R. Presynaptic inhibition in humans: a comparison between normal and spastic patients. J Physiol 1999; 93(4):379–85.

43. Hultborn H, Illert M, Nielsen J, et al. On the mechanism of the post-activation depression of the H-reflex in human subjects. Exp Brain Res 1996;108(3):450–62.

44. Aymard C, Katz R, Lafitte C, et al. Presynaptic inhibition and homosynaptic depression: a comparison between lower and upper limbs in normal human subjects and patients with hemiplegia. Brain 2000;123(Pt 8): 1688–702.

45. Hochman S, Shreckengost J, Kimura H, et al. Presynaptic inhibition of primary afferents by depolarization: observations supporting nontraditional mechanisms. Ann N Y Acad Sci 2010;1198:140–52.

46. Acebes X, Udina E. Neurofisiología de la espasticidad. Evaluación clínica y tratamiento de la espasticidad. Madrid: Médica Panamericana; 2009. p. 1–16.

47. Ibrahim IK, Berger W, Trippel M, et al. Stretch-induced electromyographic activity and torque in spastic elbow muscles. Differential modulation of reflex activity in passive and active motor-tasks. Brain 1993;116(Pt 4): 971–89.

48. Hufschmidt A, Mauritz KH. Chronic transformation of muscle in spasticity: a peripheral contribution to increased tone. J Neurol Neurosurg Psychiatry 1985; 48(7):676–85.

49. Dietz V, Quintern J, Berger W. Electrophysiological studies of gait in spasticity and rigidity. Evidence that altered mechanical properties of muscle contribute to hypertonia. Brain 1981;104(3):431–49.

50. Sinkjaer T, Magnussen I. Passive, intrinsic and reflex-mediated stiffness in the ankle extensors of hemiparetic patients. Brain 1994;117(Pt 2):355–63.

51. Malouin F, Bonneau C, Pichard L, et al. Non-reflex mediated changes in plantarflexor muscles early after stroke. Scand J Rehabil Med 1997;29(3):147–53.

52. Lieber RL, Steinman S, Barash IA, et al. Structural and functional changes in spastic skeletal muscle. Muscle Nerve 2004;29(5):615–27.

53. Smith LR, Lee KS, Ward SR, et al. Hamstring contractures in children with spastic cerebral palsy result from a stiffer extracellular matrix and increased in vivo sarcomere length. J Physiol 2011;589(Pt 10):2625–39.

54. Shah JP, Phillips TM, Danoff JV, et al. An in vivo microanalytical technique for measuring the local biochemical milieu of human skeletal muscle. J Appl Physiol 2005; 99(5):1977–84.

55. Domingo A, Mayoral O, Monterde S, et al. Neuromuscular damage and repair after dry needling in mice. Evid Based Complement Alternat Med 2013;2013: 260806.

56. Prado MA, Reis RA, Prado VF, et al. Regulation of acetylcholine synthesis and storage. Neurochem Int 2002; 41(5):291–9.

57. Hong CZ, Simons DG. Pathophysiologic and electrophysiologic mechanisms of myofascial trigger points. Arch Phys Med Rehabil 1998;79(7):863–72.

58. Nudo RJ, Plautz EJ, Frost SB. Role of adaptive plasticity in recovery of function after damage to motor cortex. Muscle Nerve 2001;24(8):1000–19.

59. Gómez L. Bases neurales de la recuperación motora en las lesiones cerebrales. Revista Méxicana de Neurociencia 2001;2(4):216–21.

60. Hsieh YL, Chou LW, Joe YS, et al. Spinal cord mechanism involving the remote effects of dry needling on the irritability of myofascial trigger spots in rabbit skeletal muscle. Arch Phys Med Rehabil 2011;92(7):1098–105.

61. Walker HW, Kirshblum S. Spasticity due to disease of the spinal cord: pathophysiology, epidemiology, and treatment. In: Brashear A, Elovic EP, editors. Spasticity. Diagnosis and management. New York: Demos Medical Publishing; 2011. p. 313–41.

62. Audette JF, Wang F, Smith H. Bilateral activation of motor unit potentials with unilateral needle stimulation of active myofascial trigger points. Ame J Phys Med Rehabil 2004;83(5):368–74.

63. Sessle BJ, Hu JW, Amano N, et al. Convergence of cutaneous, tooth pulp, visceral, neck and muscle afferents onto nociceptive and non-nociceptive neurons in trigeminal subnucleus caudalis (medullary dorsal horn) and its implications for referred pain. Pain 1986;27(2): 219–35.

64. Mense S. How do muscle lesions such as latent and active trigger points influence central nociceptive neurons? J Musculoske Pain 2010;18(4):348–53.

65. Navarro J, Herrero P, Del Moral R, et al. Cordancia electroencefálica: aplicación a la técnica de Punción Seca DNHS® en pacientes con enfermedad cerebro vascular: estudio piloto. Zaragoza, Spain: VII Encuentro de Neurociencias y Salud Mental; 2011.

66. Gracies JM. Pathophysiology of spastic paresis. I: Paresis and soft tissue changes. Muscle Nerve 2005;31(5): 535–51.

67. Dietz V, Sinkjaer T. Spastic movement disorder: impaired reflex function and altered muscle mechanics. Lancet Neurol 2007;6(8):725–33.

68. Ballyns JJ, Shah JP, Hammond J, et al. Objective sonographic measures for characterizing myofascial trigger points associated with cervical pain. J Ultrasound Med 2011;30(10):1331–40.

69. Lieber RL. Estructura del músculo esquelético, función y plasticidad. Bases fisiológicas de la fisioterapia. 2nd ed. Spain: McGraw-Hill Interamericana; 2004.

70. Mauro A. Satellite cell of skeletal muscle fibers. J Biophys Biochem Cytol 1961;9(2):493–5.

71. Reznik M. Current concepts of skeletal muscle regeneration. Baltimore, Md, USA: Williams & Wilkins; 1973.

72. Kolb B, Whishaw IQ. Neuropsicología humana. Spain: Medica Panamericana; 2006.

73. Baker SN. The primate reticulospinal tract, hand function and functional recovery. J Physiol 2011;589(Pt 23): 5603–12.

74. Rothwell JC. Overview of neurophysiology of movement control. Clin Neurol Neurosurgery 2012;114(5): 432–5.

CHAPTER 10

ACUPUNCTURE AND NEEDLING TECHNIQUES FOR SEGMENTAL DYSFUNCTION IN NEUROMUSCULOSKELETAL PAIN

Jay P. Shah • Nikki Thaker

Everything that we see is a shadow cast by that which we do not see.
MARTIN LUTHER KING, JR.

KEYWORDS

spinal segmental sensitization; neuroplastic changes; spinal facilitation; paraspinous dry needling techniques; glial cells; myofascial pain syndrome; local twitch response.

10.1 INTRODUCTION

Chronic pain states are characterized by profound changes in neuronal excitability and architecture of the pain matrix. These neuroplastic changes occur in the spinal cord, thalamic nuclei, cortical and limbic areas and may alter the threshold, intensity and affect of one's pain experience. Spinal segmental sensitization (SSS) is a hyperactive state of the dorsal horn caused by bombardment of nociceptive impulses from sensitized and/or damaged tissue. Active (i.e. spontaneously painful) myofascial trigger points (MTrPs) are a very common source of persistent nociception and sensitization of dorsal horn neurons that often results in SSS and chronic pain. Furthermore, recent studies of the biochemical milieu (using novel microanalytical techniques) and viscoelastic properties (using office-based diagnostic ultrasound) have revealed fascinating objective abnormalities of MTrPs that help explain their role in myofascial pain syndrome and SSS. The dynamic changes that occur during the initiation, amplification and perpetuation of SSS may explain the objective and reproducible segmental physical findings (e.g. dermatomal allodynia and hyperalgesia) and the effects observed following paraspinous dry needling.

10.2 CASE STUDY

Jessica is a 50-year-old woman with a complex medical history, who develops a new onset of right upper quadrant pain. She is perplexed because this episode is identical to her previous experience with gall bladder pain, despite the fact that she underwent a cholecystectomy 20 years ago. Jessica's new onset of gall bladder pain is one of the many pain complaints she has developed over the years. However, alarmed that the pain appears to be coming from an organ that is no longer there, Jessica decides to see an osteopathic physician.

Upon her first visit, her doctor collects a detailed medical history. She begins by telling him that in her teenage years, she was an elite soccer player. However, she sustained a serious sports injury during a game when an overaggressive opponent kicked the front of her right thigh, causing a noticeable limp. Jessica complained of an aching, cramping pain deep in her right knee joint that also caused the knee to buckle occasionally. Due to the pain, Jessica often had trouble sleeping at night. Since the injury, Jessica also has a mild form of patellar tracking dysfunction, in which she experiences a painful popping or grinding of the kneecap as the knee is flexed or extended. After 5 years of massage and other manual therapies, her knee joint pain completely resolved, but she was unable to return to her previous level of physical activity due to continued muscle dysfunction, weakness and a limited range of motion in her knee joint.

Over the years, doctors ruled out patellofemoral dysfunction and tendinitis of the quadriceps or patellar tendons as an explanation for her knee dysfunction. Jessica was told that there were no abnormal findings in her right knee and thigh.

Coincidentally, around this time, Jessica also developed lower-back pain and pelvic pain, which continues to persist today. Jessica obtains temporary relief from pain relievers and therapeutic massages, but has accepted that she is going to have to live with debilitating pain in her knee.

At age 35, she starts to feel immense pain radiating from her gall bladder. She finds out she has developed acute cholecystitis (gall bladder inflammation) for which she undergoes a cholecystectomy. While the surgery relieved her original gall bladder pain, now at the age of 50, she feels the same pain has returned. How is this possible?

After listening carefully to Jessica's medical history, her new physician suspects that no one has previously examined the muscles surrounding her knee joint and pelvic area for MTrPs. He conducts a thorough physical examination, palpating the soft tissue and muscles surrounding her knee and pelvic area. He finds multiple latent MTrPs in her right vastus lateralis (knee extensor muscle) and active and latent MTrPs in her lower back and pelvic area. Jessica's doctor suspects that the latent MTrPs could be responsible for her knee dysfunction, and her sports injury could have led to her other pain complaints. He goes on to explain that her chronic knee pain could have triggered her other pain complaints as a result of peripheral and central sensitization. However, there are still many unanswered questions. Why is muscle pain distinct from cutaneous and neuropathic pain? Why is myofascial pain so common and yet so often overlooked? What is the role of peripheral and central sensitization in myofascial pain? Are Jessica's pain complaints all related to one another? Are there other factors exacerbating her pain complaints? Lastly, could her pain symptoms be reversed or relieved?

10.3 DISTINCT NEUROBIOLOGY OF MUSCLE PAIN

Myofascial pain is the most common component of musculoskeletal pain conditions. As a form of muscle pain, myofascial pain can often be described as aching, cramping, deep and difficult to localize. Muscle pain is distinguished from cutaneous pain in that muscle pain involves nociceptive-specific neurons in the brainstem and spinal cord.[1,2] In addition, muscle pain activates unique cortical areas that are associated with affective or emotional components of pain.[3] Although muscle nociception is inhibited more intensely by descending pain-modulating pathways,[4,5] persistent muscle nociception, compared to cutaneous nociception, is more effective at inducing maladaptive neuroplastic changes within the dorsal horn.[6] Such neuroplastic changes underlie the clinical observation that muscle pain is often difficult to resolve.

Musculoskeletal pain is the most common manifestation of chronic pain. The term neuro-musculoskeletal pain is preferable when describing a chronic musculoskeletal pain state because it accurately implies fundamental alterations in the nervous system – sometimes irreversibly so. Myofascial pain arises from MTrPs (see chapter 8). An MTrP has been defined as a hyperirritable spot, usually within a taut band of skeletal muscle or in the muscle fascia, that is painful on compression and that can give rise to characteristic referred pain, tenderness and autonomic phenomena.[7] Active MTrPs are spontaneously painful, while latent MTrPs are not spontaneously painful, but cause local and/or referred pain upon firm palpation. Accordingly, it has been found that active MTrPs have a significantly lower pain pressure threshold than latent MTrPs and normal, uninvolved muscle tissue.[8] Diagnosis depends exclusively upon a detailed medical history and physical examination.

10.3.1 Background on sensitization

Sensitization is the lowering of the activation threshold for nociceptors, which then increases neuronal activity in the central nervous system. Through sensitization, chronic pain syndromes, such as myofascial pain syndrome, exhibit profound neuroplastic changes, altering neuronal excitability in the pain pathway (e.g. the spinal cord, thalamic nuclei, cortical areas, amygdala and periaqueductal grey area). This dynamic process can fundamentally alter pain threshold, pain intensity and emotional affect.[9] Common manifestations of sensitization are allodynia (pain to a normally non-painful stimulus) and hyperalgesia (increased pain to a normally painful stimulus).

MTrPs give rise to sensory abnormalities characterized by pain, such as the aching in the knee that Jessica experiences. Transduction of local pain sensation often begins with the activation of nociceptors. Nociceptors are receptors that upon binding to noxious substances transmit tissue damage and inflammation information into nerve impulses. These include chemoreceptors, mechanoreceptors and thermoreceptors. In Jessica's case, her fall activated the nociceptors in her vastus medialis muscle (knee extensor muscle innervated by lumbar segments L3–L4), and the subsequent nociceptive impulses bombard the dorsal horn.[10] Prolonged noxious input may lead to long-term changes in gene expression, somatosensory processing and synaptic structure. For example, a continuous barrage of noxious input into the dorsal horn (a process termed afferent bombardment) results in the co-release of L-glutamate and substance P. Released together, these two substances can lower thresholds for synaptic activation and open previously ineffective synaptic connections in wide dynamic range (WDR) neurons, thus inducing central sensitization.[10,11]

In addition, sensitization upregulates ion channel and receptor expression and increases the number of these membrane proteins on nociceptors and dorsal horn neurons. Under normal circumstances, a dynamic balance exists between facilitation and inhibition of pain signals. Neurons conveying nociceptive information are controlled by a variety of inhibitory interneurons, structures critically involved in preventing the transition from acute to chronic pain.[9]

An understanding of segmental distribution of sensory nerve fibres is a vital component in proper pain management.[12] Innervation patterns of the skin, muscles and deep structures occur at an early stage of human fetal development and little variability exists among individuals.[13] Accordingly, each spinal cord segment has a consistent segmental relationship to its spinal nerves. This allows clinicians to attribute the pattern of dermatomal, myotomal and sclerotomal hyperalgesia to dysfunction in its corresponding spinal segment.[12,14] In Jessica's case, her symptomatic pain pattern can be explained by the fact that both the knee and pelvic region are innervated by the L3–L4 segments.

SSS is a hyperactive state of the dorsal horn caused by bombardment of nociceptive impulses from sensitized and/or damaged tissue (e.g. somatic structures such as active MTrPs or visceral structures such as the gall bladder). Manifestations in the sensitized spinal segment include dermatomal allodynia and hyperalgesia in addition to sclerotomal tenderness and MTrPs within the involved myotomes.[12,14] Hyperalgesia of central origin is so prevalent that, in one study, it was found to be responsible for 61% of patients suffering from knee arthrosis. This suggests that both central and peripheral mechanisms are responsible for maintaining a chronic pain state in these individuals. Initially, hypersensitivity occurs at a local, affected site but it is likely that central mechanisms, once initiated, persist independently from the peripheral process.[15] Further, segmental sensitization occurs through neuron hypertrophy as well as upregulation of excitatory neurons, prohyperalgesic peptides and neurotransmitters at the dorsal horn. As a result, pain and inflammation occur as independent events and therefore do not necessarily correlate with one another.

KEY POINTS

Through sensitization, myofascial pain syndrome exhibits profound neuroplastic changes, altering neuronal excitability in the pain pathway, with common manifestations such as allodynia (pain to a normally non-painful stimulus) and hyperalgesia (increased pain to a normally painful stimulus).

10.3.2 Peripheral to central sensitization in muscle pain

Sensitization of both peripheral and central afferents is responsible for the transition from normal to aberrant pain perception in the central nervous system that outlasts the noxious peripheral stimulus. In animal models of pain, nociceptive input from skeletal muscle, as compared to cutaneous nociceptor activation, is much more effective at inducing neuroplastic changes in the spinal cord.[6]

As mentioned above, peripheral tissue damage arising from trauma or inflammation triggers the release of numerous substances from damaged muscle, such as adenosine triphosphate, bradykinin, serotonin, prostaglandins and potassium.[16–18] This inflammatory pool of biochemicals sensitizes local nociceptors, an event

known as peripheral sensitization, subsequently lowering the threshold for depolarization and increasing the response to noxious stimuli. The continual bombardment of primary afferent activity over time can lead to abnormal function and structural changes in the dorsal root ganglia. This is known as central sensitization,[10] an event that can lead to persistent allodynia and hyperalgesia.

A possible explanation for this phenomenon is increased synaptic efficiency through activation of previously silent (ineffective) synapses at the dorsal horn. Specifically, constant noxious input continually releases substance P and glutamate from the primary afferent fibre. These excitatory substances enter the postsynaptic cell, opening up calcium channels. The flooding of the postsynaptic neuron with calcium activates enzymes responsible for apoptosis, i.e. programmed cell death. Certain cells, like inhibitory interneurons, are more likely to undergo calcium-induced apoptosis.[19] Since large myelinated fibres dampen pain by activating inhibitory interneurons, loss of these interneurons results in increased pain intensity, leading to allodynia, hyperalgesia, temporal summation of pain[20] and expanded pain patterns.

Calcium also acts as a second messenger, initiating gene induction in the nucleus. This increases neuronal transmission, resulting in the cell firing more rapidly and the formation of new ion channel proteins. Opening of the ion channel proteins allows the neuron to hyperexcite, creating a feed-forward cycle. This results in a long-lasting, if not permanent, sensitization of dorsal horn neurons,[19] leading to allodynia and hyperalgesia. The onset of central sensitization is a hallmark in the transition from acute to chronic pain. As one can imagine, the clinical consequences may be very distressing to patients.

The concept of opening previously ineffective connections was demonstrated in a rat myositis model. Experimentally induced inflammation unmasked receptive fields remote from the original receptive field, indicating that dorsal horn connectivity expanded beyond the original neurons involved in nociceptive transmission.[21] In this study, nociceptive input resulted in central hyperexcitability and this finding helps to explain allodynia, hyperalgesia and referred pain patterns common to myofascial pain.

There is a biochemical basis to explain the development of peripheral and central sensitization in muscle pain. Studies by Shah et al.[16,18] have found that active MTrPs have a unique biochemical milieu compared to latent MTrPs and muscle without palpable MTrPs. A novel microanalytical technique was used to perform continuous, near real-time, *in vivo* sampling of biochemicals from the trapezius muscles of patients with and without neck pain, and with and without MTrPs. Results showed that patients with neck pain secondary to an active MTrP had significantly elevated local levels of endogenous substance P, calcitonin gene-related peptide (CGRP), bradykinin, serotonin/5-hydroxytryptamine, noradrenaline, tumour necrosis factor-alpha (TNF-α), interleukin-1β (IL-1β), IL-6 and IL-8 compared to carefully matched controls. These substances were considerably elevated in those with active MTrPs compared to those with latent MTrPs and those with normal tissue in the upper trapezius.[16–18] Of relevance, injection of the serotonin antagonist tropisetron was found to be more effective than lidocaine in relieving pain from MTrPs.[22,23]

Together, these studies demonstrated and confirmed that the clinical distinction between active and latent MTrPs is associated with a highly significant objective difference in the local biochemical milieu. These findings may help to explain why active MTrPs, which are associated with high concentrations of biochemicals known to cause both peripheral and central sensitization, are spontaneously painful, acutely tender and a source of referred pain. These

biochemical studies have helped to establish the clinical importance of palpating and identifying active MTrPs. They also suggest that myofascial pain is an objective entity in the spectrum of clinical pain states and may also explain why specific treatments are more effective than others.

10.3.3 Somatic and visceral input convergence

Central sensitization may also facilitate additional responses from other receptive fields as a result of convergent somatic and visceral input at the dorsal horn[24] via WDR neurons located in lamina IV and lamina V (figure 10.1). These neurons are called 'wide dynamic range' because they receive afferent input from multiple sources, including skin, muscle, viscera, periosteum and bone. In addition to activating lamina I, muscle afferents preferentially activate lamina V, where WDR neurons are predominantly located. This neuroanatomical fact explains how muscle nociception and pain can spread to seemingly unrelated structures (e.g. viscera) and, vice versa, how nociceptive input from these visceral structures can manifest as muscle pain. Furthermore, afferent fibres have the ability to sprout new spinal

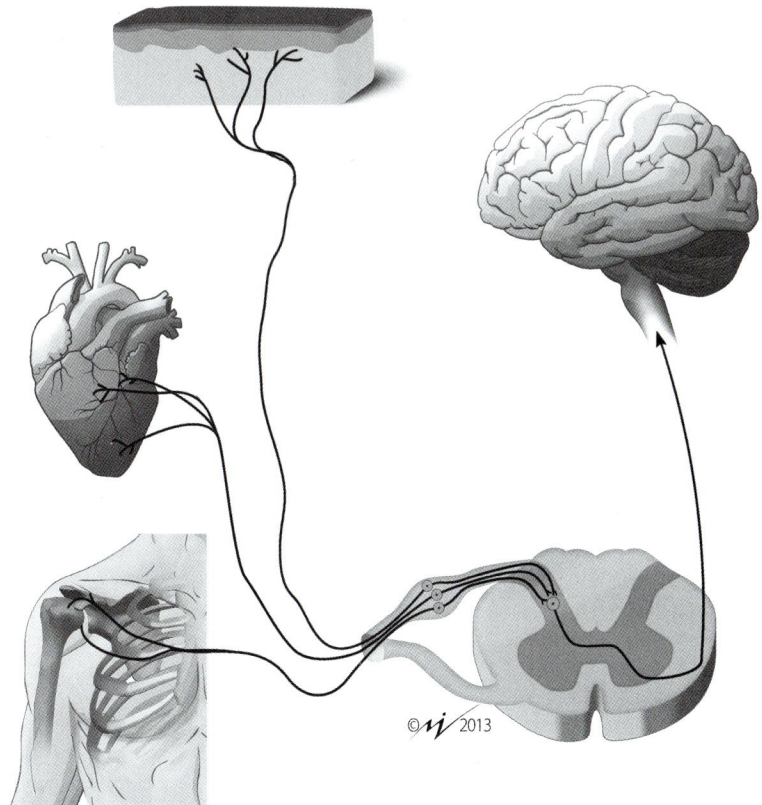

FIGURE 10.1 ■ Wide dynamic range (WDR) neuron. A WDR neuron receives convergent input from cutaneous, visceral and deep somatic afferents and subsequently sends signals to the thalamus. As such, the WDR neuron and higher-level brain centres can be driven by various inputs. Accordingly, central sensitization may facilitate responses from other structures (e.g. the shoulder, heart and skin), which share convergent input. (Adapted from Willard F. Basic mechanisms of pain. Future trends in CAM research. In: Audette JF, Bailey A (eds) Integrative Pain Medicine: The Science and Practice of Complementary and Alternative Medicine in Pain Management. Totowa: Humana Press; 2008). (Colour version of figure is available online).

terminals that broaden synaptic contacts at the dorsal horn and may also contribute to expanded pain-receptive fields.[25] This change in functional connectivity may occur within a few hours, even before metabolic and genetic alterations occur in dorsal horn neurons.[26]

KEY POINTS

Central sensitization may also facilitate additional responses from other receptive fields as a result of convergent somatic and visceral input at the dorsal horn via WDR neurons located in lamina IV and lamina V.

The convergence of somatic and visceral input at the dorsal horn could have been responsible for Jessica's onset of pelvic pain. Recall that Jessica's sports injury led to sensitization of the L3–L4 segments. The WDR neurons of these segments receiving the nociceptive input may have spread the input to her pelvic area.

10.3.4 Spinal facilitation

Spinal facilitation is an increase in activity of spinal cord neurons due to the bombardment of nociceptive stimuli into the dorsal horn (figure 10.2).[27] Under normal circumstances, activation of primary afferent nociceptors in the dorsal horn is modulated by inhibitory mechanisms either locally or via descending pathways from the cerebral cortex or brainstem. However, as mentioned above, persistent nociceptive afferent input may result in inhibitory neuronal cell death, wind-up and sensitization of secondary-order neurons in the dorsal horn. Circuits in the spinal cord (i.e. dorsal horn, ventral horn and lateral horn) may develop lowered thresholds of activation, causing them to be more easily activated by minimal or no input at all. The ensuing spinal facilitation is characterized by:

- increased ventral horn outflow that stimulates anterior motor horn cells, resulting in increased muscle tone in the myotome, corresponding to its segmental level of afferent barrage
- increased lateral horn outflow which results in autonomic reflexes that enhance nociceptive activity
- increased dorsal horn outflow that causes antidromic electrical activity along a sensory nerve (also known as dorsal root reflexes).

Dorsal root reflexes activate dorsal root ganglion cell bodies to increase production and release of vasoactive neuropeptides (substance P, CGRP and somatostatin) both centrally and peripherally. These neuropeptides have been shown to cause leaky blood vessels and trigger the liberation of inflammatory mediators into the tissue, causing inflammation *de novo*, a condition known as neurogenic inflammation.[10] However, if inflammation is already present, the release of vasoactive neuropeptides will exacerbate the condition. As a result, local tissue tenderness and mechanical hyperalgesia often ensue

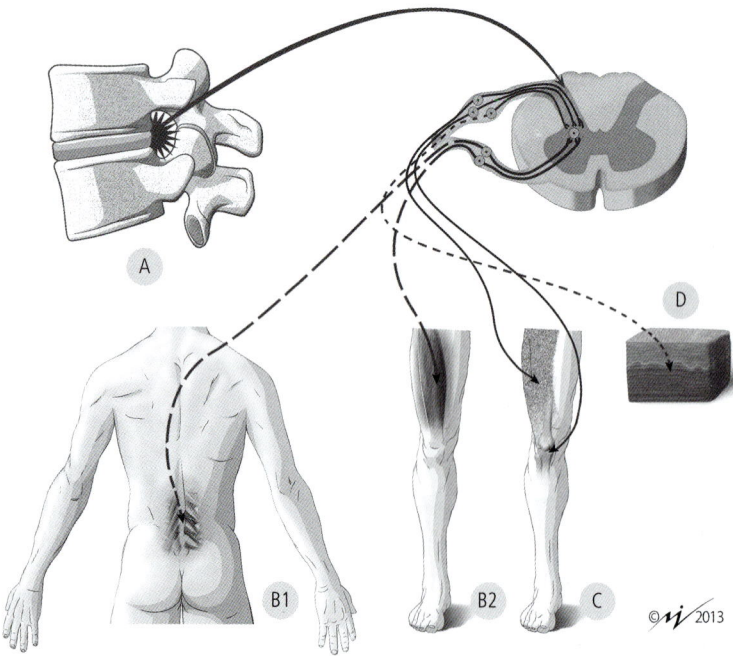

FIGURE 10.2 ■ Facilitated spinal segment. (A) Nociception originating in the L4 facet joint synapses on the dorsal horn. (B) At the L4 segmental level, a motor neuron within the ventral horn becomes activated, causing a reflex spasm of muscles innervated by the same segment such as (B1) the paraspinal muscles and (B2) the rectus femoris muscle. (C) Dermatomal and sclerotomal structures sharing the L4 segmental level may become sensitized and painful as a result of dorsal root reflexes. (D) Dorsal root reflexes in the L4 segment may also sensitize cutaneous structures, rendering them more painful. (Adapted from P. Romero Ventosilla, personal communication 2010). (Colour version of figure is available online).

(or worsen, if already present), which may underlie the clinical findings of active MTrPs.

The concept of spinal facilitation could explain the development of Jessica's back pain condition. The injury that originally started in the knee extensor muscle initiated the bombardment of noxious input via the femoral nerve (L3–L4 segments) into the dorsal horn. Depolarization of the spinal cord intensely generates dorsal root reflexes from this one location; these dorsal root reflexes diffusely release neuropeptides via several adjacent segments (above and below) into the surrounding tissue. This includes the lower thoracic segments, which innervate the lower back. This results in neurogenic inflammation, a process by which neuropeptides attract other inflammatory compounds such as inflammatory mediators, catecholamines and proinflammatory cytokines, which sensitize the lower back area. In addition, increased ventral horn outflow increases tightness of the muscles corresponding to L3–L4 segments, such as paraspinal muscles and quadriceps. Lateral horn outflow is responsible for the perpetuation of nociceptive input coming in at the L3–L4 segments via autonomic reflexes.

An underappreciated anatomical fact is that primary afferent nociceptive fibres actually trifurcate upon entering the dorsal horn (figure 10.3). That is, one branch enters the dorsal horn at that segmental level, one branch ascends and one branch descends along the dorsal margin of the dorsal horn. Furthermore, some visceral afferents have been found to span the entire length of the spinal cord.[28,29] These often-overlooked anatomical considerations have enormous implications in the initiation, perpetuation and amplification of spinal facilitation and persistent musculoskeletal and visceral pain states.

In regard to Jessica's case, recall that she had a medical history of severe acute painful cholecystitis at the age of 35. Fortunately, removal of the gall bladder completely alleviated her pain. However, the sustained noxious input caused by her cholecystitis was of sufficient intensity and duration to destroy inhibitory neurons at the segmental level of entry into the dorsal horn (T6). However, 15 years later, at the age of 50, Jessica develops a minor but acutely painful back injury while lifting heavy boxes. The resultant afferent nociceptive input immediately enters the lower thoracic/upper lumbar segments and ascends/descends the spinal cord. While ascending the cord, but prior to reaching T6, presumably intact and functional inhibitory neurons suppressed the nociceptive input and prevented the sensation of pain at those segmental levels. However, upon reaching the T6 segment, the nociceptive signals were able to activate dorsal horn neurons at this level. This is because the local inhibitory neurons became dysfunctional and/or died as a result of the original intense noxious gall bladder stimuli associated with the acute cholecystitis. In fact, Jessica now complains that she is experiencing pain in the same areas as she had years ago, when she contracted the acute gall bladder disease.

The reproduction of the identical pain pattern initiated years before is a common clinical manifestation of the trifurcation of primary nociceptive fibers. Even though Jessica knew her gall bladder had been removed, she still attributed her acute pain to her absent gall bladder, a classic example of phantom pain. Accordingly, osteopathic physicians often interpret the re-emergence of an old pain pattern as the possible harbinger of new disease. The cause of the pain pattern re-emergence could be musculoskeletal in origin (as in Jessica's case) or due to an undiagnosed visceral problem or disease (e.g. peptic ulcer disease, preclinical cardiac ischaemia).

KEY POINTS

Spinal facilitation is characterized by increased ventral horn outflow resulting in increased muscle tone in the myotome corresponding to its segmental level of afferent barrage; increased lateral horn outflow, which results in autonomic reflexes that enhance nociceptive activity; and increased dorsal horn outflow that causes antidromic electrical activity along a sensory nerve.

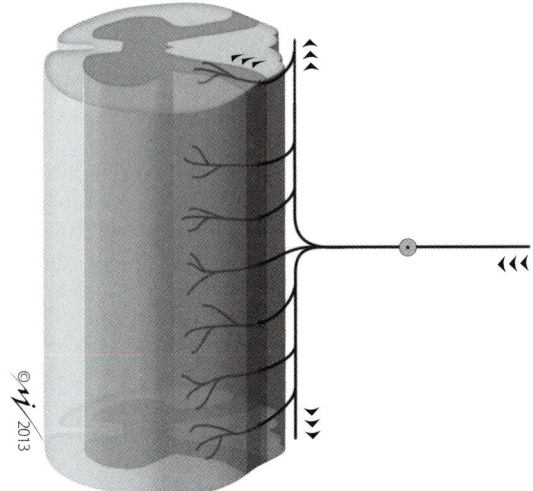

FIGURE 10.3 ■ Trifurcation of a neuron. Upon entry into the dorsal root of the spinal cord, primary afferent neurons have the ability to trifurcate; one branch enters at that segmental level while other branches may ascend and descend along the dorsal margin of the dorsal horn in Lissauer's tract. (Colour version of figure is available online).

10.3.5 Higher brain centres dynamically modulate muscle pain

The limbic forebrain and/or hypothalamus may play a role in the sequence of top-down events leading to myofascial pain syndrome. These areas are influenced by emotions and hormonal fluctuations, which then modulate the periaqueductal grey in the midbrain. The rostral ventral medulla is a relay area between the periaqueductal grey and the spinal dorsal horn. The rostral ventral medulla contains a population of on cells which can increase pain, and off cells which can decrease pain. The on/off cells are part of the descending inhibitory pain system which control pain through projections that modulate activity in the dorsal horn. Following initial tissue injury, the on cells serve a useful and protective purpose designed to prevent further damage. Under ordinary circumstances, tissue healing would lead to a decrease in on-cell activity and an increase in off-cell activity.[10] However, in chronic musculoskeletal pain conditions, there appears to be an overall shift to a decrease in inhibition, presumably due to an imbalance of on-cell and off-cell activity.[17] Thus, over time, maladaptive neuroplastic changes may develop, resulting in disinhibition in the spinal dorsal horn. As a result, dorsal root reflexes create neurogenic inflammation (and the concomitant release of sensitizing biochemicals), which leads to local tissue tenderness, even in the absence of ongoing tissue injury or nociception. Negative emotions and stress as well as hormonal changes may influence not only the perception of pain, but the clinical findings of allodynia and mechanical hyperalgesia, characteristic of myofascial pain.

During Jessica's thorough medical history and physical exam, her osteopathic physician asked many questions to understand better why her sports injury had never completely healed. In addition, he sought to investigate why there was an increased sensation of pain and sensitivity in her pelvic area, gall bladder and lower back. After determining that there were no structural or functional abnormalities in these three areas, he asked Jessica whether she was experiencing any emotional stress and whether those episodes correlated with an increased sensation of pain. Jessica admitted that a month after her sports injury, her father had passed away while she was in the midst of applying to college, and consequently she found very little time for herself. Currently, she is battling a time-consuming, difficult divorce, which has her feeling frustrated and stressed most of the time. Jessica's physician noted that these emotional stressors are likely to have exacerbated her pain symptoms.

In addition, Jessica noticed that the pain has gotten worse since she started menopause. Jessica's doctor explained that an increase in pain perception was common among many women who were experiencing changes in their menstrual cycle as a result of oestrogen and progesterone fluctuation. As discussed above, emotional stress and hormonal fluctuation may set off a cascade of neuronal activity that results in neurogenic inflammation and subsequent local tissue tenderness.

Upon confirming that Jessica has allodynia and hyperalgesia along her pelvic area, Jessica's doctor encouraged her to find ways to reduce her stress. Not only could her negative emotions and stress have influenced these clinical findings, but they could prevent her from fully recovering.

10.4 ROLE OF GLIAL CELLS

Researchers are discovering that glial cells may also be involved in the pain signalling of MTrPs. Microglia and astrocytes are activated by peripheral pathological changes, such as inflammation.[30] Since prolonged nociception activates glia, it can be hypothesized that activation of nociceptors surrounding MTrPs can increase glial activity.[31] Upon activation, glial cells release proinflammatory interleukins, TNF-α and brain-derived neurotrophic factor in the central nervous system, substances which can lead to central sensitization.[32,33] Further data from rat studies suggest that chronic muscle lesions activate microglia in the spinal cord, and the pain behaviour associated with this activation is reduced by a microglia inhibitor.[34] While no data are currently available to support the notion that MTrPs activate glia, active MTrPs are effective in central sensitization and this may in turn activate glial cells.[31] One can imagine how glial cells can exacerbate pain conditions for patients like Jessica, who are already experiencing central sensitization.

10.5 CAN LATENT MTrPs CONTRIBUTE TO CENTRAL SENSITIZATION?

Recall that Jessica's osteopathic physician found latent MTrPs during a physical examination of Jessica's right vastus lateralis muscle in the absence of any physical abnormalities in her knee joint. Her doctor suspected that Jessica may have developed active MTrPs in her vastus medialis muscle after the injury. However, the active MTrPs may have been treated coincidentally by the massage and physical therapies Jessica was receiving at the time. This would explain why the spontaneous, aching, cramping pain in Jessica's knee joint disappeared. However, because the latent MTrPs in her right thigh were never treated, Jessica continued to experience motor difficulties such as buckling of the knee and falling to the ground while walking, and being unable to extend her knee fully. Although not spontaneously painful, could latent MTrPs in the vastus lateralis muscle have played a role in Jessica's pain and knee dysfunction?

Latent MTrPs cause local and referred pain only upon firm palpation. This begs the question as to their underlying connectivity and pathophysiology. Do latent MTrPs play a role in central sensitization? How is it possible for these lesions to refer pain to distant locations? Two assumptions must be made to explain the mechanism of latent MTrPs. First, these latent MTrPs send nociceptive, subthreshold signals to the dorsal horn of the spinal cord. This would effectively sensitize the central nervous system without the perception of pain, as is characteristic of latent MTrPs. Second, ineffective synapses exist within the dorsal horn. In this way, nociceptors from muscle containing the MTrP have connections to dorsal horn neurons innervating remote muscle regions.[31]

Human studies have shown that central sensitization can occur without the experience of acute spontaneous pain. Intramuscular injection of nerve growth factor results in allodynia and hyperalgesia, both manifestations of sensitization.[35] Further, rat studies demonstrated that nerve growth factor injections activate an increased proportion of muscle nociceptors. In concordance with this finding was the presence of excitatory subthreshold potentials.[36,37] Since subthreshold potentials provide nociceptive input without subsequent action potentials into higher brain centres, there is no perception of pain.

Subthreshold potentials and ineffective synapses could serve to explain the sensory phenomenon of latent MTrPs. Taken together, it could be hypothesized that the characteristics of latent MTrPs occur due to a series of events. Latent MTrPs send excitatory, subthreshold potentials to the dorsal horn. Sensitization of the dorsal horn opens previously ineffective synapses to distant muscle sites. As a result of sensitization, normally non-noxious palpation of the latent MTrP induces pain locally and referral pain occurs upon the opening of previously ineffective synapses. Thereby, upon muscle palpation, pain is experienced at the site of the palpated latent MTrP and in distant, seemingly unrelated muscle.[31]

It is important to identify the significance of latent MTrPs because, under specific conditions, they can become active MTrPs. Excitatory subthreshold potentials from latent MTrPs can summate with subthreshold potentials from active MTrPs to surpass the threshold necessary for SSS to occur. Once the myotome is sensitized, all MTrPs in that myotome may become spontaneously painful (active).

In addition to sensitizing dorsal horn neurons, latent MTrPs may interfere with muscle performance. For example, Lucas et al. showed that patients with latent MTrPs in the scapular rotators have abnormal muscle activation patterns during shoulder abduction compared to patients with latent MTrPs, increasing a risk for developing active MTrPs.[38]

During Jessica's physical examination, her osteopathic physician measured her right-leg Q angle; this is the angle of incidence of the quadriceps muscle relative to the patella. Indeed, Jessica's Q angle was 20°, which is higher than normal (<17°), increasing the risk of patellar compression. Latent MTrPs in the vastus lateralis muscle cause shortening of the muscle, which exacerbates Jessica's patellar tracking dysfunction and further increases her Q angle. Treatment of her latent MTrPs could restore full range of motion in her knee joint. On the other hand, neglecting the latent MTrPs could lead to the return of the spontaneous knee pain if the latent MTrPs become active ones. Thus, in cases where latent MTrPs are perpetuating the sensitization or causing dysfunction, it is important to treat them.[7]

10.6 DIAGNOSIS AND IMPLICATIONS OF SPINAL SEGMENTAL SENSITIZATION IN THE CLINIC

As mentioned above, SSS is the hyperactive state of the dorsal horn caused by bombardment of nociceptive impulses from sensitized and/or damaged tissue. SSS is consistently associated with musculoskeletal pain states, underscoring its significance. For example, involvement of thoracic spinal levels (e.g. T1–T12) in SSS facilitates and perpetuates abdominal pain and somatovisceral symptoms commonly mimicking gastrointestinal conditions, such as peptic ulcer disease. The development or activation of MTrPs is one of the clinical manifestations of SSS. As mentioned above, a latent MTrP that is located along a sensitized segment (myotome) may become an active MTrP (associated with a spontaneous pain complaint).

Many treatments for myofascial pain, such as physiotherapy and trigger point injection procedures, are directed at the peripheral pain generators, e.g. active MTrPs. Often times, the segmental dysfunction is overlooked and practitioners fail to recognize the presence of SSS. As a result, many individuals may only experience temporary deactivation of MTrPs and pain frequently recurs.

An accurate diagnosis of pain distribution requires identification of the sensitized spinal segment. SSS is determined by findings of allodynia, hyperalgesia and measurable pressure pain sensitivity over the sensory, motor and skeletal areas along with viscera supplied by a particular spinal segment (the dermatome, myotome, sclerotome and viscerotome, respectively). Furthermore, these objective and quantitative findings help clinicians to identify the tissues and likely pain mechanisms involved in their patients' chronic pain. These segmental findings are not only reproducible, but they are often indicative of the severity of the sensitized state and provide important clues to the underlying pathogenesis of the pain syndrome.

The requisite examination skills are easy to learn and are of fundamental importance to the evaluation and management of a chronic pain complaint. Furthermore, their application before and after treatment, aimed at desensitizing the involved spinal segment, provides the clinician and patient with meaningful, objective and reproducible physical findings to guide treatment outcomes.

Imamura et al.[15] systematically evaluated individuals with refractory, disabling pain associated with knee osteoarthritis who were scheduled to undergo total knee replacement. The authors speculated that the pain experienced by these patients may be associated with the presence of central nervous sensitization rather than peripheral inflammation and injury. The presence of hyperalgesia was evaluated, and the impact of pressure pain threshold (PPT) measurements on pain, disability and quality of life was assessed in these patients and compared to age-matched healthy controls. PPT measurements were obtained for the subcutaneous dermatomes of the lower extremities and over the vastus medialis, adductor longus, rectus femoris, vastus lateralis, tibialis anterior, peroneus longus, iliacus, quadratus lumborum, popliteus muscles and the supraspinous ligament. The authors found that the group with knee osteoarthritis

had significantly lower PPT over all evaluated structures versus healthy control subjects. Lower PPT values were correlated with higher pain intensity, higher disability scores and poorer quality of life, except for the role-emotional and general health status. Combined PPT values over the patellar tendon, at the S2 subcutaneous dermatome and at the adductor longus muscle were the best predictors for the visual analogue scale and Western Ontario and McMaster Universities Osteoarthritis Index pain scores. The researchers concluded that patients with knee pain due to osteoarthritis who were scheduled for total knee replacement showed hyperalgesia of nervous system origin that negatively impacted pain, knee functional capacity and most aspects of quality of life.[10]

In order to determine the presence of SSS, patients are asked to identify with one finger the location of their principal pain complaint and indicate the intensity of pain from 1 to 10.

Adjacent dermatomal levels are examined paraspinally by:

- scratching the skin with the sharp edge of a paper clip or Wartenberg pinwheel – this noxious stimulus is applied across dermatomal borders and the patient is instructed to report simultaneously any sharpening or dulling in the sensation of pain during the procedure. An increased painful response is indicative of hyperalgesia
- picking up the skin between the thumb and forefinger and rolling the tissue underneath, also known as a pinch and roll test (figure 10.4) – this non-noxious stimulus is applied across dermatomal borders and the patient is instructed to report simultaneously any sensation of pain. The sensation of pain is indicative of allodynia, a finding that is the most sensitive indicator for the diagnosis of sensitization.

Adjacent myotomal levels are examined by:

- palpating segmentally related musculature for tender spots, taut bands and MTrPs
- applying a pressure algometer to measure local tenderness (PPT) along the myotome.

Adjacent sclerotomal levels are examined by:

- palpating segmentally related tendons (e.g. tendonitis), entheses (e.g. enthesitis), bursae (e.g. bursitis) and ligaments (e.g. supraspinous ligament sprain)
- applying a pressure algometer to measure local tenderness (PPT) along these sclerotomal structures.

(Note: PPT is the minimum pressure that elicits pain and is considered abnormal if it is at least 2 kg/cm^2 lower than a normosensitive control point.)

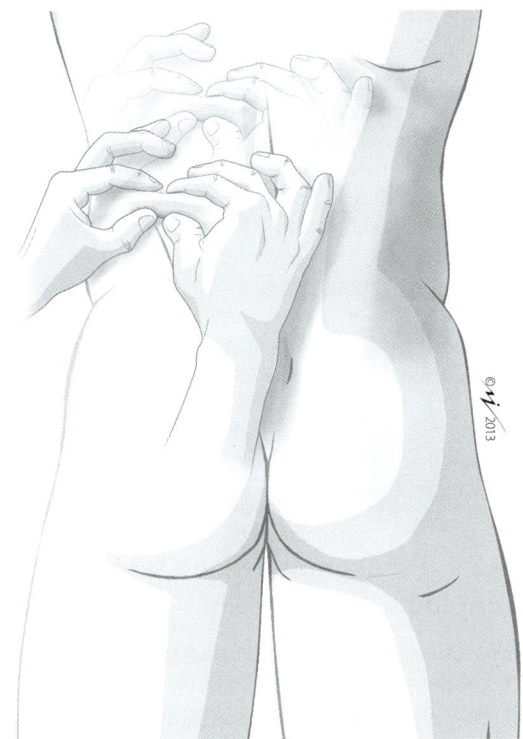

FIGURE 10.4 ■ Pinch and roll test. The skin and subcutaneous tissue are gently pinched between the thumb and forefinger and rolled vertically across dermatomal borders. Elicitation of a painful response is indicative of allodynia. (Colour version of figure is available online).

These examination techniques are used to determine the depth and breadth of the segmental manifestations of an individual's pain syndrome. Dermatomal, myotomal and sclerotomal segmental findings often overlap, making diagnosis and treatment of the sensitized segmental level relatively straightforward. However, in some cases they do not. For example, the affected dermatomal levels may be different from the affected myotomal and/or sclerotomal levels. When such differences arise, the affected segmental levels (whether dermatomal, myotomal or sclerotomal) most closely corresponding to the principal pain complaint should be treated first with paraspinous needling, a technique which addresses the centrally sensitized component of pain.

KEY POINTS

In patients with pain syndrome, dermatomal, myotomal and sclerotomal examination is used in order to determine the depth and breadth of the segmental manifestations.

If the patient experiences little or no pain relief, then the additional segmental levels may be needled paraspinally until the patient reports a decrease in pain. This subjective decrease in pain is typically accompanied by an objective improvement in the segmental findings. However, effective management involves identification and treatment of both the peripheral and central components of sensitization. Accordingly, the clinician should identify and eradicate all foci of nociceptive bombardment (i.e. peripheral sensitization) responsible for initiating and/or perpetuating the centrally sensitized segmental findings. Active MTrPs are a very common source of peripheral nociceptive bombardment which may lead to central sensitization and perpetuation of the pain complaint. If left unresolved, active MTrPs (or other peripheral pain generators) will re-sensitize the dorsal horn, resulting in the re-emergence of segmental findings (allodynia and hyperalgesia) and the reproduction of the same pain complaint even after paraspinous needling treatment.

10.6.1 Limitations of digital palpation

The gold standard for diagnosis for myofascial pain relies on palpation of MTrPs in a taut band of skeletal muscle.[7] However, proper diagnosis requires a skilled and experienced clinician. Some studies have found low interrater reliability among examiners in their attempts to identify MTrPs, an obstacle that can be overcome with standardized training of the examiners.[39–41] Unfortunately, the use of digital palpation does not: (1) provide a reliable and sensitive method of diagnosis and measurement of treatment efficacy; (2) provide quantitative comparisons of the tissue properties before and after treatment; (3) objectively differentiate among active MTrPs, latent MTrPs and palpably normal tissue; (4) objectively discriminate between superficial and deep MTrPs; and (5) permit objective study of the natural history of MTrPs. Thus, there is a need to develop objective, repeatable and reliable diagnostic tests for evaluating MTrPs and determining treatment outcome measures. Such measures can be used to diagnose MTrPs properly and understand their natural progression.

Studies by Sikdar et al.[42] have shown that ultrasound diagnostic imaging techniques can be used to measure MTrPs objectively. On ultrasound, MTrPs appear as focal hypoechoic (darker) areas with a heterogeneous echotexture. They also show reduced vibration amplitude on elastography, indicating a localized area of stiffer tissue compared to surrounding soft tissue. In addition, the use of ultrasound reveals that: (1) MTrPs have a unique vascular environment;

(2) active MTrPs have differences in microcirculation compared to latent MTrPs and normal tissue; and (3) active MTrPs have a significantly larger surface area than latent MTrPs.[8,42]

10.7 DRY NEEDLING AND THE LOCAL TWITCH RESPONSE

Dry needling is one of the effective non-pharmacological interventions used to treat MTrPs. It may be performed using either a superficial or deep dry needling technique. Elicitation of one or more local twitch responses (LTRs) is a goal of dry needling and often benefits those with pain secondary to MTrPs. Dry needling can be performed in any skeletal muscle harbouring MTrPs, including the paraspinal muscles (paraspinous dry needling). Though the mechanism of an LTR is unknown, studies suggest a biochemical component. Five minutes after the induction of a single LTR, Shah et al. found a dramatic change in the biochemical milieu of the upper trapezius muscle. For example, the initially elevated levels of substance P and CGRP within the active MTrP drastically decreased to levels approaching that of normal uninvolved muscle tissue. The reduction of these biochemicals in the local muscle area may be due to a small, localized increase in blood flow and/or nociceptor and mechanistic changes associated with an augmented inflammatory response.[16,17]

Shah et al.[8] also conducted a pilot study in which dry needling was performed on three patients presenting with active MTrPs. Two of these three patients reported a decrease in visual analogue scale with time, indicating less pain. Furthermore, there were improvements in blood flow and a decrease in the MTrP area for all three active cases.[2] Though not designed as treatment interventions, the results of these studies are provocative in that the substances analysed are known to be associated with sensitization, persistent pain and spinal facilitation in addition to findings that dry needling has been associated with symptom improvement and objective changes in the periphery. In an animal model, it appears that dry needling may, in fact, activate the descending inhibitory pain system and cause local deactivation of the MTrP.[43]

10.8 MODALITIES AND MANUAL THERAPIES

Modalities and manual therapies are often clinically effective at deactivating active MTrPs and desensitizing sensitized spinal segments and are commonly employed as a first line of treatment before attempting more invasive therapies. For example, various forms of electrical stimulation, including microcurrent, transcutaneous electrical nerve stimulation, percutaneous electrical nerve stimulation, manual therapies and spray and stretch are commonly used to treat myofascial pain and SSS. However, if pain relief is only partial or if pain persists despite using these modalities, then paraspinous dry needling and injection techniques should be considered. These techniques should be used particularly in chronic cases in which physical examination reveals severe and persistent allodynia and hyperalgesia, suggesting dense dermatomal, myotomal and sclerotomal manifestations of SSS.

10.8.1 Paraspinous block technique with local anaesthetic

Not only can paraspinal muscles be facilitated secondary to MTrPs elsewhere in the body via ventral horn outflow, but they can also act as a primary source of peripheral nociceptive input into the dorsal horn, further sensitizing it. In order to desensitize the paraspinal muscles along a specific segment, Fischer[44] developed a paraspinous block technique which traditionally utilizes a 1% lidocaine injection. A 25-gauge needle, of sufficient length to reach the deep layers up to the vertebral lamina, is inserted in the sagittal plane. Injection is performed between the levels of the spinous processes corresponding to the affected segmental levels of sensitization, as identified on physical examination. The needle is inserted through the paraspinal muscle to a maximal depth but before contacting the vertebral lamina. The needle is aspirated (in order to avoid blood vessels) and then approximately 0.1 mL of anesthetic is injected; the needle is then withdrawn to a subcutaneous level and redirected in the caudal direction, ending about 5 mm from the previous deposit of anaesthetic solution. One continues this procedure, going as far as the needle reaches. The same procedures are then repeated going in the cephalad direction. The result of this technique is multisegmental desensitization, which effectively blocks the medial branch of the posterior primary rami at affected segmental levels.[44]

10.8.2 Paraspinous dry needling and acupuncture techniques

Coincidentally, acupuncture practitioners utilize similar anatomical locations (e.g. traditional

Chinese medicine *Hua Tuo Jia Ji* points), as do clinicians performing the paraspinous block technique. According to the *Acupuncture Energetics* textbook definition, these are a collection of points on either side of the ligament attaching the transverse processes of the vertebral column, from T1 to L5, described as one-half *cun* lateral to the spinous process. These points are needled as deeply as possible into the ligaments lateral to the midline. These local acupuncture points are very useful for axial and peripheral pain problems, and to reinforce the qualities of the back *Shu* points at the same vertebral levels for needle insertion in order to achieve pain relief.[45]

Alternatively, many clinicians have adapted a technique using acupuncture needles and applied to Fischer's model of paraspinous blocks, known as paraspinous dry needling. Instead of a hypodermic syringe used traditionally in Fischer's model, these clinicians insert acupuncture needles sagitally into the paraspinal muscles (figure 10.5). The needle is manipulated by using an up-and-down (i.e. pistoning) action accompanied by clockwise and anticlockwise rotations. Traditionally, the aim of dry needling is to deactivate MTrPs, while the primary aim of paraspinous dry needling is to desensitize the SSS. However, if any active or latent MTrPs are encountered during the process of paraspinous dry needling, they can be easily deactivated and an LTR is often observed.[17]

Multiple acupuncture needles may be similarly inserted and manipulated creating a paraspinous block at each of the affected segmental levels, neuroanatomically corresponding to the principal pain complaint. Furthermore, the segmentally corresponding supraspinous ligaments may be needled using a superficial needle insertion technique accompanied by just a clockwise and anticlockwise rotation of the needle (pistoning of the needle should be avoided). The needles may be left in place for 15–20 minutes (similar to standard practice in acupuncture) while the relevant dermatomes, myotomes and sclerotomes are re-examined to determine whether the treated segments eliminate the objective signs of SSS (i.e. allodynia, hyperalgesia). This result is often accompanied by a significant reduction in pain.

There are several advantages associated with the paraspinous dry needling technique when compared with Fischer's injection technique. First, affected segments may be treated without concern for the possible side effects associated with injection of local anaesthetics. In addition, more segments may be treated in one visit with paraspinous dry needling because the number of injections is limited by the total dosage of anaesthetic that may be administered at one time. Furthermore, acupuncture needles are minimally invasive and better tolerated by patients because they have rounded tips, designed to pass painlessly around cells, blood vessels and other tissues. Conversely, hypodermic needles are bevel-edged and sharp, and are designed to cut through blood vessels (thereby damaging cells and tissues), resulting in more inflammation, bleeding and pain. Due to its fine construction and smaller diameter, an acupuncture needle provides the practitioner with superior kinaesthetic feedback when compared to a hypodermic needle. This permits more accurate manipulation and easier placement of the needle at desired tissue depths.

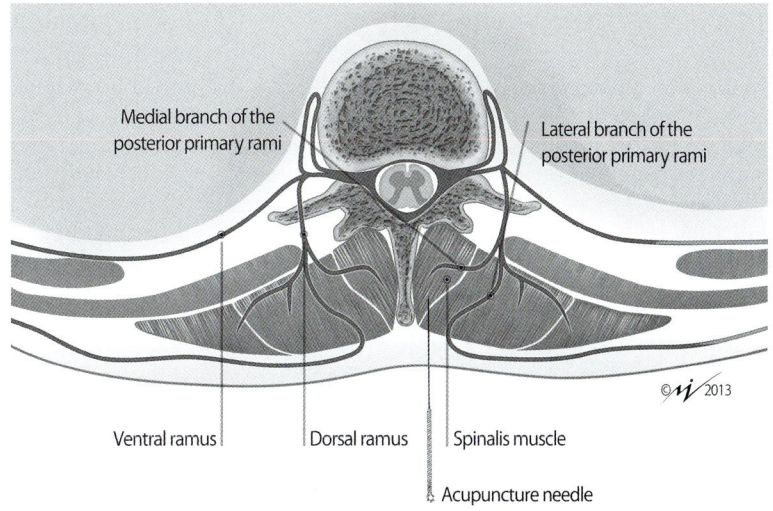

FIGURE 10.5 ■ Paraspinal dry needling. An acupuncture needle is inserted sagittally into the spinalis muscle and then manipulated as described. Multiple acupuncture needles may be inserted to create a paraspinous block at each affected segmental level. (Colour version of figure is available online).

Medial branch of the posterior primary rami

Lateral branch of the posterior primary rami

Ventral ramus

Dorsal ramus

Spinalis muscle

Acupuncture needle

10.8.3 Limitations of paraspinous block and paraspinous dry needling techniques

Though many practitioners can attest to improvement in pain levels as a result of paraspinous block and paraspinous dry needling, these merely arise from clinical observation. To date, there have been no randomized, double-blinded, placebo-controlled clinical trials examining the effects of paraspinous block and paraspinous dry needling. A recent study offers a method that may be used to determine the effectiveness of paraspinous dry needling. Mayoral del Moral[46] designed a study in which patients scheduled for total knee replacement surgery were examined several hours before surgery. They were then randomly assigned to one of two groups: true dry needling or sham dry needling. Upon the induction of general anaesthesia but before surgery began, those assigned to true dry needling of MTrPs were treated by a physiotherapist. Since subjects were unconscious at the time of true or sham treatment, they were unaware of their group assignment. Postsurgery, the true dry needling group reported less pain, demanded significantly less analgesics and rated their visual analogue scale significantly better than the sham needling group.[46] A similar protocol could be used to assess the outcome of paraspinous dry needling systematically and lend support to its use. Knee joint and related muscles are innervated by the L3–L4 segmental levels. Accordingly, it can be speculated that paraspinous dry needling within these segments prior to total knee replacement for osteoarthritis may provide better pain relief than surgery alone and could also be used as an effective and conservative first line of treatment.

10.9 CASE STUDY: TREATMENT

In order to find an effective treatment for Jessica, it was important to make detailed notes of her medical history, including any emotional aspects, and to conduct a thorough physical examination. By doing so, Jessica's osteopathic physician was not only able to organize her complex 50-year medical history into a coherent web of interconnected pain conditions, but was also able to attribute possible explanations as to their origins. Throughout her lifetime, Jessica has experienced knee, pelvic, lower-back, gall bladder, and phantom pain conditions along with patellar tracking dysfunction. All of her pain conditions started after her soccer injury. Her physician concluded that the kick to her right thigh during her soccer injury activated MTrPs in Jessica's vastus medialis and led to her initial knee joint pain. In addition, he determined that the latent MTrPs in Jessica's vastus lateralis muscle aggravated her previously inexplicable patellar tracking dysfunction.

Unbeknownst to her previous clinicians, Jessica's fall initiated noxious input from her vastus medialis muscle, sensitizing the L3–L4 segments. The convergence of somatic and visceral input at the dorsal horn via WDR neurons then created her new onset of pelvic pain despite the absence of any visceral disease or dysfunction. After initially failing to find any physical abnormalities in her knee joint, these clinicians incorrectly concluded that nothing was physically wrong with her and did not find the myofascial component of her pain and dysfunction.

Bombardment of peripheral noxious input into the dorsal horn from her sports injury likely triggered and perpetuated Jessica's back pain condition via several mechanisms, including dorsal root reflexes, neurogenic inflammation, ventral horn outflow and lateral horn outflow. The clinical consequences are increased muscle shortening, pain and tenderness of her paraspinal and quadriceps muscles (corresponding to the L3–L4 segments).

Her active MTrPs were treated with manual therapy and massage, while the latent ones in her vastus lateralis muscle went unaddressed and therefore persisted. At age 35, Jessica developed acute and exquisitely painful cholecystitis for which she underwent a cholecystectomy. Prior to surgery, the sustained noxious input from her cholecystitis was of sufficient intensity and duration to inactivate inhibitory neurons at the segmental level of entry (T6) into the dorsal horn. Fortunately, the gall bladder pain immediately resolved following surgery. However, at the age of 50, nociceptive input from a new minor, but acutely painful, injury to Jessica's lower back (an area unrelated to her sports injury) activated dorsal horn neurons upon reaching the T6 segmental level. As a result, Jessica experienced the same gall bladder pain pattern (phantom pain) as she did before her gall bladder was removed. While Jessica was alarmed by the reoccurrence of her gall bladder pain, her physician explained to her that her gall bladder symptoms likely resulted from the death and/or dysfunction of local inhibitory neurons.

In addition, it is noteworthy to mention that, while there were physical stressors that likely triggered Jessica's condition, she has also faced tremendous emotional stressors and hormonal fluctuations that may have exacerbated her condition. For example, Jessica mentioned that a month after her soccer injury, her father had passed away and that she was stressed about applying to college. At the onset of her gall bladder pain, she was in the midst of a difficult divorce and had begun menopause. The emotional stress and hormonal fluctuations as well as the activation of glial cells could certainly have aggravated Jessica's pain conditions and prevented her from recovering. Theoretically, the emotional and hormonal fluctuations could have sensitized latent MTrPs in her pelvic area and lower back, making them active and painful ones.

Considering all of Jessica's symptoms and dysfunction, what is the best course of treatment? The answer requires a comprehensive history and physical examination in addition to application of the concepts discussed in this chapter. The examination included a comprehensive neuro-musculoskeletal evaluation. First, Jessica's physician examined the affected segments corresponding to the area of pain, including the L3–L4 (pelvic and knee) and T6 segments (gall bladder) for any signs of sensitization. These include dermatomal allodynia, hyperalgesia, sclerotomal tenderness and MTrPs within the involved myotomes. To do so, he used the pinch and roll test and found allodynia in Jessica's L3–L4 and T6 segments. Next, using a Wartenberg pinwheel, the physician found hyperalgesia in Jessica's L3–L4 and T6 segments. The physician then applied a pressure algometer to measure the local tenderness (PPT) along the affected myotomes. He found active MTrPs in Jessica's pelvic area and lower back and latent MTrPs in her vastus lateralis. He explained that the best form of treatment would be dry needling in order to deactivate active and latent MTrPs in the periphery and use paraspinous dry needling to desensitize the spinal segments along her areas of pain. He also recommended that Jessica supplement dry needling treatments with biofeedback therapy, to gain greater awareness of her physiological functions and, as a result of these cognitive-emotional changes, improve in overall health and performance.

After 3 weeks of dry needling (one session per week), Jessica and her physician observed significant improvement in her knee and surrounding muscles. She no longer experienced muscle dysfunction and weakness. Upon palpation of her vastus lateralis, the physician noted that the tightness in her muscle improved and the muscle felt softer. Most notably, Jessica's range of motion around her knee joint improved. Her physician further confirmed this result by once again measuring her Q angle, which was now in the normal range (<17°), with a result of 15°.

After the paraspinous dry needling sessions in the L3–L4 and T6 segments, Jessica's pelvic pain, back pain and phantom pain decreased dramatically and her clinical findings of allodynia and hyperalgesia resolved. When an algometer was once again used to measure tenderness along the affected myotomes, there was a significant increase in PPT, suggesting that the area had become desensitized. The active and latent MTrPs in Jessica's pelvic area and lower back were also treated in order to prevent resensitization of the spinal segments. She was referred to physiotherapy to maintain and improve her range of motion, strength and flexibility. In the months following her treatment, Jessica reported that her mood improved significantly. For the first time in years, she was achieving a full night's rest without waking up in the middle of the night from pain. She was able to re-engage in sports and increase her duration of participation with regained strength. Even years after her treatment, Jessica's improvements were sustained, reinforcing the importance of identifying and treating symptoms and signs of peripheral and central sensitization commonly found in chronic pain.

10.10 CONCLUSION

Current understanding of chronic pain mechanisms, particularly the unique properties of the neuraxis, is changing rapidly as knowledge emerges in molecular and cellular biology. For example, active MTrPs function as dynamic foci of peripheral nociception that can initiate, accentuate and maintain central sensitization and chronic pain states. Continuous nociceptive input from MTrPs can increase excitability of dorsal horn neurons, leading to hyperalgesia and allodynia, and open previously ineffective synaptic connections, resulting in new receptive fields and pain referral.[17] In turn, myofascial pain syndrome may also be a result of a sequence of top-down events via the limbic forebrain and/or hypothalamus, as mentioned earlier.

Although MTrPs are a ubiquitous and underdiagnosed component of many acute and chronic pain complaints, they are also a common physical finding in asymptomatic individuals. This dichotomy challenges pain management practitioners to learn how to palpate the soft tissue carefully in order to distinguish active from latent MTrPs. Making this distinction is critical in order to identify and treat a myofascial component of pain adequately.

Histological, neurophysiological, ultrasound imaging, and somatosensory studies of MTrPs have found objective abnormalities. Novel biochemical sampling techniques demonstrate that active MTrPs have elevated levels of bradykinin, serotonin, substance P, CGRP, noradrenaline,

IL-6, IL-8, TNF-α and IL-1β. Active sites also have a more acidic pH. Together with observed motor and sensory abnormalities, these studies implicate peripheral and central mechanisms in the development of myofascial pain and associated MTrPs. These biochemical findings validate the clinical observation that active MTrPs are a source of nociceptive foci that continuously bombard dorsal horn neurons, leading to central sensitization and SSS.

Dorsal horn neurons may undergo neuroplastic changes as a result of chronic nociception. However, these changes may also occur in higher centres of the brain if pain is left unresolved for an extended period of time. Alterations in cortical areas may help to maintain and amplify the pain state and thereby create a vicious cycle that is increasingly difficult to resolve. At this point, removal of the aetiological factors may be insufficient to relieve pain.[24]

Once the presence of central sensitization has been established in a patient with chronic pain, the central nervous system should be targeted in addition to the musculoskeletal component, which is primarily treated with anti-inflammatory agents. Thorough understanding and identification of central nervous system sensitization have the ability to provide innovative and cost-effective therapeutic tools to control pain, reduce disability and improve quality of life. Comprehensive management should focus on the removal of perpetuating factors (e.g. active MTrPs) through dry needling among other treatments and by addressing SSS early in its development through methods such as electrical modalities, manual therapies, paraspinous dry needling, paraspinous blocks, centrally acting pharmacological agents, biofeedback and behavioural therapy.

SSS offers an important paradigm to explain the nature of neuro-musculoskeletal pain. Though it essentially has the same origin as peripheral sensitization, the central phenomenon is distinguished by its clinical characteristics. The presence of specific dermatomal, myotomal and sclerotomal distribution patterns is an objective, reproducible and reliable hallmark of SSS. Paraspinous dry needling provides physiotherapists and other clinicians with a clinically effective and minimally invasive treatment for neuro-musculoskeletal pain.

There is a need to develop objective, repeatable and reliable diagnostic tests for evaluation and treatment outcome measures for MTrPs. Such measures can be used to diagnose and understand properly the natural history of MTrPs and to determine the underlying mechanisms and relevance to the development and resolution of myofascial pain. They may also be used as outcome measures in treatment trials of various interventions, including manual therapies and electrical modalities.

Further studies should focus on uncovering the nature of MTrPs and surrounding soft tissue over time. For example, although painful MTrPs activate muscle nociceptors that, upon sustained noxious stimulation, initiate peripheral and central sensitization, what is their aetiology and pathophysiology? What is the mechanism by which the pain state begins, evolves and persists? What are the levels of anti-inflammatory substances, analgesic substances and muscle metabolites in the local biochemical milieu of muscle with and without MTrPs? How does a tender nodule progress to a myofascial pain syndrome? Which soft tissues are involved? Are there objective measures for assessing therapeutic outcomes? What is the mechanism by which active MTrPs contribute to SSS? What effects do local and central treatments of MTrPs have on SSS?

Future clinical research studies should focus on identifying the mechanisms responsible for the pathogenesis and pathophysiology of myofascial pain, SSS and neuro-musculoskeletal pain by linking the symptoms and objective physical findings to the physical properties and biochemical changes in the muscle tissue. The development of successful treatment approaches depends upon identifying and targeting the underlying mechanism of pain, not just the signs and symptoms.

10.11 REFERENCES

1. Sessle BJ. Acute and chronic craniofacial pain: brainstem mechanisms of nociceptive transmission and neuroplasticity, and their clinical correlates. Crit Rev Oral Biol Med 2000;11(1):57–91.
2. Arendt-Nielsen L, Graven-Nielsen T. Deep tissue hyperalgesia. J Musculoskelet Pain 2002;10(1/2):97–119.
3. Svensson P, Minoshima S, Beydoun A, et al. Cerebral processing of acute skin and muscle pain in humans. J Neurophysiol 1997;78(1):450–60.
4. XianMin Y, Mense S. Response properties and descending control of rat dorsal horn neurons with deep receptive fields. Neuroscience 1990;39:823–31.
5. Fields HL, Basbaum AI. Central nervous system mechanisms of pain modulation. In: Melzack R, Wall PD, editors. Textbook of Pain. Edinburgh.: Churchill Livingstone; 1999. p. 309–29.
6. Wall PD, Woolf CJ. Muscle but not cutaneous c-afferent input produces prolonged increases in the excitability of the flexion reflex in the rat. J Physiol 1984;356:443–58.
7. Travell JG, Simons DG. Myofascial Pain and Dysfunction: The Trigger Point Manual. VI and VII ed. Baltimore: Williams & Wilkins; 1999.
8. Ballyns JJ, Shah JP, Hammond J, et al. Objective sonographic measures for characterizing myofascial trigger points associated with cervical pain. J Ultrasound Med 2011;30:1331–40.
9. Zieglgänsberger W, Berthele A, Tölle TR. Understanding neuropathic pain. CNS Spectr 2005;10:298–308.

10. Willard F. 'Basic Mechanisms of Pain.' Future Trends in CAM Research. In: Audette JF, Bailey A, editors. Integrative Pain Medicine: The Science and Practice of Complementary and Alternative Medicine in Pain Management. Totowa: Humana Press; 2008.

11. Shah JP, Gilliams EA. Uncovering the biochemical milieu of myofascial trigger points using in-vivo microdialysis: An application of muscle pain concepts to myofascial pain syndrome. J Bodywork Mov Ther 2008; 12(4):371–84.

12. Fischer AA. Functional diagnosis of musculoskeletal pain by quantitative and objective methods. In: Rachlin ES, Rachlin IS, editors. Myofascial pain and Fibromyalgia: Trigger Point Management. St. Louis.: Mosby; 2002. p. 145–73.

13. Waldman SD. Waldman SD, editor. Physical diagnosis of pain: an atlas of signs and symptoms. Philadelphia: Saunders & Elsevier; 2006.

14. Fischer AA, Imamura M. New concepts in the diagnosis and management of musculoskeletal pain. In: Lennard TA, editor. Pain procedures in clinical practice. Philadelphia: Henley & Belfus; 2000. p. 213–29.

15. Imamura M, Imamura ST, Kaziyama HHS, et al. Impact of nervous system hyperalgesia on pain, disability, and quality of life in patients with knee osteoarthritis: A controlled analysis. Arthritis Care Res 2008;59(10): 1424–31.

16. Shah JP, Phillips TM, Danoff JV, et al. An in vivo microanalytical technique for measuring the local biochemical milieu of human skeletal muscle. J Appl Physiol 2005;99: 1977–84.

17. Shah JP, Gilliams EA. Uncovering the biochemical milieu of myofascial trigger points using in-vivo microdialysis: An application of muscle pain concepts to myofascial pain syndrome. J Bodywork Mov Ther 2008;12(4): 371–84.

18. Shah JP, Danoff JV, Desai M, et al. Biochemicals associated with pain and inflammation are elevated in sites near to and remote from active myofascial trigger points. Arch Phys Med Rehabil 2008;89:16–23.

19. Mense S. The pathogenesis of muscle pain. Curr Pain Headache Rep 2003;7:419–25.

20. Camanho LG, Imamura M, Arendt-Nielsen L. Genesis of pain in arthrosis. Revista Brasileira de Ortopedia 2011;46(1):14–17.

21. Hoheisel U, Koch K, Mense S. Functional reorganization in the rat dorsal horn during an experimental myositis. Pain 1994;59:111–18.

22. Ettlin T. Trigger point injection treatment with the 5-HT3 receptor antagonist tropisetron in patients with late whiplast-associated disorder. First results of a multiple case study. Scand J Rheumatol 2004;11(9):49–50.

23. Müller W, Stratz T. Local treatment of tendinopathies and myofascial pain syndromes with the 5-HT3 receptor antagonist tropisetron. Scand J Rheumatol 2004;11(9): 44–8.

24. Sato A. Somatovisceral reflexes. J Manipulative Physiol Ther 1995;18:597–602.

25. Sperry MA, Goshgarian HG. Ultrastructural changes in the rat phrenic nucleus developing within 2 h after cervical spinal cord hemisection. Exp Neurol 1993;120: 233–44.

26. Mense S, Hoheisel U. Central nervous sequelae of local muscle pain. J Musculoskelet Pain 2004;12:101–9.

27. Romero Ventosilla P. Consecuencias clínicas de la Estimulación Sensorial persistente: Sensibilización Espinal Segmentaria. 2010.

28. Sugiura Y, Terui N, Hosoya Y. Difference in distribution of central terminals between visceral and some somatic unmyelinated (C) primary afferent fibers. J Neurophysiol 1989;62:834–40.

29. Wall PD, Bennett DL. Postsynaptic effects of long-range afferents in distant segments caudal to their entry point in the rat spinal cord under the influence of picrotoxin or strychnine. J Neurophysiol 1994;72:2703–13.

30. Watkins LR, Maier SF. Glia: A novel drug discovery target for clinical pain. Nat Rev Drug Discov 2002;2: 973–85.

31. Mense S. How do muscle lesions such as latent and active trigger points influence central nociceptive neurons? J Musculoskelet Pain 2010;18(4):348–53.

32. Hunt SP, Mantyh PW. The molecular dynamics of pain control. Nat Rev Neurosci 2001;2:83–91.

33. Marchand F, Perretti M, McMahon SB. Role of the immune system in chronic pain. Nat Rev Neurosci 2005;6:521–32.

34. Chacur M, Lambertz D, Hoheisel U, et al. Role of spinal microglia in myositis-induced central sensitization: An immunohistochemical and behavioural study in rats. Eur J Pain 2009;13:915–23.

35. Svensson P, Cairns BE, Wang K, et al. Injection of nerve growth factor into human masseter muscle evokes long-lasting allodynia and hyperalgesia. Pain 2003;104: 241–7.

36. Hoheisel U, Unger T, Mense S. Sensitization of rat dorsal horn neurons by NGF-induced subthreshold potentials and low-frequency activation. A study employing intracellular recordings in vivo. Brain Res 2007;1169: 34–43.

37. Graven-Nielsen T, Curatolo M, Mense S. Central sensitization, referred pain and deep tissue hyperalgesia in musculoskeletal pain. In: Proceedings of the 11th World Congress on Pain. IASP Press; 2006.

38. Lucas KR, Rich PA, Polus BI. Muscle activation patterns in the scapular positioning muscles during loaded scapular plane elevation: the effects of latent myofascial trigger points. Clin Biomech (Bristol, Avon) 2010;25(8): 765–70.

39. Njoo KH, Van der Does E. The occurrence and inter-rater reliability of myofascial trigger points in the quadratus lumborum and gluteus medius: a prospective study in non-specific low back pain patients and controls in general practice. Pain 1994;58(3):317–23.

40. Wolfe F, Simons DG, Friction JR, et al. The fibromyalgia and myofascial pain syndromes: a preliminary study of tender points and trigger points in persons with fibromyalgia, myofascial pain syndrome and no disease. J Rheumatol 1992;19:944–51.

41. Gerwin RD, Shannon S, Hong CZ, et al. Interrater reliability in myofascial trigger point examination. Pain 1997;69(1–2):65–73.

42. Sikdar S, Shah JP, Gebreab T, et al. Novel applications of ultrasound technology to visualize and characterize myofascial trigger points (MTrPs) and surrounding soft tissue. Arch Phys Med Rehabil 2009;90:1829–38.

43. Hsieh YL, Chou LW, Joe YS, et al. Spinal cord mechanism involving the remote effects of dry needling on the irritability of myofascial trigger spots in rabbit skeletal muscle. Arch Phys Med Rehabil 2011;92(7): 1098–105.

44. Fischer AA. New injection techniques for treatment of musculoskeletal pain. In: Rachlin ES, Rachlin IS, editors. Myofascial pain and Fibromyalgia: Trigger Point Management. Mosby; 2002. p. 403–19.

45. Njoo KH, Van der Does E. The occurrence and inter-rater reliability of myofascial trigger points in the quadrates lumborum and gluteus medius: a prospective study in non-specific low back pain patients and controls in general practice. Pain 1994;58(3):317–23.

46. Mayoral del Moral O. Dry needling treatments for myofascial trigger points. J Musculoskelet Pain 2010;18(4): 411–16.

PART **V**

PERCUTANEOUS NEEDLE TENOTOMY (PNT)

CHAPTER 11

PERCUTANEOUS NEEDLE TENOTOMY

Todd P. Stitik · Andrew Chang · Milin Vora · John Georgy · Shounuck I. Patel

People, like wine, should improve with age.
TODD P. STITIK

KEYWORDS

percutaneous needle tenotomy (PNT), tendinopathy, ultrasound-guided percutaneous tenotomy.

11.1 INTRODUCTION

Percutaneous needle tenotomy (PNT) is a relatively new technique for treating symptomatic tendon pathology (tendinopathy). The entire topic of tendon dysfunction is rapidly evolving. Historically, pain believed to be of tendon origin was simply and in retrospect, often incorrectly, labelled as 'tendinitis'. Closer investigation led to the finding that most cases of symptomatic tendon dysfunction were not actually secondary to acute inflammation, i.e. tendinitis. Instead, the tendon dysfunction represents a more chronic process during which significant histological changes develop within tendon tissue. The term tendinopathy is now becoming increasingly used to describe pain of tendon origin, particularly for situations in which the pathology has not developed acutely.

Traditional treatments for 'tendinitis' often included measures intended to combat inflammation. These typically consisted of oral anti-inflammatory medications (especially non-steroidal anti-inflammatory drugs [NSAIDs]), ice, rest and corticosteroid injections, which were most commonly performed in a non-image-guided fashion. While patients often had temporary pain relief from this treatment regimen, pain would frequently recur and sometimes become chronic.

With the more recent recognition that true tendinitis was not necessarily involved in many cases of tendon-based pain, other theories about treatment emerged. One of these treatment strategies is known as PNT. Simply defined, PNT involves the insertion of a needle into the tendon in a plane that is parallel to the longitudinal axis of the tendon. Once placed into the tendon, the needle is directed in between the tendon fibres in a repetitive fashion within those areas of the tendon that are pathological (tendinopathic). If underlying cortical bone is also pathological, the technique ideally involves inserting the needle down to this bony attachment such that the needle is used to abrade the underlying bony surface. This technique is probably best performed under real-time image guidance using ultrasound in order to direct the needle reliably into the tendon itself and more specifically into those areas of tendinopathy as well as into areas of underlying cortical irregularity, when present. The exact technique with respect to technical details, tips and advice as well as a review of the literature examining this technique will be presented below.

11.2 TENDONS

11.2.1 Histology

Tendons are composed of 80% collagen and have the highest tensile strength of any tissue in the body. Ultrastructurally, tendons are composed of microfibrils which are grouped together into fibrils and then grouped into bundles and then into fascicles (figure 11.1). The endotenon allows sliding of the tendons whereas the epitenon contains the neurovascular bundle. Some tendons (e.g. Achilles tendon) also have an outer covering, known as a paratenon, which allows for better movement by further minimizing friction. Tendons are generally considered to be less metabolically active compared to other tissues and are thus less responsive to stressors. The nerve supply is mainly sensory and proprioceptive and is particularly concentrated at the musculotendinous junction.

11.2.2 Pathophysiology

Several different terms are used to describe the pathophysiology involving tendons, as summarized in table 11.1.[1,2] Tendinopathy is the general term describing pathological tendons and encompasses both tendinosis and tendinitis. The term tendinosis refers to intratendinous degeneration without inflammation. Aetiologies include ageing, vascular compromise and repetitive trauma. Tendinitis is the term referring to the acute inflammatory disruption of the tendon. Paratenonitis (formerly peritendinitis, tenosynovitis, tenovaginitis) by definition is inflammation of the outer tendon structures more superficial then the epitenon. Of note, paratenonitis can occur with or without tendinosis. While tendinosis can occur with or without pain, paratenonitis usually presents with pain and swelling. The

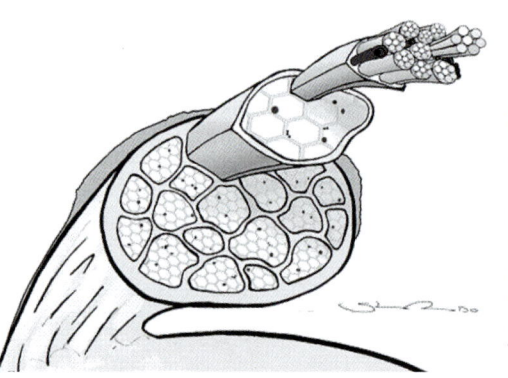

© 2013 Shounuck I. Patel, DO

FIGURE 11.1 ■ Normal tendon.

Term	Description
Tendinopathy	A broad term given to pathological tendons including, but not limited to, both tendinitis (inflammation) and tendinosis (degenerative).
Tendinosis	Chronic accumulation of degenerative processes within the tendon without the presence of inflammation. Although inflammation may be involved with initial injuries, failed or ineffective tendon repair/healing can perpetuate the pain and disability. Pain is not associated with inflammatory mediators, but other irritable biochemical substances such as lactate, glutamate or substance P.
Tendinitis	Inflammation of the tendon following acute tendon injuries causing symptomatic degeneration with vascular disruption and inflammatory repair. Tendinitis can be subdivided based on duration into acute (<2 weeks), subacute (4–6 weeks) and chronic (>6 weeks). There are three recognized histological subgroups: (1) purely inflammatory; (2) inflammatory superimposed on pre-existing degenerative changes; and (3) calcification with tendinosis in chronic conditions.
Paratenonitis (formerly: peritendinitis, tenosynovitis, tenovaginitis)	A term that refers to inflammation of the paratenon (whether synovial-lined or not). The epitenon is surrounded by a connective tissue structure called the paratenon which may or may not be lined by synovial cells. Together, the epitenon and paratenon are referred to as the peritendon.

TABLE 11.1   **Current terminology used in tendon pathology**

lack of pain sometimes associated with tendinosis explains why there can be tendon ruptures without 'advance warning' in the form of pain. This often occurs in areas of relatively low vascularity (e.g. Achilles tendon at 2–6 cm proximal to its insertion).

KEY POINTS

The term tendinosis refers to intratendinous degeneration without inflammation.

Repetitive microtrauma leads to scar tissue formation which is not as mechanically strong as normal tissue. This is an explanation as to why a rupture can occur. Scar tissue can develop with both acute trauma and repetitive overuse. Tendinosis can be thought of as failure of adaptation on the part of the cell matrix to the chronic repetitive load/trauma.

Pathophysiological changes involved with tendinopathy are becoming increasingly understood. Changes include those involving the collagen within tendon fibres when subjected to pathological forces such as repetitive activities or the opposite – i.e. disuse, which causes collagen within tendons to become irregular and uneven as well as inducing formation of dilated veins and capillaries (reducing overall weight, stiffness and tensile strength).[3] Changes within the tendon connective tissue also include the formation of calcification, which is believed to be derived from bleeding within the tendon.[4] Partial tears within the tendon itself can lead to fibrous scar tissue formation. This scar tissue collagen is weaker and less flexible than the original tendon collagen, resulting in increased risk of further damage and increased tendon stiffness.

Inflammatory-type changes (paratenonitis) can also occur within the connective tissue surrounding tendon, known as paratenon, which may or may not be lined with synovial cells. Pathological changes can occur in locations where tendons contact and rub over bony prominences. Clinically paratenonitis presents acutely with oedema and hyperaemia, reflecting the infiltration of inflammatory cells. In this acute stage a fibrinous exudate fills the tendon sheath, manifesting as crepitus on physical examination. Chronically fibroblasts, myofibroblasts and lymphocytes appear, causing new and thickened connective tissue adhesions as well as vascular proliferation.

The cortical bone on to which the tendon inserts can also undergo pathological changes. The underlying bone can remodel according to Wolf's law, which states that bone, in a healthy person, can remodel in order to adapt to stresses to which it is subjected.[5] This can result in the development of underlying cortical irregularity, particularly at points of repetitive stress. Vascular supply to the tendon can be affected. Specifically, neovascularization can occur as the tendon attempts to repair itself. Starting at the initial stages of healing and lasting throughout, angiogenesis and increased vascular permeability occur as a result of inflammatory cell migration and secretion of vasoactive and chemotactic factors (vascular endothelial growth factor and nitric oxide).

These pathological changes within the tendon, paratenon, blood supply to the tendon and underlying bone can be seen to varying degrees with diagnostic ultrasound. The ability to detect these changes is dependent upon factors such as the experience of the ultrasonographer, the depth of the tissue relative to the surface of the body, the frequency of the ultrasound probe, the quality of the ultrasound instrument and its software, the use of special parameters on the ultrasound instrument (e.g. edge artifact enhancement software for visualization of bone) and the quality of the power Doppler on the ultrasound instrument. Furthermore, the ability to detect these pathological changes is also dependent upon the severity of the pathology. Figure 11.2 illustrates typical features of tendinopathy. Figure 11.3 is an ultrasound image in a patient with chronic lateral epicondyle region tendinopathy.

11.2.3 Medication-related tendinopathy

Several medications have been implicated to varying degrees as causative factors for tendinopathy. These medications include fluoroquinolone antibiotics, the statin class of cholesterol-lowering medications, corticosteroids, NSAIDs, oestrogens and retinoids.

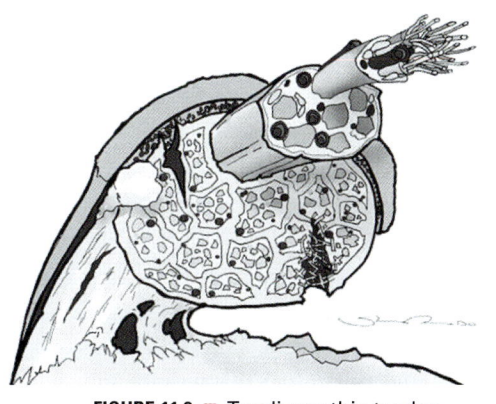

© 2013 Shounuck I. Patel, DO

FIGURE 11.2 ■ Tendinopathic tendon.

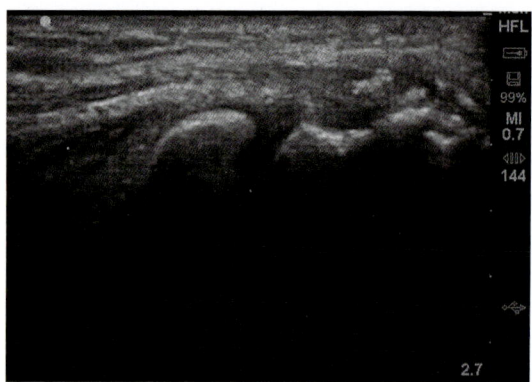

FIGURE 11.3 ■ Ultrasound image of tendinopathic tendon.

11.2.3.1 Fluoroquinolones

In the USA, the most publicized class of medications linked to tendinopathy are the floxacin (fluoroquinolones) class of antibiotics which now carry a black-box warning, as mandated by the Food and Drug Administration. This warning states that fluoroquinolones are associated with an increased risk of tendinitis/tendon rupture and that this risk occurs in all age groups but is further increased in older patients (i.e. greater than 60 years old), patients taking corticosteroids and patients with kidney/heart/lung transplants. Patients can present with symptoms of tendinopathy as early as 2 hours after the dose and as late as 6 months later (approximately 2.4 cases per 1000 patients using fluoroquinolones; 50% of cases present within the first 6 days).

The association between fluoroquinolones and tendinopathy was first reported in 1983 by Bailey et al. from New Zealand,[6] at which time they described patients with severe tendinopathy who had received fluoroquinolones and had a previous kidney transplant. This was followed by multiple case reports and then in 2003 Khaliq and Zhanel[7] published a meta-analysis in which they summarized the results of 98 cases.

Although the exact mechanism of action of fluoroquinolone-induced tendinopathy is unclear, the histological changes in this form of tendinopathy are essentially identical to that found in cases of simple overuse tendinopathy. Williams et al. studied this in a canine population, where they found an increase in matrix degradation and a decrease in matrix synthesis, which decreases the structural integrity of the tendon.[8] In 2000, Shakibaei et al.[9] studied magnesium chelation and its role in stabilizing the structural integrity of tenocytes in rats. Fluoroquinolones are in fact known to chelate cations. Thus a relative magnesium deficiency due to fluoroquinolone-induced chelation has

been suggested. Other studies have looked at fluoroquinolone-induced alterations in matrix metalloproteinase pathways as well as collagenolysis. Sendzik et al.[10] also studied induction of apoptosis as a potential fluoroquinolone-related mechanism for tendinopathy. Finally, other studies have looked at oxidative damage 'door damage', another mechanism which has led to the thought of preventing oxidative damage by giving antioxidants such as vitamin E and coenzyme Q10.

Clinically, fluoroquinolone-induced tendinopathy usually presents as acute pain and swelling, often bilaterally and particularly affecting the Achilles tendon, common wrist extensors, finger flexors and patellar tendon. Fluoroquinolones are a very commonly prescribed class of antibiotics whose use has been also called into question in young athletic patients who perform a lot of repetitive tendon-loading activities.[11] Anecdotally, one of the authors (TPS) recalls his training as a resident in internal medicine and the antibiotic Levaquin® being commonly referred to as 'vitamin L'. To this day, the fluoroquinolones remain the number-one class of antibiotics prescribed for adults in the USA.

11.2.3.2 Statin class of cholesterol-lowering medications

Another medication class strongly implicated in the pathogenesis of tendinopathy is the statin class of cholesterol-lowering medications. Unlike the fluoroquinolones, which appear to have variations with respect to the likelihood of causing tendinopathy, the statin effect on tendinopathy appears to be a class phenomenon, i.e. these medications cause tendinopathy and switching from one agent to another is of no benefit with respect to potentially decreasing the chance of tendinopathy production. As opposed to the fluoroquinolones, statins also do not have a dose-dependent relationship. In a review published in France,[12] 96 cases of statin-induced tendinopathy were analysed. The study concluded that 2–13% of patients exposed to statins develop tendinopathy and that the Achilles tendon was the most commonly affected tendon, followed by the quadriceps tendon, wrist extensors and then biceps brachii tendon. The onset was as soon as 4 hours after the dose to as late as several years after. Bilaterality was described in 41% of patients. Symptom resolution within 1–2 months of discontinuing the statin was typical.

The proposed mechanism of action was that blocking of cholesterol synthesis decreased cholesterol within the tenocyte cell membrane, destabilizing the tenocyte. This ultimately alters the tendon's structural integrity. Statin-induced vascular apoptosis can have a detrimental effect on vascular smooth muscle, which can then lead to apoptosis of the tenocyte. Statins are also believed to reduce the level of regulatory proteins, particularly metalloproteinases. The exact prevalence is unknown: it is felt to be higher than that reported, as most patients have mild to moderate symptoms and thus there may be under-reporting. Males are more commonly affected (2.1:1 ratio), with age of onset most commonly in the 50s. Comorbid illnesses – in particular, diabetes and hyperuricaemia – increase the risk of statin-induced tendinopathy.

KEY POINTS

Fluoroquinolone antibiotics, the statin class of cholesterol-lowering medications, corticosteroids, NSAIDs, oestrogens and retinoids can cause tendinopathy.

11.2.3.3 Corticosteroids

Corticosteroid-induced tendinopathy has also been reported. The mechanism is believed to be due to a decrease in local vascularity induced by the steroid. Most of the studies on corticosteroid-induced tendinopathy have involved the injectable corticosteroids. The issue of tendon rupture as it relates to injectable corticosteroids has been examined in some detail. Because of this potential, alternative treatment techniques such as PNT and EPI® have been developed. Oral steroids have been examined as part of concomitant use with fluoroquinolones. This combination is believed to cause a synergistic effect on tendinopathy. In contrast, there is little evidence that oral steroids when used alone can cause tendinopathy.

11.2.3.4 Non-steroidal anti-inflammatory drugs

There is less evidence that NSAIDs per se can cause tendinopathy. This is a major potential issue as many physicians still treat tendinopathy as though it is tendinitis and therefore prescribe NSAIDs. There is some animal evidence in rat studies[13] which suggests that NSAIDs reduce tendon healing. Specifically, reduced healing of the supraspinatus tendon in rats has been demonstrated as it relates to NSAID use. An inhibition of tendon cell migration and proliferation was found. Ibuprofen is the NSAID that is most highly correlated with the development of tendinopathy.

11.2.3.5 Oestrogens

Oestrogens have also been somewhat implicated in the development of tendinopathy. This is an important issue as oestrogens are now widely used as part of oral contraceptives and oestrogen replacement therapy. The data however are unclear as to whether or not oestrogens are actually deleterious to tendons or in fact protective. Oestrogen playing a protective role in tendinopathy was raised as an issue given the increased rates of tendinopathy in postmenopausal women. In contrast, Holmes et al.[14] in 2006 examined oestrogens as part of oral contraceptives and suggested that these may be a causative factor for tendinopathy development. Oestrogen receptors are found on tenocytes, suggesting that a reduction in collagen synthesis due to oestrogens could be a mechanism for tendinopathy production.

11.2.3.6 Retinoids

Retinoids, a form of vitamin A synthetic derivatives, have been found to produce skeletal changes, including premature closure of the proximal tibial epiphysis, ossification and hyperostosis of the spine and calcification of the anterior and posterior longitudinal ligaments. The first case of tendinopathy due to retinoids was described in 1983.[15,16] The only current data at the time of writing are available in the form of case reports and descriptive case series. Most of the case reports have described enthesopathy.[17] Enthesopathy can develop as soon as 5 weeks after treatment initiation or become symptomatic after many years. No specific risk factors have been identified.

11.3 PERCUTANEOUS NEEDLE TENOTOMY GOALS

Goals of treatment with PNT are really twofold: (1) to reduce pain and any other symptoms; (2) to restore normal tendon architecture. Simply reducing or temporarily eliminating a patient's pain is not adequate with respect to the 'big picture'. Perhaps the main problem with corticosteroid injections for tendinopathy in general is the very temporary pain relief that they often provide. Without treating the underlying pathology directly and addressing any risk factors why the problem to have developed, the symptoms will probably return. PNT attempts to correct directly the underlying pathophysiology, described in detail above. In doing so, it is expected that the tendinopathy-associated pain will eventually cease. For any weakness that may have developed due to the pain, rehabilitation

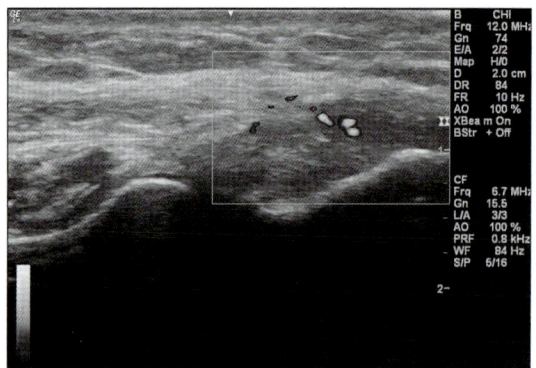

FIGURE 11.4 ■ Increased power Doppler signal at lateral epicondyle tendon insertion.

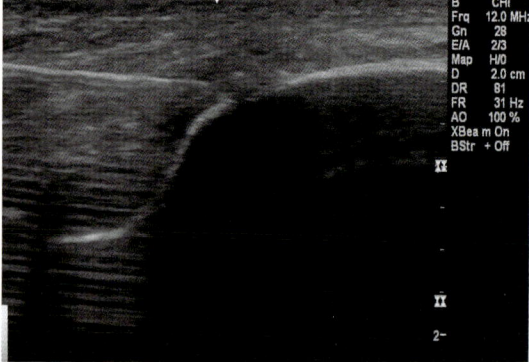

FIGURE 11.5 ■ Percutaneous needle tenotomy procedure: lateral epicondyle.

should be ideally prescribed as an adjunctive measure to correct muscular atrophy. Thus, a combined treatment approach is advocated, in which the symptoms are managed, the underlying pathophysiology is corrected, risk factors for development of the condition in the first place are modified or ideally eliminated, and any strength and/or functional deficits that have developed are corrected. If all of these goals can be accomplished, then one would anticipate that the patient has been cured of the tendinopathy and its sequelae. In contrast, if any of these goals are not met, then the potential for symptomatic recurrence is a reality.

In some circumstances, corticosteroid injections and PNT will need to be combined sequentially. For example, I managed a patient with chronic lateral epicondylosis who suffered an activity-related flare of her lateral epicondyle symptoms. Evaluation under ultrasound using colour power doppler (CPD) signal was consistent with an acute flare of true epicondylitis (figure 11.4). She was managed with a corticosteroid injection in order to 'cool off' her acute lateral epicondylitis. This was followed approximately 6 weeks later by PNT. The CPD signal after the corticosteroid injection at a follow-up visit approximately 1 month later had significantly decreased. Her symptoms had also decreased, but she continued to have chronic low-grade symptomatology that was more consistent with her chronic epicondylosis. PNT was performed in light of her symptoms in the setting of chronic tendinopathy, including a lateral epicondyle spur (figure 11.5). Subsequent follow-up revealed a marked improvement in overall symptoms. This was an example of how an appropriately timed corticosteroid injection with subsequent PNT was used to manage an acute-on-chronic flare of tendinopathy successfully.

A modification of PNT which the senior author (TPS) has coined a 'mini-tenotomy' can

be performed during a local anaesthetic injection targeting a calcification within a tendon. A typical scenario is a patient with a discrete calcification within a tendon. Sonopalpation may suggest that the calcification is painful. In order to help with the diagnosis of symptomatic tendinopathy, a small amount of local anaesthetic can be injected adjacent to the calcification. During the injection procedure the needle can be moved through the tendon containing the calcification in a manner analogous to tenotomy. One given example of this is a patient who had been performing repetitive exercises using a 'total gym' machine. While there were no overt signs of tendinopathy other than the minor calcification, his response to the injection both acutely and over time is indicative of how a focal defect can be quite painful. The decision was made not to inject corticosteroid at his time of presentation in an attempt to see if prolonged relief could be achieved through the lidocaine injection. The patient subsequently reported prolonged pain relief.

11.4 PERCUTANEOUS NEEDLE TENOTOMY TECHNIQUE

11.4.1 Detailed description

Box 11.1 gives a detailed step-by-step description of a typical PNT procedure. This description is used within a patient's procedure note as part of the medical record to document the procedure.

11.5 LITERATURE REVIEW

A limited number of articles have been published in journals both domestically and internationally documenting the safety and effectiveness of PNT using sonographic guidance.

Step-by-step description of a typical percutaneous needle tenotomy procedure

- Written/signed informed consent was obtained after the potential benefits and side effects of the procedure, including tendon rupture, were explained to the patient, and after opportunity for questions was provided

PREPARATION

- The patient was positioned appropriately on the procedure table
- The overlying skin was prepped with 30-second scrub with chlorhexidine and allowed to dry
- The ultrasound probe was sterilized with a PDI wipe and sterile ultrasound gel was applied to the probe
- The procedure needle was bent at the base with bevel down in order to facilitate insertion parallel to tendon fibres (figure 11.6)

PROCEDURE

- During the procedure, local anaesthesia was maintained by intermittently injecting the following solution through the spinal needle: 1% preservative-free lidocaine
- Using direct ultrasound visualization, a 22-gauge spinal needle of appropriate length was guided to the target tendon
- The needle was adjusted accordingly throughout the procedure so that aspiration was negative for blood return
- Tenotomy: 20–30 needle passes were made through the abnormal region of the tendon under ultrasound guidance
- A Band-Aid was placed over the needle entry site

RECOMMENDATIONS

- Patient was advised to avoid icing the area, anti-inflammatory medications and excessively strenuous activities of that body region
- We discussed likelihood of increased postprocedure pain as localized inflammation is induced
- Contact me with any questions/concerns

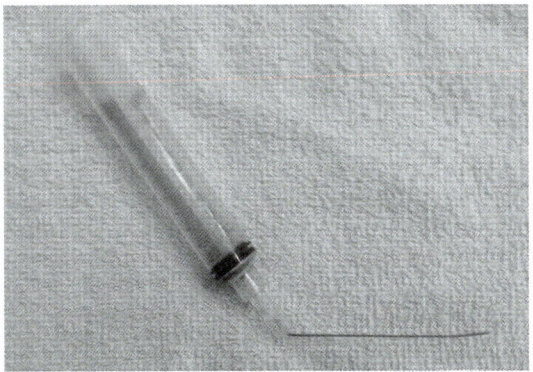

FIGURE 11.6 ■ Needle bent at base for percutaneous needle tenotomy procedure.

In one of the first publications[18] documenting PNT as a procedure, the long-term results of ultrasound-guided percutaneous longitudinal tenotomy of the Achilles tendon were reported. Athletes with unilateral Achilles tendinopathy underwent ultrasound-guided PNT under local anaesthetic infiltration after failure of conservative management. There were 75 subjects in the study, in which 63% of patients were reviewed at least 36 months after the procedure. The recorded outcomes included 35 patients who were rated as excellent, 12 good, 9 fair and 7 poor. Nine of the 16 patients with a fair or poor result underwent a formal exploration of the Achilles tendon 7–12 months after the procedure. The operated tendons remained thickened and the ultrasonographic appearance of operated tendons remained abnormal even 8 years after the operation, without interfering with physical training. Isometric maximal muscle strength and isometric endurance gradually returned to values similar to their contralateral unoperated tendon. The authors concluded that percutaneous longitudinal ultrasound-guided internal tenotomy is simple, can be performed on an outpatient basis, requires minimal follow-up care, does not hinder further surgery if it is unsuccessful and, in their experience, has produced no significant complications. It should be considered in the management of chronic Achilles tendinopathy after failure of conservative management. However, patients should be advised that, if they suffer from diffuse or multinodular tendinopathy or from pantendinopathy, a formal surgical exploration with stripping of the paratenon and multiple longitudinal tenotomies may be preferable.

In a research article by McShane et al.,[19] the authors reported pain relief and improved functionality of the common extensor tendon using PNT. Sonographically guided PNT was given to 58 consecutive patients with persistent pain from tendinosis of the common extensor tendon. All patients with recalcitrant symptoms and who had findings on sonography of tendinopathy were offered the procedure after failing multiple non-surgical treatments. The results showed that 35 (63.6%) of 55 respondents reported excellent outcomes, 16.4% good, 7.3% fair and 12.7% poor. It was concluded that sonographically guided PNT for lateral elbow tendinosis is a safe, effective, and viable alternative for patients in whom all other non-surgical treatments failed. A better way to evaluate outcomes in this study may have been to assess specific functional abilities both before and after the procedure.

The authors published a second study[20] in which they evaluated the efficacy of a corticosteroid injection in conjunction with PNT.

Patients were similarly treated and the results showed that, of the 52 patients who agreed to participate. 30 (57.7%) reported excellent outcomes, 18 (34.6%) good, 1 (1.9%) fair and 3 (5.8%) poor. The authors concluded that sonographically guided PNT for a lateral elbow tendinosis is a safe and effective treatment even without subsequent corticosteroid injections and on the basis of this study they no longer inject corticosteroids when performing PNT.

KEY POINTS

Sonographically guided PNT is a safe and effective treatment for tendinopathy.

A study done at Shanghai Jiao Tong University, China by the Department of Ultrasound Medicine was published[21] which evaluated the efficacy of PNT under sonography in treating lateral epicondylitis ('tennis elbow'). Ultrasound-guided percutaneous needle puncture was performed on 76 patients presenting with persistent elbow pain. Under a local anaesthetic a needle was advanced to the calcification foci, which were mechanically fragmented. This was followed by a local injection of 25 mg prednisone acetate and 1% lidocaine. A visual analogue scale (VAS) was used to evaluate the degree of pain pre-and posttreatment at 1 week and 24 weeks. The results showed that, of the 76 patients, 55% were rated as excellent outcome, 32% good, 11% average and 3% poor. From 3 weeks posttreatment VAS scores were significantly reduced compared with pretreatment scores and continued to decline up to 24 weeks posttreatment. Sonography demonstrated that the calcified lesions disappeared completely in 13% of patients, were reduced in 61% of patients and did not change in 26%. Colour Doppler flow signal used to assess haemodynamic changes showed improvement in most patients. It was concluded that ultrasound-guided percutaneous needle puncture is an effective and minimally invasive treatment of tennis elbow and sonography can be used to identify the puncture location accurately and monitor tendon morphology.

A publication by Housner et al.[22] confirms initial reports showing that PNT without corticosteroid injection is effective for the treatment of tennis elbow. This case series report described the effectiveness of this procedure on various tendons throughout the body. In this report, 14 tendons in 13 patients were identified as having a greater than 6-month history of clinical presentation consistent with tendinopathy that had failed treatment with physical therapy. All the patients were treated with sonography-guided PNT and a local anaesthetic. A VAS pain score measurement was obtained before the procedure and at 4- and 12-week follow-up visits. The 14 tendons in the study included patellar (5), Achilles (4), proximal gluteus medius (1), proximal iliotibial tract (1), proximal hamstring (1), common extensor elbow (1) and proximal rectus femoris (1). The composite VAS score was significantly lower at both 4 weeks (mean ± SEM, 2.4 ± 0.7) and 12 weeks (2.2 ± 0.7) compared with the baseline (5.8 ± 0.6; $P < 0.001$). The results of this study imply that PNT is effective in reducing pain in patients with chronic tendinopathy, without complications.

A 2013 publication by Kanaan et al.[23] reported on a study to determine whether any sonographic features of patellar tendinosis (jumper's knee) can predict the outcome after sonographically guided percutaneous patellar tendon fenestration (tenotomy). A retrospective sonogram interpretation to characterize patellar tendon changes was documented on the basis of length, width, anteroposterior dimension, definition (well-defined or poorly defined) of the focal tendinosis (hypoechoic abnormality), ratio of the abnormal tendon echogenicity to the entire thickness of the tendon measured in the anteroposterior dimension, distance of the focal tendinosis from the patella, patellar cortical irregularity, presence of calcification within the patellar tendon (echogenic foci with possible shadowing) and the presence of increased vascularity. The study included 45 patellar tendons in patients with an average preprocedure functional pain score of 3.6 (range, 2–5), and an average postfenestration pain score of 1.4 (range, 0–5) 4 weeks after the procedure. The authors concluded that the presence of a well-defined area of tendinosis at the patellar tendon correlated significantly with clinical improvement of patients with jumper's knee 4 weeks after songraphically guided patellar tendon fenestration (tenotomy). After the procedure, 76% (34 of 45) showed clinical improvement, 24% (11 of 45) showed no change and 0% (0 of 45) had worse symptoms after 4 weeks. The authors also documented that other sonographic findings, such as increased vascularity, did not correlate with clinical improvement. Some of the limitations to this study include small sample size and selection bias.

In addition to the growing trend of PNT, researchers have tested the efficacy of platelet-rich plasma (PRP) injection in conjunction with PNT. PRP has emerged as a treatment alternative for many musculoskeletal conditions. Although concentrated platelet therapy, which includes PRP, has been used for 20 years, it has been popularized by the media after its positive effects were reported to be responsible for an American professional football player's accelerated return to play and subsequent victory in the 2009 Super Bowl.[24]

PRP injections following PNT, resulting in pain reduction, functional improvement or structural alterations in patients with chronic, recalcitrant tendinopathy were the main finding of the study.[25] Participants were required to have chronic (>3 months) recalcitrant tendinopathy. The design was done in two parts, with part A being a retrospective observational study in which subjects completed a survey obtaining data. Subjects' platelet, haemoglobin and white blood cell concentrations from their whole-blood and PRP samples were also obtained. There were 51 subjects who met the inclusion criteria, of which 41 participated in part A and 34 subjects participated in part B, a prospective observational study. Part B had subjects return to the clinic after PNT and PRP injection for a diagnostic ultrasound, which was compared with their pre-procedure diagnostic ultrasound. The tendinopathy location was in the upper extremity in 10 subjects, the lower extremity in 31 subjects, and had been present for an average of 40 months. Results showed that the mean postprocedure follow-up was 14 months, and the maximum benefits occurred 4 months after the procedure. There were functional and worst-pain improvements of 68% and 58%, respectively, and 83% of patients were satisfied with their outcomes and would recommend the procedure to a friend. Although no tendons demonstrated a normal sonographic appearance after the procedure, 84% of subjects had an improvement in echotexture, 64% had a resolution of intratendinous calcification and 82% had a decrease in intratendinous neovascularity. The authors of the study found ultrasound-guided PNT followed by PRP injection to be safe and effective treatment of chronic, recalcitrant tendinopathy, and this treatment was associated with sonographically apparent improvements in tendon morphology. Some limitations of this study include the intrinsic nature of the design and heterogeneity of treated tendons.

11.6 SUMMARY

Tendinopathy is being increasingly recognized as a major cause of musculoskeletal pain. Risk factors have been identified and the basic science behind the pathophysiology of tendinopathy is being elucidated. The traditional treatment of tendon pathology in general has typically included NSAIDs, ice and rest. Results using this treatment approach for chronic tendinopathy have been largely disappointing, with short-term benefit the typical result. PNT has been shown to be a relatively straightforward outpatient procedure that usually requires minimal follow-up care, does not preclude the performance of subsequent surgery if required, and has produced no significant complications. Literature on ultrasound-guided PNT, although limited, has shown consistent overall beneficial outcomes with respect to effectiveness and safety in the clinical setting. PNT is now being explored in combination with other treatments. For instance, PRP injections in conjunction with PNT have shown significant benefit in the treatment of tendinopathy. Eccentric strengthening is another potentially very useful treatment that warrants study in conjunction with PNT and PRP.

11.7 REFERENCES

1. O'Brien M. Functional anatomy and physiology of tendons. Clin Sports Med 1992;11:505–20.
2. Clancy WG. Tendon trauma and overuse injuries. In: Leadbetter WB, Buckwalter JA, Gordon SL, editors. Sports-Induced Inflammation. Park Ridge, IL: AAOS; 1990.
3. Wang JH. Mechanobiology of tendon. J Biomech 2006; 39(9):1563–82.
4. Codman EA (n.d.). Calcified deposits in the supraspinatus tendon. Calcified Deposits in the Supraspinatus Tendon. Retrieved May 05, 2013, from http://www.shoulderdoc.co.uk/article.asp?article=921.
5. Wolff J. The Law of Bone Remodeling. Berlin: Springer; 1986 (translation of the German 1892 edition).
6. Bailey RR, Kirk JA, Peddie BA. Norfloxacin-induced rheumatic disease. N Z Med J 1983;96(736):590.
7. Khaliq Y, Zhanel GG. Fluoroquinolone-associated tendinopathy: a critical review of the literature. Clin Infect Dis 2003;36(11):1404–10.
8. Williams RJ 3rd, Attia E, Wickiewicz TL, et al. The effect of ciprofloxacin on tendon, paratenon, and capsular fibroblast metabolism. Am J Sports Med 2000;28(3): 364–9.
9. Shakibaei M, Pfister K, Schwabe R, et al. Ultrastructure of Achilles tendons of rats treated with ofloxacin and fed a normal or magnesium-deficient diet. Antimicrob Agents Chemother 2000;44(2):261–6.
10. Sendzik J, Shakibaei M, Schäfer-Korting M, et al. Fluoroquinolones cause changes in extracellular matrix, signalling proteins, metalloproteinases and caspase-3 in cultured human tendon cells. Toxicology 2005;212(1): 24–36.
11. Hall MM, Finnoff JT, Smith J. Musculoskeletal complications of fluoroquinolones: guidelines and precautions for usage in the athletic population. PM R. 2011;3(2): 132–42.
12. Marie I, Delafenêtre H, Massy N, et al. Tendinous disorders attributed to statins: a study on ninety-six spontaneous reports in the period 1990–2005 and review of the literature. Arthritis Rheum 2008;59(3): 367–72.
13. Cohen DB, Kawamura S, Ehteshami JR, et al. Indomethacin and celecoxib impair rotator cuff tendon-to-bone healing. Am J Sports Med 2006;34(3):362–9.

14. Holmes GB, Lin J. Etiologic factors associated with symptomatic achilles tendinopathy. Foot Ankle Int 2006;27:952–9.

15. Brandt JR, Mick TJ. Extraspinal enthesopathy caused by isotretinoin therapy. J Manipulative Physiol Ther 1999;22(6):417–20.

16. Rodriguez-Guzman M, Montero JA, Santesteban E, et al. Tendon-muscle crosstalk controls muscle bellies morphogenesis, which is mediated by cell death and retinoic acid signaling. Dev Biol 2007;302(1):267–80.

17. Stitik TP, Nadler SF, Foye PM, et al. Greater trochanter enthesopathy: an example of 'short course retinoid enthesopathy': a case report. Am J Phys Med Rehabil 1999;78(6):571–6.

18. Testa V, Capasso G, Benazzo F, et al. Management of Achilles tendinopathy by ultrasound-guided percutaneous tenotomy. Med Sci Sports Exerc 2002;34(4):573–80.

19. McShane JM, Nazarian LN, Harwood MI. Sonographically guided percutaneous needle tenotomy for treatment of common extensor tendinosis in the elbow. J Ultrasound Med 2006;25:1281–9.

20. McShane JM, Nazarian LN, Harwood MI. Sonographically guided percutaneous needle tenotomy for treatment of common extensor tendinosis in the elbow. J Ultrasound Med 2006;25(10):1281–9.

21. Zhu J, Hu B, Xing C, et al. Ultrasound-guided, minimally invasive, percutaneous needle puncture treatment for tennis elbow. Adv Ther 2008;25(10):1031–6.

22. Housner JA, Jacobson JA, Misko R. Sonographically guided percutaneous needle tenotomy for the treatment of chronic tendinosis. J Ultrasound Med 2009;28(9): 1187–92.

23. Kanaan Y, Jacobson JA, Jamadar D, et al. Sonographically guided patellar tendon fenestration: prognostic value of preprocedure sonographic findings. J Ultrasound Med 2013;32(5):771–7.

24. Schwarz A. A promising treatment for athletes, in blood. New York Times. 16 Feb. 2009. Web. 6 May 2013.

25. Finnoff JT, Fowler SP, Lai JK, et al. Treatment of chronic tendinopathy with ultrasound-guided needle tenotomy and platelet-rich plasma injection. PM R. 2011;3(10):900–11.

PART **VI**

PERCUTANEOUS NEEDLE ELECTROLYSIS (PNE)

CHAPTER 12

MOLECULAR MECHANISMS OF INTRATISSUE PERCUTANEOUS ELECTROLYSIS (EPI® TECHNIQUE)

**José Manuel Sánchez Ibáñez • Fermín Valera Garrido •
Francisco Minaya Muñoz • Soralla Vallés Martí • José María Estrela Ariguel •
Sergio García Herreros • Patricio Paredes Bruneta •
Diana Marcela Aguirre Rueda • Pilar García Palencia •
Francisco Valderrama Canales • Ferrán Abat González • Fernando Polidori**

*He who can no longer pause to wonder and stand rapt in awe,
is as good as dead; his eyes are closed.*
ALBERT EINSTEIN

CHAPTER OUTLINE

KEYWORDS

Intratissue Percutaneous Electrolysis; galvanic current; invasive physical therapy; liquefaction; basic research.

12.1 INTRODUCTION

12.1.1 Intratissue percutaneous electrolysis (EPI®)

12.1.1.1 Concept

EPI® is an invasive physiotherapy technique consisting of the ultrasound-guided application of a galvanic continuous current (CC) via a puncture needle that acts as a negative electrode (cathode). This provokes an electrochemical reaction in the degenerated region of the tendon[1,2] which consists of a non-thermal electrochemical and local ablation that induces cellular necrosis via an electrolytic reaction produced by the cathode flow (CF). A local inflammatory response is then produced in the soft tissue, thus enabling phagocytosis and repair of the affected tissue.[1]

The galvanic electric current applied onto the body is characterized as being continuous, uninterrupted and of constant intensity. This has primarily two basic effects: electrochemical and electrophysical.

The electrochemical effect of EPI® is based on the use of the cathode as an active electrode. The human body, which is composed of more than 80% water and electrolytes, displays similar behaviour to a solution of sodium chloride with the passage of an electrical current. When an electric current is applied to an electrolytic conductor, such as that formed by all interstitial and bodily fluids, electrolytic dissociation is produced. Liberation of sodium hydroxide ($2NaOH$) is also produced on the negative electrode. This triggers immediate activation of the inflammatory response necessary to re-establish repair of the altered soft tissue and tissue liquefaction with a liberation of hydrogen (H_2).

$$2Na + 2H_2O = 2NaOH + H_2 \text{ (alkaline)}$$

Together with this, the electrophysical effect consists of the migration of the electrically charged molecules (e.g. proteins, lipoproteins) towards one of the poles. The main consequence of this ionic movement is activation of analgesic endogenic mechanisms and vascular responses.

The following definition of EPI® reflects these facts:

- Electrolysis: the flow of a continuously applied electrical current causes sodium chloride and water in our bodily tissues to decompose into their basic chemical elements. These then rapidly regroup and form completely new substances. This process is called electrolysis.
- Percutaneous: this refers to the fact that the application is performed through the skin, using a needle. The needle acts as a passageway for the electrical current, in the same way as the cork electrodes or superficial adhesive electrodes work in other electrotherapy techniques.
- Intratissue: the galvanic electrical current is directed straight on to the affected tissue within the body using a local application

that is supported by musculoskeletal ultrasound (ultrasound-guided applications) or palpation (manual applications). The galvanic current is applied to the inside of the tissue. This is unlike other applications that use this type of electrical current from the surface, such as iontophoresis.

KEY POINTS

EPI® under ultrasound guidance consists of the application of a CC through a puncture needle which acts as a negative electrode (cathode) and which triggers an electrochemical reaction in the degenerated area of the tendon. The main objective of percutaneous electrolysis is to produce electrolytic ablation of the degenerated tissue.[3]

12.1.1.2 History

EPI® is a technique developed by the Spanish physiotherapist José Manuel Sánchez Ibáñez in Barcelona. Since he completed his physiotherapy studies in 1991, his clinical work and line of research have consistently been related to sport injuries. In 1992 his participation as a volunteer physiotherapist at the Barcelona Olympic Games proved a decisive moment, as he witnessed, at first hand, the number of athletes who suffered from chronic tendinopathy. Many were forced to compete while on non-steroidal anti-inflammatory drugs (NSAIDs) treatment or corticosteroid infiltrations. These athletes had tried all types of treatment but their hope for eventually finding a cure was fading fast. Conventional treatments were not sufficiently effective to resolve many lesions, which, due to their clinical and histopathological relevance, were forcing many athletes to retire from competition.

The main problem was how best to treat chronic tendinopathies. It was not until the year 1997 when the first studies on the histopathological causes of tendinopathies were published by authors such as Cook, Jòzsa, Järvinen Davis and Woo (1997), Almekinders (1998), Khan (2000)[4] and Alfredson (2002)[5], whose clear line of research changed the therapeutic approach model in these types of condition. From then on, everything began to fall into place. The chronicity of many tendon lesions was not due to chronic inflammation (tendinitis) but was rather associated with a degenerative process of the tendon (tendinosis). At that point Sánchez Ibáñez understood why many of the 'tendinitis' cases he had seen did not improve after the supposedly correct anti-inflammatory based treatment. This was simply because it was not the appropriate treatment.

In 1998 Sánchez Ibáñez began studying the subject of chronic patellar tendinopathies in depth, covering all areas of knowledge: basic science, clinical symptoms, histopathology, image diagnosis and treatment interventions. Between 1998 and 2000 he dedicated his time almost exclusively to working and developing a new approach for tendinopathies: EPI®. The need to achieve precise localization of the focus of the lesion in tendinopathies, plus the requirements for safety and effectiveness, led to the technique being applied with ultrasound guidance.

From the year 2008, Sánchez-Ibáñez began sharing his knowledge and experience with the rest of the scientific community, and also began training physiotherapists via postgraduate courses. Currently (2015) EPI® training courses are organized by different private and public institutions, universities and professional boards, which are accredited by the Commission of Continued Training of the Health Professions of the National Health System in Spain. Currently, more than 1500 physiotherapists are trained in Spain; the remainder are based in Europe and South America.

12.1.2 Theoretical model of the effect of EPI®

12.1.2.1 Physiotherapy background

At present, the role of physiotherapy in the treatment of tendinopathies is still unclear and, according to scientific evidence, it is impossible to reach any real conclusion regarding its effectiveness.[6] Initial treatment usually includes a programme of rest, ice, electrotherapy, manual therapy, anti-inflammatory drugs or cortisone injections. However, there is not enough scientific evidence on the effectiveness of any of these in the treatment of tendinopathies.[7,8] In the last decade, research has evolved, suggesting novel paths of treatment for tendinopathies, especially in relation to the use of new conservative or non-surgical treatments. Currently, there are a series of medical and physiotherapy interventions that show promising results for the treatment of this condition, although it is still too soon to draw any conclusions.[9]

From the mid-1960s, the level of research has increased, with the aim of assessing the effects of exogenous electric currents on the healing of chronic soft-tissue lesions. In contrast to acute lesions, chronic soft-tissue lesions fail to heal spontaneously within a predictable time frame and frequently fail to respond to conventional treatment.[10] The practice of percutaneous electrostimulation techniques using acupuncture needles in physiotherapy has been around for more than two decades.[11] These techniques are known as percutaneous electrical nerve stimulation, and currently the results are divergent for particular pathological entities.[11–15]

For a long time, it has been known that the application of CC in a solution of salty water produces a chemical reaction: the CC causes the sodium chloride (NaCl) and water (H_2O) to decompose into their basic chemical elements (figure 12.1), which regroup to form completely new substances. This process is called electrolysis.[10] The content of the ground substance, which is rich in electrolytes and water, undergoes an electrochemical reaction with the passing of the CC, and produces a dissociation of the basic elements of H_2O and NaCl. The CC causes the charged ions, Na^+ and Cl^-, to migrate towards the cathode and the anode respectively. At the cathode, the Na^+ ion reacts with the H_2O, forming sodium hydroxide (NaOH) and H^+, whereas at the anode, the Cl^- reacts with H_2O, forming hydrogen chloride (HCl) and OH^-. Therefore, when these therapeutic doses of CC are used in soft tissues, the caustic end-products

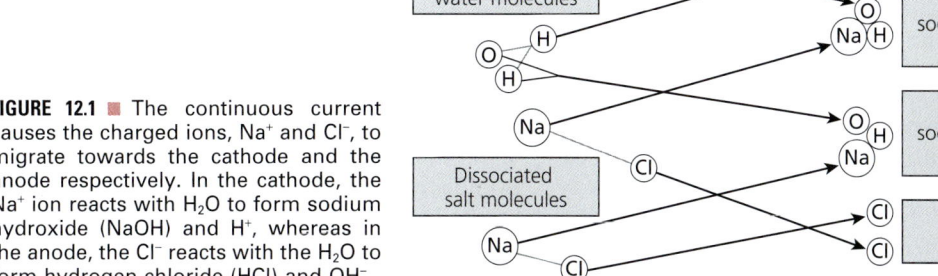

FIGURE 12.1 ■ The continuous current causes the charged ions, Na^+ and Cl^-, to migrate towards the cathode and the anode respectively. In the cathode, the Na^+ ion reacts with H_2O to form sodium hydroxide (NaOH) and H^+, whereas in the anode, the Cl^- reacts with the H_2O to form hydrogen chloride (HCl) and OH^-.

BOX 12.1	The effects of EPI® (cathode needle)

Reduced concentration of H^+ in the intervention area

Modification of pH in the intervention area

Destruction of fibrotic and necrosed tissue

No effect on the needles

Production of electrochemical neurolysis

Activation of the necessary inflammatory response for renovation of degenerated tissue

Softening and relaxation of the tissue. Tissue remodelling is facilitated

Germicide

which are formed in the electrode/tissue interphase can create acid or alkaline pH, depending on whether the cathode or anode is used.[10] If the dose of CC (width of the current in milliamps multiplied by the time in seconds) is allowed to flow within the pathological tendinous tissue, at a specific width and for long enough, the changes in pH in the electrode/degenerated tissue interphase would produce tissue irritation. This irritation is manifested by a liquefying effect (with the material of the myxoid substance passing from the gel state to a sol state, i.e. much more fluid) and an electrochemical reaction secondary to the change of pH. This electrochemical reaction is an effective ablation instrument when performed in the region where the degenerated collagen tissue and myxoid substance are present.[16]

These electrically charged electrolytes are called ions and, as a consequence of ionic instability, the ions generate the formation of sodium hydroxide molecules, which modify pH and cause an increase in PO_2 beneath the active electrode or cathodic needle. This enables phagocytosis and biological activation of the repair/regeneration of the tendon (box 12.1), which is altered due to the chronicity of the degenerative process.[1,17,18]

12.1.2.2 Medical background

Within the various medical specialities there are several scientific studies that have demonstrated that CC is an effective method for the treatment of several types of cancer.[19,20] In particular, for the treatment of tumour tissue a low-frequency CC is used with two or more electrodes placed within or around the tumour. This treatment is characterized by its effectiveness, minimally invasive nature, local action and low cost.[21] Nordenström[20] describes the possible associated

mechanisms of this type of therapy and highlights the change in pH, the electro-osmotic transport of water and the effects on the flow of transmembrane ions as mechanisms that are partially responsible for the effectiveness of this procedure.[22] In a histological study performed on tumours of the liver in pigs, it was observed how, in the tumours treated with electrolytic ablation, necrosis of the cancerous cells occurred, surrounded by an infiltration of lymphocytes. This local inflammatory reaction (after ablative electrolysis) could favour the development of a local and systemic immune response.[3]

The inhibition of tumour growth induced by treatment with CC has been described in other models, which suggests that one of the mechanisms responsible for the antitumoural effects of CC is the generation of reactive types of oxygen, known as chloramines.[23] CCs can destroy the tumour cells via two different mechanisms: apoptosis or necrosis. These mechanisms are associated with the polarity of the current; the cells exposed to anodic flow (AF) are primarily subject to apoptosis, whereas those exposed to CF die almost in their entirety as a consequence of necrosis. These studies attribute cellular death by apoptosis to reactive types of chlorine (Cl^-, Cl_2, $HClO$) that are generated by the AF, and that react with amino acids to produce oxidating apoptosis, inducing molecules called chloramines.[24] Other studies, developed with reactive types of oxygen, have demonstrated that the oxidants, hypochlorous acid and chloramines, induce cell death by apoptosis as a consequence of the reaction between reactive types of chlorine with free amino acids present in the cellular suspension.[25]

In another study[26] the influence of the different amino acids was compared (taurine, arginine, lysine, glutamic acid, glutamine and isoleucine) as regards viability of lymphoma cells in the presence of oxidizing compounds. This study found that, depending on the type of amino acids, cellular death was caused by either necrosis or by apoptosis. In this experimental model, the formation of chloramines, generated by the reaction of hydrogen peroxide (H_2O_2) with glutamine and arginine, would include apoptosis and necrosis, respectively.[26] In fact, in 2005, Veiga et al.[24] confirmed this hypothesis by adding L-glutamine into the electrolytic medium during exposure of the leukaemic cells to the AF generated by the CC. The greatest cytotoxic effect, induced by the chloramines generated by CC stimulation, has been obtained in the presence of the L-tyrosine amino acid.

The main damage to tumoural cells induced by a CC has been linked to the formation of electrolytic byproducts that are capable of killing these cells.[27] However, in these studies, death of the tumoural cells though CC is not only attributed to the effects of the acidification of the pH and the alkalinization induced by the AF and the CF, but also due to the oxidizing compounds produced by the AF. In fact, the acidification or alkalinization of the medium, produced by the action of the AF and the CF respectively, cannot be considered responsible for cell death, as the variations in pH induced by anodic and cathodic reactions are not significant.[24] Furthermore, when pH is artificially mimicked via incorporation of hydrogen chloride, cellular viability does not decrease at an equivalent rate as that detected with exposure of the AF generated by the CC. This suggests that the role of the electrolysis products (figure 12.1), such as chlorine and the reactive types of oxygen, is key in elimination of the tumour.[24]

12.1.3 The use of animal models in research

Several studies point out the need for research on animals in order to understand the pathogenesis and management strategies of chronic tendinopathy.[28] These studies highlight that all the relevant criteria regarding the known characteristics of human tendinopathies at the clinical, functional and histopathological level must be found, if possible, in the animal model. The presence of a valid animal model allows for the performance of detailed studies on the aetiology, molecular mechanisms and possible effects of the treatments available for tendinopathies. This is due to the fact that the animal samples are more homogeneous and easier to control than human beings.

On the other hand, there is controversy regarding the validity of the studies in the animal model, when considering whether a pathogenesis of tendinopathy (similar to that in humans) can be recreated based on animal models.[29]

At present, the reviews on this subject are unclear regarding certain aspects, such as the true pathogenesis of patellar tendinopathy[30]; repeated overload of the tendon seems to have the most solid scientific support regarding its pathogenesis.[31] Other findings, however, offer alternative explanations, such as ageing of the extracellular matrix, oxidative stress, alteration in metabolic turnover of the tendon and degradation of collagen due to the activity of certain enzymes.[30] In a study by Sánchez-Ibáñez et al.,[32] injection of collagenase was chosen to induce patellar tendinopathy in an animal model, and followed the criteria of authors reviewed in the scientific bibliography.[33,34]

In any case, as these are studies performed on animals, it is important to exercise caution when extrapolating the results to humans. For this reason, there is a need for future research based on biopsies of human tendons, molecular microdialysis studies[35] and histological studies in human tendons,[36] which could shape the direction of future studies. In essence, histological studies of the tendon must be performed to gather further information regarding the behaviour of the tendon tissues treated with EPI®. This would enable more detailed analysis of the changes and histological cycles that occur during the repair process.

KEY POINTS

Basic research using animal models is fundamental in order to understand the molecular and histological mechanisms of tendinopathies, as well as for gaining better knowledge of the effectiveness of the EPI® technique.

12.2 MACROSCOPIC STUDIES AND THE MOLECULAR MECHANISMS OF EPI® APPLIED TO THE TENDON

12.2.1 Macroscopic study of the effect of EPI®

Various studies have demonstrated the effects of the galvanic current (which is the basic current used in EPI®) on the healthy tendon[37] and the molecular mechanisms involved in patellar tendinopathies in rats and their recovery via EPI®.[38,39]

Recently, Minaya et al.[40] analysed the immediate effect of EPI® and dry needling (DN) on rat tendon (figure 12.2), in an experimental

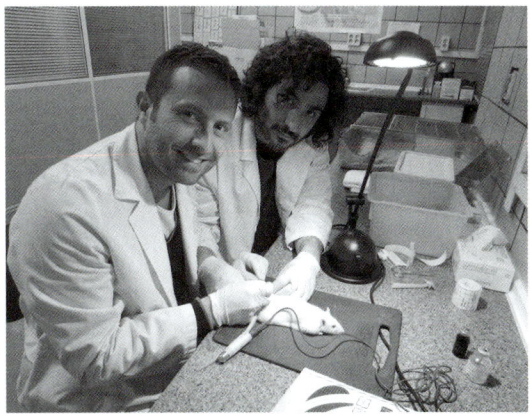

FIGURE 12.2 ■ EPI® and dry needling on the body of the tendon and the tendon-periosteum area of the Achilles tendon of the rat. (Colour version of figure is available online).

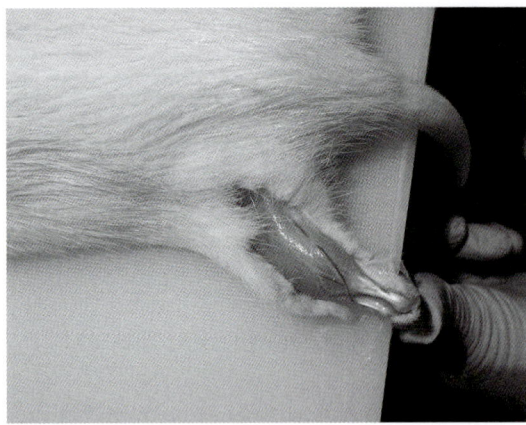

FIGURE 12.3 ■ Macroscopic image of the Achilles tendon of the rat. A haemorrhagic response is observed. (Colour version of figure is available online).

laboratory study with male Sprague–Dawley rats. EPI® was applied on one of the Achilles tendons of the rat and DN was applied on the contralateral side, in order to determine the isolated mechanical effect of DN alone and in combination with an electrical current (EPI®). After the intervention, the animal was immediately sacrificed by asphyxia with CO_2 and a macroscopic study of the tendon was performed. Of the tendons studied, 100% presented a haemorrhagic response and oedema of the tendinous and surrounding tissue, compared with the control (figure 12.3) as a consequence of the mechanical procedures with the needle, whether or not combined with galvanic current (DN as opposed to EPI®), with a greater response observed in the EPI® group.

12.2.2 The healthy tendon

By definition, the electrochemical non-thermal ablation that occurs with the application of EPI® will produce a local inflammatory response in the soft tissue, enabling the onset of the tissue repair process.

In a recent study by Valera et al.,[41] the main aim was to assess the effect of EPI® on the healthy tendon, in relation to possible changes in its structure and immunohistochemical response and in order to corroborate the theoretical local inflammatory response, as well as posterior tissue repair.

12.2.2.1 EPI® produces an acute inflammatory response in the first 72 hours

Initial repair of the tendon included an important inflammatory infiltration (days 1 and 3) in the Achilles tendons treated with EPI® compared to the tendon stimulated with isolated DN (figure 12.4).

12.2.2.2 EPI® triggers an elevated proliferative response

Figure 12.4 shows how, in the Achilles tendons of rats treated with EPI®, a significant increase in cellular proliferation is noticeable. This is due to the infiltration of fibroblasts as well as alteration in the phenotypes of collagen tissue (especially on day 8 poststimulation). Subsequently, the tendon begins a phase of synthesis, during which the deposit of extracellular matrix in tendons treated with EPI® is more mature than in those stimulated via isolated puncture (day 14). This phase was accompanied by a remodelling and maturation phase during which the tensile force of the treated tendons recovered in a similar manner – both those tendons treated with EPI® as well as those treated with needling alone.

KEY POINTS

The EPI® technique causes an acute inflammatory response and a proliferative repair response.

12.2.3 The pathological tendon

The traditional model of 'tendinitis' understood as an inflammatory process is currently in disuse, since several publications have described the pathological process of the tendon mainly as a degenerative process (tendinosis), due to the absence of inflammatory cells and the presence of areas of collagen degeneration, myxoid degeneration and increase in ground substance, combined with a failed process of tendon repair.[35,42,43] However, other experts believe that the degenerative and inflammatory changes are not isolated to the histopathology of the tendon but, rather, these changes commonly coexist with changes in the neighbouring regions.[44]

Considering the scientific publications and the clinical experience to date, it is now known that EPI® produces positive effects in the treatment of tendinopathies.[45–49] The application of EPI®, together with the performance of eccentric exercise, noticeably improves tendinopathy, both in tendon structure as well as in function. Thus, physiotherapy provided at this point could be the most effective type of therapy to resolve this situation. However, despite its positive results, few studies have assessed the molecular

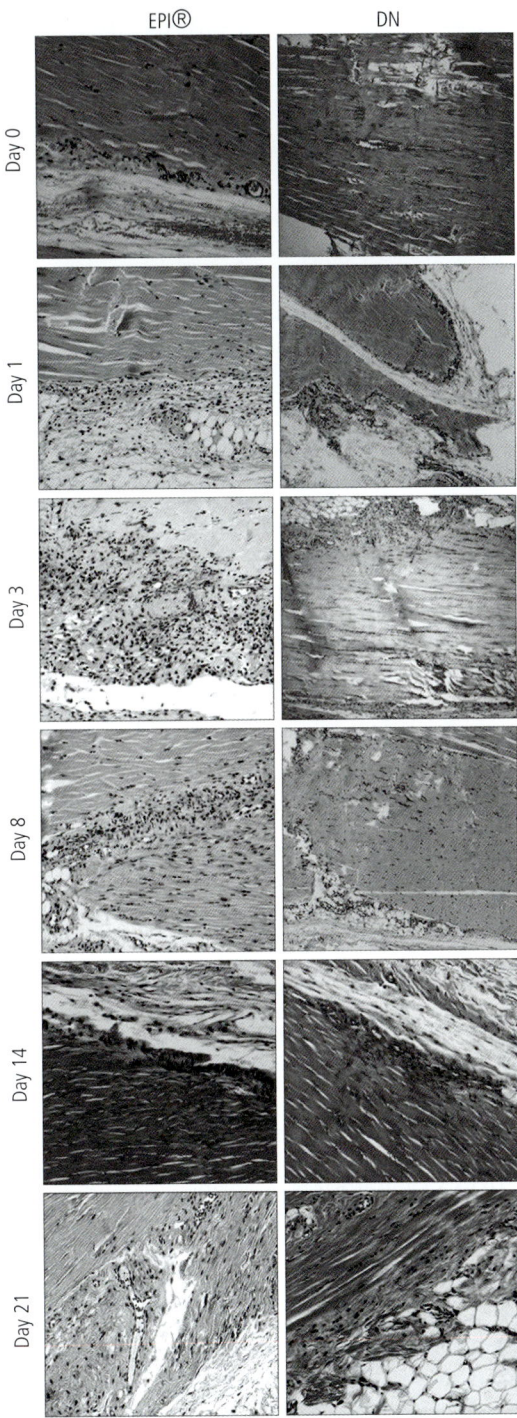

EPI®   DN

Day 0
Day 1
Day 3
Day 8
Day 14
Day 21

FIGURE 12.4 ■ Micrographs illustrating the histological sections of the Achilles tendon of the Sprague–Dawley rat treated with haematoxylin and eosin. DN, dry needling. (Colour version of figure is available online.)

mechanisms with regard to the application of the different physiotherapy techniques or the biological therapies available for the treatment of tendinopathies, and no studies are available on the use of EPI® in humans.

In a recent study by Sánchez-Ibáñez et al.,[32] the main objective was to corroborate the results obtained in humans performing research with female Sprague–Dawley rats to analyse the molecular mechanisms underlying the recovery of the tendinopathies and the use of EPI® technology. The hypothesis of the mechanism of action of EPI® is based on the inflammatory effects and oxidative stress which accompany the tendinopathies and which may also be the recovery mechanism. A working hypothesis suggested that EPI® may have a repairing effect on the damage induced by collagenase in the patellar tendon of the rat. For this purpose, collagenase type I was injected into the patellar tendon of the rat and, 3 days later, it was treated with EPI® in order to analyse recovery of the tendinopathy. One week later, the animals were sacrificed and the tendons were extracted for their subsequent use in electrophoretic techniques and for immunodetection.

In order to achieve the general goal, different and specific objectives were established:

- to determine the effect of the collagenase on the patellar tendon of the rat
- to determine the effect of the collagenase on cellular oxidative stress
- to determine the effect of the collagenase at the level of proinflammatory and anti-inflammatory proteins
- to determine the effect of EPI® on cellular oxidative stress after the application of collagenase
- to determine the effect of EPI® and the level of proinflammatory and anti-inflammatory proteins after the application of collagenase.

Seven days later (collagenase causes a tendinopathy that becomes chronic in the rat at the 7th day posttreatment), EPI® was administered to the predetermined group of rats. Two EPI® interventions were performed (figure 12.5) with different doses at the level of the proximal insertion of the patellar tendon.

It was also confirmed that EPI® increases cytochrome C in the patellar tendon of rats. Figure 12.6 shows how, in the patellar tendons of rats that were injected with collagenase type I for 3 days and treated with EPI® at 3–6 mA for 4 seconds, an increase in cytochrome C occurred, which was greater in the 6 mA group.

12.2.3.1 EPI® increases the expression of Smac/DIABLO proteins in the patellar tendon of rats

The underlying mechanisms responsible for the effect of collagenase-EPI® have been researched

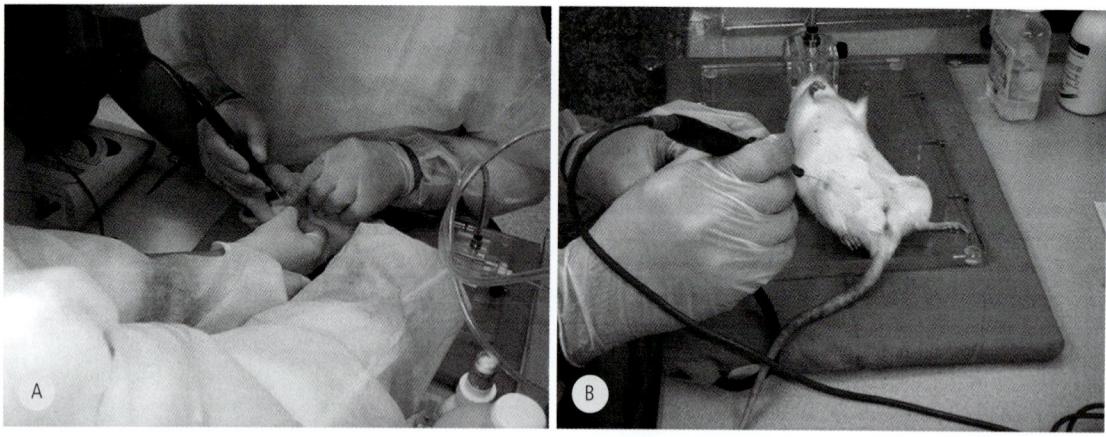

FIGURE 12.5 ■ EPI® (3 mA or 6 mA) applied on the patellar tendon of the rat. (A) Identification of the area to be treated. (B) Application of EPI®. (Colour version of figure is available online).

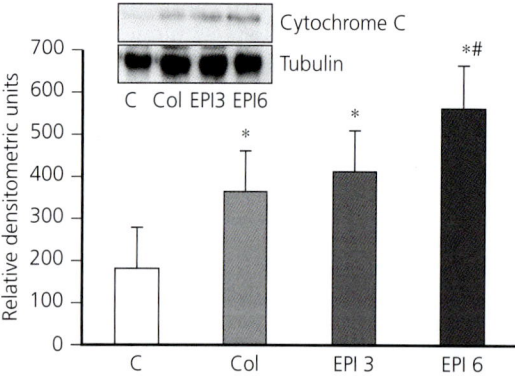

FIGURE 12.6 ■ EPI® 3, EPI® 6 and collagenase increase the expression of cytochrome C in the patellar tendon of the rat. A representative immunoblot is shown above the histogram. The histogram represents the average ± SD. *$p < 0.05$ compared to control cells; #$p < 0.05$ compared to collagenase cells. C, control; Col, collagenase.

FIGURE 12.7 ■ EPI® 3, EPI® 6 and collagenase increase the expression of the Smac/DIABLO protein in the rat patellar tendon. A representative immunoblot is displayed above the histogram. The histogram quantifies the average ± SD. *$p < 0.05$ compared to control cells; #$p < 0.05$ compared to collagenase cells.

and it has been evaluated whether this technique could produce alterations in the induced apoptosis process due to the activity of the Smac/DIABLO protein. Figure 12.7 displays a significant increase in expression of Smac/DIABLO after treatment with EPI, when compared to the control and to rats treated with collagenase. In the rats with collagenase an increase in proteins was observed compared with the tendons of the control rats, but this occurred at a lower level than in those treated with EPI®. This indicates the existence of a relation between the alteration of homeostasis of the cholesterol and the activation of apoptosis via the Smac/DIABLO process.

On the other hand, the bibliography[50] suggests that the apoptosis associated with cytochrome C and Smac/DIABLO, and that associated with liberation of the mitochondria, responds to different mechanisms. Smac/DIABLO apoptosis is performed through induction of caspase, which is exported from the mitochondria to the cellular cytosol and is produced as a consequence of cytotoxic drugs and damage to the DNA, as well as from its union with the death receptor, CD95. For this reason, the induction of apoptosis during treatment with EPI® has to be made via the caspase route.

12.2.3.2 EPI® increases the expression of VEGF proteins in rat tendons

Figure 12.8 displays a significant increase in vascular endothelial growth factor (VEGF) in the patellar tendon treated with collagenase type I and with EPI®. It is not possible to establish statistically significant differences between collagenase and EPI®. On the other hand,

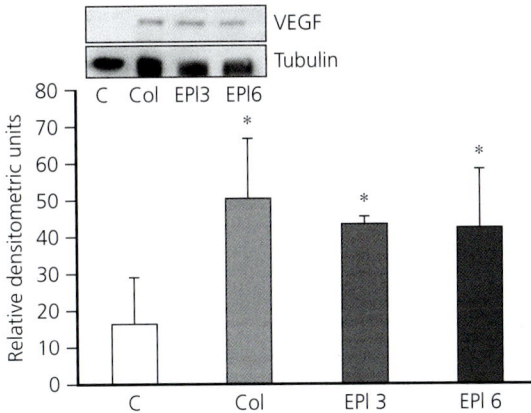

FIGURE 12.8 ■ EPI® 3, EPI® 6 and collagenase increase the expression of vascular endothelial growth factor (VEGF) in the patellar tendon of the rat. A representative immunoblot is displayed above the histogram. The histogram quantifies the average ± SD. *$p < 0.05$ compared to control cells.

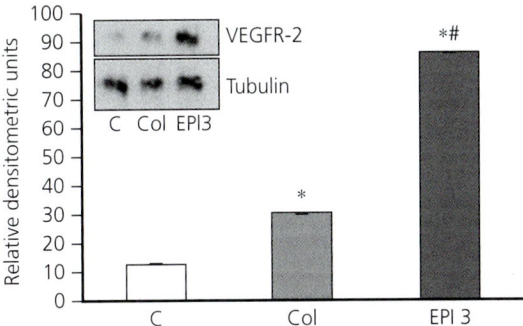

FIGURE 12.9 ■ EPI® 3 and collagenase increase the expression of vascular endothelial growth factor receptor-2 (VEGFR-2) expression in the patellar tendon of the rat. A representative immunoblot is displayed above the histogram. The histogram quantifies the average ± SD. *$p < 0.05$ compared to control cells; #$p < 0.05$ compared to collagenase cells.

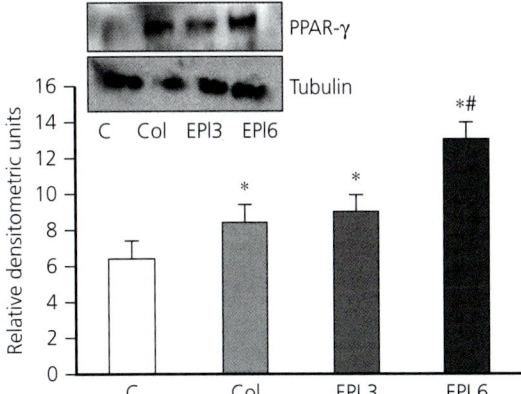

FIGURE 12.10 ■ EPI® 3, EPI® 6 and collagenase increase the expression of the peroxisome proliferator-activated receptor-γ (PPAR-γ)protein in the patellar tendon of the rat. A representative immunoblot is displayed above the histogram. The histogram quantifies the average ± SD. *$p < 0.05$ compared to control cells; #$p < 0.05$ compared to collagenase cells. C, control; Col, collagenase.

an increase in expression of protein of VEGF type 2 receptor (VEGFR-2) has been demonstrated (figure 12.9), thus demonstrating the existence of a process different to that of cellular apoptosis.

12.2.3.3 EPI® increases the expression of the PPAR-gamma protein in the patellar tendons of the rat

Figure 12.10 indicates a significant increase in the peroxisome proliferator-activated receptor-γ (PPAR-γ) protein in the patellar tendon treated with EPI® compared to the patellar tendons of rats treated with collagenase. As an anti-inflammatory protein, PPAR-γ is induced after treatment with EPI®; this is something that

does not occur after damage with collagenase. This demonstrates a recovery mechanism that occurs after treatment with EPI® in which activation of PPAR-γ takes place.

The activation of PPAR-γ and the increase in expression of VEGF and VEGFR-2 demonstrate an increase in anti-inflammatory and angiogenic mechanisms.[51,52] The inflammatory and oxidative stress mechanisms begin after the damage caused by the collagenase and produce an increase in cell death and the angiogenesis.

KEY POINTS

Considering the *in vivo* findings related to the use of EPI®, one can establish that, after treatment with EPI®, an increase in the apoptotic Smac/DIABLO pathway takes place, together with an induction of VEGF via VEGFR-2.

12.3 MOLECULAR MECHANISMS OF EPI® IN THE MUSCLE

Injuries affecting the soft tissues are recurrent in sports, whether produced by traumatic events or due to tissue overload from exceeding the response capacity of the tissues involved in the movement. Within the multiple types of sports lesions, special importance is given to those affecting the musculoskeletal system, particularly muscle tissue. This is because approximately 30% of injuries suffered by athletes involve the muscles.[8] When these injuries affect

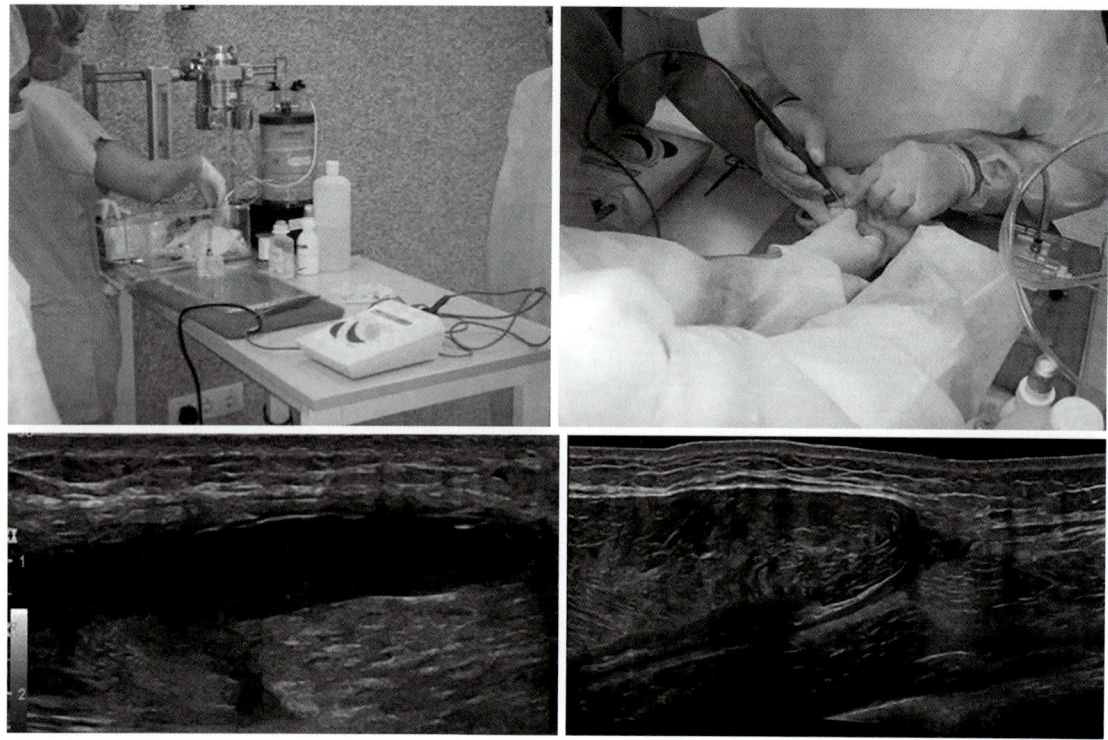

FIGURE 12.11 ■ Anaesthesia and handling of rats prior to EPI® in a lesion induced with notexin in the rectus femoris muscle. (Colour version of figure is available online).

professional athletes, due to their numerous social and economic implications, it is important to provide a reliable and precise prognosis of the length of time the person will be unable to take part in sports. Return to competition too soon could cause a relapse and worsening of the lesion; however, therapy that is too conservative conflicts with economic and sports interests.

In chapter 14 other characteristics related to the physiopathology of muscular injury, the resolution process and fibrosis are explained.

12.3.1 EPI® in regeneration of the muscle lesion

The application of EPI® in the soft tissue in general, and in the muscle lesion in particular, is a treatment technique that can be performed concurrently with other techniques. Considering the variability in anatomical localization of muscle lesions, and the variability in tissue dimensions between patients, the effectiveness and safety of the application are greater if the procedure is performed with ultrasound guidance in real time, as this allows the needle to be introduced directly into the lesional area. Currently, due to its recent incorporation into the

clinical practice of the physiotherapist, there is no research regarding the effects of the application of this treatment on muscle tissue.[19]

In a recent study by Sánchez-Ibáñez et al.[53] performed with female Sprague–Dawley rats, the main objective was to analyse the molecular mechanisms underlying recovery of muscular injuries and the application of EPI®. For this purpose, notexin was injected (figure 12.11) in the rectus femoris muscle and, 7 days later, treatment with EPI® ensued. Twenty-one days after the lesion and prior to sacrifice of the experimental animals, an ultrasound examination was performed on all rats involving both extremities with the purpose of assessing both the evolution of the lesion and the treatment applied through image analysis. The muscle tissue of the treatment area was extracted in all rats, both lesioned and control, and the samples were analysed using an electrophoretic and immunodetection technique in order to identify the metabolic mediators of the inflammatory process and determine whether treatment with EPI® generates changes with regard to the induced lesion and the control group. In addition, blood was extracted from the rats in each group in order to evaluate the presence of cytokines. A plasma control group was used to avoid the systemic effect of the induced injury influencing the control levels.

12.3.2 EPI® stimulates recovery of liberation of TNF-α to basal levels

A significant difference was observed in the concentration of tumour necrosis factor-α (TNF-α) between the group treated with notexin+ EPI® and the group treated only with notexin. On the other hand, the application of the EPI® to induced muscular lesions elicits recovery of the liberation of TNF-α to basal levels (figure 12.12) and, therefore, to normal conditions.

This finding is believed to be indicative of a possible regeneration process that is reinforced by EPI®.

Figure 12.13 shows a significant decrease in the concentration of interleukin-1β in the

notexin + EPI® group when compared to the notexin group. The application of EPI® and notexin to the injured muscle produces a decrease in concentration of interleukin-1β in plasma compared to the notexin group.

12.3.3 EPI® applied after muscle lesion increases the expression of VEGF

The application of EPI® elicited a significant increase in the protein expression of VEGF compared to the control group. Application of EPI® to the induced muscular lesion increased expression of VEGF, with no significant differences found between this group and the group of only notexin and/or only EPI® (figure 12.14).

12.3.4 EPI® increases expression of VEGF type 1 receptor after muscular lesion

The application of EPI® induced a significant increase in the type 1 receptor of the VEGFR-1 (figure 12.15), indicating that EPI® could be influencing the elimination of the receptor and/or its transcription. It is important to highlight that the application of EPI® with notexin 7 days after the lesion produced a highly significant increase in VEGFR-1 compared to the control group and that subsequently, an increase compared to the notexin group was observed.

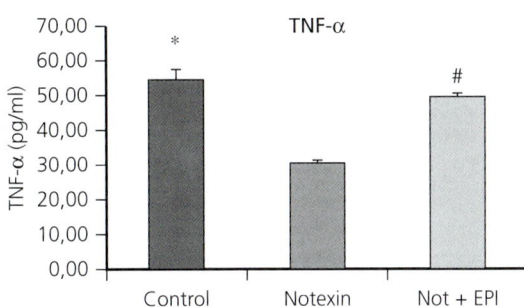

FIGURE 12.12 ▪ Levels of tumour necrosis factor-α (TNF-α) in pg/mL at 21 days post induced lesion. The application of notexin + EPI® does not reduce the levels of TNF-α. The histograms represent quantifications of the concentration of TNF-α in plasma of $n = 6$ for each group (average, SD). *$p \leq 0.05$ compared to control cells; #$p \leq 0.05$ compared to notexin using a one-way analysis of variance test.

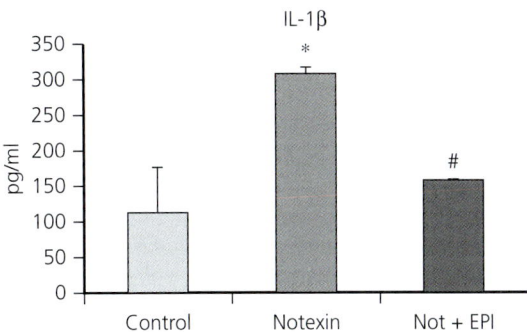

FIGURE 12.13 ▪ Levels of interleukin-1β (IL-1β) in pg/mL (enzyme-linked immunosorbent assay) at 21 days after the induced lesion in the different groups. The histogram quantifies the concentration of IL-1β in plasma for $n = 6$ in each group (average, SD). *$p \leq 0.05$ for the differences compared to the control and #$p \leq 0.05$ compared to notexin using a one-way analysis of variance test.

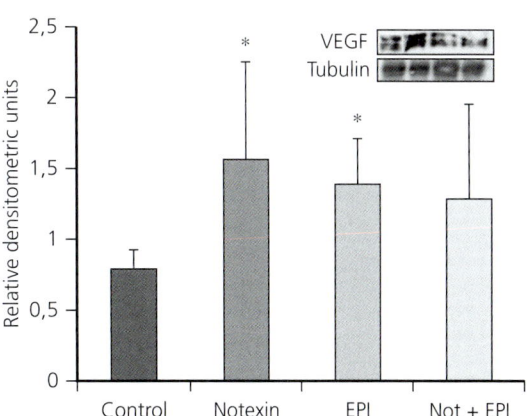

FIGURE 12.14 ▪ Expression of vascular endothelial growth factor (VEGF) in densitometric units relative to the muscle of the rat 21 days after inducing a muscular lesion. The histogram quantifies the concentration of the expression of VEGF. *$p \leq 0.05$ for differences compared to control using a one-way analysis of variance test.

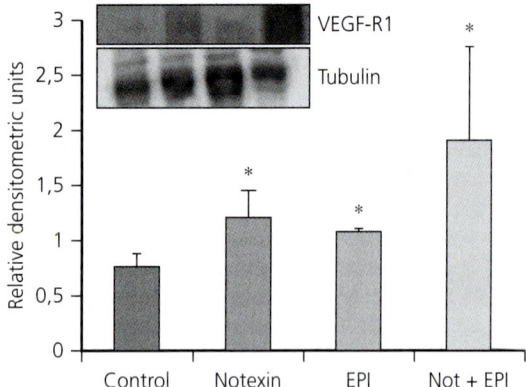

FIGURE 12.15 ■ Expression of vascular endothelial growth factor receptor-1 (VEGFR-1) in densitometric units relative to the muscle of the rat 21 days after the induced muscle lesion. The application of EPI® increases the expression of VEGFR-1 in the muscle. The histogram represents the quantification of the concentration of the protein expression of VEGF in the muscular tissue of the different groups (average, SD) *$p \leq 0.05$ for the differences compared to control using a one-way analysis of variance test.

KEY POINTS

The application of EPI® in the muscle of the rat previously injured with notexin caused a reduction in the amount of fibrosis and calcification nuclei and extension of the induced lesion, as well as a significant increase in plasma TNF-α, VEGF and VEGFR-1. There was also a decrease in the levels of IL-1β in plasma and a reduction of the effects of the inflammatory process on the muscle tissue with the induced lesion, which positively influenced neovascularization of the injured site.

12.4 REFERENCES

1. Sánchez-Ibáñez JM. Fisiopatología de la regeneración de los tejidos blandos. In: Vilar E, Sureda S, editors. Fisioterapia del aparato locomotor. Madrid: Mc Graw Hill; 2005.
2. Sánchez-Ibáñez JM, García-Herreros S, Aguirre-Rueda D, et al. Molecular mechanisms induced by patellar tendinopathy in rats: protection by percutaneous electrolysis intra-tissue (EPI®). In: XXI International conference on sport rehabilitation and traumatology. Football medicine strategies for Knee injuries. London: 2012.
3. Hinz S, Egberts JH, Pauser U, et al. Electrolytic ablation is as effective as radiofrequency ablation in the treatment of artificial liver metastases in a pig model. J Surg Oncol 2008;98(2):135–8.
4. Khan KM, Cook JL, Taunton JE, et al. Overuse tendinosis, not tendinitis part 1: a new paradigm for a difficult clinical problem. Phys Sportsmed 2000;28:38–48.
5. Alfredson H, Lorentzon R. Chronic tendon pain: no signs of chemical inflammation but high concentrations of the neurotransmitter glutamate. Implications for treatment? Curr Drug Targets 2002;3(1):43–54. Review.
6. Maffulli N, Longo UG. Conservative management for tendinopathy: is there enough scientific evidence? Rheumatology (Oxford) 2008;47(4):390–1.
7. Fredberg U, Bolvig L. Jumper's knee. Review of the literature. Scand J Med Sci Sports 1999;9(2):66–73.
8. Peers KH, Lysens RJ. Patellar tendinopathy in athletes: current diagnostic and therapeutic recommendations. Sports Med 2005;35:71–87.
9. Rees JD, Maffulli N, Cook J. Management of tendinopathy. Am J Sports Med 2009;37:1855–67.
10. Zhao M. Electrical fields in wound healing. An overriding signal that directs cell migration. Semin Cell Dev Biol 2009;20(6):674–82.
11. Proctor ML, Smith CA, Farquhar CM, et al. Transcutaneous electrical nerve stimulation and acupuncture for primary dysmenorrhoea. Cochrane Database Syst Rev 2002;1:CD002123.
12. Ahmed HE, Craig WF, White PF, et al. Percutaneous electrical nerve stimulation (PENS): a complementary therapy for the management of pain secondary to bony metastasis. Clin J Pain 1998;14(4):320–3.
13. Ghoname ES, Craig WF, White PF, et al. The effect of stimulus frequency on the analgesic response to percutaneous electrical nerve stimulation in patients with chronic low back pain. Anesth Analg 1999;88(4):841–6.
14. Hamza MA, Ghoname EA, White PF, et al. Effect of the duration of electrical stimulation on the analgesic response in patients with low back pain. Anesthesiology 1999;91(6):1622–7.
15. Yokoyama M, Sun X, Oku S, et al. Comparison of percutaneous electrical nerve stimulation with transcutaneous electrical nerve stimulation for long-term pain relief in patients with chronic low back pain. Anesth Analg 2004;98(6):1552–6.
16. Assimacopoulos D. Low intensity negative electric current in treatment of ulcers of leg due to chronic venous insufficiency: preliminary report of three cases. Am J Surg 1968;115:683–7.
17. Danielson P, Alfredson H, Forsgren S. Distribution of general (PGP 9.5) and sensory (substance P/CGRP) innervations in the human patellar tendon. Knee Surg Sports Traumatol Arthrosc 2006;14(2):125–32.
18. Alfredson H, Cook J. A treatment algorithm for managing Achilles tendinopathy: new treatment options. Br J Sports Med 2007;41:211–16.
19. Miklavcic D, An D, Belehradek J Jr, et al. Host's immune response in electrotherapy of murine tumors by direct current. Eur Cytokine Netw 1997;8(3):275–9.
20. Ciria HC, Quevedo MS, Cabrales LB, et al. Antitumor effectiveness of different amounts of electrical charge in Ehrlich and fibrosarcoma Sa-37 tumors. BMC Cancer 2004;4:87.
21. Nordenström BE. Biologically closed electric circuits: activation of vascular interstitial closed electric circuits for treatment of inoperable cancers. Bioelectromagnetics 1984;3:137–53.
22. Nordenström BE, Eksborg S, Beving H. Electrochemical treatment of cancer. II: effect of electrophoretic influence on Adriamycin. Am J Clin Oncol 1990;13(1):75–88.
23. De Campos VE, Teixeira CA, da Veiga VF, et al. L-tyrosine-loaded nanoparticles increase the antitumoral activity of direct electricurrent in a metastatic melanoma cell model. Int J Nanomedicine 2010;5:961–71.
24. Veiga VF, Nimrichter L, Teixeira CA, et al. Exposure of human leukemic cells to direct electric current: generation of toxic compounds inducing cell death by different mechanisms. Cell Biochem Biophys 2005;42(1):61–74.
25. Englert RP, Shacter E. Distinct modes of cell death induced by different reactive oxygen species: amino acyl

chloramines mediate hypochlorous acid-induced apoptosis. J Biol Chem 2002;277(23):20518–26.

26. Wagner BA, Britigan BE, Reszka KJ, et al. Hydrogen peroxide-induced apoptosis of HL-60 human leukemia cells is mediated by the oxidants hypochlorous acid and chloramines. Arch Biochem Biophys 2002;401(2):223–34.

27. Nilsson E, von Euler H, Berendson J, et al. Electrochemical treatment of tumours. Bioelectrochemistry 2000;51(1):1–11.

28. Longo UG, Forriol F, Campi S, et al. Animal models for translational research on shoulder pathologies: from bench to bedside. Sports Med Arthrosc 2011;19(3):184–93.

29. Warden SJ. Development and use of animal models to advance tendinopathy research. Front Biosci 2009;14:4588–97.

30. Riley G. The pathogenesis of tendinopathy. A molecular perspective. Rheumatology (Oxford) 2004;43(2):131–42.

31. Lui PP, Maffulli N, Rolf C, et al. What are the validated animal models for tendinopathy? Scand J Med Sci Sports 2011;21(1):3–17.

32. Sánchez JM, Vallés SL, García S, et al. Mecanismos moleculares implicados en la tendinopatía rotuliana en ratas y su recuperación mediante la técnica de Electrólisis Percutánea Intratisular(EPI®). In: I Congreso Internacional de Electrólisis Percutánea Intratisular(EPI®). Madrid: Libro de comunicaciones y ponencias; 2011.

33. Carpenter JE, Thomopoulos S, Flanagan CL, et al. Rotator cuff defect healing: a biomechanical and histologic analysis in an animal model. J Shoulder Elbow Surg 1998;7(6):599–605.

34. Dahlgren LA, van der Meulen MC, Bertram JE, et al. Insulin-like growth factor-I improves cellular and molecular aspects of healing in a collagenase-induced model of flexor tendinitis. J Orthop Res 2002;20(5):910–19.

35. Alfredson H, Ljung BO, Thorsen K, et al. In vivo investigation of ECRB tendons with microdialysis technique – no signs of inflammation but high amounts of glutamate in tennis elbow. Acta Orthop Scand 2000;71(5):475–9.

36. Maffulli N, Testa V, Capasso G, et al. Similar histopathological picture in males with Achilles and patellar tendinopathy. Med Sci Sports Exerc 2004;36(9):1470–5.

37. Sánchez-Sánchez J. Estudio comparativo de un tratamiento fisioterápico convencional con uno que incluye la técnica de Electrólisis Percutánea Intratisular (EPI®) en pacientes con tendinopatía crónica del tendón rotuliano (doctoral thesis). Salamanca: Universidad de Salamanca; 2011.

38. Sánchez JL, Martín AM, Calderón L, et al. Efecto de la Electrólisis Percutánea Intratisular (EPI®) a nivel histológico en el tendón sano de la rata. In: I Congreso Internacional de Electrólisis Percutánea Intratisular (EPI®). Madrid: Libro de comunicaciones y ponencias; 2011.

39. Vallés S, Sánchez JM, Valera F, et al. Mecanismos moleculares implicados en la tendinopatía rotuliana en ratas y su recuperación mediante la técnica de Electrólisis Percutánea Intratisular (EPI®). In: I Congreso Internacional de Electrólisis Percutánea Intratisular

(EPI®). Madrid: Libro de comunicaciones y ponencias; 2011.

40. Valera F, Minaya F, García P, et al. Estudio macroscópico del tendón de la rata tras la aplicación de la Electrólisis Percutánea Intratisular vs. Punción seca (Premio a la mejor comunicación oral). In: XIV Congreso Nacional de Fisioterapia. Madrid: Asociación Española de fisioterapeutas (AEF); 2012.

41. Valera-Garrido F, Minaya-Muñoz F, Sánchez-Ibáñez JM, et al. Comparison of the acute inflammatory response and proliferation of dry needling and Electrolysis Percutaneous Intratissue (EPI®) in healthy rat Achilles tendons. In: 2nd International scientific tendinopathy symposium. Vancouver: Department of Physical Therapy, University of British Columbia; 2012.

42. Cook JL, Purdam CR. Is tendon pathology a continuum? A pathology model to explain the clinical presentation of load-induced tendinopathy. Br J Sports Med 2009;43:409–16.

43. Fu SC, Rolf C, Cheuk YC, et al. Deciphering the pathogenesis of tendinopathy: a three-stages process. Sports Med Arthrosc Rehabil Ther Technol 2010;2:30.

44. Abate M, Gravare-Silbernagel K, Siljeholm C, et al. Pathogenesis of tendinopathies: inflammation or degeneration? Arthritis Research & Therapy 2009;11(3):1–15.

45. Sánchez-Ibáñez JM. Ultrasound guided percutaneous electrolysis (EPI®) in patients with chronic insertional patellar tendinophaty: a pilot study. Knee Surg Sports Traumatol Arthrosc 2008;16:220–1.

46. Sánchez-Ibáñez JM. Tratamiento mediante Electrólisis Percutánea Intratisular (EPI®) ecoguiada de una tendinopatía de Aquiles en un futbolista profesional. Rev Podologia Clínica 2008;9(4):118–27.

47. Sánchez-Ibáñez JM. Fascitis plantar: tratamiento regenerativo mediante Electrólisis Percutánea Intratisular (EPI®). Rev Podologia Clinica 2010;2(1):22–9.

48. Valera F, Minaya F, Sánchez JM. Efectividad de la Electrólisis Percutánea Intratisular (EPI®) en las tendinopatías crónicas del tendón rotuliano. Trauma Fund MAPFRE 2010;21(4):227–36.

49. Minaya F, Valera F, Sánchez JM. Uso de la Electrólisis Percutánea Intratisular (EPI®) en la epicondilagia crónica: caso clínico. Fisioter calid vida 2011;14(1):13–16.

50. Ghavami S, Hashemi M, Ande SR, et al. Apoptosis and cancer: mutations within caspase genes. J Med Genet 2009;46:497–510.

51. Nakama LH, King KB, Abrahamsson S, et al. VEGF, VEGFR-1, and CTGF cell densities in tendon are increased with cyclical loading: An in vivo tendinopathy model. J Orthop Res 2006;24:393–400.

52. Sahin H, Tholema N, Petersen W, et al. Impaired biomechanical properties correlate with neoangiogenesis as well as VEGF and MMP-3 expression during rat patellar tendon healing. J Orthop Res 2012;30:1952–7.

53. Sánchez JM, Paredes P, Valles-Martí S, et al. Análisis molecular de la Electrólisis Percutánea Intratisular (EPI®) en la lesión muscular de la rata. In: I Congreso Internacional de Electrólisis Percutánea Intratisular (EPI®). Madrid: Libro de comunicaciones y ponencias; 2011.

CHAPTER 13

INTRATISSUE PERCUTANEOUS ELECTROLYSIS (EPI® TECHNIQUE) IN TENDON INJURIES

Fermín Valera Garrido • José Manuel Sánchez Ibáñez • Francisco Minaya Muñoz • Fernando Polidori • Ferrán Abat González

What would life be if we had no courage to attempt anything?
VINCENT VAN GOGH

KEYWORDS

Intratissue Percutaneous Electrolysis (EPI®); tendinitis; tendinopathy; tendinosis: tendon; healing process.

13.1 INTRODUCTION

13.1.1 The present model of tendinopathy

13.1.1.1 Histopathological findings

The traditional model of tendinitis, understood as an inflammatory process, is currently in disuse, following several research publications that have described the pathological process of the tendon mainly as being degenerative due to the absence of inflammatory cells and the presence of areas of collagen and myxoid degeneration, as well as the increase in ground substance. These processes are associated with a failure in the healing process of the tendon.[1-5] Therefore, the concept of tendinitis is being replaced by the term tendinopathy or tendinosis, in reference to this degenerative process. These research findings have challenged the more traditional therapeutic approaches, historically based on the theory of inflammation, towards incorporating the treatment of degeneration processes.[6]

Macroscopically, it has been observed that tendinopathies are characterized by the presence of a tendon of a soft consistency with disorganized and brownish-yellow coloured collagen fibres.[7-9] Some authors propose the existence of a transition process from the normal tendon towards a tendinosis[1] via a prior stage of inflammatory tendinitis. However, there are studies that prove that there is no presence of inflammatory cells in an overuse tendinopathy. This suggests that if there really is a transitory tendinitis stage, it is very short.[7,8]

KEY POINTS

Different studies confirm that the concept of tendinitis refers to a non-inflammatory condition and, therefore, the use of the term with the suffix 'itis' is incorrect.

However, the degenerative changes are not isolated and frequently coexist with signs of inflammation. In a study performed on patients with symptoms of patellar tendinosis who were undergoing knee surgery (and were examined via fluid cytometry and immunohistochemical techniques), the presence of inflammatory mediators such as prostaglandins, interleukins and cyclooxygenase-2 (COX-2) was observed.[9] These findings could play a key role in helping to understand the development of tendinopathy, as well as the mediation of pain and the ultimate recovery of the tendon.[10]

There are few prospective, randomized controlled trials that have analysed all aspects of tendinopathies, and, in particular, few studies that have researched the initial stages of the tendinopathy and its repair process.[9] Some authors describe four histological findings that are characteristic of tendinopathy. These are globally known as angiofibroblastic hyperplasia and are: (1) functional changes in the tenocytes (tendon cells); (2) degradation of the collagen; (3) hypervascularization (also known as vascular hyperplasia); and (4) proliferation of the ground substance.[9,11]

All these disorders are essential components of the tendon lesion and, considering that the cellular integrity is necessary for maintenance of the connective tissue, it is also possible that the changes in the cellular metabolism (synthesis and degradation of the extracellular matrix) may influence the structural properties of the tendon. Histopathological studies have demonstrated that in these tendon disorders there is an alteration of the extracellular matrix, combined with an increase in type III collagen, compared with type I collagen (the latter is more dense and resistant) mainly in calcifying tendinopathy. Type III collagen is deficient in the number of cross-links,[12] presenting a decreased consistency of its fibrils and a decreased density of branching, as well as a less regular undulation, associated with ruptures of the intramolecular and intermolecular bridges.[7,13,14] The degraded and degenerated collagen fibres are sometimes replaced by calcifications or by the accumulation of lipid cells (tendolipomatosis).[15]

The increase in proliferation of the ground substance is the main cause of the mucoid or myxoid, cystic and hyaline appearance of the tendinopathy.[16] The aggrecan is overexpressed, altering the balance with the decorin; aggrecan forms chondroitin sulphate, which constitutes the ground substance of the cartilaginous tissue.[17] Less frequently, the presence of calcifications and metaplasia of the fibrocartilage and bone are observed.[9] The mechanisms for degeneration are represented by an increase in the expression of matrix metalloproteinases (MMP-3). This favours degradation of the extracellular matrix and the overproduction of inflammatory cytokines such as endothelial growth factor, and the growth factor derived from platelets, leukotrienes and prostaglandins E_2.[18] The synthesis and degradation of the matrix are important for the maintenance and repair of the tendon.

The tenocytes are active throughout the lifespan, and express a great variety of proteins and enzymes. One of these proteins is collagen type I, which is highly resistant to enzymatic degradation and has a prolonged lifespan. With repeated overload, collagen experiences greater glycation with the accumulation of pentosidine. The degradation of the collagen is extracellular and mediated by proteases. The collagenases, members of the MMP family, are able to keep the collagen type I molecule intact. This action occurs in a specific site of the molecule and is the limiting factor in replacement of collagen, generating fragments that are susceptible to the action of other proteinases, such as gelatinases.[9] In studies of supraspinatus tendons undergoing degenerative processes, a discrete reduction of the total content of collagen was observed and a greater proportion of collagen type III was found in relation to collagen type I. The cross-bridges of hydroxyproline and lysyl-pyridinoline were significantly increased.[19] Similar findings were obtained in chronic tendinopathies in animals and after acute lesions were induced via surgical trauma or collagenase injection. Other studies revealed the increase of various proteoglycans in tendons undergoing degeneration, a phenomenon which is still not completely understood. The glycoproteins, such as tenascin-C, have been found to increase in the ruptured supraspinatus tendon, with differences in expressed isoforms. An accumulation of necrotic tissue and fibrin has also been observed. These changes in the matrix are compatible with a scarring process present in the tendon undergoing degeneration, although with incomplete remodelling.

In 2007, Scott et al.[20] carried out a histological study with pathological patellar tendons compared with normal tendons. A significant increase in proteoglycans and versican was found in the extracellular matrix of the pathological tendons. Versican plays a major role in the structural transformation of the molecules. The presence of versican is a highlighted characteristic of normal and pathological fibrocartilaginous tissues, although its production is regulated by an excess of mechanical loading. In this study it was hypothesized that the increase in content of versican may, in fact, weaken the tendon, decreasing its resistance module, especially in the tissue regions that are more vulnerable to tensile load. Furthermore, an increase in versican deposit can promote the formation of neovascularization, although it is still unclear whether these molecular changes represent a positive or pathological adaptation.[20]

These findings represent small pieces of a great histopathological puzzle and pose a possible key to future treatment approaches.

KEY POINTS

Histologically, tendinopathies are characterized by so-called angiofibroblastic hyperplasia, in which the tissues display a series of fundamental changes in the tenocytes, a degrading of collagen (discrete reduction in the total quantity of collagen and a greater proportion of collagen type III in comparison to type I), hypervascularization and, finally, proliferation of ground substance.

13.1.1.2 Pathogenesis

There are several theories regarding the aetiopathogenesis of tendinous lesions. Some refer to the forces supported by the tendon, and others to the processes of tendon repair. With regard to the forces supported by the tendon, these are signalled as factors that influence the force that the tendon supports, the cyclic charge secondary to repetitive submaximal forces, the overload of the tendon due to muscular weakness and the viscoelastic deterioration which will affect the tendon's shock-absorbing capacity.[16] Direct compression is understood to be another causal mechanism, mainly affecting the patellar and supraspinatus tendons, which are vulnerable to the forces of entrapment. Regarding the theories concerning the factors that influence the repair process of the tendon, currently the most accepted are the iceberg theory[10] and the theory of failed healing, in which an insufficient recovery time is cited, together with an accumulation of microlesions.[21]

13.1.1.3 Iceberg theory

The pathogenesis of the tendinopathy is a continuum from the physiology of the tendon to the clinical patient presentation. This sequence of events can be compared with an iceberg (figure 13.1). The base of the iceberg represents what occurs under physiological conditions. Once damage to the tissue appears, two phases begin: the asymptomatic and the symptomatic phases, in which pain is usually the alarm symptom. Indeed it is infrequent, except for in the case of highly demanding athletes who undergo routine screenings, for changes in tendon structure to be identified via musculoskeletal ultrasound prior to the appearance of pain. It is important to highlight, however, that the actual moment that these events appear can vary considerably due to various individual factors.

13.1.1.4 Failed healing theory

The understanding of the pathogenesis of tendinopathy is based on fragmentary evidence, similar to the pieces of a puzzle. The failed healing theory (figure 13.2) is proposed in order to join these pieces together in an attempt to understand the pathogenesis.

This theory is based on the pathological changes within the tendon, with the main feature being the collagenolytic lesions associated with active healing processes, together with focal hypervascularization and metaplasia of the tissue. This theory considers that overload lesions and lesions caused by repetitive microtrauma could be the main agents of the pathological process (table 13.1). The typical clinical, biochemical and histopathological presentation refers to a

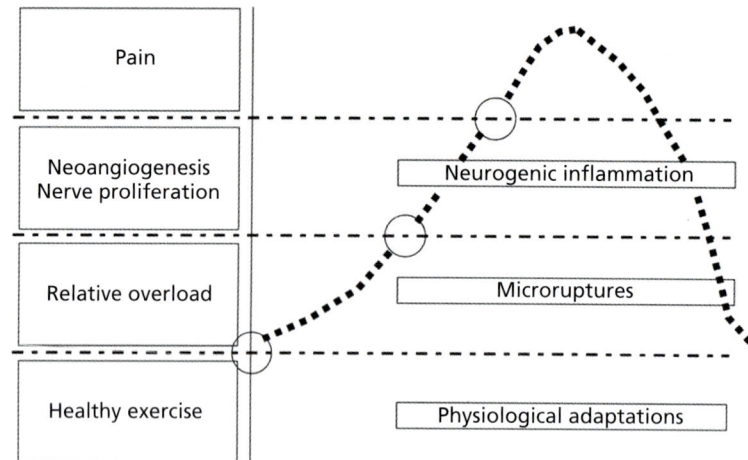

FIGURE 13.1 ■ The iceberg theory. (Reproduced from Abate M, Gravare-Silbernagel K, Siljeholm C et al. Pathogenesis of tendinopathies: inflammation or degeneration? Arthritis Res Ther 2009; 11(3):1–15, with permission).

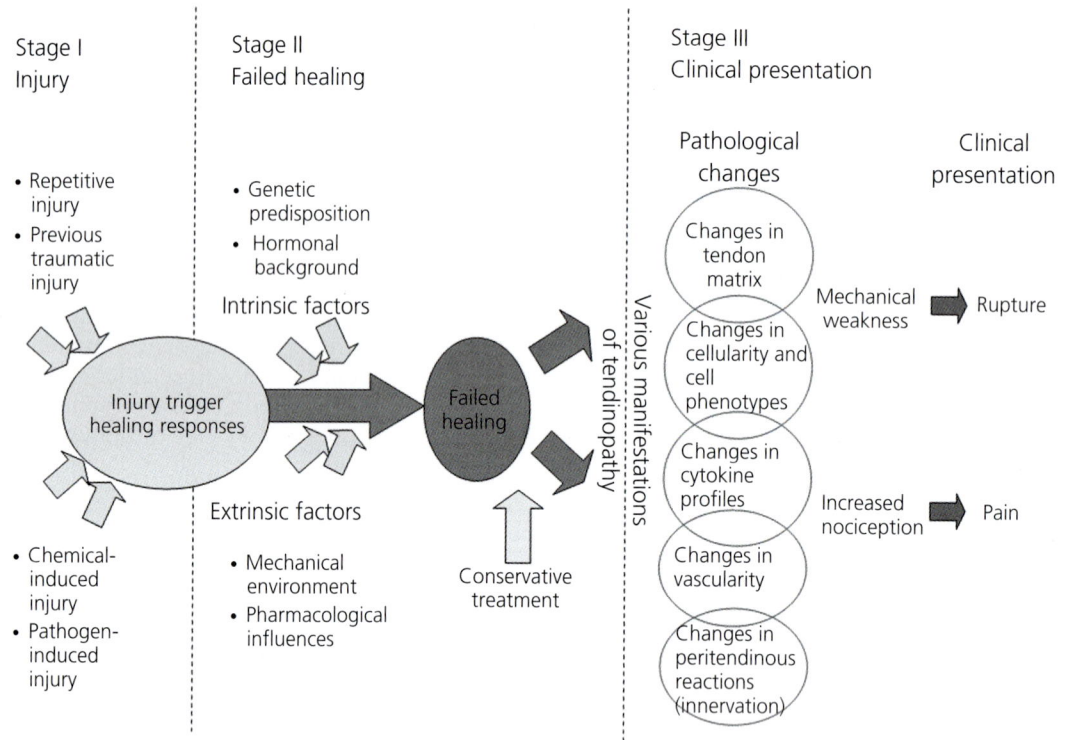

FIGURE 13.2 ■ The failed healing theory. (Reproduced from Fu SC, Rolf C, Cheuk YC et al. Deciphering the pathogenesis of tendinopathy: a three-stages process. Sports Med Arthrosc Rehabil Ther Technol 2010; 2:30, with permission).

condition of chronic localized pain that can lead to rupture of the tendon attributed to mechanical weakness.[5]

The epidemiological observations indicate that the initial determining cause of tendinopathy is an excessive use of the tendon. Indeed, tendinopathies represent conditions that mainly affect athletes who practise a repetitive activity, such as jumping (volleyball, basketball), kicking (football), quick starts and stops (tennis, squash) or running (short or long distances), as reflected by up to 40% of basketball and volleyball players affected by this condition.[21] It is believed that the mechanical stimulus that the tendon is subjected to is one of the most important factors in the development of tendinopathy – a theory that is justified by the fact that the tendons which are exposed to higher mechanical demands are those

TABLE 13.1	**Implication of failed healing in different tendinopathy manifestations**				
Lesion	**Healing response**	**Failed healing**	**Histopathological changes**	**Clinical presence**	**Different manifestations**
Overuse	Inflammation	→	Presence of proinflammatory cytokines	Increased nociception Mechanical weakness	Tendinitis Paratendinitis Overuse lesions Spontaneous rupture Pain related to the activity Calcifying tendinopathy
Prior trauma Xenobiotics	Neovascularization Innervation	→ →	Hypervascularization Increase in neuropeptides and hyperinnervation		
Pathogen agents	Cellular recruitment/ apoptosis	→	Hypercellularity, increase in apoptosis		
	Synthesis of the extracellular matrix Tenogenic differentiation/ apoptosis	→	Mucoid and lipid degeneration		
	Extracellular matrix remodelling	→	Collagenolysis, tendon adhesions		

that are more frequently injured (for example, the patellar tendon or the Achilles tendon). However, it has subsequently been observed that Achilles tendinopathy can also appear in sedentary subjects. Thus, this overuse theory alone cannot explain the pathogenesis of tendinopathy.[22]

When the tendon is overloaded and subject to repetitive stress, the collagen fibres begin to slide one over another, breaking their cross-links and provoking denaturalization of the tissue. These cyclic and accumulative microtraumas not only weaken the collagen cross-links, but also affect the extracellular matrix, as well as the vascular elements of the tendon. It is well known that well-structured physical exercise practised in the long term and within a physiological range does not damage the tendon, but rather strengthens it via stimulating the production of new collagen fibres. Studies on collagen renovation and the components of the extracellular matrix, via molecular microdialysis techniques performed on human subjects, have demonstrated that, after different types of exercise, synthesis and degradation of collagen increases, although synthesis prevails over degradation.[23,24] On the other hand, biochemical adaptation to exercise is characterized by the liberation of substances or molecular mediators of inflammation and growth factors. This takes place both in the general circulation as well as the local circulation of tendons, like interleukin-1ß, which, at the same time, increases the expression of COX-2 and MMP.

These enzymes are important, both for regulation of cellular activity as well as for degradation of the extracellular matrix, and have functions in the growth and development of the collagen fibre.[25] However, when the tendon is subjected to extenuating and cyclical exercise, extremely high temperatures are reached in its interior. The lack of control over hyperthermia induced by extenuating exercise can cause the death of tendon cells.[26–28]

KEY POINTS

Factors that can, supposedly, cause tendinopathy include:
- forces supported by the tendon: submaximal repetitive forces, muscular weakness, viscoelastic deterioration, direct compression and high temperatures caused by extenuating exercise
- repair processes: repair time and the accumulation of microlesions.

13.1.2 Chronic pain in tendinopathy

Although various studies have tried to explain the causes of pain in tendinopathy, the mechanisms that underlie chronic tendinous pain are not completely clear. The traditional theories on tendinitis, which assumed an inflammatory process as the cause of pain, have been disre-

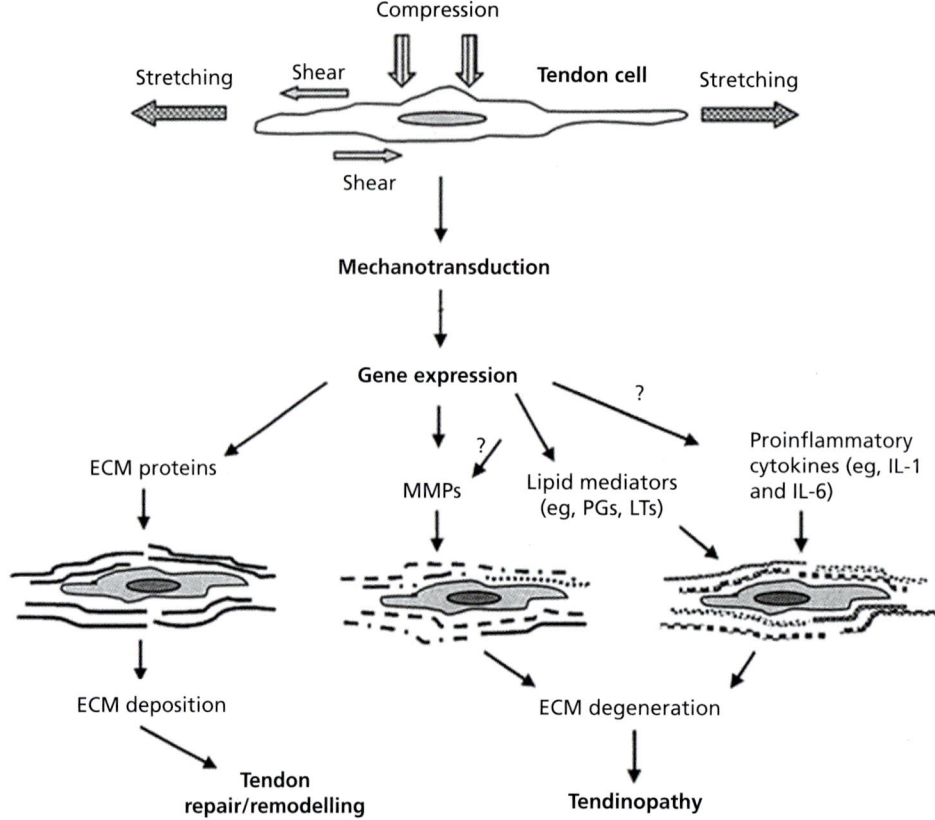

FIGURE 13.3 ■ Biological response from the fibroblasts in conditions of repetitive mechanical loading. MMPs, matrix metalloproteinases; PGs, prostaglandins; LTs, leukotrienes; ECM, extracellular matrix; IL-1, interleukin-1; IL-6, interleukin-6. (Reproduced from Wang JH, Iosifidis MI, Fu FH. Biomechanical basis for tendinopathy. Clin Orthop Relat Res 2006; 443: 320–332, with permission).

garded. In short, there are many theories regarding the cause of pain in tendinopathy as well as increasing data pointing towards a more neurochemical rather than structural cause.[7]

13.1.2.1 Biomechanical model

There have been attempts to explain tendon pain via a biomechanical model, which attributes pain to different conditions. These are tissue compression (figure 13.3) and lesion of the collagen fibres.

The authors who defend the theory of compression or entrapment attribute the presence of pain in tendinopathy to entrapment and compression of the tendon between the adjacent structures.[29–31]

The authors who support the theory that pain arises as a consequence of lesions in the collagen fibres are basing this on the fact that these could be the origin of the pain when they break, due to the fact that pain is not present when they are intact. However, if collagen disorganization were the origin of the pain, it should be present in all types of tendinopathy. In this sense, the removal

of large fragments of collagen rarely causes pain in the tendon, for example, when extracting tendinous tissue from the patellar tendon for a bone–tendon–bone ligamentoplasty. In the same way, there is no correlation between the changes observed with imaging techniques after tendon surgery, and symptoms.[32] Imaging studies have demonstrated that there is also no correlation between the amount of disorganized collagen fibres and pain, as ultrasound lesions with ample collagen tissue disorganization have been detected that are asymptomatic and tendons which on ultrasound appear to be normal may in fact be painful.[33]

KEY POINTS

There is no clear correlation between the collagenous alterations and the presence of pain in tendinopathy.

Furthermore, recent studies on the patellar tendon and the Achilles tendon[7,22] have identified low levels of load in deep regions of the tendon associated with changes compatible with tendinopathy. This suggests that those areas exposed to low load can predispose specific regions of the tendon to developing a structural weakness, thus making them more susceptible to overload. On the other hand, different authors[7] have maintained that insertion tendinopathy can be a result of lesions that are not only produced by a mechanism of increased tension, but rather compression and shear forces can also be implicated (as occurs, for example, during wrist extension movements with the elbow in pronation).

13.1.2.2 Biochemical model

The biochemical model is presented as an alternative with regard to the previous model. This model proposes that the cause of pain in tendinosis is a consequence of a chemical irritation due to general hypoxia and lack of phagocyte cells to eliminate anabolites. Furthermore, the damaged tenocytes and blood vessels liberate toxic chemical substances that have an impact on the intact neighbouring cells.

The chondroitin sulphate that is liberated when the tendon is injured can stimulate the nociceptors of the peritenon. It is possible that the nociceptors of other structures may also be stimulated; for example, in patellar tendinopathy, those found in the lateral and medial patellar wings, the infrapatellar fat pad, the synovial fat pad and the periosteum.

Recent studies have detected an increase in the concentration of glutamate and lactate neurotransmitters in patients with patellar tendinopathy.[9,33] Glutamate produces a well-known process known as excitotoxicity; this overstimulates the tenocytes and allows for the entrance of large amounts of calcium ions (Ca^{2+}), causing destructive processes. Alfredson et al.[32] found statistically significant differences in glutamate using molecular microdialysis in a group with Achilles tendinopathy when compared to a control group, whereas there was no difference in the concentration of type E_2 prostaglandins, which suggests the absence of inflammation. In another study, the same group, via the technique of microdialysis and immunohistochemical analysis of the tendon tissue in patients with patellar tendinopathy, found a high concentration of glutamate and N-methyl-D-aspartate-1 (NMDA-R1) receptors, without inflammatory substances (prostaglandin E_2). In the biopsies, inflammatory cells were not found, although there was an immunoreaction by the glutamate receptor (NMDA-R1) associated with the proliferation of nervous structures in the tendons.[9] For this reason, the presence of glutamate and

its receptor NMDA-R1 in tendinopathy is interpreted as an amplifier of the pain signal.

Other studies on animals have shown an increase in messenger ribonucleic acid (mRNA) of the glutamate in supraspinatus muscle tendinopathy.[34] However, some studies challenge these observations as they have noted that, in previously painful tendons (after treatment and becoming painfree), they then fail to show significantly different glutamate concentrations compared to when they were painful.[35]

KEY POINTS

Different substances have been found that provide an explanation for the presence of pain in tendinosis. These are chondroitin sulphate, lactate and, especially, glutamate.

Neural damage and hyperinnervation have been poorly studied despite possibly representing one of the physiopathological mechanisms of pain in tendinopathy. In several studies, a correlation between tendinopathy and hyperinnervation was found. In these it is claimed that the production of neural growth factor and the corresponding hyperinnervation could be induced by repetitive ischaemic crisis. This growth of nerve fibres, which would justify the chronic pain, could form part of a process of anomalous tissue repair preceded by repetitive microtraumas.[36]

There are few studies that describe the innervation of the different tendons, and fewer still that describe the innervation of their corresponding blood vessels. In a study from 2006, a marked overexpression of substance P (SP) and of calcitonin gene-related peptide (CGRP) was found in the innervation of the capillaries at the level of the osteotendinous junction, compared to the rest of the patellar tendon structure. The presence of para-arterial innervation in the lax connective tissue of the paratenon suggests that there is a marked neurovascular relation at this level.[37] The presence of this perivascular innervation is of great relevance in the ultrasound assessment via Doppler, as it enables one to distinguish between hypovascular tendinosis and neovascular tendinosis, as well as allowing for the performance of ablation treatments of these neurochemical alterations via different techniques.

The presence of pain in symptomatic hypovascular tendinosis may be due to an energetic crisis affecting the mechanisms regulating the tendon metabolism (an increase of lactate, hypoxia inducible factor-1 [HIF-1]), produced by local ischaemia with an increase in free radicals and

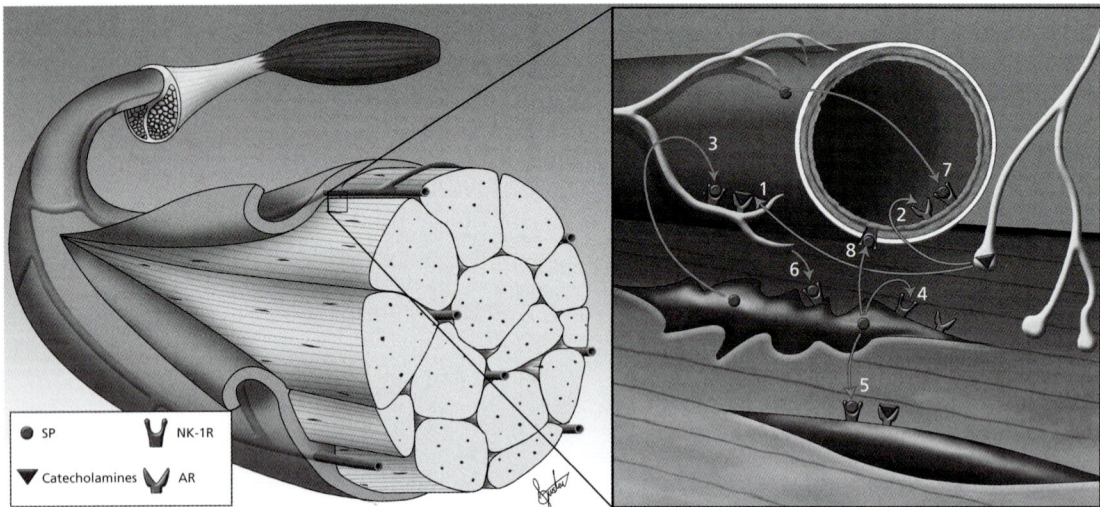

FIGURE 13.4 ■ Drawing of the Achilles tendon displaying the possible pathways for substance P (SP) in the tendon structure, as well as a summary of the possible influences and interactions of the paratendinous innervations. AR: adrenergic receptor; NK-1R: neurokinin receptor 1. (Reproduced from Andersson G. Influences of paratendinous innervations and non-neuronal substance P in tendinopathy – studies on human tendon tissue and an experimental model of Achilles tendinopathy (PhD thesis). Chapter 20, figure 8, with permission). (Colour version of figure is available online).

excitatory nociceptive neurotransmitters. These mechanisms sensitize the nervous branches that are able to maintain a secondary hyperalgesia.[38]

Patients suffering from symptomatic hypervascular tendinosis are characterized for presenting mechanical allodynia. In other words, a banal mechanical stimulus is capable of producing pain. This phenomenon can be explained by neurogenic inflammation that occurs at the level of the neocapillarization with an oedematous presentation of the capillaries and an increase in neurotransmitters and nociceptive neuropeptides, such as glutamate, SP, catecholamines and acetylcholine (figure 13.4).[39,40] This sensitization could be explained as being due to the permanent accumulation of glutamate in the synaptic region, which produces an increase in the NMDA-R receptors of the postsynaptic membrane.[9]

The cellular mechanisms of chronic pain in tendinopathy are little known. It has been suggested that the close relation of the mast cells with the vessels in the connective tissue could influence the development of the hypervascularization and oedema present in tendinopathy. One study examined the distribution of mastocytes in patients with patellar tendinopathy and discovered an overexpression of these cells.[41] These mastocytes proliferate in the lesion area, liberating an important range of growth factors and profibrotic cytokines, such as transforming growth factor-beta, interleukin 1 and interleukin 4. In the same way, the tryptases liberated by the mastocytes can act directly upon the tenoblasts, triggering the activation of receptors activated

by protease and inducing the fibrotic proliferation dependent upon the COX-2 enzyme. Tryptases are powerful angiogenic agents that may explain the neovascularization present in some tendinopathies.[42] The mastocytes are also capable of producing powerful neurotrophins, such as neural growth factor, possibly implicated in neurovascular angiogenesis and hyperinnervation and that, according to recent findings, characterize tendinosis and could justify the chronic pain being suffered.[36] The mastocytes can play a significant role in the symptomatology of tendinopathy, as they could be associated with the abnormality of autonomic vascularization and sensory innervation that is potentially implicated in the chronic pain of tendinopathy.[43] Therefore, it seems plausible that the mast cells play an important proangiogenic and neurotrophic role in chronic tendinopathy, as there are many possibilities of paracrine interaction between mast cells, nerves, endothelial cells and tenocytes.

KEY POINTS

Knowledge of the molecular and biological mechanisms of pain in tendinopathy is fundamental from a clinical point of view, as any treatment must be aimed at alleviating pain. There are several theories that attempt to explain the cause of pain in tendinosis. The available evidence points to biochemical processes (neurovascular hyperinnervation) rather than biomechanical processes (lesion of the collagen fibres, tissue compression).

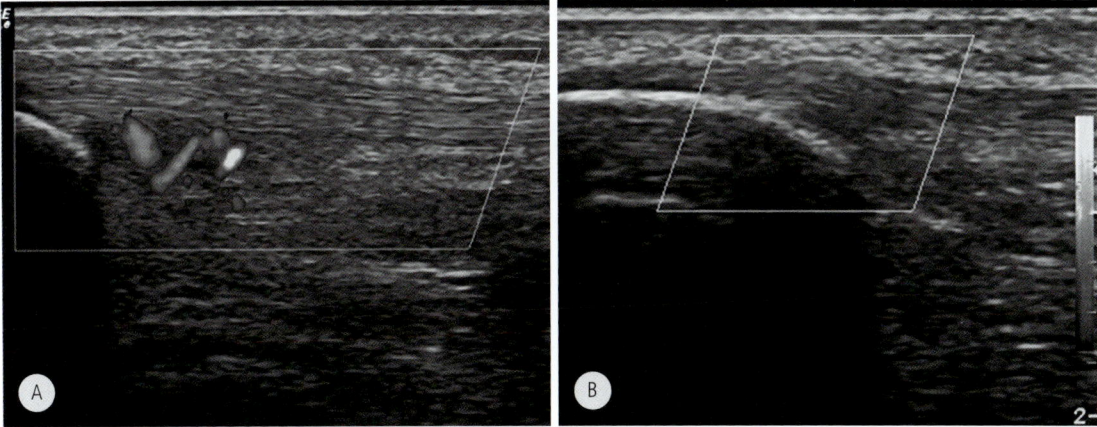

FIGURE 13.5 ■ Ultrasound power Doppler image. (A) Hypervascularization. (B) Hypovascularization.

13.1.3 Clinical classification of tendinopathy

After the onset of tendon symptoms (whether associated with an internal or external traumatic agent), it has been observed that a high percentage of subjects continue with symptoms that become chronic. This is explained by the failure of an initial repair or healing process, after which the tendon begins a progressive degeneration cycle which is defined as tendinosis.[1,5,6] The acute tendon lesion and, therefore, the painful symptoms must not continue beyond the 3 first weeks postlesion, which is the duration of the total inflammatory response.

From a clinical point of view, according to physiopathological criteria and ultrasound image findings, the tendinosis can be classified as hypovascular or hypervascular, as well as symptomatic or asymptomatic (figure 13.5).

13.1.3.1 Hypovascular symptomatic tendinosis

Hypovascular symptomatic tendinosis is characterized by the presence of pain that may be due to an energetic crisis in the mechanism of tendon metabolism regulation (increase of lactate, HIF-1), when produced by local ischaemia with increases in free radicals and excitatory nociceptive neurotransmitters that sensitize the nerve branches able to maintain secondary hyperalgesia.[5]

13.1.3.2 Hypovascular asymptomatic tendinosis

Hypovascular asymptomatic tendinosis is characterized by the absence of symptoms. In the case of the Achilles tendinopathy, it is associated with non-traumatic or minimally traumatic rupture.

13.1.3.3 Hypervascular tendinosis or symptomatic neovascular tendinosis

Hypervascular tendinosis or symptomatic neovascular tendinosis is characterized by the presence of pain with mechanical allodynia. In other words, the mechanical innocuous stimulus is capable of producing pain. This phenomenon can be explained by a neurogenic inflammation at the level of the neocapillarization with an oedematous presentation of capillaries and an increase in nociceptive neurotransmitters and neuropeptides, such as glutamate and SP.[37] The sensitization can be explained by the permanent accumulation of glutamate in the synaptic region, which produces an increase of NMDA-R receptors in the nervous synapse.[38]

13.1.3.4 Hypervascular tendinosis or asymptomatic neovascular tendinosis

This occurs in subjects that do not present pain in a situation of hypervascularization, despite the presence of a greater degradation of the tendon. At present, the scientific evidence cannot explain these anatomopathological differences.[12]

13.2 BASIC PRINCIPLES OF INTRATISSUE PERCUTANEOUS ELECTROLYSIS (EPI®) IN TENDON INJURIES

13.2.1 The effects of continuous current on the soft tissues

Since the mid-1960s there has been an increase in research directed at assessing the effects of exogenous electrical currents for the healing of chronic soft-tissue lesions that, unlike acute lesions, do not heal spontaneously within a predicable time frame and that frequently fail to respond to conventional treatments.

Studies in human and animal models have demonstrated that continuous currents (CC) favour the healing of injuries, particularly when these are applied together with conventional care. The mechanisms by which the CC favours the healing of tissues include an increase in synthesis of proteins, improvement in oxygenation of the tissues, attraction of the appropriate cell types for the area, activation of these cells due to the alteration of membrane function, the modification of endogenous electric potential of the tissue according to healing potential, the reduction of oedema, the enhancement of microbial activity and the promotion of blood circulation.[44]

13.2.2 Ionic effects

Most electric currents that are used with therapeutic purposes present balanced biphasic-type waves that do not leave an electric charge in the tissue and, therefore, do not have ionic effects. In contrast, the CC, the monophasic pulsed currents and the unbalanced biphasic waveforms leave a net charge in the tissue. This charge can produce ionic effects: the negative electrode (cathode) attracts the positively charged ions and repels the negatively charged ions, whereas the positive electrode (anode) attracts the negatively charged ions and repels the positively charged ions. These ionic effects can be taken advantage of from a therapeutic point of view. For example, the CC can be used to repel ionized pharmacological molecules and, therefore, can provide a strength that increases the penetration of transdermal drugs. Similarly, the ionic effects of the electricity can be used to treat inflammatory states, to facilitate tissue healing and reduce the formation of oedema.[45]

13.2.3 Galvanotaxis/electrotaxis

Galvanotaxis or electrotaxis is the directional migration of the cells within an electrical field. Studies have demonstrated that some types of cells migrate actively towards a specific pole (the anode or the cathode).[46] Indeed, many cells implicated in tissue healing migrate towards the anode or the cathode when exposed to an electrical field of CC.[45,47]

Cells such as neutrophils, macrophages, fibroblasts, endothelial cells and nervous cells respond to the electrical field. Indeed, several in vitro studies have demonstrated improvement in the mobility of different cells towards either pole.[48] The activated neutrophils that are present in an acute soft-tissue lesion are attracted to the cathode pole, whereas the inactive ones move towards the positive pole. The tenoblasts, fibroblasts, lymphocytes, mast cells and platelets are attracted towards the negative pole. Generally, it is recommended that, to attract more appropriate cell types, a negative electrode should be used, while a positive electrode should only be used when the lesion is in the proliferative stage.[49,50]

Stimulation with CC will not only attract cells from the injured area, but will also strengthen replication of the fibroblasts and increase DNA synthesis and collagen on behalf of the fibroblasts.[49,51] The fibroblasts and collagen that are produced are essential for the proliferation phase of healing in the injured soft tissue. The proposed mechanism for improvement of cellular function is based on the pulse of the electrical field causing the calcium channels in the membrane of the fibroblast to open. The opening of the calcium channels allows the calcium to flow towards the interior of the cells, increasing the cellular concentration of calcium, which induces exposure of additional insulin receptors on the cellular surface. Insulin can join on to the exposed receptors, stimulating the synthesis of DNA and collagen within the fibroblasts.[51]

If the histopathological findings related to the tendinosis (understood as a degenerative process) are considered, the therapeutic intervention must differ from the treatment of an inflammatory process. In this circumstance, treatment should favour the inflammatory response necessary for healing mechanisms and/or repair of the soft tissue to be reactivated.[6]

The EPI® technique, when applied to the focal tendinopathy lesion, triggers an electrochemical reaction, which leads to destruction of fibrotic and necrosed tissue. Likewise, the passage of the CC in the needle/target tissue interphase provides liquefaction of the myxoid substance, facilitating migration of the inflammatory cells (neutrophils and macrophages) towards the intervening area.[52] The macrophages play an essential part in tissue healing, as they not only phagocytose but also promote migration of the fibroblasts, thus liberating growth factors and facilitating synthesis of collagen. The cathodic action of the CC will facilitate the attraction of the tenoblasts towards the area, stimulating their proliferation and the synthesis of new collagen.[51]

13.3 DESCRIPTION OF THE EPI® TECHNIQUE IN TENDON INJURIES

13.3.1 Procedure

The procedure for the application of the EPI® technique on the tendon comprises various elements.

13.3.1.1 Ultrasound-guided application

The use of ultrasound in physiotherapy is still in its beginnings, although related applications that go far beyond those traditionally used in radiology (see chapters 4, 6 and 7) have been developed. The possibility of monitoring the patient's response to treatment together with a thorough assessment of function and of the dynamic interaction among the anatomical structures are very important aspects which are highly valued by physiotherapists.[53]

The use of ultrasound guidance combined with the EPI® technique in the treatment of tendinopathy is essential in order to avoid producing an iatrogenic effect, such as a lesion of the nerves or the vessels.[54] Furthermore, it guarantees the application of the technique upon the target tissue, thereby improving the effectiveness of the intervention.

In addition, it is important to consider that the application of the EPI® technique generates a hyperechogenic well-defined image as a consequence of the density of hydrogen gas produced by the electrochemical reaction from the cathode flow.[55] This enables a clearer needle visualization (see chapter 7) and improved ability to determine the area of electroporation, thus better quantifying the effect of the EPI® technique.

13.3.1.2 Target tissue

The areas that are most frequently affected in tendinopathy are the tendon–periosteum junction, the deep fascicle[56,57] of the tendon and the adjacent structures, such as Hoffa's fat pad or the bursa.

Ultrasound analysis of the tendon enables identification of the affected tissue associated with focal hypoechoic areas, cortical irregularities, a loss of continuity of the tendinous tissue or areas of hypervascularization.[58] Despite the ample area of degeneration frequently associated with the tendon matrix in this type of clinical presentation (with a loss of echotexture), the clinically relevant area is usually 2–3 mm next to the tendon–periosteum junction, and is one of the targets of the EPI® technique. Together with

this, the areas of degeneration of the deep tendon fascicle and the relevant neovascularization sites constitute the most frequent target tissue. In this sense, the EPI® technique has been demonstrated to be effective for absence of hypervascularization areas in the short term.[59]

Once the different intervention areas are determined, it is necessary to verify the destruction of the tissue. Note that this takes place when the needle does not come across viscoelastic resistance in the intratendinous region where the electrolytic ablation was performed.

13.3.1.3 Dosage

The EPI® technique frequently employs intensities of 3–4 mA for tendinous processes and more than 4 mA where there is dense fibrotic tissue, plus time intervals of 3–4 seconds which are applied along different points of the affected tendon area. In any case, it is necessary to establish the dosage for each subject, which is determined by the algogenic response and the tissue. For this purpose, specific equipment has been developed that allows for perfect adjustment of the parameters and guarantees their safe application.

It is necessary to differentiate between tendons with and without a synovial sheath, as two separate biological routes are believed to be involved in the healing of these tendons. The intrinsic healing pathway involves cells of the endotenon and the epitenon that migrate towards the tendon lesion area. In the intrinsic pathway, it is the non-originating cells of the tendon that participate in the regeneration process. In these, the stem cells can be included as well as cells from other tissue compartments. Biomechanically, the intrinsic pathway produces a complete repair at the intratendon level, resulting in a stronger and more elastic tendon. The extrinsic pathway contributes to the formation of a scar callus and adherences during the healing process. In all tendons the repair occurs via the fibroblasts pertaining to the tendon (tenoblasts) and the cells located around the sheath, the paratenon and even in the neighbouring soft tissue. In this manner, one can conclude that the repair mechanisms are different depending on the morphological characteristics of the tendon. For example, healing for the extrinsic pathway of the hand flexors is relatively limited. This is due to the presence of synovial liquid which physically inhibits how growth factors can extrinsically reach the intrinsic cells,[60] and which determines that, for those tendons with a sheath, the EPI® technique is applied in minimal doses.

13.3.1.4 Frequency

The application of EPI® is usually performed every 7–10 days, in order to respect the entire phagocytosis phase, which lasts approximately 5–6 days until returning to basal level. It would be equally justifiable to consider respecting the complete inflammatory cycle of approximately 14–15 days.

KEY POINTS

The commonly used dosage for application of EPI® is 3–4 mA and the inflammatory phase of tissue repair must be respected.

13.3.1.5 Postintervention care
(see chapter 11)

After each EPI® intervention it is essential to educate patients by teaching them to stay in the optimal range of functional load, thereby avoiding any sports activities that lead to the appearance of injury or pain.[61]

13.3.2 Results

The EPI® technique acts upon the affected area by triggering the biological process of collagen repair and achieving rapid improvement in function. The changes in the structure of the tendon itself, however (i.e. thickening, hypoechoic images) take longer to occur, as they require a biomechanical process that involves remodelling and maturation of the tendon.

In the short term, at the time of the patient's discharge (at an average of 4 weeks from the start of the programme) various studies have shown significant changes in tendon function via the use of orthopaedic tests and functional assessment questionnaires, such as Disabilities of the Arm, Shoulder and Hand (DASH) or the Victorian Institute of Sports Assessment Patellar (VISA-P), and in the quantification of pain via the visual analogue scale (VAS) and digital algometry. Regarding the structure of the tendon itself, changes have not been observed (i.e. changes in thickening, the presence of hypoechoic areas, calcifications, bone cortical irregularities), with the exception of the presence of hypervascularization in the area. In this sense, in contrast to results published on the effectiveness of EPI® on patellar tendinopathy,[62] the hypervascularization of the common extensor tendon displayed significant modifications in the short term.[59] The hypothesis that may justify these differences is based on the structure of the patel-

lar and common extensor tendon themselves and the pattern of neovascularization found in these patients. The affected common extensor tendon has a lesser volume while the hypervascularization areas, when present, are much smaller and more localized than that of the patellar ligament. These are circumstances that could facilitate elimination or significant decrease in neovascularization using EPI® in the short term and in just a few sessions. A programme of eccentric exercise and stretching would help guide the orientation of the collagen tissue, resulting in a less thickened tendon, and the absence of other degenerative changes.

In the mid and long term, one of the frequent problems of tendinopathy is relapse, which varies between 34% and 72%.[63,64] In these cases, patients usually improve with conventional physiotherapy programmes commonly associated with sports rest and the use of braces; however, on return to sports or exercise of equal or greater intensity, the symptoms are always present. In the published studies available, such as in the case of epicondylalgia,[59] 6-week follow-up did not reveal any relapses in the group of patients, despite the fact that 75% practised some type of sports activity. Only 16.7% of cases needed a final session of EPI® in order to treat the odd localized point of residual pain. Ultrasound analysis in the mid and long term (6 and 12 months), after finalizing the EPI® cycle, revealed changes in the structure of the tendon.[65]

Apart from the use of EPI®, the physiotherapy programme includes eccentric-type exercises and stretches of the affected muscles carried out at home. Our hypothesis is that EPI® stimulates the biology of the tendon by provoking an initial inflammatory repair phase with the addition of early mechanical and controlled loading (eccentric exercise and stretching), which facilitates the process of collagen tissue proliferation. This thereby improves the biomechanical properties of the stimulated tendon. In this sense, the effect of platelet-rich plasma has been studied in the Achilles tendon of a rat that was subjected to loading and posterior unloading.[66] This study found that, after 14 days postprocedure, the effects of platelet-rich plasma disappeared in the unloaded group, with the mechanical properties of the stimulated tissue being reduced by at least half compared with the healthy tissue.

On the other hand, the type of exercise (mechanical load) plays a crucial role in the healing process. According to the available evidence, eccentric training seems to be the exercise of choice in these types of patient.[67–70] Furthermore, based on clinical experience, in the case of chronic tendinopathy, the isolated application of eccentric exercise and stretching is not enough to achieve an optimal functional result.[71] Along the same lines as the proposed programme (EPI® + eccentric exercise + stretching), other authors are achieving good results with the use of other interventions on the common extensor tendon (for example, platelet-rich plasma) as well as combining similar programmes of eccentric training and stretching.[72]

13.3.3 Indications and contraindications

13.3.3.1 Indications

Related to injuries affecting the tendon:
- extrasynovial tendinopathy
- intrasynovial tendinopathy.

13.3.3.2 Contraindications

Absolute contraindications
- Endoprosthesis and osteosynthesis: avoid electrolytic reactions in the implant, as they can trigger a rejection response.
- Pacemakers: avoid any electrical interference that may affect a pacemaker. Many pacemaker covers are metallic, and EPI® may cause electrolytic effects.
- Heart disease: the heart can be influenced by electric fields such as EPI®, which may alter the rhythm and cause the appearance of extrasystoles or arrhythmia.
- Pregnancy: as a precautionary measure and due to a lack of knowledge about what occurs in the fetal dissolutions (with high metabolism and high mitosis), do not apply EPI® during pregnancy.
- Cancer processes: malignant tumours are cells that have lost functional control over their metabolism and reproduction, therefore electrochemical influences may contribute to uncontrolled mitogen activation.
- Thrombophlebitis: in this case EPI® is contraindicated, due to the possible destruction of vessels. Patients with this disorder have a reduced turnover of soft tissues.
- Endocrine glands: avoid directly influencing the endocrine glands, as this can lead to the triggering of undesired general effects.
- Skin disorders: if abrasions or pressure ulcers are present in the region, an important deficiency of skin resistance will be encountered and there will be an excessive concentration of electrical energy that can cause a burn. However, the galvanic currents applied around these ulcers may improve their trophism with small doses with the cathode, as

this alkalizes the environment of the tissues surrounding the ulcer.
- Neurosensitive disorders: when patients are unable to respond (due to either motor or sensitive paralysis) with defence mechanisms towards their electrochemical alterations, there is a serious risk of a burn.

Relative contraindications
- Corticoids: scientific bibliography already indicates that treatment with non-steroidal anti-inflammatories or corticoid infiltrations inhibits the migration process of inflammatory cells (i.e. neutrophils, macrophages) necessary to activate the process of phagocytosis.[73–77] The depressed response of these cells will avoid activation of the fibroblasts in order to generate new collagen and products of the ground substance (prostaglanding, glycosaminoglycans).
- Steroids: the use of steroids is equally associated with an inhibition in the healing response of the tissue.[78]

13.4 THE EPI® TECHNIQUE APPLIED TO DIFFERENT TENDINOPATHIES

13.4.1 Patellar ligament

The tendinopathy of the patellar ligament, also known as jumper's knee, causes pain in the inferior pole of the patella.[79] This is considered to be one of the most frequent lesions in athletes,[80,81] with a clear degenerative (i.e. non-inflammatory) component associated with what is known as overuse injuries.[82,83]

13.4.1.1 Assessment protocol

Within the process of assessment and diagnosis in physiotherapy of the patellar ligament, it is necessary to perform an analysis of the structure and function of this ligament. For analysis of the tendon structure, a musculoskeletal ultrasound test is recommended, following the protocol described by the European Society of Musculoskeletal Radiology.[84] The ultrasound exploration consists of a longitudinal sequence from the proximal origin of the tendon to the distal insertion and transverse sections over the pole of the patella, the tendon body and the insertion in the anterior tibial tuberosity. This is performed bilaterally, with the subject in supine, with 20° knee flexion and a small wedge under the popliteal fossa. The presence of degenerative signs compatible with the medical

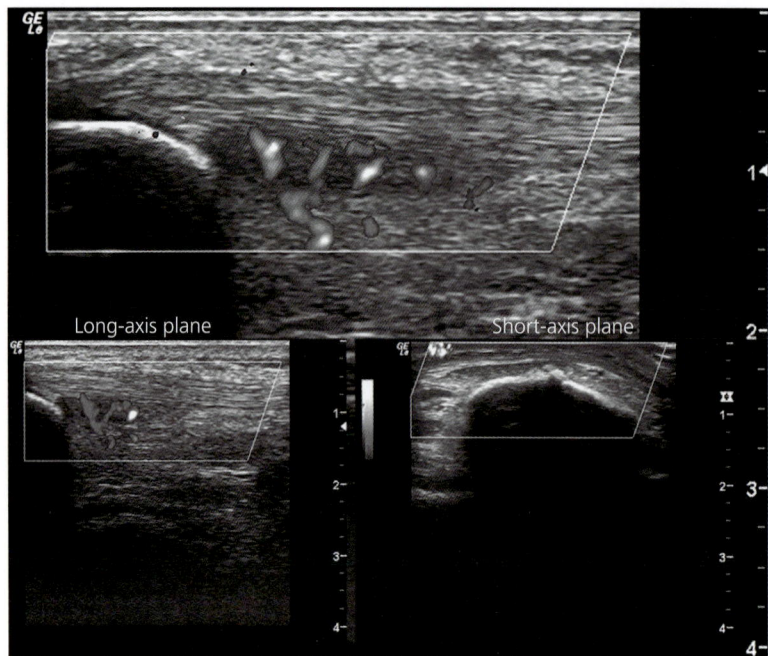

Long-axis plane

Short-axis plane

FIGURE 13.6 ■ Ultrasound power Doppler image sections in which different hypervascularization patterns are visible, indicating an alteration in the structure of a patellar ligament with tendinosis.

diagnosis of chronic tendinopathy is assessed (thickening of the tendon, hypoechoic images, cortical irregularities, calcifications), as these are important elements that influence the planning of the physiotherapy programme and follow-up.

Likewise, the power Doppler test (figure 13.6) is performed to analyse the presence of hypervascularization in the area, as it has been observed in vivo that neovascularization frequently occurs in subjects suffering pain in the patellar ligament.[85–88] The test is performed with the subject in supine, and the knee totally extended and relaxed. The image study can be completed with sonoelastographic analysis of the tendon.

The assessment of the patient is completed with the VISA-P scale in order to assess individual function (score 0–100 points)[89] and VAS. Depending on the results of the VISA-P scale in the first assessment, subjects can be classified into two groups: group 1 and group 2, scoring less or more than 50 points, respectively (patients with poorer or better function).

13.4.1.2 Clinical forms

According to the information obtained, different clinical forms of patellar tendinopathy can be established:

- depending on the presence of neovascularization (figure 13.5):
  - *hypovascular*: absence of new vessels
  - *neovascular*: presence of angioblastic hyperplasia – the most frequent.

- according to anatomical localization (figures 13.6 and 13.7):
  - deep interphase – patellar pole
  - deep interphase – Hoffa's fat pad.

The structural characteristics that predominate are: alteration of the deep fascicle with the presence of focal hypoechoic regions upon the patellar pole and cortical irregularities, tendon thickening with altered echotexture (figure 13.7) and neovascularization (over the pole of the patella or a greater distribution upon the tendon and in relation to Hoffa's fat pad) (figure 13.6). From a clinical point of view patellar tendinopathies are associated with longer evolution and worsening of the symptoms (VISA-P < 50 points) with the presence of hypervascularization.[62]

13.4.1.3 Procedure

This procedure consists of ultrasound-guided application of EPI® according to the following commonly used approaches (video 13.1):

- intratendon distal-proximal approach to the area of the pole of the patella (figure 13.8) with an orientation of 45° on the long axis and accessing the deepest area of the tendon penetrating into the cortex and a fan-shaped application (see chapter 3). This is in order to reach the deep medial and lateral tendon fibres
- deep interphase approach from medial to lateral between the tendon and Hoffa's fat

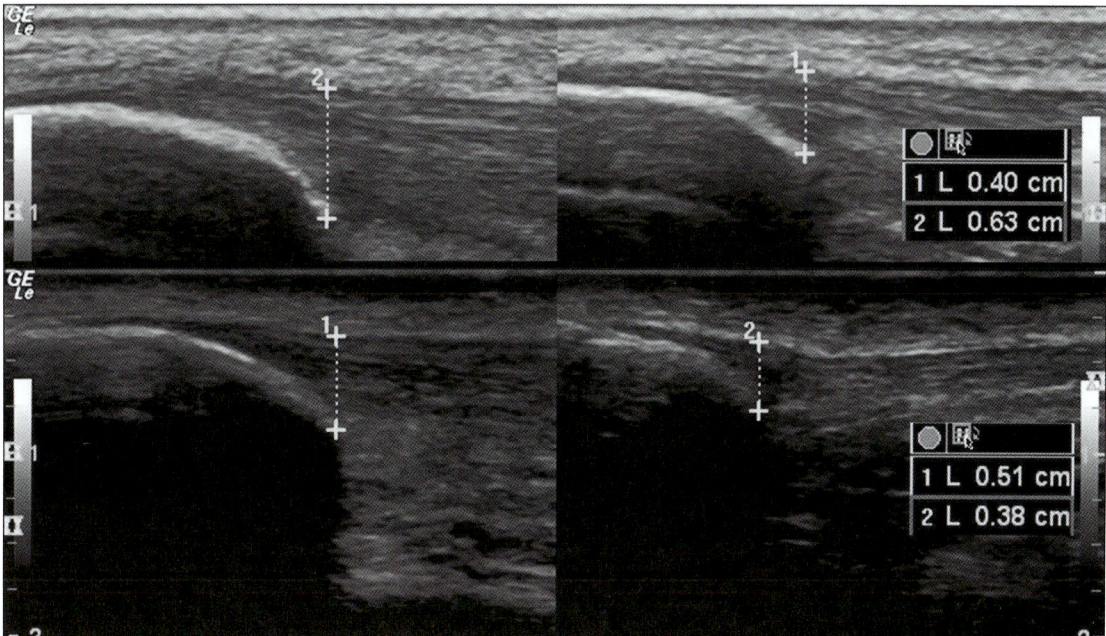

FIGURE 13.7 ■ Ultrasound image sections showing signs of structural alteration in a patellar ligament with tendinosis (left) compared to a healthy tendon (right).

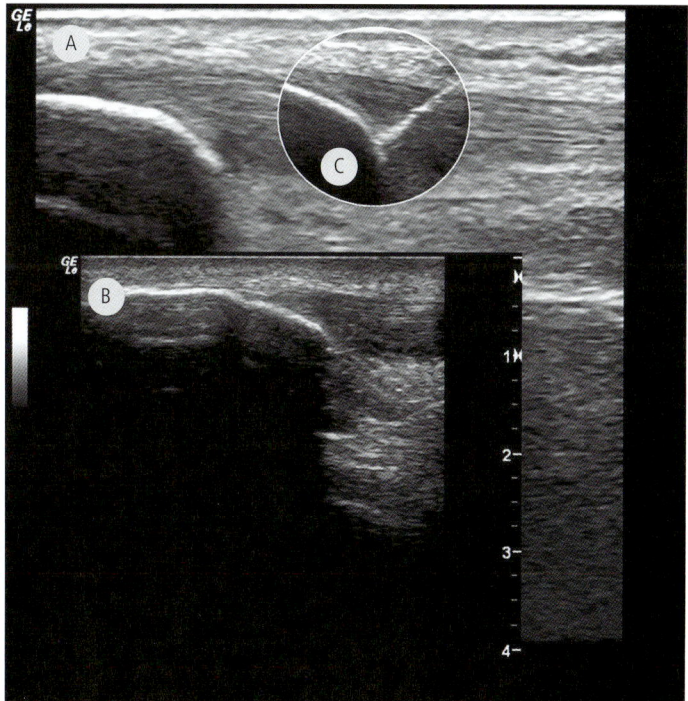

FIGURE 13.8 ■ EPI® treatment approach to the inferior patellar pole. (A) Focal hypoechoic region on the pole of the patella. (B) Needle on the pole of the patella with a 45° orientation. (C) Hyperechoic area on the pole of the patella after EPI® application which covers the initial hypoechoic area.

pad (figure 13.9). Fan-shaped application eliminating the neovascular connexion between Hoffa's fat pad and the deep tendon (see chapter 3)

• treatment approach focused on the relevant hypervacularization area.

The treatment approach to the superficial fascicle of the patellar ligament is infrequent, in contrast to the pattern involved, for example, in the Achilles tendon.

The intensity applied commonly ranges between 4 and 6 mA for 3–4 seconds.

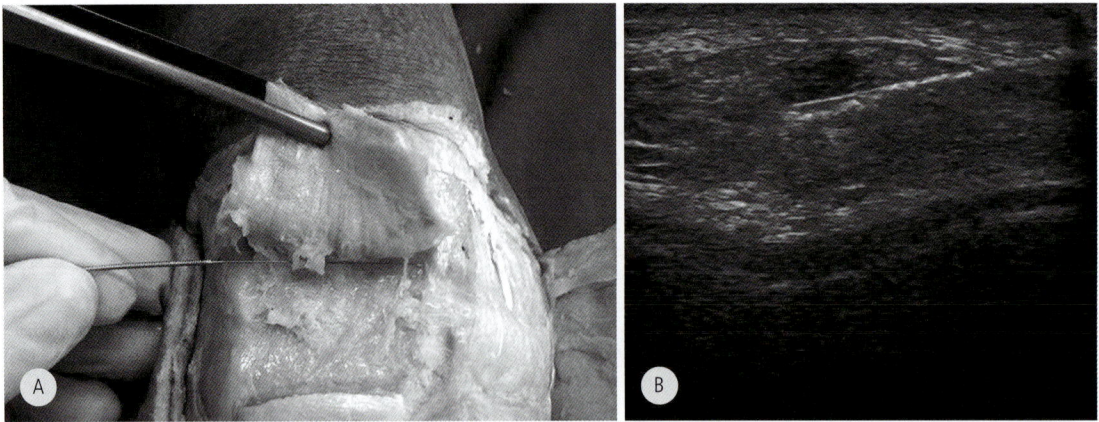

FIGURE 13.9 ■ EPI® treatment approach to the deep interphase of the patellar ligament and Hoffa's fat pad. (A) Simulated cadaver approach. (B) Ultrasound image of the long-axis approach over the deep interphase of the patellar ligament and Hoffa's fat pad in a transverse section. (Colour version of figure is available online).

13.4.1.4 Scientific and clinical results: evidence

Studies by Sánchez-Ibáñez et al.,[90] Valera et al.[62] and Sánchez-Sánchez[91] obtained similar results in the short term. The follow-up period in the study by Valera et al. obtained results in the mid term (6 weeks) and in the long term (6 and 12 months).

13.4.1.5 Short-term findings

After the treatment period (4–6 weeks on average) there were no significant changes in the structure of the tendon itself (as regards thickening, hypoechoic areas or hypervascularization) as this requires a greater process of biomechanical remodelling and maturation.

Important changes were found in analysis of function; the average score obtained in the total 32 subjects with the VISA-P scale was 80 points (SD 12; 27 points more than at the beginning), with a difference of 69 points (SD 7; 36 points more at the beginning, which represents more than 100% of the initial score) in group 1 (VISA-P with less than 50 points) and 88 points (SD 7; 20 points more than at the beginning) in group 2 (VISA-P with more than 50 points).

13.4.1.6 Mid- to long-term findings

The follow-up performed on patients confirmed changes in the tendon matrix (figures 13.10 and 13.11).

13.4.2 Common extensor tendon

Epicondylitis (lateral epicondylalgia or 'tennis elbow') is one of the most frequent clinical entities affecting the elbow, affecting 1–3% of the population.[92,93] However, the physiopathological changes that are behind this clinical picture still do not seem to be very clear, and their management by health professionals has yet to be conclusively determined.

Traditionally, epicondylitis has been defined, diagnosed and treated as an inflammatory process of an insertional nature. However, several studies have demonstrated[94,95] that this is in fact a degenerative process. Chen et al.[96] identified high cellular apoptosis and cellular autophagic death while other authors, using microdialysis, were able to identify in vivo an excessive concentration of neurotransmitters, such as glutamate, and neuropeptides, such as SP, CGRP and neurokinin A. These concentrations were found especially in the tendon of the extensor carpi radialis brevis (ECRB)[97] muscle, plus there was thickening at the capsule of the humeroradial joint, as well as in the lateral ulnar collateral ligament, the radial collateral ligament and the annular ligament.[98]

13.4.2.1 Assessment protocol

The assessment protocol for the tendon of the epicondyle muscles is defined using the *Musculoskeletal Ultrasound Technical Guidelines: Elbow* of the European Society of Musculoskeletal Radiology.[84] The ultrasound examination consists of a longitudinal sequence from the proximal origin of the tendon to the muscle and of transverse sections over the head of the radius, the body of the tendon and the insertion on the lateral epicondyle of the humerus, bilaterally, with the subject seated, the forearm supported on the plinth and the elbow at 90° flexion and maximal pronation.

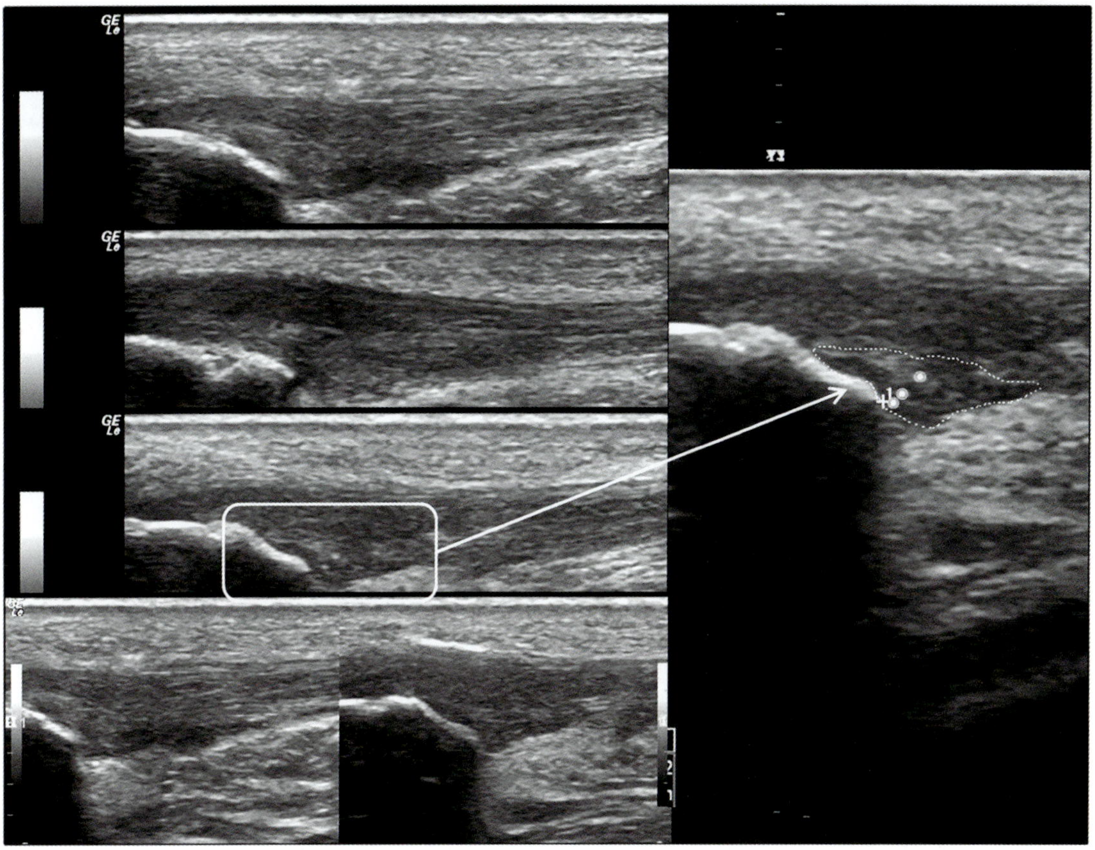

FIGURE 13.10 ■ Changes in structure of the patellar ligament in the mid and long term. The image on the right-hand side shows the formation of proliferation nuclei in the collagen tissue.

Likewise, the power Doppler test is recommended in order to analyse the presence of hypervascularization in the area, as it has been observed in vivo that neovascularization is frequent in subjects with lateral epicondylalgia.[99,100] The test is performed with the subject seated, the forearm supported on the plinth and elbow at 90° flexion and maximal pronation.

The process of assessment and diagnosis in physiotherapy is completed with the functional assessment via orthopaedic tests, such as the Cozen test, the Thomson test, the Mills test, the DASH questionnaire[101] (0–100 points) and the assessment of pain using the VAS and pressure values using digital algometry on the lateral humeral epicondyle.

According to published studies, such as that by Clarke et al.,[102] the affected areas identified using musculoskeletal ultrasound correlate with the patient's clinical findings.

13.4.2.2 Clinical presentations

The most frequent clinical presentations in lateral epicondylalgia are:

- depending on the presence of neovascularization:
  - hypovascular (most frequent)
  - neovascular.
- depending on anatomical localization (figure 13.12):
  - ECRB – deep fascicle
  - at the insertion of the common tendon in the lateral margin of the lateral epicondyle
  - ECRB – articular capsule of the humero-radial joint.

The structural characteristics that predominate are: alteration of the ECRB with presence of focal hypoechoic regions, loss of intratendon continuity, irregularities in the bone cortex and changes in the insertion to the epicondyle.

13.4.2.3 Procedure

The procedure consists of ultrasound-guided application of EPI® via the following commonly used approaches (video 13.2 and figure 13.12):

- Intratendon approach of the ECRB in the deepest plane to the lateral epicondyle. The

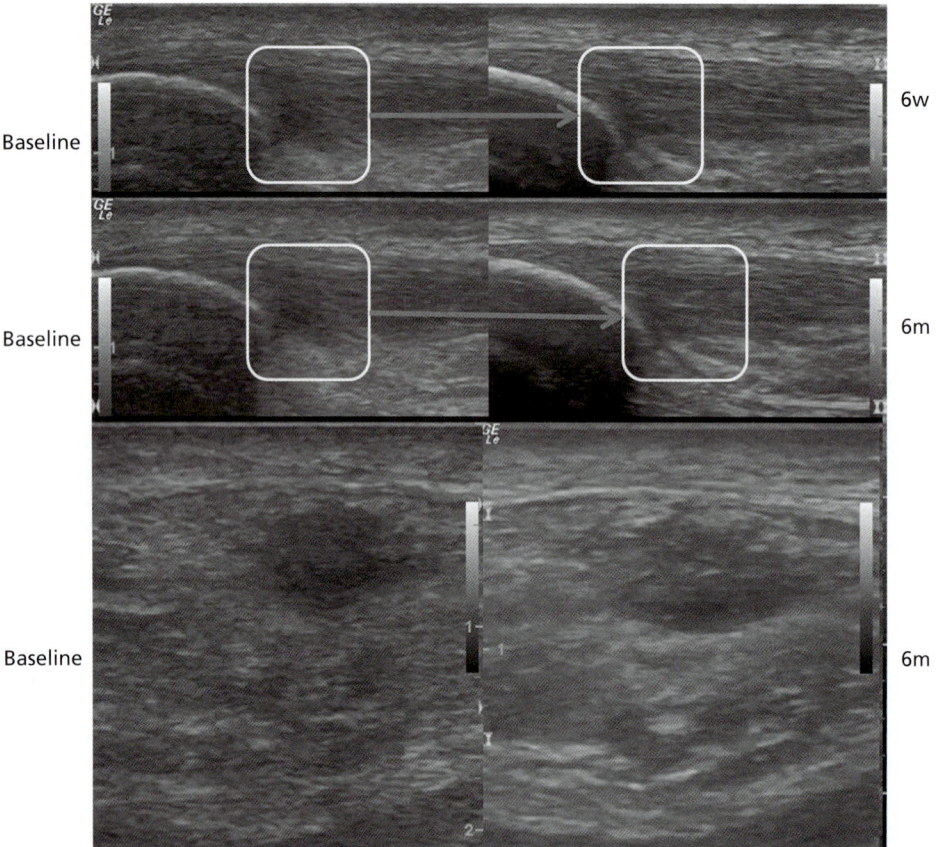

FIGURE 13.11 ■ Changes in the structure of the patellar ligament in the mid and long term. (Colour version of figure is available online).

needle is inserted in the long axis with an orientation of 45–60° from caudal to cranial and slightly from anterior to posterior, seeking the insertion point of the deep fascicle of the tendon.

- Procedural approach on to the insertion of the common extensor tendon. The needle is inserted in the long axis with an orientation of 30° from caudal to cranial, seeking the insertion of the tendon on the lateral epicondyle.
- Procedural approach on to the deep fascicle of the ECRB tendon in relation to the articular capsule of the humeroradial joint in the short axis, entering perpendicularly.

13.4.2.4 Results: scientific and clinical evidence

In a study by Minaya et al.[59] 36 subjects were included (52.8% men and 47.2% women), with an average age of 38 years (SD 6.4). A total of 88.9% of subjects performed a work-related activity with maintained postures or repeated gestures that affected common extensor tendon (such as, for example, administrative workers, plumbers, waiters and firemen) and 75% practised some kind of sport with a mechanical use of these muscles, such as tennis. The duration of the symptoms ranged from 4 to 24 months (average 9.6 months; SD 4.6 months).

13.4.2.5 Short-term findings

After four sessions, 80.5% of subjects ended the initial intervention programme with no pain (score of 2 or less) on the VAS. In 86.2% of subjects, pain was not reproduced in the Cozen or Thomson test and algometric values were significantly raised, with pressure upon the lateral epicondyle changing from 7.9 kg to 29.3 kg. The analysis of functionality according to the DASH questionnaire showed important changes. The average score obtained in all 36 subjects was 37.4 points, which means that an improvement of more than 40% was obtained in functional capacity. None of the subjects abandoned the treatment and no complications or adverse reactions were reported during the application of EPI®.

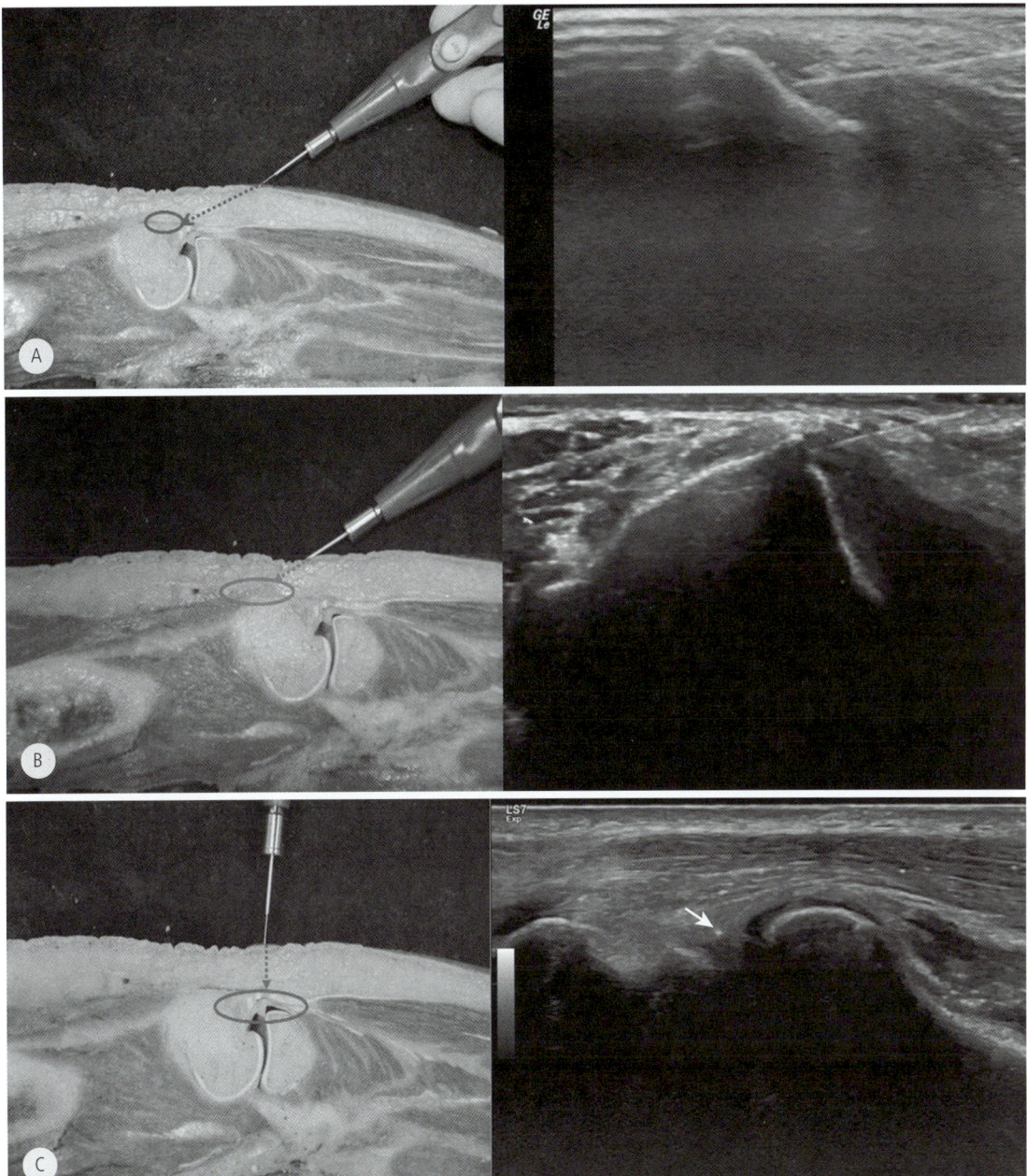

FIGURE 13.12 ■ EPI® technique approaches to the lateral epicondyle region. (A) Tendon of the extensor carpi radialis brevis (ECRB) muscle – deep fascicle. (B) Insertion of the common extensor tendon along the lateral aspect of the lateral epicondyle. (C) ECRB – joint capsule of the humeroradial joint. (Colour version of figure is available online).

Changes in structure were not identified, except regarding hypervascularization; this was eliminated or significantly reduced.

13.4.2.6 Mid- and long-term findings

Analysis in B-mode, Doppler colour and elastography evidenced changes in tendon structure (figures 13.13 and 13.14).

13.4.3 Supraspinatus tendon

Currently, it has been said that one in three people experiment shoulder pain at least once in their life, and approximately half the population experiences shoulder pain at least once a year. The incidence of shoulder pain increases substantially with age, and, for people over 65 years old, shoulder pain is the most common

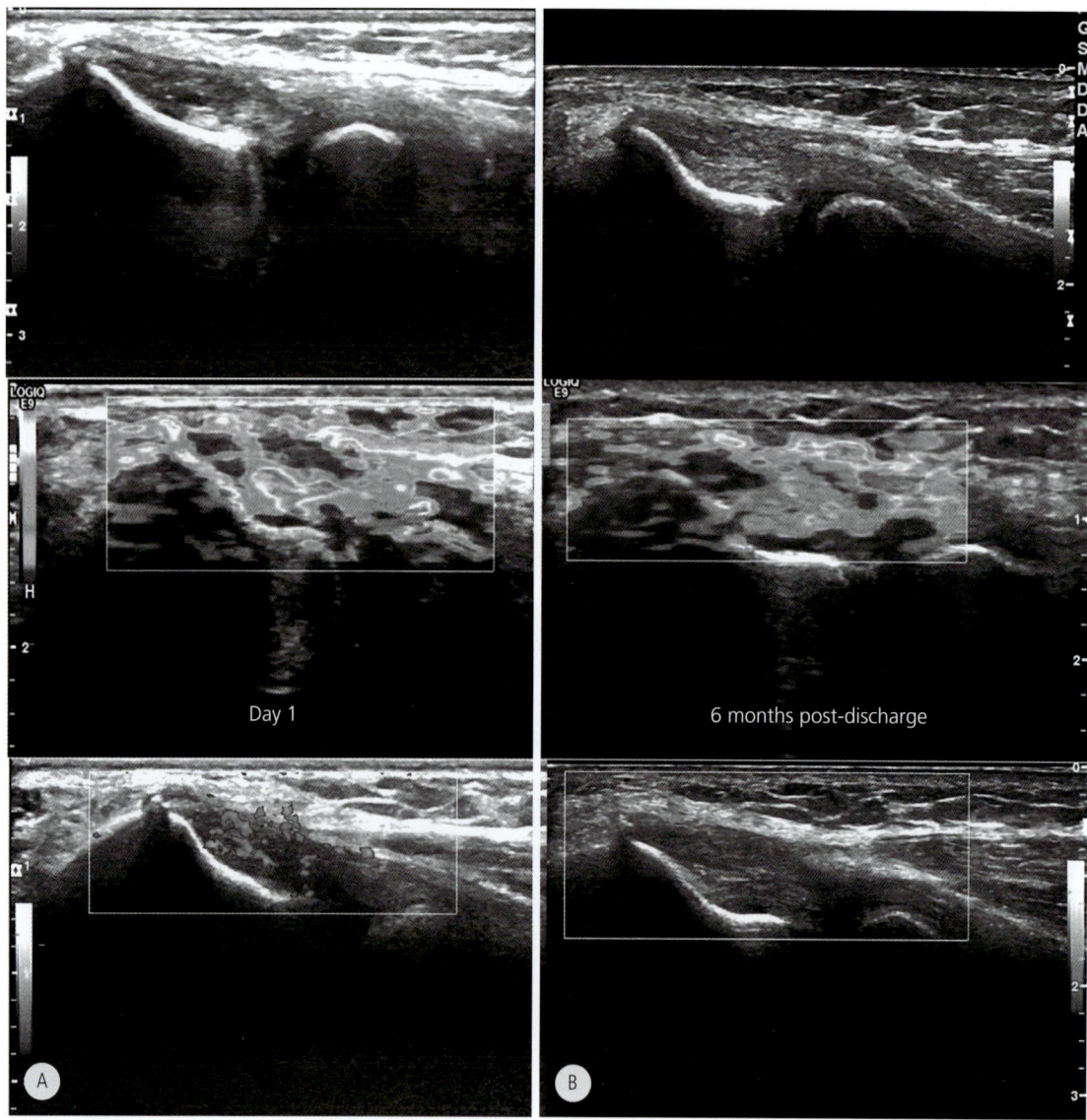

FIGURE 13.13 ■ Changes in the structure of the common extensor tendon in the mid term. (A) B-mode image, sonoelastography and power Doppler at baseline. (B) B-mode image, sonoelastography and power Doppler at 6 months postdischarge.

musculoskeletal problem. The dysfunction in the shoulder is often persistent and recurrent, with 54% having relapses in the following 3 years, postlesion.[102,103]

In relation to the structures implicated in shoulder pain, the rotator cuff and the subacromial bursa are considered the main structural sources of pain. Hashimoto et al.[104] identified diffuse degenerative changes associated with microscopic ruptures in the tendon and infiltration of fibroblasts, vascular hyperplasia-hypervascularization, disorganization of the collagen fibres, calcification and fat infiltration. With the exception of fat infiltration and hypervascularization, the changes were highly evident in the middle and deep planes. On the other hand, in patients with shoulder pain and a degenerated rotator cuff, the presence of collagen type III was observed and deposits of amyloids were found,[104] which could justify the mechanical weakness and irreversible changes of the tendinous tissue. Other authors also found that injuries of the rotator cuff begin where the forces are greater, in other words, in deeper planes, implicating the tendon of the biceps brachii muscle with lesions and patterns of tendon instability affecting the long head of the biceps brachii muscle[105,106] and provoking specific lesions of the biceps pulley (figure 13.15) and the rotator interval (figure 13.16).[106]

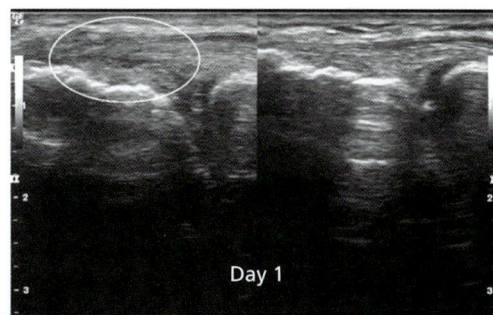

Day 1

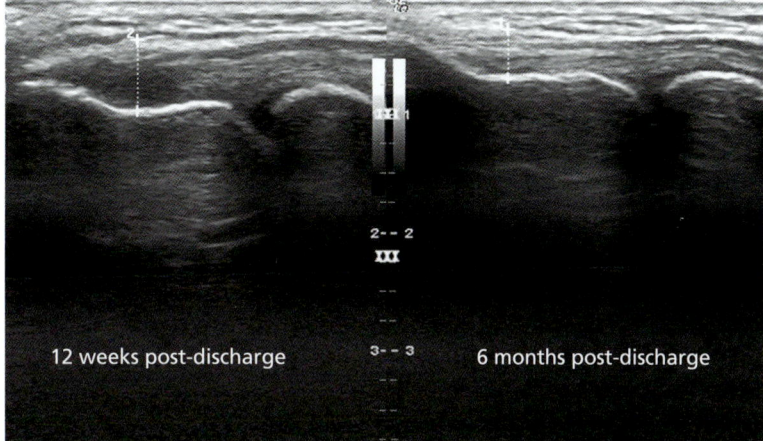

12 weeks post-discharge   6 months post-discharge

FIGURE 13.14 ■ Changes in the structure of the common extensor tendon in the mid and long term.

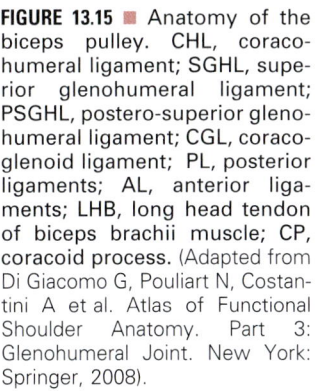

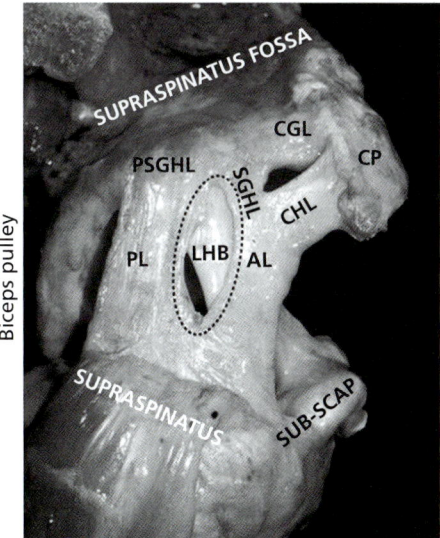

FIGURE 13.15 ■ Anatomy of the biceps pulley. CHL, coracohumeral ligament; SGHL, superior glenohumeral ligament; PSGHL, postero-superior glenohumeral ligament; CGL, coracoglenoid ligament; PL, posterior ligaments; AL, anterior ligaments; LHB, long head tendon of biceps brachii muscle; CP, coracoid process. (Adapted from Di Giacomo G, Pouliart N, Costantini A et al. Atlas of Functional Shoulder Anatomy. Part 3: Glenohumeral Joint. New York: Springer, 2008).

13.4.3.1 Assessment protocol

The assessment protocol for the rotator cuff, according to the *Musculoskeletal Ultrasound Technical Guidelines: Shoulder* of the European Society of Musculoskeletal Radiology,[84] consists in a longitudinal sequence from the proximal origin of the supraspinatus tendon to its insertion in the humerus and transverse sections for assessment of the rotator interval. The subject is seated, with the arm in extension, adduction and external rotation, and the palm of the hand is placed upon the posterior iliac crest.

Similarly, the power Doppler test is recommended in order to assess the presence of hypervascularization in the area.

Complete the patient assessment by testing function via orthopaedic tests such as Neer,

Rotator interval

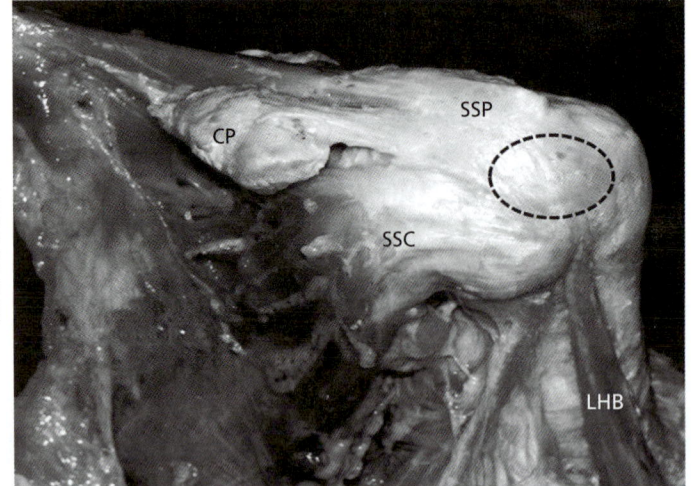

FIGURE 13.16 ■ Anatomy of the rotator interval. CP, coracoid process; LHB, long head tendon of biceps brachii muscle; SSC, subscapular muscle; SSP, supraspinatus muscle; dashed line: rotator interval (pillars anchor the long head tendon of biceps brachii muscle, fibres of the supraspinatus tendon, fibres of the subscapularis tendon and joint capsule). (Adapted from Di Giacomo G, Pouliart N, Costantini A et al. Atlas of Functional Shoulder Anatomy. Part 3: Glenohumeral Joint. New York: Springer, 2008).

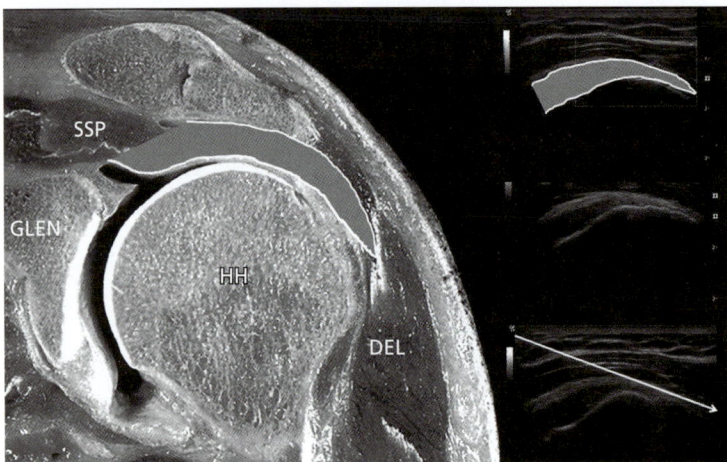

FIGURE 13.17 ■ EPI® treatment approaches on the deep interphase, intratendon and superficial interphase of the supraspinatus tendon. DEL, deltoid muscle; GLEN, glenoid; HH, humerus; SSP, supraspinatus muscle. (Courtesy of Drs Fermín Valera and Francisco Minaya; cadaveric image adapted from Di Giacomo G, Pouliart N, Costantini A et al. Atlas of Functional Shoulder Anatomy. Part 3: Glenohumeral Joint. New York: Springer, 2008).

Hawkins and Kennedy and functional assessment scales such as the Shoulder Pain and Disability Index (SPADI) at baseline and discharge.

13.4.3.2 Clinical presentations

The most frequent clinical presentations in the tendinopathy of the rotator cuff are:
- depending on the presence of neovascularization:
  - hypovascular (most frequent)
  - neovascular.
- depending on the anatomical localization (figure 13.17):
  - supraspinatus
  - rotator interval.

Predominant structural characteristics include alteration in the echotexture of the supraspinatus tendon with hypoechoic focal regions, the presence of calcifications and changes in the enthesis.

13.4.3.3 Procedure

The most frequently used approaches are (video 13.3):
- Approach into the deep interphase, intratendon and superficial interphase of the supraspinatus tendon (figure 13.17). The needle is inserted from the anterosuperior approach with a 40° orientation in a lateral and caudal direction.
- Approach over the rotator interval. Using a fan-shaped application over the fibres of the supraspinatus, the long portion of the biceps and subscapularis (figures 13.18 and 13.19), puncture from cranial to caudal, perpendicular to the structure, or from medial to lateral, or lateral to medial, depending on the tissue affected (see chapter 3).

The application is always performed with ultrasound guidance and the intensity of the

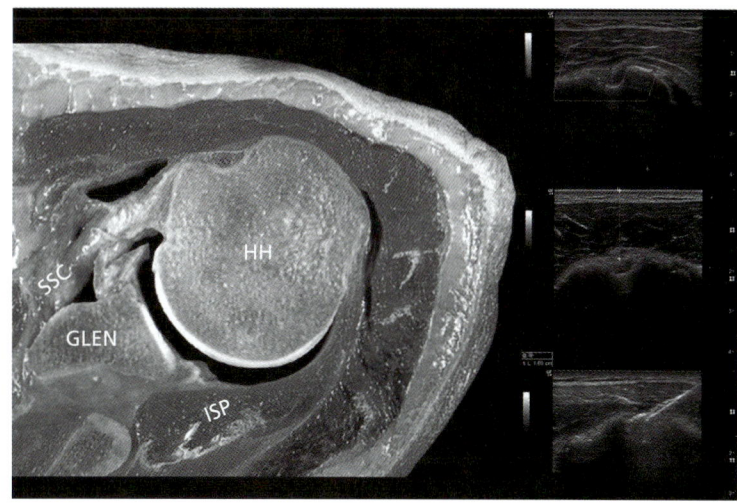

FIGURE 13.18 ■ EPI® treatment approaches on long-head of biceps brachii tendon. CP, coracoid process; SSC, subscapular muscle; SSP, supraspinatus muscle. (Courtesy of Drs Fermín Valera and Francisco Minaya; cadaveric image adapted from Di Giacomo G, Pouliart N, Costantini A et al. Atlas of Functional Shoulder Anatomy. Part 3: Glenohumeral Joint. New York: Springer, 2008).

FIGURE 13.19 ■ EPI® treatment approaches on the rotator interval. SSC, subscapular muscle; GLEN, glenoid; HH, humerus; ISP, infraspinatus. (Courtesy of Drs Fermín Valera and Francisco Minaya; cadaveric image adapted from Di Giacomo G, Pouliart N, Costantini A et al. Atlas of Functional Shoulder Anatomy. Part 3: Glenohumeral Joint. New York: Springer, 2008).

application commonly ranges between 4 and 6 mA for a period of 3–4 seconds.

13.4.3.4 Results – clinical evidence

In a sample of patients from the Valera et al. study,[58] patients were included who had a medical diagnosis of tendinitis of the rotator cuff of more than 3 months' duration, and who had previously performed a conventional physiotherapy treatment programme which had failed to provide adequate functional recovery. Twenty-four subjects were included (70.8% males and 29.2% females). The average age was 42 years. The most frequent clinical localization of degenerative changes (thickening, fibrosis, focal hypoechoic regions, calcifications) was upon the rotator interval and the insertion of the suprasp-

inatus. Hypervascularization was present in 20.8% of cases.

13.4.3.5 Short-term findings

Significant functional improvement was reported in 71% of subjects after three sessions of EPI® (Neer test 83.3% to 16.7%, Hawkins and Kennedy 91.7% to 20.8%, SPADI 78% to 12%) together with a reduction in hypervascularization of the area. No further changes in the structure were identified.

13.4.3.6 Mid- and long-term findings

The analyses in B-mode, Doppler colour and elastography evidenced important changes in the structure of the tendon.

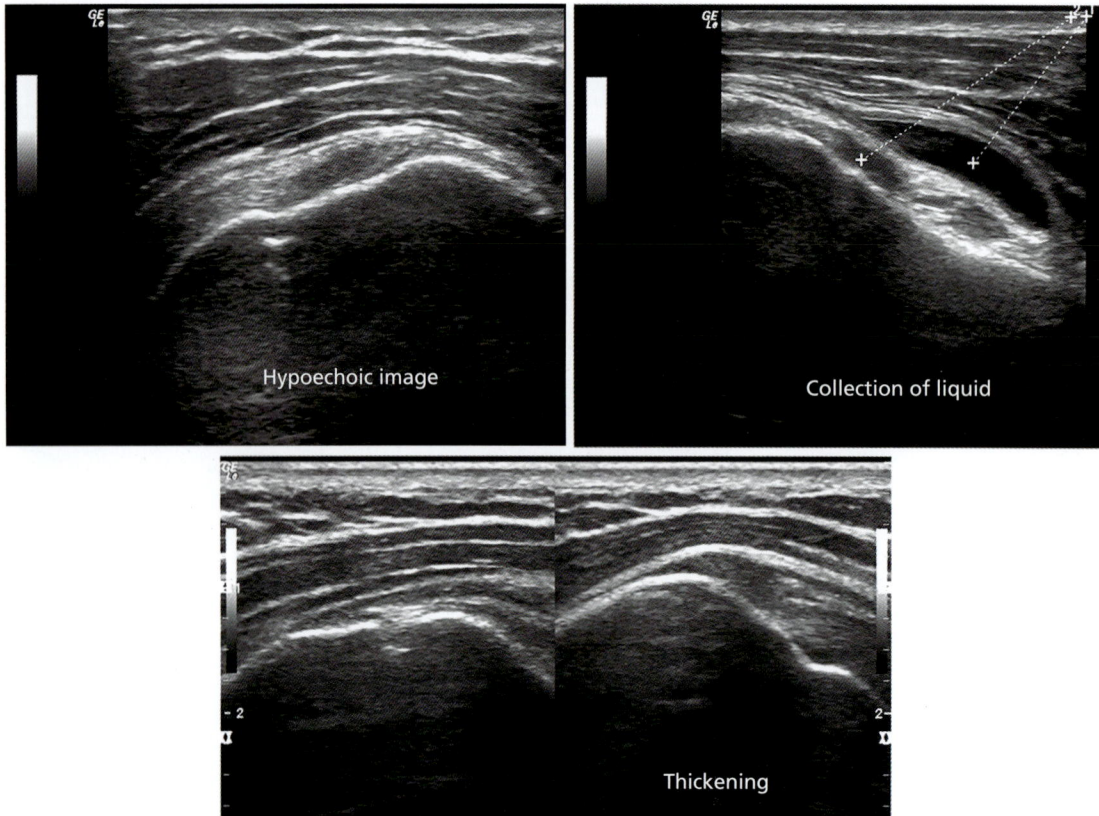

FIGURE 13.20 ■ Rupture of the supraspinatus tendon and tenosynovitis of the long-head tendon of the biceps brachii muscle.

KEY POINTS

The EPI® technique for the treatment of tendinopathy provokes changes in function in the short term and changes in tendon structure in the mid and long term.

13.5 CLINICAL CASE

This case involved treatment of rupture of the supraspinatus tendon and tenosynovitis of the long head tendon of the biceps brachii muscle using EPI®[105] (figure 13.20).

Injuries affecting the rotator cuff are highly frequent and prevalent in the workplace and sports and are characterized by frequent relapses that can easily become chronic. Traditionally, alterations in the rotator cuff have been defined, diagnosed and treated as an inflammatory process affecting the tendon insertions. However, several studies have now demonstrated that these are, in fact, associated with a degenerative process in microscopic ruptures in the tendon and infiltration of fibroblasts, vascular hyperplasia-hypervascularization and disorganization of the collagen fibres, compatible with the concept of tendinosis. This change of paradigm requires modification of the conventional approach from an inflammatory perspective towards treatment of the degenerative condition.

Reason for consultation: the patient has a medical diagnosis of partial rupture of the supraspinatus tendon and tenosynovitis of the long head of the biceps brachii muscle who attends the physiotherapy service of MVClinic-Madrid for assessment and treatment due to the presentation of a case resistant to any type of treatment and as a last treatment option before considering surgery.

History of the problem: male, 34 years, right-handed, fireman, who regularly trains doing body building at a gym with a case of pain in the right shoulder which he has suffered for 18 months and which he associates with the performance of a push-up during which an audible click was heard in the anterior aspect of the shoulder. Prior to his visit, he had attended various conventional physiotherapy programmes (e.g. therapeutic ultrasound, laser, Cyriax massage), tried pharmacological treatment and received three corticoid infiltrations (the last one more than 6 months previously with a minimal improvement in pain), without reaching adequate functional recovery.

Diagnostic tests: the patient brought a magnetic resonance image scan with the result of 'partial tendon rupture of the supraspinatus and tenosynovitis of the long head tendon of the biceps brachii muscle'.

Physiotherapy diagnosis: at the first visit, an analysis of the structure and function of the patient was performed. The structure of the rotator cuff and the biceps brachii was assessed with musculoskeletal ultrasound (portable ultrasound Logiq-E® by General Electric with a linear 12L-RS, 5–13 MHz probe), which showed signs of degeneration in the insertion of the supraspinatus tendon (thickening of the tendon and hypoechoic areas), plus a considerable collection of liquid in the pathway of the biceps brachii tendon of the biceps brachii muscle, at the level of the bicipital groove, with signs of hypervascularization at this level. Patient function was assessed with the SPADI questionnaire, the Neer orthopaedic test (+), the Hawkins and Kennedy test (+) and pain was found on palpation of the insertion area of the supraspinatus tendon, with a limitation of the internal rotation of the arm affecting the last 15° in the frontal plane. The asymptomatic tendon (contralateral) was considered the control.

(Clinical case continued on pages 489-490)

13.6 REFERENCES

1. Cook JL, Purdam CR. Is tendon pathology a continuum? A pathology model to explain the clinical presentation of load-induced tendinopathy. Br J Sports Med 2009;43:409–16.
2. Alfredson H, Ljung BO, Thorsen K, et al. In vivo investigation of ECRB tendons with microdialysis technique – no signs of inflammation but high amounts of glutamate in tennis elbow. Acta Orthop Scand 2000; 71(5):475–9.
3. Puddu G, Ippolito E, Postacchini F. A classification of Achilles tendon disease. Am J Sports Med 1976;4(4): 145–50.
4. Maffulli N, Khan KM, Puddu G. Overuse tendon conditions: time to change a confusing terminology. Arthroscopy 1998;14(8):840–3.
5. Fu SC, Rolf C, Cheuk YC, et al. Deciphering the pathogenesis of tendinopathy: a three-stages process. Sports Med Arthrosc Rehabil Ther Technol 2010; 2:30.
6. Khan KM, Cook JL, Kannus P, et al. Time to abandon the 'tendinitis' myth. BMJ 2002;324(7338):626–7.
7. Coombes BK, Bisset L, Vicenzino B. A new integrative model of lateral epicondylalgia. Br J Sports Med 2009; 43:252–8.
8. Khan KM, Cook JL, Bonar F, et al. Histopathology of common tendinopathies. Update and implications for clinical management. Sports Med 1999;27:393–408.
9. Alfredson H, Forsgren S, Thorsen K, et al. In vivo microdialysis and immunohistochemical analyses of tendon tissue demonstrated high amounts of free glutamate and glutamate NMDAR1 receptors, but no signs of inflammation, in Jumper's knee. J Orthop Res 2001; 19(5):881–6.
10. Abate M, Gravare-Silbernagel K, Siljeholm C, et al. Pathogenesis of tendinopathies: inflammation or degeneration? Arthritis Res Ther 2009;11(3):1–15.
11. Lian Ø, Dahl J, Ackermann PW, et al. Pronociceptive and antinociceptive neuromediators in patellar tendinopathy. Am J Sports Med 2006;34(11): 1801–8.
12. Fredberg U, Stengaard-Pedersen K. Chronic tendinopathy tissue pathology, pain mechanisms, and etiology with a special focus on inflammation. Scand J Med Sci Sports 2008;18:3–15.
13. Kader D, Saxena A, Movin T, et al. Achilles tendinopathy: some aspects of basic science and clinical management. Br J Sports Med 2002;36(4):239–49.
14. Józsa L, Kannus P. Human tendon: anatomy, physiology and pathology. Champaign: Human Kinetics; 1997.
15. Józsa L, Kannus P. Histopathological findings in spontaneous tendon ruptures. Scand J Med Sci Sports 1997; 7(2):113–18.
16. Kannus P. Etiology and pathophysiology of chronic tendon disorders in sports. Scand J Med Sci Sports 1997;7(2):78–85.
17. de Mos M, Koevoet W, van Schie HT, et al. In vitro model to study chondrogenic differentiation in tendinopathy. Am J Sports Med 2009;37(6):1214–22.
18. Langberg H, Boushel R, Skovgaard D, et al. Cyclooxygenase-2 mediated prostaglandin release regulates blood flow in connective tissue during mechanical loading in humans. J Physiol 2003;551(Pt 2):683–9.
19. Kumagai J, Uhthoff HK, Sarkar K, et al. Collagen type III in rotator cuff tears: An immunohistochemical study. J Shoulder Elbow Surg 1992;1(4):187–92.
20. Scott A, Lian Ø, Roberts CR, et al. Increased versican content is associated with tendinosis pathology in the patellar tendon of athletes with jumper's knee. Scand J Med Sci Sports 2008;18(4):427–35.
21. Seitz AL, McClure PW, Finucane S, et al. Mechanisms of rotator cuff tendinopathy: intrinsic, extrinsic, or both? Clin Biomech (Bristol, Avon) 2011;26(1):1–12.
22. Lyman J, Weinhold PS, Almekinders LC. Strain behavior of the distal Achilles tendon: implications for insertional Achilles tendinopathy. Am J Sports Med 2004; 32(2):457–61.
23. Khan KM, Maffulli N, Coleman BD, et al. Patellar tendinopathy: some aspects of basic science and clinical management. Br J Sports Med 1998;32(4): 346–55.
24. Birch HL, Rutter GA, Goodship AE. Oxidative energy metabolism in equine tendon cells. Res Vet Sci 1997; 62(2):93–7.
25. Wren TA, Lindsey DP, Beaupré GS, et al. Effects of creep and cyclic loading on the mechanical properties and failure of human Achilles tendons. Ann Biomed Eng 2003;31(6):710–17.
26. Langberg H, Ellingsgaard H, Madsen T, et al. Eccentric rehabilitation exercise increases peritendinous type I collagen synthesis in humans with Achilles tendinosis. Scand J Med Sci Sports 2007;17(1):61–6.
27. Ying M, Yeung E, Li B, et al. Sonographic evaluation of the size of Achilles tendon: the effect of exercise and dominance of the ankle. Ultrasound Med Biol 2003; 29(5):637–42.
28. Corps AN, Jones GC, Harrall RL, et al. The regulation of aggrecanase ADAMTS-4 expression in human Achilles tendon and tendon-derived cells. Matrix Biol 2008;27(5):393–401.

29. McLoughlin RF, Raber EL, Vellet AD, et al. Patellar tendinitis: MR imaging features, with suggested pathogenesis and proposed classification. Radiology 1995; 197(3):843–8.

30. Wang JH, Iosifidis MI, Fu FH. Biomechanical basis for tendinopathy. Clin Orthop Relat Res 2006;443: 320–32.

31. Khan KM, Visentini PJ, Kiss ZS, et al. Correlation of ultrasound and magnetic resonance imaging with clinical outcome after patellar tenotomy: prospective and retrospective studies. Victorian Institute of Sport Tendon Study Group. Clin J Sport Med 1999;9(3): 129–37.

32. Cook JL, Khan KM, Harcourt PR, et al. Patellar tendon ultrasonography in asymptomatic active athletes reveals hypoechoic regions: a study of 320 tendons. Victorian Institute of Sport Tendon Study Group. Clin J Sport Med 1998;8(2):73–7.

33. Alfredson H, Thorsen K, Lorentzon R. In situ microdialysis in tendon tissue: high levels of glutamate, but not prostaglandin E2 in chronic Achilles tendon pain. Knee Surg Sports Traumatol Arthrosc 1999;7(6): 378–81.

34. Molloy TJ, Kemp MW, Wang Y, et al. Microarray analysis of the tendinopathic rat supraspinatus tendon: glutamate signaling and its potential role in tendon degeneration. J Appl Physiol 2006;101(6):1702–9.

35. Jelinsky SA, Lake SP, Archambault JM, et al. Gene expression in rat supraspinatus tendon recovers from overuse with rest. Clin Orthop Relat Res 2008;466(7): 1612–17.

36. Bagge J, Lorentzon R, Alfredson H, et al. Unexpected presence of the neurotrophins NGF and BDNF and the neurotrophin receptor p75 in the tendon cells of the human Achilles tendon. Histol Histopathol 2009; 24(7):839–48.

37. Danielson P, Alfredson H, Forsgren S. Distribution of general (PGP 9.5) and sensory (substance P/CGRP) innervations in the human patellar tendon. Knee Surg Sports Traumatol Arthrosc 2006;14(2):125–32.

38. Alfredson H, Bjur D, Thorsen K, et al. High intratendinous lactate levels in painful chronic Achilles tendinosis. An investigation using microdialysis technique. J Orthop Res 2002;20(5):934–8.

39. Bjur D, Danielson P, Alfredson H, et al. Presence of a non-neuronal cholinergic system and occurrence of up- and down-regulation in expression of M2 muscarinic acetylcholine receptors: new aspects of importance regarding Achilles tendon tendinosis (tendinopathy). Cell Tissue Res 2008;331(2):385–400.

40. Andersson G, Danielson P, Alfredson H, et al. Presence of substance P and the neurokinin-1 receptor in tenocytes of the human Achilles tendon. Regul Pept 2008; 150(1–3):81–7.

41. Scott A, Lian Ø, Bahr R, et al. Increased mast cell numbers in human patellar tendinosis: correlation with symptom duration and vascular hyperplasia. Br J Sports Med 2008;42(9):753–7.

42. Duchesne E, Tremblay MH, Côté CH. Mast cell tryptase stimulates myoblast proliferation; a mechanism relying on protease-activated receptor-2 and cyclooxygenase-2. BMC Musculoskelet Disord 2011; 12:235.

43. Danielson P, Andersson G, Alfredson H, et al. Marked sympathetic component in the perivascular innervation of the dorsal paratendinous tissue of the patellar tendon in arthroscopically treated tendinosis patients. Knee Surg Sports Traumatol Arthrosc 2008;16(6):621–6.

44. Assimacopoulos D. Wound healing promotion by the use of negative electric current. Am Surg 1968;34(6): 423–31.

45. Huttenlocher A, Horwitz AR. Wound healing with electric potential. N Engl J Med 2007;356(3): 303–4.

46. McCaig CD, Rajnicek AM, Song B, et al. Controlling cell behavior electrically: current views and future potential. Physiol Rev 2005;85(3):943–78.

47. Jaffe LF, Vanable JW Jr. Electric fields and wound healing. Clin Dermatol 1984;2(3):34–44.

48. Soong HK, Parkinson WC, Sulik GL, et al. Effects of electric fields on cytoskeleton of corneal stromal fibroblasts. Curr Eye Res 1990;9(9):893–901.

49. Cheng N, Van Hoof H, Bockx E, et al. The effects of electric currents on ATP generation, protein synthesis, and membrane transport of rat skin. Clin Orthop Relat Res 1982;171:264–72.

50. Kloth LC. Electrical stimulation for wound healing: a review of evidence from in vitro studies, animal experiments, and clinical trials. Int J Low Extrem Wounds 2005;4(1):23–44.

51. Bourguignon GJ, Jy W, Bourguignon LY. Electric stimulation of human fibroblasts causes an increase in Ca2+ influx and the exposure of additional insulin receptors. J Cell Physiol 1989;140(2):379–85.

52. Franke K, Gruler H. Galvanotaxis of human granulocytes: electric field jump studies. EurBiophys J 1990; 18(6):335–46.

53. Cook JL, Khan KM, Kiss ZS, et al. Asymptomatic hypoechoic regions on patellar tendon ultrasound: A 4-year clinical and ultrasound follow up of 46 tendons. Scand J Med Sci Sports 2001;11(6):321–7.

54. Hoksrud A, Bahr R. Ultrasound-guided sclerosing treatment in patients with patellar tendinopathy (jumper's knee). 44-month follow-up. Am J Sports Med 2011;39(11):2377–80.

55. Hinz S, Egberts JH, Pauser U, et al. Electrolytic ablation is as effective as radiofrequency ablation in the treatment of artificial liver metastases in a pig model. J Surg Oncol 2008;98(2):135–8.

56. Hägglund M, Zwerver J, Ekstrand J. Epidemiology of patellar tendinopathy in elite male soccer players. Am J Sports Med 2011;39(9):1906–11.

57. Cook JL, Khan KM, Kiss ZS, et al. Patellar tendinopathy in junior basketball players: a controlled clinical and ultrasonographic study of 268 patellar tendons in players aged 14–18 years. Scand J Med Sci Sports 2000;10(4):216–20.

58. Valera F, Minaya F, Sánchez JM, et al. Mitos y realidades en fisioterapia. Tendinitis vs. Tendinosis. In: I Congreso Internacional EPI®: Ponencias y Comunicaciones. Madrid: 2011. p. 100–1.

59. Minaya F, Valera F, Sánchez JM, et al. Estudio de coste-efectividad de la electrólisis percutánea intratisular (EPI®) en las epicondialgias. Fisioterapia: revista de salud, discapacidad y terapéuticafísica 2012;34(5): 208–15.

60. Gott M, Ast M, Lane LB, et al. Tendon phenotype should dictate tissue engineering modality in tendon repair: a review. Discov Med 2011;12(62):75–84.

61. Dye SF. Functional morphologic features of the human knee: an evolutionary perspective. Clin Orthop Relat Res 2003;410:19–24.

62. Valera F, Minaya F, Sánchez JM. Efectividad de la Electrólisis Percutánea Intratisular (EPI®) en las tendinopatías crónicas del tendón rotuliano. Trauma Fund MAPFRE 2010;21(4):227 36.

63. Tonks JH, Pai SK, Murali SR. Steroid injection therapy is the best conservative treatment for lateral epicondylitis: a prospective randomised controlled trial. Int J Clin Pract 2007;61:240–6.

64. Barr S, Cerisola FL, Blanchard V. Effectiveness of corticosteroid injections compared with physiotherapeutic

interventions for lateral epicondylitis: a systematic review. Physiotherapy 2009;95(4):251–65.

65. Minaya-Muñoz F, Valera-Garrido F, Sánchez-Ibáñez JM, et al. Short- and long-term outcomes of Intratissue Percutaneous Electrolysis (EPI® technique)in lateral epicondylitis. In: 2nd International Scientific Tendinopathy Symposium. Vancouver: Department of Physical Therapy, University of British Columbia; 2012.

66. Virchenko O, Aspenberg P. How can one platelet injection after tendon injury lead to a stronger tendon after 4 weeks? Interplay between early regeneration and mechanical stimulation. Acta Orthop 2006;77:806–12.

67. Finestone H, Rabinovitch DL. Tennis elbow no more: practical eccentric and concentric exercises to heal the pain. Can Fam Physician 2008;54(8):1115–16.

68. Stasinopoulos D, Stasinopoulou K, Stasinopoulos I, et al. Comparison of effects of a home exercise programme and a supervised exercise programme for the management of lateral elbow tendinopathy. Br J Sports Med 2010;44(8):579–83.

69. Malliaras P, Maffulli N, Garau G. Eccentric training programmes in the management of lateral elbow tendinopathy. Disabil Rehabil 2008;30(20–22):1590–6.

70. Croisier JL, Foidart-Dessalle M, Tinant F, et al. An isokinetic eccentric programme for the management of chronic lateral epicondyle artendinopathy. Br J Sports Med 2007;41(4):269–75.

71. Minaya F, Valera F, Sánchez JM. Uso de la electrólisis percutánea intratisular (EPI®) en la epicondilagia crónica: caso clínico. Fisiotercalidvida 2011;14(1):13–16.

72. Thanasas C, Papadimitriou G, Charalambidis C, et al. Platelet-rich plasma versus autologous whole blood for the treatment of chronic lateral elbow epicondylitis: a randomized controlled clinical trial. Am J Sports Med 2011;39:2130–4.

73. Haraldsson BT, Aagaard P, Crafoord-Larsen D, et al. Corticosteroid administration alters the mechanical properties of isolated collagen fascicles in rat-tail tendón. Scand J Med Sci Sports 2009;19:621–6.

74. Haraldsson BT, Langberg H, Aagaard P, et al. Corticosteroids reduce the tensile strength of isolated collagen fascicles. Am J Sports Med 2006;34:1992–7.

75. Haraldsson BT, Aagaard P, Krogsgaard M, et al. Region-specific mechanical properties of the human patella tendon. J Appl Physiol 2005;98:1006–12.

76. Halpern AA, Horowitz BG, Nagel DA. Tendon ruptures associated with corticosteroid therapy. West J Med 1977;127:378–82.

77. Wong MW, Tang YN, Fu SC, et al. Triamcinolone suppresses human tenocyte cellular activity and collagen synthesis. Clin Orthop Relat Res 2004;277–81.

78. Papaspiliopoulos A, Papaparaskeva K, Papadopoulou E, et al. The effect of local use of nandrolonedecanoate on rotator cuff repair in rabbits. J Invest Surg 2010;23(4):204–7.

79. Ramos L, Teixeira de Carvalho R, Garms E, et al. Prevalence of pain on palpation of the inferior pole of the patella among patients with complains of knee pain. Clinics 2009;64(3):199–202.

80. Blazina ME, Kerlan RK, Jobe FW, et al. Jumper's knee. Orthop Clin North Am 1973;4:665–78.

81. Lian OB, Engebretsen L, Bahr R. Prevalence of jumper's knee among elite athletes from different sports: a cross-sectional study. Am J Sports Med 2005;33:561–7.

82. Khan KM, Cook JL, Taunton JE, et al. Overuse tendinosis, not tendinitis part 1: a new paradigm for a difficult clinical problem. Phys Sports Med 2000;28(5):38–48.

83. Ferretti A, Papandrea P, Conteduca F. Knee injuries in volleyball. Sports Med 1990;10:132–8.

84. Beggs I, Bianchi S, Bueno A, et al. ESSR Ultrasound Group Protocols. Musculoskeletal Ultrasound Technical Guidelines: Knee. 2012. <http://www.essr.org/html/img/pool/knee.pdf>; [Accessed: 1 sept. 2012.].

85. Gisslen K, Alfredson H. Neovascularisation and pain in jumper's knee: a prospective clinical and sonographic study in elite junior volleyball players. Br J Sports Med 2005;39:423–8.

86. Cook JL, Ptazsnik R, Kiss ZS, et al. High reproducibility of patellar tendon vascularity assessed by colour Doppler ultrasonography: a reliable measurement tool for quantifying tendon pathology. Br J Sports Med 2005;39:700–3.

87. Cook JL, Malliaras P, De Luca J, et al. Neovascularization and pain in abnormal patellar tendons of active jumping athletes. Clin J Sports Med 2004;14(5):296–9.

88. Malliaras P, Purdam C, Maffulli N, et al. Temporal sequence of greyscale ultrasound changes and their relationship with neovascularity and pain in the patellar tendon. Br J Sports Med 2010.

89. Visentini PJ, Khan KM, Cook JL, et al. The VISA score: an index of severity of symptoms in patients with jumper's knee (patellar tendinosis). J Sci Med Sport 1998;1:22–8.

90. Sánchez-Ibáñez JM. Ultrasound guided percutaneous electrolysis (EPI®) in patients with chronic insertional patellar tendinopathy: a pilot study. Knee Surg Sports Traumatol Arthrosc 2008;16:220–1.

91. Sánchez-Sánchez J. Estudio comparativo de un tratamiento fisioterápicoconvencional con uno que incluye la técnica de Electrólisis Percutánea Intratisular (EPI®) en pacientes con tendinopatía crónica del tendón rotuliano (doctoral theis). Salamanca: Universidad de Salamanca; 2011.

92. Scher D, Wolf J. Lateral epicondylitis. Orthopedics 2009;32(4):276–82.

93. Faro F, Wolf JM. Lateral epicondylitis: review and current concepts. J Hand Surg [Am] 2007;32:1271–9.

94. Jobe FW, Ciccotti MG. Lateral and medial epicondylitis of the elbow. J Am Acad Orthop Surg 1994;2:1–8.

95. Bishai SK, Plancher KD. The basic science of lateral epicondylosis: update for the future. Tech Orthop 2006;21:250–5.

96. Chen J, Wang A, Xu J, et al. In chronic lateral epicondylitis, apoptosis and autophagic cell death occur in the extensor carpi radialis brevis tendon. J Shoulder Elbow Surg 2010;19:355362.

97. Smith J, Wright A. The effect of selective blockade of myelinated afferent neurons on mechanical hyperalgesia in lateral epicondylalgia. Pain Clin 1993;6:9–16.

98. Sasaki K, Tamakawa M, Onda K, et al. The detection of the capsular tear at the undersurface of the extensor carpi radialis brevis tendon in chronic tennis elbow: the value MRI and CTA. J Shoulder Elbow Surg 2011;20:420–5.

99. Beggs I, Bianchi S, Bueno A, et al. ESSR Ultrasound Group Protocols. Musculoskeletal Ultrasound Technical Guidelines: Knee. <http://www.essr.org/html/img/pool/knee.pdf>; [Accessed: 1 sept. 2012.].

100. Poltawski L, Jayaram V, Watson T. measurement issues in the sonographic assessment of tennis elbow. J Clin Ultrasound 2010;38(4):196–204.

101. Hervás M, Navarro Collado MJ, Peiró S, et al. Versión española del cuestionario DASH. Adaptación transcultural, fiabilidad, validez y sensibilidad a los cambios. Med Clin (Barc) 2006;127(12):441–7.

102. Clarke AW, Ahmad M, Curtis M, et al. Lateral elbow tendinopathy. Correlation of ultrasound findings with

pain and functional disability. Am J Sports Med 2010; 38(6):1209–14.

103. Lewis JS. Rotator cuff tendinophaty. Br J Sports Med 2009;43:236–41.

104. Hashimoto T, Nobuhara K, Hamada T. Pathologic evidence of degeneration as a primary cause of rotator cuff tear. Clin Orthop Relat Res 2003;415:111–20.

105. Cole AS, Cordiner-Lawrie S, Carr AJ, et al. Localised deposition of amyloid in tears of the rotator cuff. J Bone Joint Surg Br 2001;83:561–4.

106. Minaya F, Valera F, Sánchez JM. Tratamiento de la rotura del tendón del supraespinoso y la tenosinovitis del bíceps braquial con Electrólisis Percutánea Intratisular (EPI®): caso clínico. In: II Congreso Regional de fisioterapia de la Universidad de Murcia. Libro de comunicaciones y ponencias. Murcia; 2012.

INTRATISSUE PERCUTANEOUS ELECTROLYSIS (EPI® TECHNIQUE) IN MUSCLE INJURIES

José Manuel Sánchez Ibáñez • Fernando Polidori • Ferrán Abat González •
Francisco Minaya Muñoz • Fermín Valera Garrido

Secret science is no science.
WARREN BURKETT

KEYWORDS

Intratissue Percutaneous Electrolysis (EPI®); eccentric exercise; muscle injury; healing process; myofascial trigger point.

14.1 INTRODUCTION

There are four fundamental types of tissues in the human body: epithelial, connective, muscular and nervous. All of these body tissues can be described as soft tissues, except for bone. Soft tissue is defined as the matrix of the human body, composed of cellular elements within a ground substance. The soft tissue is the most common site of functional impairment in the musculoskeletal system and, therefore, most sports injuries affect these tissues.[1]

However, why do muscle injuries occur? Scientific research has attempted to respond to this question, but with little overall consensus. Inadequate training and warm-up, prior injuries followed by inadequate recovery, prior injuries with the formation of a fibrous scar, fatigue, lack of flexibility and prolonged exposure to cold seem to be the most documented variables in the scientific literature to date.[2]

Ekstrand et al.[3] performed a study with 51 UEFA football teams, with a sample of $n = 2299$ and follow-up from 2001 to 2009. This study found that muscle injuries represent up to 31% of all sports lesions. Of these, 92% affect the four large muscle groups of the lower limb. These are: hamstring muscles (37% of all injuries), adductors (23%), quadriceps (19%) and triceps surae (13%) muscles. Relapses are responsible for extending the total rest period and the incidence of muscle injuries increases with age. When the different muscle groups were analysed, an increase in the incidence of muscle injuries with ageing was only found in injuries of the triceps surae muscle, and not for the quadriceps and hamstring muscles or for the muscles of the hip and pelvis.

In this chapter, the physiopathology of healing will be described, together with the different mechanisms of repair and regeneration of skeletal muscle injury. The aim of this chapter is for physiotherapists to be able to design, apply and supervise a functional recovery programme based on the physiological response of the tissues to the lesion and its healing mechanisms.

In order to achieve optimal patient recovery, the following general objectives must be considered (figure 14.1):

- control of the inflammatory process
- alleviation of pain
- optimization of the regeneration/repair process
- maintenance of cardiovascular resistance
- restoration of joint mobility
- restoration of the flexibility of the soft tissues
- recovery of muscular strength
- increased muscular resistance
- improvement of proprioception and neuromuscular control
- increased functionality of the individual (walking, jumping, running)
- development of biomechanical patterns related to the sport technique.

On the other hand, in order to achieve a correct evolutive healing process, it is important to design a series of specific objectives that should be prioritized when planning a physiotherapy intervention for muscular lesions. These are:

- improvement of symptoms
- promotion of early restoration of the individual's function
- achievement of regeneration versus repair
- prevention of relapses.

14.1.1 Repair versus regeneration

Repair of the biological tissue is the restoration or replacement of the tissue which has lost its original architecture or function. This is a transformation that occurs spontaneously and the final result is formation of a scar or a fibrous scar. As the tissue does not completely recover to its original state, its mechanical and physical properties become inferior. On the other hand, regeneration is restoration of the tissue with the development of properties that are indistinguishable from that of the original tissue. The capacity for regeneration is limited to only select tissues.

Considering these two distinctions, the physiotherapist must seek to promote regeneration over repair, although both processes occur simultaneously in the presence of a soft-tissue injury.

One of the main issues to be dealt with in physiotherapy is the identification of the cellular and molecular differences that exist between regeneration (new tissue) and repair (scarring). The circumstances under which a tissue scars instead of regenerating depend on the content of the cells and the presence of stimulating cells necessary for regeneration.

One prerequisite for regeneration is the potential for cell division. This depends on the type of cell according to its capacity for division (unstable, stable and permanent), and therefore not all differentiated cell populations are subject

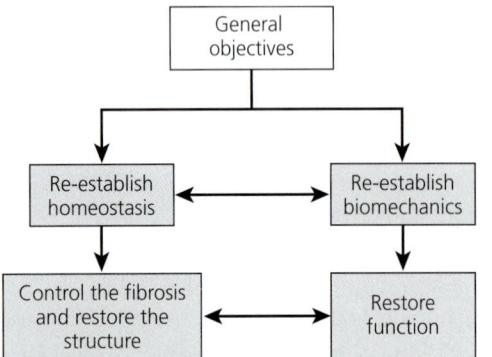

FIGURE 14.1 ■ General objectives for achieving optimal patient recovery.

TABLE 14.1   **The different growth factors have a specific action on the cell depending on specific cell receptors**

Growth factor	Fibroblast proliferation	Extracellular matrix synthesis	Neovascularization
Vascular endothelial growth factor (VEGF)	?	–	++
Platelet-derived growth factor (PDGF)	++	+	*
Transforming growth factor-beta (TGF-beta)	+/–	++	*
Type 1 insulinic growth factor (IGF-I)	+	++	–

? uncertain; – no effect or negative effect; +: increase; ++ substantial increase; * indirect effect.
Adapted from Anitua.[7]

to regeneration. For example, permanent cells cannot be substituted if they are lost. They have a long life, which is why they live in protected environments (which is the case for most nervous cells). However, most differentiated cells are not permanent but rather are periodically renewed. The new cells can originate in two ways: either by simple duplication of pre-existing cells (which divide, forming child cells of the same type), or via a process of differentiation from undifferentiated mother cells, which implies a change in cellular phenotype.[4] The renovation time varies according to the type of tissue, and can be as short as 1 week or as long as 1 year. Many tissues with very slow renewal kinetics can be stimulated in order to produce new cells at a higher speed. An example of this is the endothelial cells of the blood vessels. These cells renew themselves via duplication and their turnover is very slow; however they can regenerate rapidly when damaged. In other words, the cell loss stimulates proliferation via a haemodynamic mechanism. The new capillaries are formed via gemmation (angiogenesis) and growth of the capillary network is controlled by the factors liberated by the neighbouring tissues.

The bone medulla is the source of precursor cells that are capable of differentiating themselves into the different cell types: osteoblasts, chondroblasts and myoblasts. The different types of differentiated cells must maintain the correct proportions and the correct position and, in order to maintain this order, there must be communication signals between the different cells. The cellular signs are determined by certain cytokines and growth factors.[5] These proteins are sent from one cell to another in order to transmit a correct migration signal, differentiation and/or activation signal. From a functional point of view, these growth factors can be differentiated into two types:

- autocrine growth factors: these interact with the autoreceptors of the same cell that synthesizes them

- paracrine growth factors: these act upon another adjacent or distant cell.

The growth factors are the main biological mediators that regulate key occurrences in tissue repair, such as cell proliferation, chemotaxis (directed cellular migration), cellular differentiation and synthesis of the extracellular matrix. The union of the growth factors with their specific membrane receptors triggers biological actions, transforming this extracellular event (the union of the ligand with its receptor) into an intracellular event. A stimulus is transmitted into the interior of the cell, where the signal is amplified and specifically channelled.[6] The amplification of the signal implies a large spectrum of enzymes with specialized functions.

Currently growth factors are recognized as being multifunctional. In other words, they can, on the one hand, stimulate the proliferation of certain cells, and on the other, inhibit the proliferation of others. They can also cause undesirable effects, unrelated to the proliferation, in other types of cells[7] (table 14.1).

14.1.2 Physiological regeneration mechanisms

The process of healing takes place in the following phases: inflammatory response, fibroblastic repair and remodelling/maturation. Although these phases are presented as three separate entities, the process of healing is actually a continuous progression. The phases overlap and they do not have fixed beginning/end points.[8]

14.1.2.1 Inflammatory response

The destruction of the tissue produces a lesion of the cells and this, in turn, causes alteration in the basal metabolism and liberation of chemical substances that initiate the inflammatory response. This inflammatory response is a process via which cells of an inflammatory nature reach the site of the lesion (neutrophils

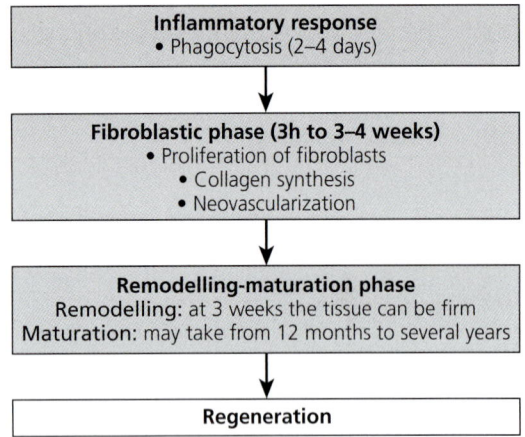

FIGURE 14.2 ■ Evolutive phases of muscular regeneration. It is essential to respect the inflammatory response in order to allow for the process of proliferation and remodelling of the destroyed cells and essential elements of the extracellular matrix.

and macrophages), producing oedema. This inflammatory response has a protective function over the injured tissue and tends to eliminate the elements or substances resulting from the lesion via phagocytosis. This process also prepares the ground for tissue regeneration (figure 14.2).

Once the inflammation is in place, there is a series of local vascular effects that occur, comprising alterations of the haemodynamics and diapedesis of the leukocytes. The vascular reaction implicates formation of a platelet plug and growth of fibrous tissue. The immediate response to the injury is a capillary vasoconstriction that lasts 5–10 minutes, in order to continue with a vasodilation that progresses later towards stagnation and stasis. The histamine liberated by injured cells causes vasodilation and increase in permeability of the endothelial vascular cells. The leukotaxine facilitates alignment of the leukocytes along the wall of the blood vessels, enabling separation of the endothelial cells in order to facilitate the diapedesis or migration of the leukocytes to the injured area. The necrosis is in charge of the phagocytic action and the degree of swelling that occurs in the area is related to the seriousness of the injury. The clot is formed by conversion of fibrinogen to fibrin, so that the injured area remains isolated during the inflammatory phase. The leukocytes (neutrophils and macrophages) not only phagocytose most of the waste products, but also liberate necessary growth factors in order to activate the fibroblasts.

The inflammatory response lasts between 2 and 4 days after the formation of the injury.[9]

14.1.2.2 Fibroblastic repair

The period of fibroblastic repair begins a few hours after the injury and can last 4–6 weeks.

During this period many symptoms and signs of inflammation decrease or disappear while the scarring advances.[10] During this phase the decrease in PO_2 also stimulates proliferation of the capillaries towards the site of the injury and, therefore, the injury is able to heal under aerobic conditions. With the increase in blood an increase in the administration of O_2 and the necessary nutrients occurs in order to facilitate fibroblastic proliferation and, therefore, the synthesis of the constituting elements of the extracellular matrix.

On the sixth or seventh day, the fibroblasts begin to synthesize collagen fibres, which are randomly arranged. At this point, it is vital to provide the optimal mechanical stimulus in order to favour the correct alignment and remodelling of the newly formed collagen tissue. According to the degree to which the tension force of the collagen tissue increases, the number of fibroblasts decreases and this indicates the onset of the maturation phase.

In some cases, when the inflammatory response is excessive, a continuous fibroplasia occurs, which results in increased fibrogenesis that creates the appearance of a fibrosis.

14.1.2.3 Remodelling phase/maturation phase

In this phase, the reorganization or remodelling of the collagen fibres takes place, and this will constitute the scar tissue.

With an increase in tension, the collagen fibres arrange themselves in parallel, following the vectors of the traction forces. The tissue will begin to take on a normal appearance and functioning and, 3 weeks later, a resistant and avascular scar will form; the maturation phase can last up to several years.[11]

14.1.2.4 Factors affecting healing

There are a series of factors[12] that can alter the healing process:

- The nature of the injury: in the case of muscular grade II–III injuries, there may be an imbalance in the repair mechanisms compared to the regeneration mechanisms.
- Deficiency in the blood supply: those injured tissues with a deficient vascular supply heal more slowly and with more difficulty. This is related to precarious activation of the phagocyte and fibroblast cells.

- Excessive tension upon the injured tissue: it is fundamental for there to be optimal mechanical stimulus in order to improve the mechanical and physical qualities of the collagen tissue. If this tension is excessive and repeatedly goes beyond the supraphysiological limit, intermittent injuries of collagen tissue will occur together with cyclic ischaemia, which will prolong the healing period.
- Atrophy and muscle spasm: the weakness of the muscle tissue favours proliferation of the scar tissue surrounding the muscle fibres. This creates stiffness and a decrease in muscular extensibility. Similarly, the muscle spasm can result in local ischaemia, which hampers cellularity and maturation.
- Corticosteroids: the use of steroids in the first stages of healing inhibits the inflammatory cellular response and, in a similar way, fibrogenesis. It has been demonstrated that, due to the early administration of corticosteroids, a decrease in collagen synthesis occurs and the tension vectors of the collagen are decreased.[13]

14.1.3 Muscle injury and regeneration

Muscle injuries, contusions, distensions or tears are common traumas in sports physiotherapy and their incidence represents 10–55% of all sports lesions.[1]

Muscles can be injured by direct trauma that provokes an excessive compression force, in other words, a contusion. With the application of great tensile strength, distension occurs. From an aetiological point of view, muscle injuries are classified into:

- injuries produced by extrinsic mechanisms or direct impact, including muscular contusions
- injuries due to intrinsic mechanisms and secondary to an intramuscular trauma.

These are a consequence of ballistic movements and stretches with an eccentric action that originate from excessive tension within the muscle, causing its injury.

On the other hand, it is important to stress the risk factors[2] that may favour the appearance of these types of lesions:

- people of a short and broad or hypermuscular phenotype
- biarticular muscles: associated with a higher risk of injury
- excessive or deficient training, inadequate warm-up and accumulated fatigue
- environmental factors such as cold and humidity that notably influence the appearance of these types of muscle injury.

14.1.3.1 Muscle injuries with an extrinsic cause: muscle contusion

Muscle contusion occurs as a consequence of a direct impact upon the muscle. The muscle is subjected to a compressive force against the subjacent bone causing a rupture with a profound haemorrhage.

Muscle contusions are most frequently located in the deep muscle areas close to the bone, but they may also be superficial and can appear in any part of the muscle. The intensity of these injuries is determined depending on the limitation of mobility arising from the affected joints. A contusion is mild when it causes a loss of less than a third of normal mobility, whereas serious contusions cause limitations of more than a third of normal articular mobility.[14]

In order to assess the prognosis and speed of recovery, the classification by Jackson and Feagin is very useful[15] (table 14.2).

As soon as a muscle is subjected to a hard impact, a haemorrhage occurs, and this may be intra- or intermuscular. In the first case, swelling occurs secondary to an increase in intramuscular pressure. This compresses the blood vessels and prevents them from continuing to

TABLE 14.2	**Classification of quadriceps contusions**		
Intensity	**Symptoms**	**Knee motion range**	**Functional capacity**
Mild	Localized tenderness	>90°	Normal gait Normal flexion
Moderate	Swollen tender muscle mass	<90°	Antalgic gait Pain going up stairs Pain getting up
Severe	Marked tenderness and swelling	<45°	Severely antalgic (crutches are necessary)

Adapted from Jackson and Feagin.[15]

bleed. A tumefaction occurs that lasts for more than 48 hours, accompanied by pain and decreased mobility. The extravasated blood attracts the liquid of the neighbouring tissues via osmosis. This increases the oedema even further, causing a secondary hypoxic lesion. The uninjured cells that managed to escape the damage caused by the trauma or contusion will suffer metabolic problems due to lack of oxygen as a consequence of the reduced blood circulation produced by the inflammatory reaction. The cells can die in areas where there is extensive lack of oxygen.

The haematoma (i.e. bruising) increases in volume as a consequence of the accumulation of more tissue remains produced in the affected area due to secondary hypoxic injury. As the cells are being destroyed by the inflammatory process they liberate more free proteins, causing oedema and producing a secondary additional injury. The insufficient oxygen supply to the cells can cause acidosis, causing the cells to expand and burst and, finally, be digested by the enzymes of the destroyed lysosomes. Both the rupture of the cellular membrane together with the intracellular liberation of the lysosome enzymes lead to cell death and the debris resulting from this process is aggregated to the contents of the haematoma. In this manner, the total mass of the damaged muscle tissue increases.

An intermuscular haematoma is characterized by injury of the aponeurosis that surrounds the muscle, enabling extravasation of the haemorrhage between the muscles. The effect of gravity makes the haematoma and the tumefaction appear in an area distal to the injury after 24–48 hours. If there is no elevation in pressure and the oedema is transitory, the muscle rapidly recovers its function.

All muscle injuries should be considered to be potentially serious during the first 2–3 days, and an immediate exploration of the injured area should be performed and repeated in order to try and distinguish whether the haemorrhage is intermuscular or intramuscular. Between 48 and 72 hours after the muscle injury, it is important to try to respond to the following questions:

- Has the tumefaction passed?
- Has the haemorrhage disseminated and caused the appearance of haematomas at a distance from the injured area?
- Has the contractile capacity of the muscle normalized or improved?

If the response to these three questions is negative, then it is probable that the injury corresponds with a case of intramuscular haemorrhage. Likewise, it is important to define how serious an injury it is in order to provide the sports

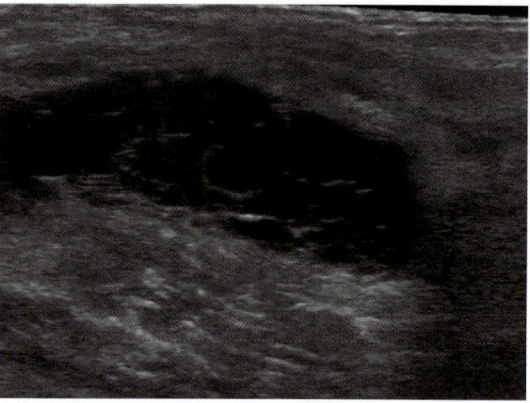

FIGURE 14.3 ■ Transverse ultrasound section of a rectus femoris muscle contusion. An anechoic image is observed in the interior of the muscle, indicating the presence of the haematoma produced by the injury.

player with both the correct and appropriate treatment.[14]

The muscular contusion is visible under ultrasound because of the presence of one or various cavities with an echoic content and irregular borders, accompanied by small hypoechoic images that correspond to areas of disorganization located within the muscle structure or small well-defined haematomas (figure 14.3).

With regard to recovery programmes, athletes who have suffered a muscular contusion progress faster than those who have suffered a distension or partial muscle tear. In the case of a mild muscular contusion, the recovery time does not exceed 7 days, while a moderate contusion should last approximately 15 days, and a serious contusion 3–4 weeks. Obviously, this chronology of recovery will depend on the extent of the injury, the rapidness of the intervention by the physiotherapist and respect for the biological repair/regeneration processes of the muscle tissue. Under musculoskeletal ultrasound, it is possible to guarantee that healing is complete when a decreased size and echogenicity of the haematoma are observed, with increased echogenicity and size of the borders of the rupture (figure 14.4). Immediate treatment of muscular contusions and distensions is of utmost importance as this helps to limit the haematoma and, therefore, favours an earlier return to sports.

14.1.3.2 Muscle injuries with an intrinsic cause

Within muscle injuries with no apparent involvement of the structure and no alteration under ultrasound, we can include muscle cramps, contractures and delayed-onset muscle soreness. In this section we will only describe the structural

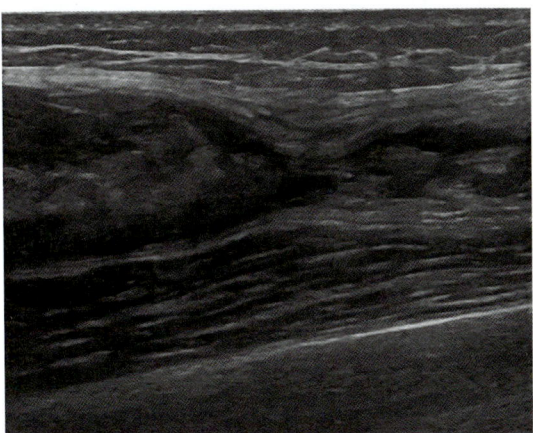

FIGURE 14.4 ■ Panoramic ultrasound image displaying a longitudinal section of a complete rupture of the myotendinous junction of the rectus femoris muscle. The echogenicity of the borders of the tear, the decrease in the haematoma and the re-establishment of the muscle architecture are ultrasound signs of healing.

muscle injuries presenting with ultrasound alteration, as these are considered more important from an anatomopathological and clinical point of view. These are muscle elongation, partial tears or muscle distension and total ruptures.

Muscle elongation occurs as a consequence of an excessive stretch of the muscle fibres without causing a rupture. The patient complains of acute pain and functional impairment and there is no haematoma (or bruising), ecchymosis or tumefaction, but there is pain under palpation.

Distensions or ruptures of muscle fibres occur more frequently in biarticular muscles (quadriceps, hamstring and calf muscles) as a consequence of a momentary neuromuscular incoordination.[14] The most frequent distensions are not complete ruptures but partial ruptures of the muscle tissue (mainly in the myotendinous junction).

The clinical classification of muscle injuries depends on the intramuscular or intermuscular nature of the haematoma or the seriousness of the injury[16]:

- Grade I: a few fibres are torn, although the aponeurosis is intact. If there is an intramuscular haematoma, it is usually smaller than 1 cm.
- Grade II: a moderate number of fibres are torn, whereas the aponeurosis is intact, although a localized haematoma is apparent. The fibrillar rupture is less than a third of the muscle surface, the accompanying haematoma is less than 3 cm and occasionally, a small interfascial haematoma may be present.

- Grade III: many muscle fibres are torn with a partial rupture of the aponeurosis. The fibre rupture affects more than a third of the muscle surface and the haematoma is greater than 3 cm. This is always accompanied by a large interfascial haematoma.
- Grade IV: this corresponds with total muscle rupture. The muscle appears retracted and hyperechogenic and is accompanied by a large haematoma. On ultrasound it is typical to see the image of a 'bell clapper', which is a lack of continuity with the retractile fibres within the haematic cavity.

Regeneration of the contractile elements begins with activation of the satellite cells. In adults, these cells are inactive and are located between the basal lamina and the sarcolemma of the muscle fibre, and a greater quantity of satellite cells are found in type I muscle fibres. When the basal lamina ruptures after an injury, the mitotic capacity of these cells is activated. When an injury occurs, the affected muscle fibres retract, forming a gap between the broken ends, which leads to hypertrophy of the sarcomeres in order to avoid the approach of inflammatory cells in the healthy muscle fibres. The trauma causes rupture of the blood vessels and the space that remains in between the muscle fibres is filled with blood. This is when cytokines are liberated; this attracts leukocytes and macrophages to the site of the injury. During these first days the macrophages phagocytose the necrosed muscle tissue, which is found in the space between the proximal and distal ends of the torn muscle fibres. It has also been noted that the macrophages liberate growth factors, which favour the proliferation of satellite cells. The quantities of leukocytes and macrophages decrease considerably between the fifth and seventh day after the lesion. Elimination of the necrosed cellular debris marks the beginning of regeneration due to the fact that satellite cells are activated and transformed into myoblasts.[9]

In a matter of days after the injury, the myoblasts fuse among themselves in order to form a myotube, which itself fuses among others to form a new muscle fibre (fast or slow). Coinciding with muscular regeneration, the haematoma is gradually substituted by fibroblasts and components of the extracellular matrix, restoring the integrity of the connective tissue. These two repair processes support one another, although they also compete with each other. Maturation of the myotubes to myofibres takes place approximately 14 days postlesion. A few hours after the trauma, the presence of fibronectin is found at the site of the injury, and this substance attaches to the fibrin, forming the shell on to which the fibroblasts will attach. The fibroblasts synthesize type I and type III collagen and, as the repair process advances, type I collagen starts becoming more predominant, reaching its maximal critical point 3 weeks later.[17]

During the first week, the site of the injury is the weakest point during passive stretches. After the first week, the tendency to rupture is displaced towards the proximal aspect of the injury. For this reason, it is necessary to provide a rest period immediately after the injury as this will favour a decrease in the quantity and density of the scar tissue and the regenerating myofibrils will be able to cross the tissue with greater ease.[18]

14.1.4 Muscle regeneration via EPI®

Over recent years the number of muscle injuries in sports players has increased due to a range of factors, such as the increase in number of competitions, overtraining, lack of adequate recovery periods and influence of environmental factors. The development of novel therapeutic methods for the treatment of these injuries must be based on the study of the muscle's biological and biomechanical basis. To this end, EPI® has proved to be very effective in the regeneration of muscle injuries.[19]

Since 1982, there have been no methodologically sound studies on the influence of bioelectrical currents in the regeneration of non-neural tissues. Owoeye et al.[20] published the first work on this matter, in which the authors applied an electric current directly over the tendon with the hope of promoting healing. It was found that the tendons treated with anodal currents were mechanically stronger than those that were left to heal without any stimulation. Furthermore, the absence of stimulation produced stronger tendons than those treated with the cathode.

Although the first studies were performed on nerves, it was subsequently discovered that other tissues, such as muscles, tendons and ligaments, had endogenous currents when faced with injury. It has been observed that the electric current induced in the tissue has a direct effect on the cell membrane, modifying the flow of cations and favouring the opening of the transmembrane channels, becoming voltage-dependent on the cell. This creates a change in the concentration of cations within the cell, facilitating the proliferation of myoblasts and, therefore, the formation of muscle fibre.[21]

Considering the role of monocytes, macrophages, fibroblasts and myoblasts and the multitude of cells that mediate the regeneration/ repair process, and, likewise considering the importance of optimal ionic strength, temperature and pH, the question to ask is: how do the electric fields and the modulated currents applied directly upon the muscle tissue facilitate the process of regeneration? It is known that the application of electric fields directly to the muscle does not necessarily produce an increase in proliferation of myoblasts, but it does produce an elevated synthesis of muscle fibre, via modulation of the cyclic adenosine monophosphate (cAMP) of the internal cell membrane. The modulation of cAMP metabolism increases the synthesis of myotubes and DNA, increasing the concentration of intracellular Ca^{2+} and, therefore, raising the insulin level.

Litke and Dahners[22] observed that the direct application of electric current to the muscle at an intensity of 1–20 μA caused a faster recovery and a significant improvement with regard to muscle strength and resistance (higher doses produced tissue damage). Becker[23] conducted studies based on the assumption that within living beings there is a continuous electric current responsible for the correct function of the tissues. When a lesion occurs, this electrical balance is altered and, in the words of the author, a so-called 'lesional current' appears which is responsible for initiation of the healing process.

Sánchez-Ibáñez et al.[19] carried out an original study in which they proved that the use of EPI® provokes a reduction in fibrosis and calcification nuclei and extension of the secondary lesion due to hypoxia (see chapter 12). These data correlate with the clinical results in humans.[24] Also, these results indicate the need to initiate treatment with EPI® as soon as possible after injury, thus enabling better control over the reabsorption of the haematoma and improvement in the tissue homeostasis which is necessary for correct regeneration (video 14.1).

EPI® acts in a direct manner, impacting upon the following physiopathological processes:

- At the time of the muscle tear, a modification in pH occurs as well as a modification in oxygen tension, which has the effect of inhibiting bioelectric regeneration mechanisms.
- The predominance of the inhibitory bioelectric potentials favours the permanence of the fibrin clot located at the ends of the muscle tear.
- The chronological extension of this clot will alter the regeneration mechanisms to favour fibroblasts. This produces an increase in connective tissue with regard to muscle tissue. Stimulation of the myoblasts close to the membrane will allow activation

of the transmembrane integrins and second messengers that stimulate the transcription of DNA from the nucleus. The result is a larger proliferation of myotubes and elements from the ground substance and muscle.

- The early haematoma reduction, intra- or intermuscular, favours optimal muscle regeneration, avoiding an excess of fibrin and the formation of connective tissue which would increase adherences, fibrosis and muscle rigidity.

The mechanisms for which muscle regeneration is activated via the direct action of EPI® are exempt from many of the inconveniences of the current conservative treatments. The risk of fibrosis and adherences is decreased and the improved resistance and muscle strength achieved allow for rapid return to competitive sports.[25]

14.2 EPI® IN THE MUSCLE TISSUE

Ultrasound analysis of the muscle enables identification of the affected tissue, which is commonly associated with any of the following signs: focal anechoic-hypoechoic areas, breakdown of muscle echotexture, lack of continuity of muscle tissue or hypervascularized areas, changes in the elasticity pattern via sonoelastographic analysis and the presence of myofascial trigger points (MTrPs). Despite the ample lesion area, the EPI® technique is minimally invasive, making use of the fluid's dynamic movement for its hydrolysation (figure 14.5).

Once the different intervention areas are determined, the liquefaction of the tissue is verified when the gas density occupies the total intervention area. An important consideration for the safety of EPI® is the possibility of directly visualizing the needle via ultrasound guidance. The well-delimited hyperechogenic image generated during EPI® is a consequence of the density of hydrogen gas produced by the electrochemical reaction of cathodic flow.

On the other hand, it is important to highlight that the muscle is regenerated in electronegative regions and reabsorbed in electropositive regions. The potentials thus generated are derived from the piezoelectric properties of the effects of the collagen matrix and electrokinetics. This property is known as current potential. The electric fields are also generated in the injury sites, soft tissues and bone (injury induced by potentials) and in the areas of active muscle formation. It is possible that the faradic products of the electrochemical reaction produced by the cathode increase the expression of growth factors. Likewise, it has been noted that prostaglandins, which are known to stimulate muscle formation, are implicated in the pH increases of the cytoplasm of the myoblastic cells.

The electrochemical reaction that occurs in the cathode may also contribute to the mechanism of action of EPI® stimulation. It is observed that the decrease in oxygen concentration is essential in order to improve myoblastic activity, whereas the increase in pH increases the fibroblastic activity. Also, hydrogen peroxide stimulates macrophages in order to liberate vascular endothelial growth factor, which is an essential angiogenic factor for muscle regeneration.[19]

14.2.1 Target tissue

In acute injuries of the skeletal muscle, the most affected areas are frequently the myotendinous, myoconnective or myoaponeurotic junctions. In chronic injuries, the most common complications are due to fibrotic scar tissue.

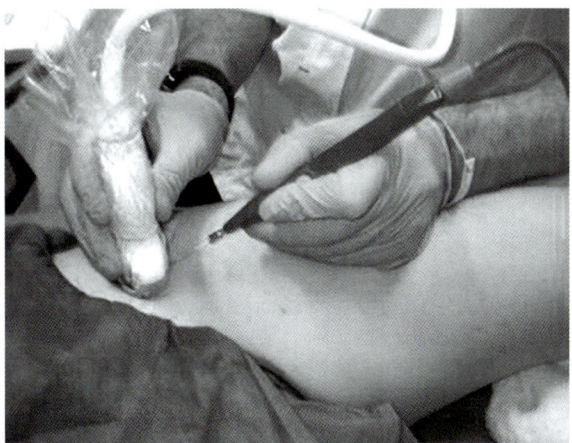
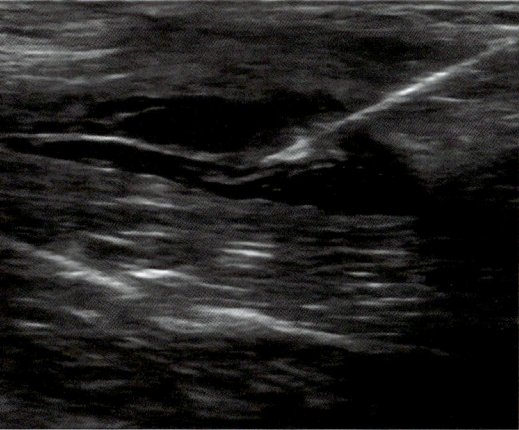

FIGURE 14.5 ■ Ultrasound-guided EPI® treatment of a muscle injury. (Colour version of figure is available online).

Intratissue percutaneous electrolysis is demonstrated to be highly effective in the treatment of the myofascial pain syndrome via the treatment of MTrPs, with the advantage of eliciting a high number of local twitch responses with a minimal number of punctures (video 14.2). Activation of the local twitch response is decisive, not only for the diagnosis of MTrPs, but also for their treatment, producing bimolecular modifications and re-establishing homeostasis of the muscle tissue. On the other hand, the postpuncture pain is less than with traditional dry needling, and the regenerative effects are superior.[26]

14.2.2 Application of the technique

It is important to note that EPI® is always applied under ultrasound guidance (figure 14.5) in order to avoid producing iatrogenic effects, such as nerve or vessel lesions. Furthermore, this favours an improved physiotherapy diagnosis of the various muscle injuries, especially if performed with Doppler and sonoelastography. Ultrasound assessment with colour Doppler enables study of the direction and speed of blood flow and the performance of a clinical classification, according to whether or not hypervascularization is detected. Only the flow rates can be registered. In this way, one can identify whether it is a muscle injury, as this is a significant indicator in the treatment and prognosis of muscle injuries.

In the distension type of muscle injuries, decreased echogenicity is observed; this appears as a hypoechoic image and the muscle, rather than appearing homogeneous, is seen as a heterogeneous image.

Once the different intervention areas have been determined, liquefaction of the fibrous scar tissue is considered to be achieved when the needle does not find viscoelastic resistance in the intrafibrotic region where electrolytic ablation has been performed.

The maximal peak in inflammatory response induced by EPI® in muscular injuries occurs on the fifth day postintervention. Also, it is safe to say that at 15 days postintervention there will no longer be signs of inflammatory cellular infiltration in the intervention area.

The EPI® technique, when applied to muscular injuries, employs current widths of 0.2–6 mA and time intervals of 3–4 seconds, applied at different points within the area of affected muscle. After each EPI® intervention it is essential to educate the patient to keep within an optimal range of functional loading in order to avoid any sports activity that involves pain.

KEY POINTS

Ultrasound-guided EPI® is a novel, effective and safe technique that promotes an inhibition of the fibrotic response due to its direct action upon control of the expression of interkeukin-1, which activates the corresponding muscle regeneration mechanisms.

14.2.3 Postintervention care for EPI®

Immediately after intervention with EPI®, the patient is advised not to apply cryotherapy due to the possibility of negatively influencing the inflammatory response induced by EPI®.[27] In the case of the needle accidentally puncturing a capillary, digital haemostatic pressure is advised, without gliding or massaging (see chapter 1). To finish off, the intervention area is cleaned with povidone-iodine and patients are controlled and supervised during the 10–20 minutes after intervention to prevent any vagal reaction.

On their first visit, all patients should be informed that the EPI® procedure activates an acute inflammatory response postintervention, that usually causes pain lasting for up to 48 hours and that, for this purpose, and always under medical prescription, they may choose to take some type of analgesia. In this case, the caveat is that the analgesic of choice must not produce great anti-inflammatory effects. This makes drugs such as paracetamol preferable as, although non-steroidal anti-inflammatory drugs are not contraindicated in application of the technique, they may alter the muscle tissue properties and inhibit the inflammatory response.[28]

McConnell-type taping is recommended for all patients for at least 48 hours postprocedure, corresponding with the acute phase of the inflammatory response induced by EPI®. The objective is to avoid ischaemia within the muscle that may negatively affect the healing mechanisms. It is also important to inform patients that they may carry out physical activity as long as no pain is elicited in the muscle; in other words, they must stay within the functional range or the homeostasis described by Dye.[29]

All patients are provided with a telephone number so that they can consult with any questions that may arise.

KEY POINTS

After treatment with EPI® on the muscle tissue, it is important to avoid situations of muscle ischaemia that could negatively affect the healing mechanisms.

14.3 ULTRASOUND ASSESSMENT IN INTERVENTIONS USING EPI®

There are studies in both animals and humans that confirm that musculoskeletal ultrasound is a valid tool for observing changes in muscle injuries during the process of regeneration, based on ultrasound criteria such as the degree of echogenicity or echotexture or the localization and behaviour of vascularization using Doppler.[24,30]

During the first visit, it is important to perform a correct physiotherapy diagnosis, including a correct assessment and clinical examination of the injured muscle. After the clinical examination, assessment with ultrasound will enable identification of ultrasound signs of muscle injury, such as the presence of intramuscular haematoma, loss of ultrasound homogeneity, increase in muscle volume, hypervascularization and calcifications.

These ultrasound signs, which are characteristic of muscle injuries due to tears or contusion, are important considerations in order to explain these complications. On the other hand, the hypoechoic or anechoic image usually appears after the fifth day of the injury, generally associated with the finding of anechoic areas and, if functionality has worsened, hypervascularization is present (figure 14.6).

In this sense, ultrasound constitutes an exceptional tool for the physiotherapist, as it enables analysis of muscle deficiencies. Likewise, it enables dynamic assessments when combined with the performance of joint movements and active muscle contraction. Perhaps what is most noteworthy is that it allows for treatment of the EPI® technique under ultrasound guidance, ensuring the intervention is exactly on the injury site.

In patients who are administered with EPI® under ultrasound guidance, the injury site is determined by measuring square grid lines in a transverse section. On inspection of the grid squares, not all the muscles have the same degree of lesion in their transverse section and it is observed that the destruction of muscle tissue is not homogeneous. There are regions with a significant degree of injury and other, less affected areas. Therefore, via the grid technique (figure 14.7), only the regions presenting more significant ultrasound lesion signs (as described previously) are selected as EPI® intervention regions.

On the other hand, the physiotherapist can use anisotropy (see chapter 5) to visualize the magnitude of the electromagnetic field provoked by EPI® (figure 14.8), and thus the intervention area that is exposed to the therapeutic effects of

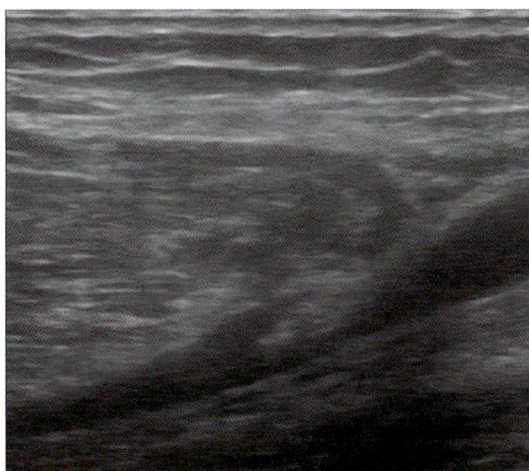

FIGURE 14.6 ■ Longitudinal ultrasound section of a complete tear of the myotendinous junction of the rectus femoris muscle. A hypoechoic image is observed which corresponds to the intramuscular haematoma.

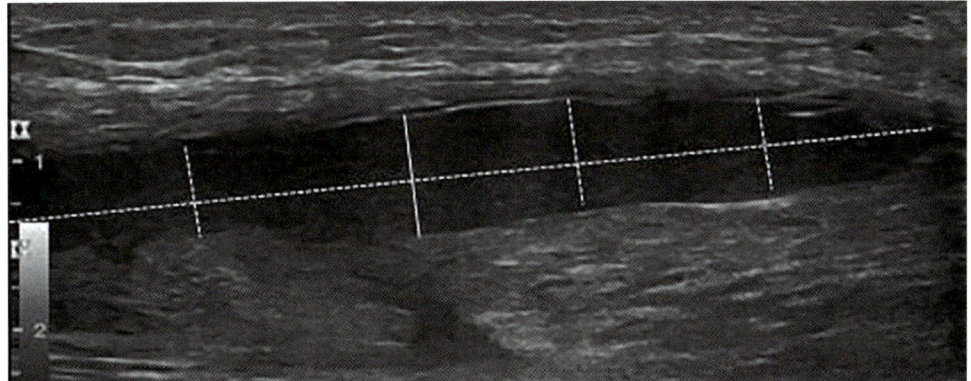

FIGURE 14.7 ■ Transverse ultrasound section of a tear of the biceps femoris muscle. Application of the grid technique in order to select the field of intervention using the EPI® technique.

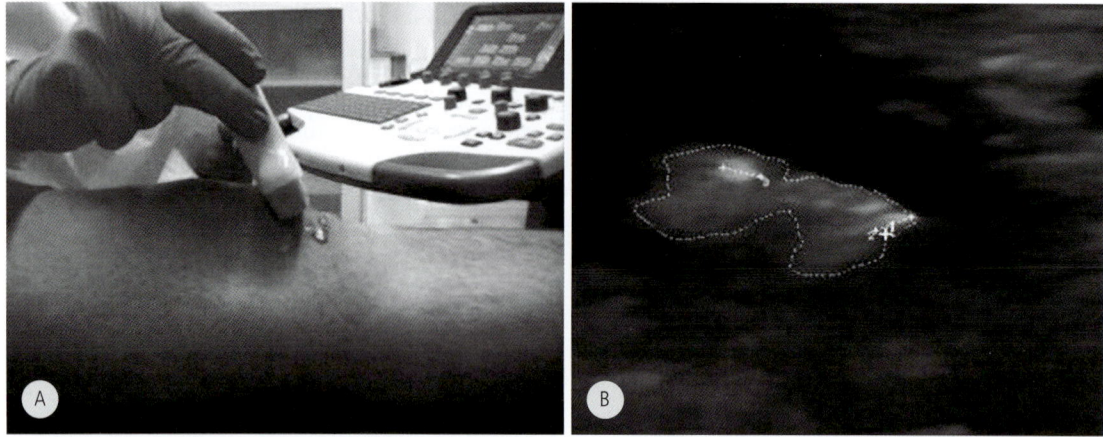

FIGURE 14.8 ■ Use of the anisotropy effect for visualization of the EPI® technique's electric field in the soft tissue. (A) Placement of the ultrasound transducer more obliquely to the perpendicular axis in the direction of the fibres in order to provoke the anisotropy effect. (B) The hyperechoic points correspond to the effect of EPI® on the needle tip (0.9 mm) and the electromagnetic field produced by EPI® is visible (the more hypoechoic area of 19.2 mm), increasing its effects on the neighbouring tissue. (Colour version of figure is available online).

EPI® can be calculated. The hyperechoic points represent the electrochemical ablation area of the needle tip, although the electric field created by the EPI® technique also acts in the area peripheral to the intervention. The width of the electromagnetic field widens in the intervening area, and therefore the adjacent tissue is also subject to the effects of EPI®, thus avoiding a secondary hypoxic lesion due to inhibition in the expression of interleukin-1 and hypoxia-inducible factor-1.[19]

A 7-day interval is commonly used between EPI® sessions in order not to interfere with the complete cycle of inflammatory response caused by EPI®, which is estimated to last approximately 14 days. The grid squares that are treated do not always coincide in each session, in order to avoid repeating the treatment in the exact same degenerated foci.

14.3.1 Sonoelastography of muscle injuries

Muscle fascicle and its perimysium can be identified under ultrasound, whereas the myofilaments, basement membrane and muscle fibres are unidentifiable with this technique. Regarding the echogenicity of the different muscular elements, the muscle strands present a hypoechoic image, the subcutaneous tissue is isoechoic and the perimysium or fibroadipose septum, the epimysium, the fascia, the intermuscular planes and tendons all appear as hyperechoic images.

The indications for ultrasound in muscular injuries are based on:

- detection of alterations in muscle structure
- assessment of the magnitude of these structural changes

- assessment of the healing process
- use of haematoma aspiration when this is indicated
- intervention with ultrasound guidance using the EPI® technique.

As previously noted, conventional ultrasound (B-mode) is able to display and detect significant changes in muscle structures. Changes in echostructure can be revealed, pertaining to both the muscle fascicles as well as to the connective component.

The new technological advances in musculoskeletal ultrasound have enabled incorporation of techniques such as sonoelastography which uses compression of the soft tissues to produce displacement within the tissue. Tissues that are more rigid provoke less displacement than those that are softer (see chapter 6).[31,32] The quality unique to sonoelastography is that it allows for detection of different degrees of rigidity within a biological tissue such as the muscle. This provides the physiotherapist with a great tool to establish physiotherapy diagnostic criteria (degrees of change in the muscle structure), control the evolution of the healing and detect different areas that are vulnerable to relapse (figure 14.9).

A fundamental aspect observed in clinical practice is that, while performing EPI® in the soft tissue, and examining its effect in real time with sonoelastography, an increase in tissue rigidity occurs. This is explained by the action of the extracellular adhesion proteins, thus facilitating the interconnection between the cell and the matrix and optimizing the space for intercellular diffusion necessary for tissue regeneration. This effect can be explained via activation of the expression of the stress proteins. The stimulation of stress proteins is elevated by endogenous

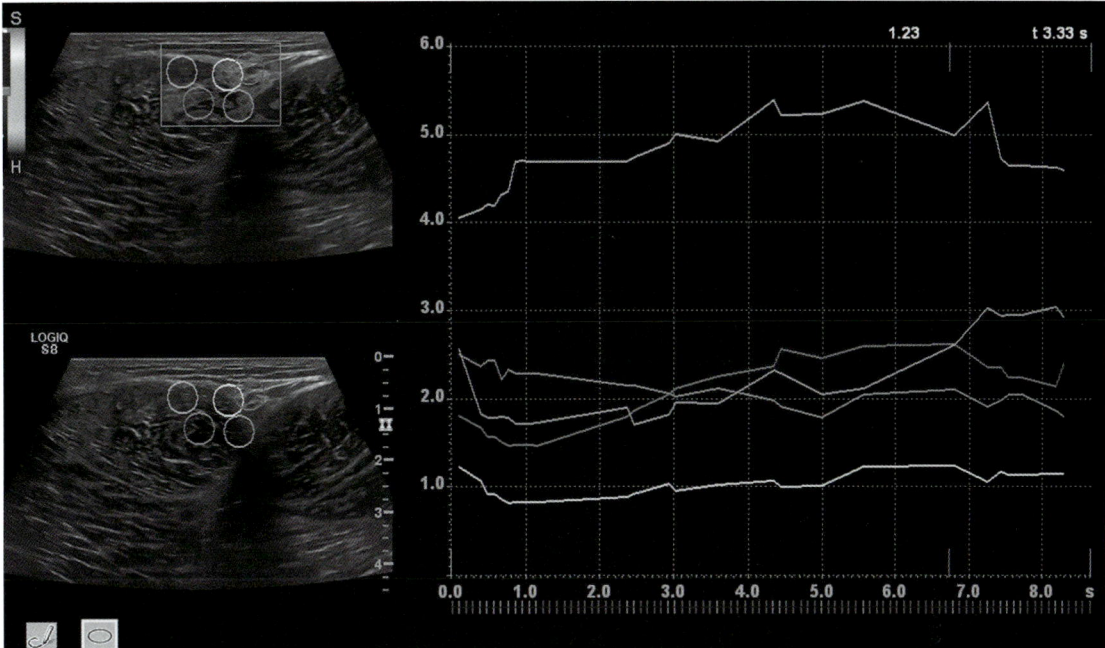

FIGURE 14.9 ■ Sonoelastography of an injury to the myotendinous junction of the biceps femoris muscle. Quantitative data and spectral colour analysis. (Colour version of figure is available online).

agents, such as the electrochemical action of EPI®. The typical function of a chaperone (stress protein) is to assist in newly formed chains of polypeptides in order for them to reach their functional conformation as a new protein and subsequently aid that protein to reach the site of the cell where it will act. This biological phenomenon is a result of the stimulus produced by EPI® for the cells, the result of the adaptive response on the mechanisms of maintenance, repair and regeneration in order to maintain haemodynamics in a situation of small magnitude and stress.[33]

14.3.2 Ultrasonographic signs of musculoskeletal healing

A large spectrum of distensions or muscular tears exists, of variable severity (mild, moderate and serious), as they can range from a small contusion to total rupture. The exam and continued evaluation via ultrasound are very useful in order to appreciate the evolution of the healing process. It can also influence the active physiotherapy protocol in establishing the most suitable course of treatment according to the evolution of the injury. The ultrasound signs of muscle healing are as follows (table 14.3):

- decreased size of the haematoma followed by complete resolution
- increased echogenicity along the margins of the tear

TABLE 14.3	Ultrasound characteristics of muscle healing	
Normal healing	**Abnormal healing**
Decreased size and echogenicity of the haematoma	Formation of scar tissue with variable presentation: linear, nodular or star-like
Increased echogenicity of the tear margins	Hyperechoic scar tissue (linear, nodular or star-like)
Increased width of margins	Muscular cyst which manifests as a small anechoic structure and which may contain septa
Return to normal muscle architecture	

- increased width of the margins
- reorganization of the muscular architecture
- return to normality in the muscular architecture.

Two frequent complications in the healing process of the muscle are:

1. the formation of scar tissue, which can present various appearances (nodular, linear or star-like)
2. muscular cyst, which manifests as a small anechoic structure that can contain septa.

The accumulation of intramuscular liquid is easily detected with ultrasound. The intramuscular accumulations are generally round, whereas the intermuscular ones are fusiform. Their content can be:

- anechoic
- hypoechoic, with posterior non-significant shadow
- echoic, due to the presence of debris that moves freely within the liquid
- a liquid–liquid level, with debris piled up on the most dependent part.

When the injury compromises the epimysium, the accumulation is also visible from the inter-muscular space as an anechoic structure. In the same way, it is important to remember that the echogenicity of the haematoma depends on the duration of its instauration.

14.4 THE APPLICATION OF EPI® IN DIFFERENT MUSCLE INJURIES

The actions of EPI® in muscle tissue can be summarized as follows:

- In myoconnective injuries, it enables the thickening of collagen by the action of thermal shock via the chaperones (heat shock protein 47).
- It decreases intramuscular pressure via evaporation and, therefore, the ectopic nociceptive depolarization.
- It balances the relation between metallo-proteinases and their inhibitors.
- It acts upon inhibition of the proinflamma-tory cytokines (tumour necrosis factor-alpha, interleukin-1) as a consequence of an increase in PO_2 and regulation of pH.
- It reduces kinetic hyperactivity and overex-pression of the proinflammatory macro-phages and optimizes expression of the anti-inflammatory macrophages, thus allowing for a correct control of the scar.
- It favours liquefaction of fibrotic and mature muscle tissue, permitting reinitia-tion of the remodelling process.

Specialists in sports injuries are aware that there are mainly four muscle groups that are most vulnerable to muscle injury (which some authors call the 'top 10' muscle injuries in sports players). These muscles are the quadriceps (mainly the rectus femoris muscle), the hamstrings (mainly the biceps femoris muscle), gastrocnemius and adductor muscles.

14.4.1 Rectus femoris muscle injuries

Acute injuries (due to tears of the quadriceps muscle) occur most frequently in competitive sports such as football, rugby, hockey and

TABLE 14.4 Classification of quadriceps muscle injury due to strain or tear

Grade	Pain	Strength	Physical exam
1	Mild	Minimal loss of strength	Non-palpable muscle defect
2	Moderate	Moderate loss of strength	Small palpable muscle defect
3	Severe	Complete loss of strength	Clearly palpable muscle defect

athletics. These sports require regular eccentric-type muscle activation to control both knee flexion and hip extension. If these strength vectors of the eccentric action go over the resistance threshold of the fibres of the myo-tendinous junction, a tear injury occurs, mainly in the rectus femoris muscle. On the other hand, a maximal or excessive passive stretch or activa-tion of the muscle may cause a muscle strain.[34]

Various factors predispose the rectus femoris muscle to sustaining a strain injury:

- polyarticular muscles
- muscles with a high percentage of type II fibres
- muscles with a complex architecture of the myotendinous junction
- muscular fatigue (especially in relation to acute lesions).

Various classifications for quadriceps injuries have been proposed. Perhaps the most widely used is the one that incorporates assessments of pain, the quality of strength and a physical exam-ination (table 14.4).[35]

Treatment with EPI® in the acute phase has been demonstrated to produce great control and optimization of matrix regulation due to inhibition of interleukin-1 and increase in ang-iogenesis, mainly due to overexpression of the type 2 receptors of vascular endothelial growth factor. These recent data are highly significant and novel, representing a great advance in mus-cular regeneration.[19] In figure 14.10 a complete rupture of the myotendinous junction of the rectus femoris muscle is observed; EPI® is being applied with ultrasound guidance over the intra-muscular haematoma.

14.4.2 Vastus intermedius muscle contusions

The aetiology of this type of injury is contu-sion of the vastus lateralis, which reaches the

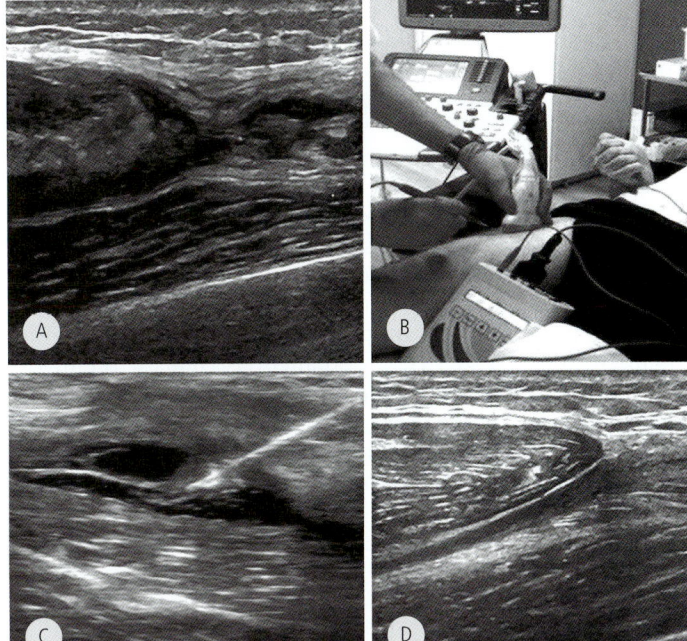

FIGURE 14.10 ■ Regeneration process of the rectus femoris muscle based on treatment using EPI®. (A) Total tear of the myotendinous junction (MTJ) distal to the rectus femoris muscle. (B) EPI® ultrasound-guided treatment. (C) Gas density (hyperechoic line) at the level of the intramuscular haematoma. (D) Day of discharge: an optimal repair of the rectus femoris MTJ is observed. (Colour version of figure is available online).

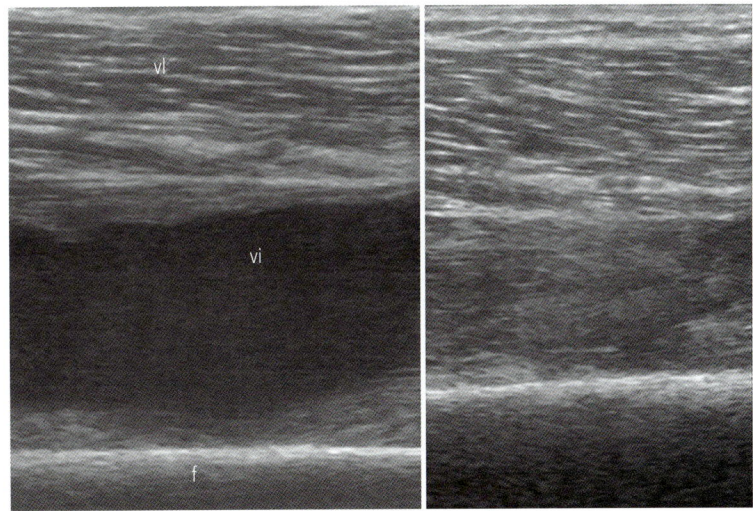

FIGURE 14.11 ■ Intramuscular haematoma due to contusion of the vastus intermedius quadriceps muscle. The ultrasound image on the right displays reabsorption of the haematic effusion due to EPI®. f, femur; vi, haematoma in vastus intermedius muscle; vl, vastus lateralis muscle.

juxtaosseous muscle region in a manner that produces a breakdown of the muscle fibres of the vastus intermedius and a vascular injury.

If there is no injury of the intermuscular aponeurosis, the haematoma remains confined to the intramuscular level, as seen in figure 14.11. In this figure the depth of the injury is found at around 4 cm. In order to improve the effectiveness of EPI®, the transducer is focused exactly on the region of maximal haematic volume. Immediately after the EPI® procedure, an elastic compressive tape is applied on the muscle.

14.4.3 Biceps femoris muscle injuries

The injury of the hamstring muscles represents 30–37% of all muscle injuries. Up to 57–60% of all hamstring injuries occur during pre-season due to the higher intensity of the training sessions.[16] The greatest incidence is in sports such as football and athletics, with 34% relapses, which makes this the muscle injury that produces the most relapses. Most relapses occur 2 weeks after return to competitive sports.[36] Orchard and Seward[37] observed that injuries of the hamstrings represent 15% of all injuries occurring in Australian football players during a whole season, with a high recurrence rate of 34%. The accumulative risk of relapse during the whole season was 30.6%.

In recent years, many football clubs have suffered a period of injuries related to the biceps femoris. Furthermore, there is a series of predisposing factors (innate in the sportsperson) that, when associated with some determining factors (environmental) and in a situation of physical activity of risk, favour the appearance of this type of muscle injury. Note that a footballer has 1000 times more risk of suffering an injury than someone carrying out a more dangerous profession, such as a miner. Furthermore, it is known that prior injuries in the vertebral spine and prior injuries in this muscle group are considered to be significant risk factors.

A series of clinically essential variables have been identified in relation to the injury of this muscle group in sportspeople. The biceps femoris mainly acts in eccentric contraction in order to decelerate the tibia in its anterior displacement. The mechanism via which it ruptures (figure 14.12) is not conditioned by a direct trauma, but rather it is a consequence of a sudden stretch that occurs while the muscle is in eccentric contraction, during which the leg is positioned in hip flexion and the knee in eccentric extension. In other words, an 'interruption of the neuromuscular control' of the biceps femoris muscle will cause the appearance of the injury.

Factors associated with an increased risk of injury to the biceps femoris muscle include:

- anatomy of the hamstring muscles and insertion areas
- poor lumbopelvic control
- muscle fatigue
- inadequate warm-up
- optimal position or range of the hamstrings' peak torque
- critical deficit of the hamstrings. Deficit in strength is the most important risk factor and there is a relation between the muscle injury and the strength deficit attributed to inadequate recovery
- alteration of the hamstrings/quadriceps ratio. A hamstrings/quadriceps ratio of less than 0.6 and an asymmetry of the flexors of 5% are considered to be risk factors for the appearance of an injury in the biceps femoris muscle.

It is important to verify, assess, control and modify, if necessary, an anomaly and alteration of the factors mentioned above. A series of controls should be performed throughout the season in order to reduce the risk of injury significantly. The most important aspect is the recurrence factor, as recurrent injury is known to involve a longer absence period and recovery.

Injury of the hamstrings commonly implies a prolonged absence from competition due to the slow healing process. The musculotendinous junctions of the hamstring muscles extend along most of the muscle length and therefore it is difficult to differentiate between injuries of the muscle belly and the musculotendinous junction based on clinical assessment. Injuries that affect the myotendinous and osteotendinous junctions require more recovery time than those that affect muscle tissue (Garret 1984).[49] They also entail a greater risk of compromising the sciatic nerve.

With regard to treatment of biceps femoris muscle injury, the first factor worth mentioning is that there is little consensus regarding which is the most effective treatment. Correction of the critical deficit parameters of the hamstrings and the hamstrings/quadriceps ratio by increasing muscle strength decreases the rate of hamstring injuries from 7.6% to 1% and the rate of recurrence from 31.7% to 0% in footballers.[38]

On the other hand, repetitive microfibrosis is one of the main causes in both the appearance of the biceps femoris injury, as well as its relapse. Football is a sport that continuously implicates this muscle group, and the repetitive eccentric action to which the biceps femoris muscle is exposed causes a series of ultrastructural microlesions that trigger inflammatory responses and often induce poor-quality repair processes. The deficit in recovery time with a stable hypoxia-inducible factor-β favours the appearance of fibrosis in the myotendinous junctions. If these critical fibrosis regions are not released, the risk of injury is very high.[25]

According to both scientific and clinical evidence, EPI® is the therapy of choice in muscle injuries. A great infiltration of inflammatory cells is observed 48 hours after the application of EPI®, together with an increase in cytokines, membrane receptors and growth factors necessary for the regeneration of muscle tissue.[19] The activation of these membrane receptors, when they form a ligand with growth factors, causes hyperactivity of the P13-kinase, with a consequent increase in proliferation, migration and cellular metabolism.[39] EPI® is able to stimulate poor-quality fibrous tissue in order to achieve a connective tissue of greater elastic resistance and viscoelasticity (figure 14.13). Currently, it is possible to affirm that EPI® not only guarantees greater recovery but is also a preventive technique in muscular lesions.

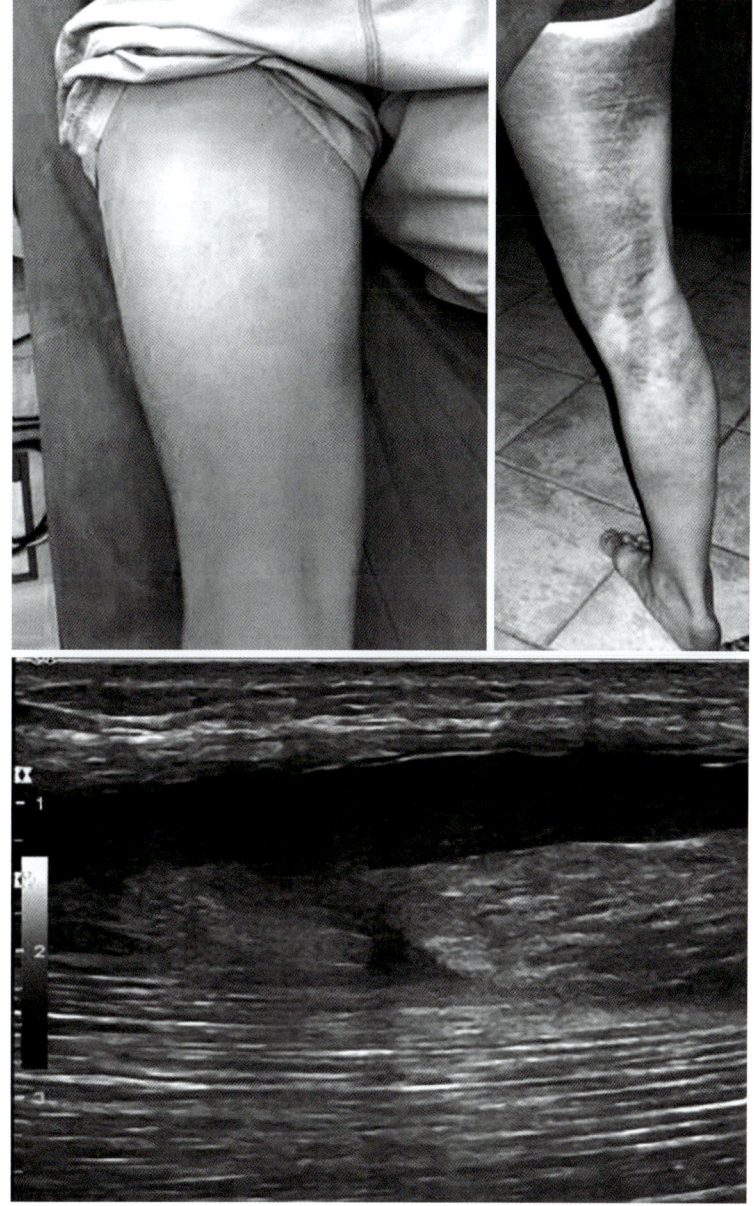

FIGURE 14.12 ■ Grade III tear of the biceps femoris muscle. The ultrasound image displays a haematic intramuscular fluid collection due to a tear of the distal biceps femoris muscle. (Colour version of figure is available online).

14.5 ECCENTRIC OVERLOAD TRAINING FOR MUSCLE REGENERATION

Together with EPI®, patients need a planned programme of eccentric training to perform each time they come to the consultation (twice a week) and before starting intervention with EPI®.

Eccentric exercises are performed after warm-up of the agonistic and antagonistic muscles with a stationary bicycle and associated with analytical stretches in active tension (isometric contraction for 6 seconds and progressive relaxation for 12 seconds) of the quadriceps and hamstring muscles.

The scientific literature offers several different protocols for the performance of eccentric exercise in the treatment of muscle injuries.[38,40,41] It is considered that the eccentric exercises proposed by some authors, based on the performance of a series of 15 repetitions, twice daily, for 7 days a week,[42,43] which are also those that are used most in tendinopathy, may negatively

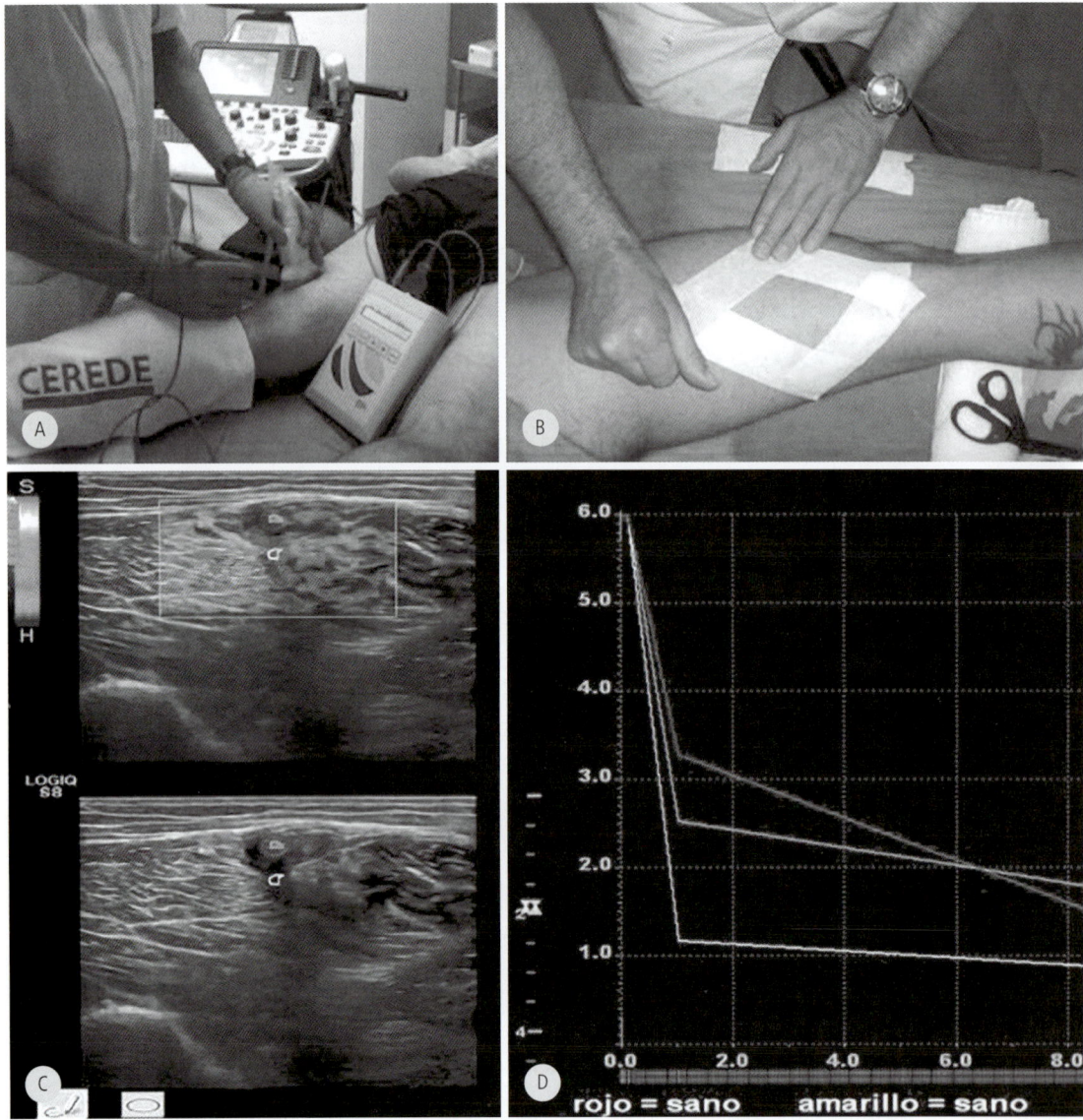

FIGURE 14.13 ■ Treatment of a biceps femoris muscle tear injury using EPI®. (A) Ultrasound-guided EPI®. (B) Taping for relaxation of the muscle tissue treated with EPI®. (C) and (D) Assessment and sonoelastographic control of the regeneration of the biceps femoris muscle treated with EPI®. (Colour version of figure is available online).

interfere with the acute inflammatory response produced by EPI®, which is a response that is important to respect in order to avoid any failure in the healing response. For this reason, a personal protocol is selected based on the biomechanical and biological criteria of each muscle group.

The individual protocol that is proposed consists of the performance of eccentric exercises based on the following points:

- The tension in the injured muscle varies according to the joint range of the joint/s in which it crosses.[44]

- The eccentric exercises are set as a protocol following the optimal criteria of functional load (table 14.5).

- Eccentric work is recommended to be performed in closed kinetic chain rather than open kinetic chain for two fundamental reasons: firstly, due to the fact that it is an exercise that bears more similarity with the functional use of the joint, and secondly, because closed kinetic chain work offers a decreased ischaemic compression in the injury area,[45] which could negatively influence treatment with EPI®.

- Eccentric overload training has been demonstrated to increase the level of strength and resistance of the muscle significantly, as well as the expression of cytokines and hormones related to the synthesis of muscle regeneration proteins.[46]

TABLE 14.5 **Optimal range of functional loading in tear injuries of the rectus femoris muscle**

Range of movement	Open kinetic chain	Closed kinetic chain
0–30°	+++	–
30–60°	–	–
60–90°	–	++
90–120°	++	+++

– less ischaemic tension; ++ moderate tension; +++ greater ischaemic tension.
Reproduced from Sánchez-Ibáñez.[25]

- The biomechanics of the joint are considered in order to avoid any iatrogenesis and greater tension strengths for both closed and open chain kinetics.[44] For this reason the optimal sector of load is respected, as shown in table 14.5.
- For the performance of eccentric exercises, there are commercially available devices designed by NASA, among which we can highlight the leg-press, yo-yo squat, leg curl, leg extension and multigym yo-yo[47] based on isoinertial eccentric work (YoYo Technology, Stockholm, Sweden) (figure 14.14).
- All isoinertial devices have computerized programs, including dynamometry, electronic goniometry, speed execution control and electromyography (Muscle-Lab), which provide an objective control of improvement in muscle strength, neuromuscular coordination and muscle speed

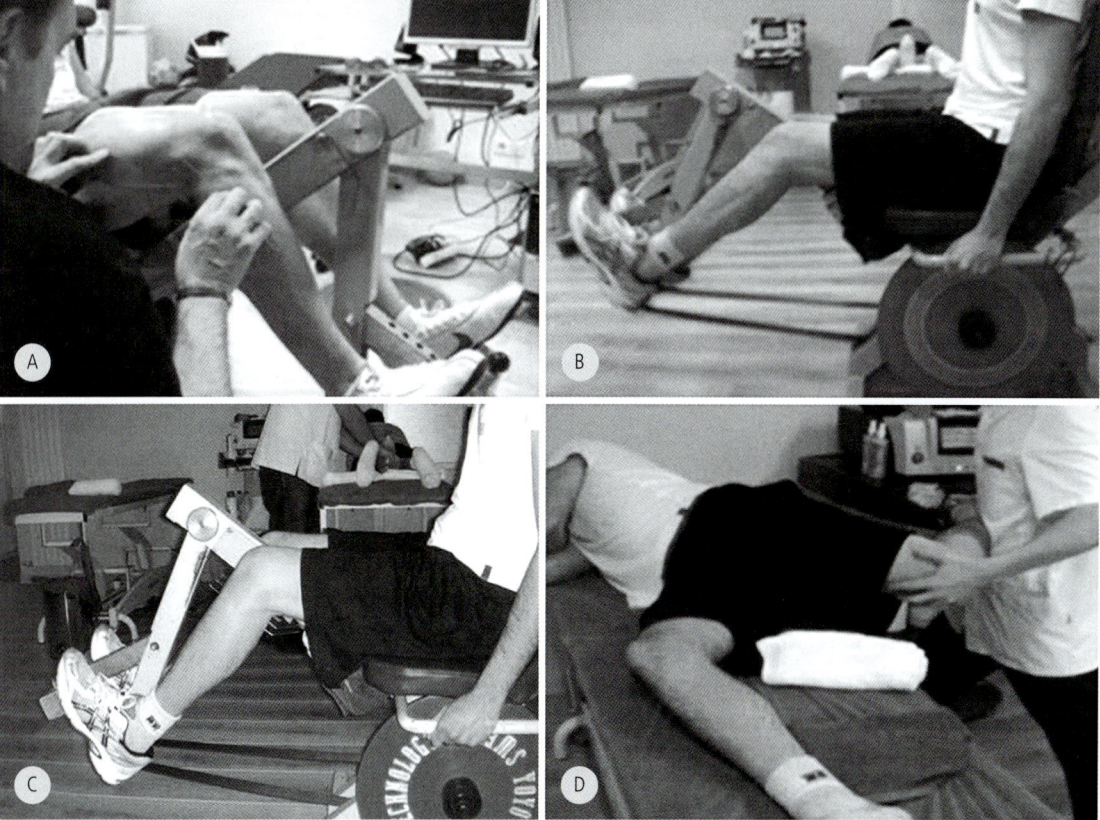

FIGURE 14.14 ■ Isoinertial eccentric exercise protocol for injuries of the rectus femoris muscle. (A) Determine the optimal range of loading using a goniometer. (B) Concentric phase performed with both legs. (C) Eccentric phase of the affected leg. (D) Quadriceps muscle stretch. (Reproduced from Sánchez Ibáñez JM. Fisiopatología de la regeneración de los tejidos blandos. In: Vilar E, Sureda S. Fisioterapia del aparato locomotor. Madrid: McGraw Hill, 2005). (Colour version of figure is available online).

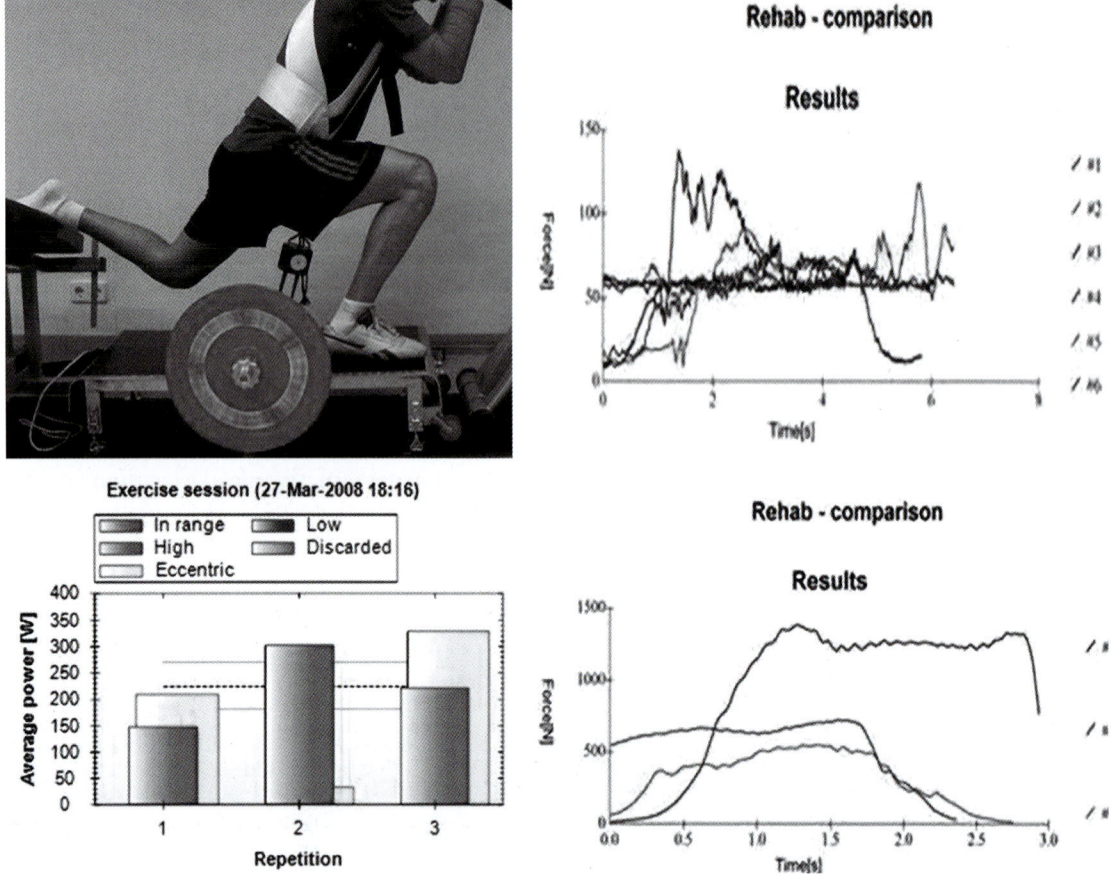

FIGURE 14.15 ■ Eccentric overloading using an isoinertial device. Electromyographic control charts regarding the eccentric/concentric strength and comparison of results. (Reproduced from Sánchez Ibáñez JM. Fisiopatología de la regeneración de los tejidos blandos. In: Vilar E, Sureda S. Fisioterapia del aparato locomotor. Madrid: McGraw Hill, 2005). (Colour version of figure is available online).

of both agonist as well as antagonist muscles (figure 14.15).

- All the patients must be previously taught the correct performance of three series of 10 repetitions, following the proposal of pioneer authors of these devices.[38,40,47,48]
- After eccentric overload exercises, stretches of a moderate intensity involving the same muscle groups are performed, consisting of five stretches with 6-second cycles of isometric contraction and 12 seconds' relaxation.

Eccentric training combined with EPI® has been demonstrated to be highly effective in the process of remodelling and maturation of the muscle injury, mainly with isoinertial computerized systems, which provide an objective control of the mechanical and neuromuscular characteristics of the injured muscle.

14.6 CLINICAL CASE

14.6.1 The effect of EPI® in acute muscle ruptures: tennis leg injury[24]

The most frequent injuries suffered by professional and amateur sports players are muscular injuries. These injuries, depending on their location, are especially important due to relapses; such is the case with muscle ruptures that affect the septum of the rectus anterior, the hamstrings and the medial gastrocnemius. In this last case, rupture of the distal portion of the medial gastrocnemius is also known as 'tennis leg' injury, and this pathology is frequently associated with rupture of the soleus or the plantaris muscle.

Reason for consultation: patient with a medical diagnosis of muscle rupture of the medial gastrocnemius.

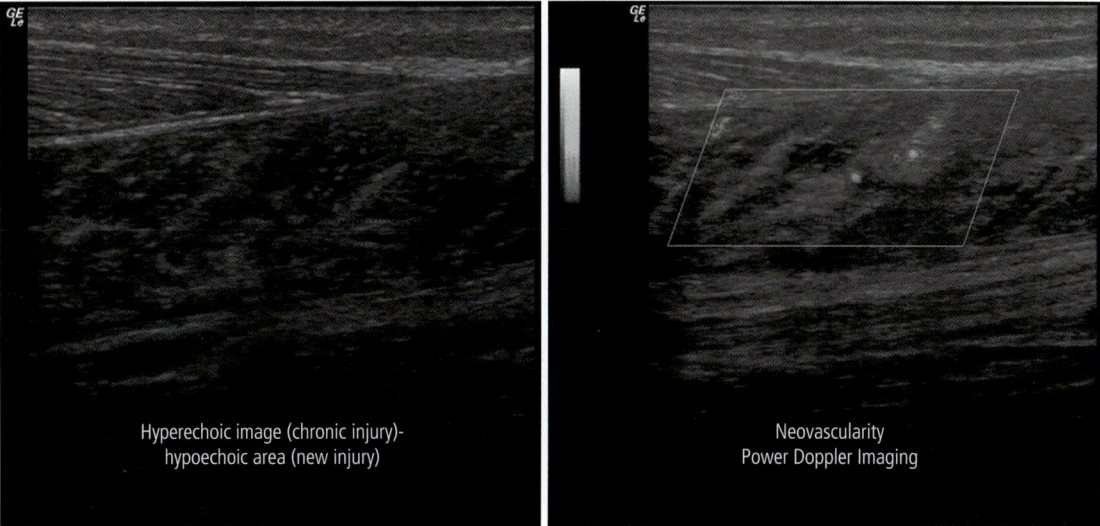

Hyperechoic image (chronic injury)-
hypoechoic area (new injury)

Neovascularity
Power Doppler Imaging

FIGURE 14.16 ■ Ultrasound image of the myoaponeurotic septum between the soleus and the medial gastrocnemius muscles. Power Doppler imaging. (Colour version of figure is available online).

History of the problem: 34-year-old male, right-handed, professional sportsman, with a case of recurrent muscle rupture affecting the medial gastrocnemius of the left leg. Six weeks earlier, the player suffered from the first muscle tear which was treated conservatively until he was discharged and allowed to return to training and competition. Four days after discharge, the patient suffered a re-rupture affecting the same area after performing another lesional movement and was referred to the clinic.

Diagnostic tests: the patient provides a nuclear magnetic resonance scan performed 24 hours after the appearance of the injury with the result of 'partial fibrillar rupture of the soleus with persistence of oedema'.

Physiotherapy diagnosis: at the first visit, the structure and function of the gastrocnemius and soleus muscles were analysed with musculoskeletal ultrasound (figure 14.16) (portable ultrasound device Logiq-E® by General Electric with a linear transducer 12L-RS [5–13 MHz]), showing signs compatible with poorly scarred tissue together with a flare-up of the process. Manual strength tests of the gastrocnemius and soleus evoked pain. There was selective pain on palpation of the muscle lesion area and a mild loss of continuity in the tissue ('dent' or 'gap' sign).

(Clinical case continued on page 490)

14.7 REFERENCES

1. Zarins B, Ciullo JV. Acute muscle and tendon injuries in athletes. Clin Sports Med 1983;2(1):167–82.
2. Dvorak J, Junge A, Chomiak J, et al. Risk factor analysis for injuries in football players. Possibilities for a prevention program. Am J Sports Med 2000;28(5 Suppl.):S69–74.
3. Ekstrand J, Hägglund M, Waldén M. Epidemiology of muscle injuries in professional football (soccer). Am J Sports Med 2011;39(6):1226–32.
4. Yao L, Heuser-Baker J, Herlea-Pana O, et al. Bone marrow endothelial progenitors augment atherosclerotic plaque regression in a mouse model of plasma lipid lowering. Stem Cells 2012;30:2720–31.
5. Mizrahi K, Stein J, Yaniv I, et al. TNF-α has tropic rather than apoptotic activity in human hematopoietic progenitors: involvement of TNF receptor-1 and caspase-8. Stem Cells 2013;31:156–66.
6. Kushida S, Kakudo N, Suzuki K, et al. Effects of platelet-rich plasma on proliferation and myofibroblastic differentiation in human dermal fibroblasts. Ann Plast Surg 2013;71:219–24.
7. Anitua E. Un nuevo enfoque en la regeneración ósea. Plasma rico en factores de crecimiento (PRGF). Puesta al díapublicaciones SL; 2000.
8. Fernandez A, Finley JM. Wound healing. Helping a natural process. Postgrad Med 1983;74(4):311–17.
9. Serhan CN, Chiang N, Van Dyke TE. Resolving inflammation: dual anti-inflammatory and pro-resolution lipid mediators. Nat Rev Immunol 2008;8(5):349–61.
10. Riley WB Jr. Wound healing. Am Fam Physician 1981; 24(5):107–13.
11. Darby IA, Hewitson TD. Fibroblast differentiation in wound healing and fibrosis. Int Rev Cytol 2007;257:143–79.
12. Mori R, Shaw TJ, Martin P. Molecular mechanisms linking wound inflammation and fibrosis: knockdown of osteopontin leads to rapid repair and reduced scarring. J Exp Med 2008;205(1):43–51.
13. Metcalfe D, Achten J, Costa ML. Glucocorticoid injections in lesions of the achilles tendon. Foot Ankle Int 2009;30(7):661–5.
14. Renström P, Peterson L. Groin injuries in athletes. Br J Sports Med 1980;14(1):30–6.
15. Jackson DW, Feagin JA. Quadriceps contusion in young athletes. J Bone Joint Surg 1973;55A:95–105.

16. Woods C, Hawkins RD, Maltby S, et al. The Football Association Medical Research Programme: an audit of injuries in professional football – analysis of hamstring injuries. Br J Sports Med 2004;38(1):36–41.

17. Järvinen TA, Järvinen TL, Kääriäinen M, et al. Muscle injuries: optimising recovery. Best Pract Res Clin Rheumatol 2007;21(2):317–31.

18. Järvinen TA, Järvinen TL, Kääriäinen M, et al. Muscle injuries: biology and treatment. Am J Sports Med 2005; 33:745–64.

19. Sánchez JM, Paredes P, Valles-Martí S, et al. Análisis molecular de la Electrólisis Percutánea Intratisular (EPI®) en la lesión muscular de la rata. In: I Congreso Internacional de Electrólisis Percutánea Intratisular (EPI®). Libro de comunicaciones y ponencias. Madrid: 2011.

20. Owoeye I, Spielholz NI, Fetto J, et al. Low-intensity pulsed galvanic current and the healing of tenotomized rat achilles tendons: preliminary report using load-to-breaking measurements. Arch Phys Med Rehabil 1987; 68(7):415–18.

21. Zhao Y, Zeng H, Nam J, et al. Fabrication of skeletal muscle constructs by topographic activation of cell alignment. Biotechnol Bioeng 2009;102(2):624–31.

22. Litke DS, Dahners LE. Effects of different levels of direct current on early ligament healing in a rat model. J Orthop Res 1994;12(5):683–8.

23. Becker RO. The bioelectric factors in amphibian limb regeneration. J Bone Joint Surg 1961;43-A:643–56.

24. Valera F, Minaya F, Sánchez JM. Efecto de la Electrólisis Percutánea Intratisular (EPI®) en las roturas musculares agudas. Caso clínico de la lesión de 'tennisleg'. En: II Congreso Regional de fisioterapia de la Universidad de Murcia. Libro de comunicaciones y ponencias. Murcia: 2012.

25. Sánchez Ibáñez JM. Fisiopatología de la regeneración de los tejidos blandos. In: Vilar E, Sureda S, editors. Fisioterapia del aparato locomotor. Madrid: McGraw Hill; 2005.

26. Minaya F, Valera F, Sánchez JM. Efectividad de la Electrólisis Percutánea Intratisular (EPI®) versus punción seca en los puntos gatillo miofasciales del antebrazo. In: X Jornadas Sociedad Española de Traumatología Laboral. Libro de comunicaciones y ponencias. Toledo: 2010.

27. Nemet D, Meckel Y, Bar-Sela S, et al. Effect of local cold-pack application on systemic anabolic and inflammatory response to sprint-interval training: a prospective comparative trial. Eur J Appl Physiol 2009;107:411–17.

28. Haraldsson BT, Aagaard P, Crafoord-Larsen D, et al. Corticosteroid administration alters the mechanical properties of isolated collagen fascicles in rat-tail tendon. Scand J Med Sci Sports 2009;19(5):621–6.

29. Dye SF. Functional morphologic features of the human knee: an evolutionary perspective. Clin Orthop Relat Res 2003;410:19–24.

30. Jiménez-Díaz F, Jimena I, Luque E, et al. Experimental muscle injury: correlation between ultrasound and histological findings. Muscle Nerve 2012;45(5):705–12.

31. Ginat DT, Destounis SV, Barr RG, et al. US elastography of breast and prostate lesions. Radiographics 2009; 29(7):2007–16.

32. Lalitha P, Reddy MCH, Reddy KJ. Musculoskeletal applications of elastography: a pictorial essay of our initial experience. Korean J Radiol 2011;12(3):365–75.

33. Sankhala RS, Damai RS, Swamy MJ. Correlation of membrane binding and hydrophobicity to the chaperone-like activity of PDC-109, the major protein of bovine seminal plasma. PLoS ONE 2011;6(3):e17330.

34. Cross TM, Gibbs N, Houang MT, et al. Acute quadriceps muscle strains: magnetic resonance imaging features and prognosis. Am J Sports Med 2004;32(3): 710–19.

35. Young JL, Laskowski ER, Rock MG. Thigh injuries in athletes. Mayo Clin Proc 1993;68:1099–106.

36. Heiderscheit BC, Sherry MA, Silder A, et al. Hamstring strain injuries: recommendations for diagnosis, rehabilitation, and injury prevention. J Orthop Sports Phys Ther 2010;40(2):67–81.

37. Orchard J, Seward H. Epidemiology of injuries in the Australian Football League, seasons 1997–2000. Br J Sports Med 2002;36(1):39–44.

38. Tous-Fajardo J, Maldonado RA, Quintana JM, et al. The flywheel leg-curl machine: offering eccentric overload for hamstring development. Int J Sports Physiol Perform 2006;1(3):293–8.

39. Leadbetter WB, Buckwalter JA, Gordon SL. Sports induced inflammation. Rosemont, IL: American Academy of Orthopaedic Surgeons; 1990.

40. Romero-Rodriguez D, Gual G, Tesch PA. Efficacy of an inertial resistance training paradigm in the treatment of patellar tendinopathy in athletes: a case-series study. Phys Ther Sport 2011;12(1):43–8.

41. Paulsen G, Mikkelsen UR, Raastad T, et al. Leucocytes, cytokines and satellite cells: what role do they play in muscle damage and regeneration following eccentric exercise? Exerc Immunol Rev 2012;18:42–97.

42. Alfredson H, Pietilä T, Jonsson P, et al. Heavy-load eccentric calf muscle training for the treatment of chronic Achilles tendinosis. Am J Sports Med 1998;26(3): 360–6.

43. Purdam CR, Jonsson P, Alfredson H, et al. A pilot study of the eccentric decline squat in the management of painful chronic patellar tendinopathy. Br J Sports Med 2004;38(4):395–7.

44. Grelsamer RP, Klein JR. The biomechanics of the patellofemoral joint. J Orthop Sports Phys Ther 1998;28(5): 286–98.

45. Nakamura K, Kitaoka K, Tomita K. Effect of eccentric exercise on the healing process of injured patellar tendon in rats. J Orthop Sci 2008;13(4):371–8.

46. Kalliokoski KK, Langberg H, Ryberg AK, et al. Nitric oxide and prostaglandins influence local skeletal muscle blood flow during exercise in humans: coupling between local substrate uptake and blood flow. Am J Physiol Regul Integr Comp Physiol 2006;291(3):R803–9.

47. Tesch PA, Berg HE, Bring D, et al. Effects of 17-day spaceflight on knee extensor muscle function and size. Eur J Appl Physiol 2005;93(4):463–8.

48. Askling C, Karlsson J, Thorstensson A. Hamstring injury occurrence in elite soccer players after preseason strength training with eccentric overload. Scand J Med Sci Sports 2003;13(4):244–50.

49. Garrett WE Jr, Califf JC, Bassett FH 3rd. Histochemical correlates of hamstring injuries. Am J Sports Med 1984; 12(2):98–103.

PART VII

ACUPUNCTURE

CHAPTER 15

CLINICAL ACUPUNCTURE

Antonio García Godino · Roberto Sebastián Ojero · Francisco Minaya Muñoz

The wise man seeks all that he wants in himself; the common man seeks all that he wants from others.
CONFUCIUS

KEYWORDS

acupuncture; dermatome; acupuncture meridian; classic acupuncture points; segmental response; algogenic substances; intra-articular technique; tendinomuscular meridian technique; Western acupuncture.

15.1 INTRODUCTION

This chapter is not intended to be a treaty on traditional Chinese medicine (TCM) but rather seeks to demonstrate to the therapist the necessary knowledge in order to integrate acupuncture within a more global approach. Acupuncture is an ideal complement to the rest of the techniques available, and offers the possibility of notably improving therapeutic effectiveness with highly satisfactory results for patients.

Acupuncture is considered a complex type of medicine as it offers, on the one hand, an empirical-philosophical concept and, on the other, a scientific concept with regard to its theories and application.

Throughout this chapter, we will try to integrate both these modalities or concepts (philosophical and scientific) in order to develop a clinical model of acupuncture as applied to common patient pathologies within the field of physiotherapy.

15.2 FROM MILLENARY WISDOM TO SCIENTIFIC EVIDENCE

Acupuncture is an invasive technique in which needles are inserted into determined points on the body with the goal of re-establishing the energetic balance of the meridians, improving and/or recovering the patient's state of health. It is considered to be one of the basic pillars of TCM together with moxibustion (biological heat), herbal medicine, *tui-na* (manual therapy) and *Qi-gong* (exercises for cultivating energy).

Through acupuncture, a therapeutic procedure is established which is able to prevent and treat different illnesses via stimulation with needles or via other means at precise, predetermined points.

This is a thousand-year-old technique that was originally performed using instruments made of different materials (i.e. Bian stones) in order to stimulate these points or areas with the purpose of healing. Thereafter, other types of materials have been used, such as fishbone, bone or bamboo, until the first metallic needles were produced.

According to various sources, there are acupuncture texts written more than 2000 years ago, while others support the theory that acupuncture dates back to around the third century BC (475–221 BC). There is also an ancient descriptive reference text that states the principles of TCM for the first time with a diversity of data regarding the beginning of this millenary practice. The classic text of reference is undoubtedly *The Medical Classic of the Yellow Emperor*, by Huang di Neijing Suwen[1] (which dates from 500–300 years BC) and which describes conversations between the emperor and the doctors of the court. In this work the fundamental basis of acupuncture is described. Thereafter, during the ensuing Chinese dynasties, different evolutionary phases took place which have enriched, developed and perfected this technique and whereby the various theories are gathered together with a description of the meridians and different clinical experiences. At the end of the 17th century, acupuncture methods arrived in Europe thanks to Jesuit missionaries, but it was during the 19th century that the French ambassador Soulié de Morant led its dissemination and consequent development in the West.[2]

During the last two decades, acupuncture has spread throughout the world, and has been both widely supported and perfected. In particular, studies have taken place from a medical perspective and, using modern research techniques, have obtained highly relevant and significant results. Not only has acupuncture been studied in various illnesses that affect people in different therapeutic fields (e.g. the musculoskeletal system, internal medicine, dermatology, gynaecology, otorhinolaryngology, the respiratory system), but also the acupuncture points have been subject to detailed study, together with the network of channels or meridians, for the purpose of clinical practice.

15.3 MECHANISMS OF ACTION

15.3.1 General concepts

Acupuncture has always provided knowledge as an empirical therapy based on facts, observations and experiments, and has been perfected throughout history. The concepts of the taoist *yin–yang* philosophy are considered, and nomenclature forms are used that distinguish between pathology and pathogenesis, as well as the attack of the different pathogens and their impact on the body. Often, supernatural practices are intermingled with medicine. Acupuncture closely considers phenomena that usually go unnoticed in Western medicine, such as the influence of perverse climatic factors (e.g. wind, cold, heat, dryness, humidity), emotions, the seasons or conducting an anamnesis structured by body organ. All these factors can provide definitive information in order to formulate a diagnosis and provide the appropriate treatment.

Notwithstanding, in the world of contemporary medicine there can be no doubts concerning the clinical and scientific effectiveness of acupuncture for a great variety of medical conditions, as well as the influence of the biological cycles of TCM and its empiricism.

15.3.2 The effects of acupuncture

The effects of acupuncture can be classified into: local effects (see chapter 2) and distal effects (segmental and extrasegmental).

15.3.2.1 Distal effects

- Segmental response: after the puncture, a stimulus is produced in one to three dermatomes. A parallel can be established between the metameric pathway and that of the acupuncture meridian. The segmental structure (metameres) of the body performs a key role in internal disorders.[3,4] For example, the gall bladder (GB) meridian corresponds with the S1 territory, while that of the small intestine (SI) corresponds with the territory of C6.
- Extrasegmental response: after the puncture, activity is produced in the central cerebral mechanisms, regulating and balancing the internal homeostasis. This acts on different levels of the nervous system: peripheral, medullar and central. Apart from triggering neurohormonal mechanisms (including the immune and endocrine systems), it produces a cascade of biological repair elements with the release of endogenous opioids that modulate and control pain, specifically in the midbrain periaqueductal grey mattet.[5] Furthermore, the organism's capacity for self-regulation and self-repair is stimulated, thus neutralizing pain-causing agents.[6]

Regarding the mechanisms of action of acupuncture, not only are the effects on the segment and corresponding metameres highlighted, but also notable neurochemical mechanisms are triggered. In addition, blood circulation is stimulated and there is a regulation of the vegetative nervous system, as well as a stimulation of the self-regulation systems, the endocannabinoid system, 'local' effects, the mechanotransduction and influences on the function of the brain.[7]

15.3.3 The neurophysiology of pain

The clinical practice of acupuncture influences different levels of the nervous system (figure 15.1)[7–9]:

- activation and sensitization of the peripheral nociceptors

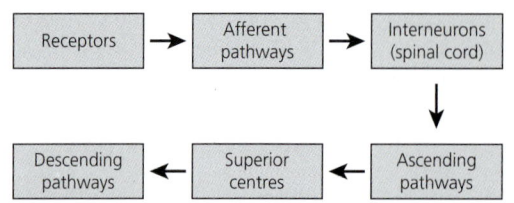

FIGURE 15.1 ■ Acupuncture mechanisms of transmission and action.

- transmission of nociceptive stimuli by the primary afferents
- modulation and integration of the nociceptive response at the level of the spinal dorsal horn: first level of integration of information from sensory afferents into the central nervous system
- transmission through ascending pathways
- integration of the response in the higher centres (brain structures)
- control through the descending pathways.

15.3.3.1 Peripheral nociceptors

Via the acupuncture needling technique, afferent fibres of the peripheral nerves are activated – A-β (type II) and A-δ (type III), producing the so-called 'Qi flow' in TCM.[10]

On the other hand, the local concentration of algogen substances activated by the peripheral tissue lesion is reduced and changes are produced in circulation, temperature and chemical effects.

15.3.3.2 The medullary level and ascending pathways

The stimulus caused by the needle will reach the spinal cord. This is the first synaptic station and the filter that permits elimination of unnecessary messages while amplifying the most important one towards the higher centres.

Neuromodulation occurs in the posterior horn of the grey matter of the spinal cord via modulator interneurons. This, in turn, produces the gate control phenomenon, blocking the entrance of pain at the spinal level, thus inhibiting transmission of nociceptive information towards higher nervous centres.[11] The afferent neurons of the dorsal horn synapse directly (synapsis between the first and second neuron via the liberation of neurotransmitters) and indirectly (synapsis between the first neuron and the modulatory interneurons) with the motor neurons of the anterior horn. This synapsis is responsible for the reflex muscular activity (normal or pathological) that is associated with pain.

The information pathway circulates along the anterolateral quadrant of the white matter of the spinal cord, after having crossed the commissure (the axons of the neurons of the dorsal horn form the ascending pathways) until arriving at the thalamus, prefrontal zone and limbic system (somatosensory cortex)[12] through the following ascending pathways:

- spinothalamic pathway: carries the most information and nociception: pain and temperature

- spinoreticular tract: in relation to affective phenomena. some axons terminate in the reticular formation of the pons and the brainstem
- spinomesencephalic tract: collateral pathway to the midbrain periaqueductal grey matter.

The main neurotransmitters released are:

- Endogenous opioid peptides: their action is similar to morphine. Endogenous opioid peptides participate in the modulation of nociception and the perception of pain. They have an analgesic action: e.g. enkephalins, endorphins, dynorphins.
- Endogenous non-opioid peptides: their action is not very clear, e.g. calcitonin, cholescystokinin, neurotensin, somatostatin.
- Neuromodulators: these come from the superior nuclei that descend to the spinal cord and have an inhibitory action, e.g. serotonin, catecholamines (noradrenaline).
- Gamma-aminobutyric acid: this is a spinal inhibitor.
- Excitatory amino acids: glutamate and aspartate.

15.3.3.3 Higher nervous centres

These areas of the central nervous system participate in the transmission of information and in the analysis of stimulus, in relation to the duration, intensity and localization of the information. Furthermore, they project to cortical areas or elaborate motor and emotional reactions.

Shen demonstrated that the dorsomedial part of the bulbar reticular formation, which comprises the posterior group of the raphe nuclei, is the most important nervous structure in the supraspinal modulation caused by acupuncture.[12]

KEY POINTS

The axons, after crossing the midline at the spinal level, ascend on the contralateral side and carry the information to the reticular formation, the nucleus raphe magnus, the periaqueductal grey, the nuclei of the thalamus, the limbic system and hypothalamus and the somatosensory cortex.

15.3.3.4 Descending pathways

At this level, an endogenous modulation of pain is produced which is expressed using inhibition systems of nociceptive impulses. The final balance determines the magnitude and duration of the painful sensations triggered by a painful stimulus.

The descending component courses through the dorsolateral fascicle of the spinal cord, as the most important control system that connects the periaqueductal grey, the reticular formation, the nucleus raphe magnus and the thalamic nuclei of the rostroventromedial bulbar reticular formation, (the 'relay station' between the midbrain and the dorsal horns) and the dorsolateral pontine tegmentum.

The principal mediators that act upon the descending system are serotonin and noradrenaline.

15.4 THE CLINICAL CORRELATION AND CORRESPONDENCE BETWEEN ACUPUNCTURE POINTS

Many authors have described a clinical correspondence between the classical acupuncture points and the most relevant myofascial trigger points (MTrPs).

According to Dorsher and Fleckenstein[13], there is a 93% anatomical correspondence between regions of MTrPs and classic acupuncture points. Furthermore, these authors assert that highly evident anatomical and clinical correspondences exist, as the acupuncture points are firmly based on the anatomy of the nervous and muscular systems. There are also clinical correlations between both systems regarding pain disorders and their treatment (97%) and somatovisceral disorders (93.3%). This provides clinical support for the fact that MTrPs and acupuncture points may, in fact, reflect the same physiological phenomena. In contrast, only 7–9% of the point pairs showed a poor or null correspondence between patterns of referred pain and acupuncture meridians.

According to Melzack[14], there is an anatomical correspondence of approximately 94–97% between the classical acupuncture points and the MTrPs traditionally used for the treatment of pain syndromes in general. As a result, in pain with clinical and anatomical similarities, both treatments have shown positive results. For example, the MTrP of the masseter muscle (superior, posterior, middle, anterior portions and superficial and deep layers) for the treatment of posterosuperior dental pain, tinnitus or pain in the upper incisors corresponds with the number 6 acupuncture point of the stomach meridian (ST6) and the acupuncture points ST36, ST37 and ST39 correspond with the MTrP of the tibialis anterior muscle and are used

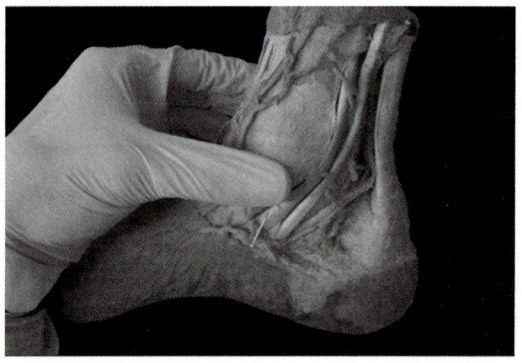
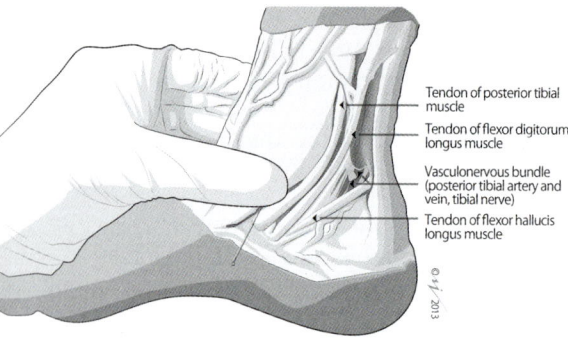

Tendon of posterior tibial muscle

Tendon of flexor digitorum longus muscle

Vasculonervous bundle (posterior tibial artery and vein, tibial nerve)

Tendon of flexor hallucis longus muscle

FIGURE 15.2 ■ The KID6 point and its correspondence with the medial retromalleolar vasculonervous bundle (posterior tibial artery and vein, tibial nerve) and dependent musculoskeletal structures, such as the tendon of tibialis posterior muscle, tendon of flexor digitorum longus muscle and tendon of flexor hallucis longus muscle. (Cadaver image courtesy of F. Valderrama, F. Valera and F. Minaya). (Colour version of figure is available online).

in neurophysiological studies in order to test the deep fibular nerve, as accessory branches dependent on the common fibular nerve, such as in the case of drop foot.

On the other hand, these authors support the existence of a clinical correlation between the pathway of the meridian within which the acupuncture points are found and the MTrPs that are anatomically correlated[15] in the description of patterns of referred pain. For example, the most common pattern of referred pain for the latissimus dorsi muscle corresponds with the pathway of the small-intestine meridian.

The correspondence of some of the acupuncture points with MTrPs[13–17] are presented below:

- SI15, TB14: deltoid (anterior, medial and posterior fibres)
- LI12: brachioradialis
- LI11: extensor carpi radialis longus
- SI3: abductor digiti minimi
- LI4: adductor hallucis
- SI11: infraspinatus
- HE3: pronator teres
- LI8: extensor carpi radialis brevis
- TB23: orbicularis oculi.

Furthermore, numerous authors have demonstrated that a close relationship exists between the classic acupuncture points and structures such as fat, subcutaneous cellular tissue, fascia, the connective tissue system and cutaneous nerves. Furthermore, they have studied the correspondence of acupuncture points/meridians with the connective tissue, as acupuncture points are usually located within fascial planes (subcutaneous cellular tissue, between bones and muscles).

The relation of the acupuncture points with cutaneous nerves is detailed below:

- TB10, SI8, HE7, HE6, HE5, HE4: ulnar nerve
- LU9, LI5: radial nerve

- BL36, BL37, BL40, BL55: sciatic nerve
- KID1: lateral plantar nerve
- TB5: posterior interosseous nerve
- GB20: greater occipital nerve.

Another example is the acupuncture point KID6 (figure 15.2), which is found below the maximal prominence of the medial malleolus of the ankle and which has special relevance due to its relation with the innervation path of the posterior tibial artery and vein or acupuncture points KID6 and KID7. The latter are more commonly and traditionally used in the West for stimulation of the posterior tibial artery and vein, and tibial nerve (and its symptoms), while in the East these are traditionally used for tonification of the functional sphere of the kidney (*yin*), due to the correspondence with the cycle of the five elements.

KEY POINTS

In TCM the scientific concept is integrated with the philosophical-empirical concepts. An example are the ST36, ST37 and ST39 points, which are motor points of the tibialis anterior and which, furthermore, are used in both acute and chronic illnesses of the gastrointestinal system as special points of action for unblocking the stomach, the large intestine and the small intestine.

15.5 NOTIONS OF BIONERGETICS

15.5.1 Basic description of the energies

Acupuncture, as previously defined, is an energy technique. Thus, in this section, we shall present a brief description of the fundamental energies that enable the system to function and which will provide the therapist with a therapeutic strategy when approaching the patient. These energies are divided as follows.

15.5.1.1 Ancestral Qi

This is the ancestral energy or the essence with which we are born and is due to the sum of *yuangqi* or the original energy of each species with *zhongqi*, which is the energy inherited from our parents and related to the reproductive processes of the cellular formation. The genetic predisposition of the person to fall ill depends on this latter energy.

15.5.1.2 Acquired Qi

This is the energy obtained from the relation of individuals with their surroundings via teluriccosmic processes. Within acquired *Qi* we can find:

- *Rong Qi:* this is the energy obtained from simple metabolic processes from the energy extracted from food and air. This energy circulates within channels called principal acupuncture meridians during a 24-hour cycle and is responsible for the dynamics of functional organic activities, such as intestinal peristalsis and respiratory function.
- *Wei Qi:* this is a type of energy that also arises from complex metabolic processes, resulting in an energy that is more *yang*, and which carries a defensive function. This energy circulates through more superficial channels called the tendinomuscular meridians (TMM). These are responsible for energetic nutrition of the musculoskeletal system and defensive processes.

15.5.2 Concepts of energy physiology

In the following section, the two fundamental theories upon which TCM is based will be explained: the *yin–yang* theory and the theory of the five elements. These provide an explanation for the human body, its physiology and its physiopathology. These theories introduce the reader to the related diagnosis and physiotherapy treatment.[18,19]

15.5.2.1 Yin–yang theory

The *yin–yang* theory states that everything in nature is formed by two polarities, one called *yin*, and another, *yang*. These are opposites, but they complement each other and one cannot exist

without the other. They form a single unit that is known as the vital *tao*.

Humans are considered to be a vital *tao*, formed of a *yin* part, which is the matter and the physiological processes, and a *yang* part, which is the energy needed to perform these processes (adenosine triphosphate), so that matter cannot exist without energy, and vice versa.

This concept of bipolarity in the vital *tao* must be in harmony, and is fundamental in order to maintain the balance between the internal processes and the external surroundings, and body homeostasis is reliant on this.[20,21]

On the other hand, this *yin–yang* concept is described as being integrated within a law of relativity: 'The *yin* and *yang*[22] are antagonists; they mutually control one another; each is considered the basis of the other; they reciprocally transform into their inverse and both the increase and the decrease of the *yin–yang* are in balance'. For this reason, an absolute *yin* or *yang* cannot exist; everything is relative according to a framework of comparison.

An example of the *yin–yang* law of relativity is that, within the body, the head would be the *yang*, as opposed to the feet, which would be *yin*. However, within the head, the eyes would be *yang*, as opposed to the mouth, which would be *yin* (table 15.1).

KEY POINTS

The yin and yang are antagonists, they control one another mutually, each is considered the basis of the other, they reciprocally transform into their inverse and both the increase or the decrease of the yin-yang are in balance.

As previously noted, the concept of health is established on the basis of the balance between *yin* and *yang* (figure 15.3). If one becomes imbalanced with regard to the other, either by excess or defect, the body loses its capacity for adaptation and begins a process which, if the body is

TABLE 15.1	*Yin–yang* characteristics
Yin	**Yang**
Woman	Man
Dark	Light
Night	Day
Earth	Sky
Matter	Energy
Organ	Viscera
Deficiency	Excess
Parasympathetic	Sympathetic
-osis (wasting)	-itis (inflammation)
Xue	*Qi*

not able to resolve on its own, would result in the appearance of the first symptoms of illness depending on the affected meridian (figures 15.4 and 15.5).

An example of this is a patient who attends a consultation with inflammation, pain and redness in a knee. Apparently, the patient presents *yang*-type symptoms, but the cause could be an acute process with a predominance or plentitude of *yang* (arthritis) or the acute spike of a chronic process with waste and a lack of *yin* (arthrosis).

15.5.2.2 Theory of the five elements

TCM describes a series of elements or energetic movements based on the observation of nature and for which a series of characteristics are assigned, such as colours, tastes, emotions and climatic factors. A series of interrelations are also established between all of these and this allows for the explanation, diagnosis and treatment of a large number of pathologies.

These elements are: wood (table 15.2), fire (table 15.3), earth (table 15.4), metal (table 15.5) and water (table 15.6).

Once these five elements and their characteristics are described, an image is created of the penta-coordination and their relations are established, thereby developing what are known as physiological and pathological cycles.

15.5.2.3 The physiological cycles

The physiological cycles are the interdependent interrelations that are established between the

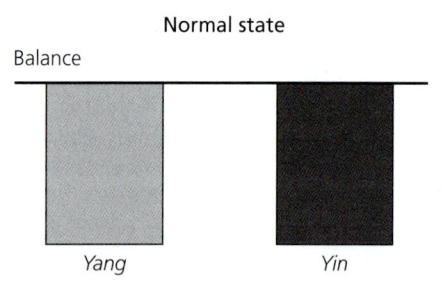

Normal state

Balance

Yang   Yin

FIGURE 15.3 ■ State of balance between *yin* and *yang*.

TABLE 15.2	**Wood element correspondences**
Organ	Liver
Viscera	Gall bladder
Sense	Sight
Colour	Green
Taste	Acid
Season	Spring
Emotions	Imagination/anger
Nourishes	Muscles/tendons/nails
Climatic factor	Wind

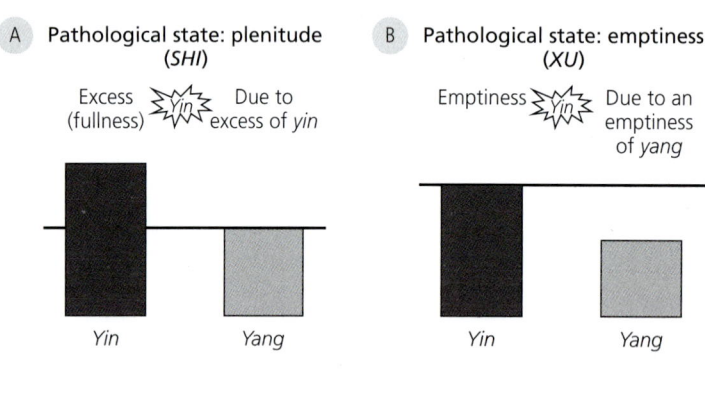

A Pathological state: plenitude (*SHI*)

Excess (fullness) → *Yin* ← Due to excess of *yin*

Yin   Yang

B Pathological state: emptiness (*XU*)

Emptiness → *Yin* ← Due to an emptiness of yang

Yin   Yang

FIGURE 15.4 ■ (A) Pathological state of plenitude or excess (*Shi*) of *yin*. (B) Pathological state of deficiency or emptiness (*Xu*) of *yang*.

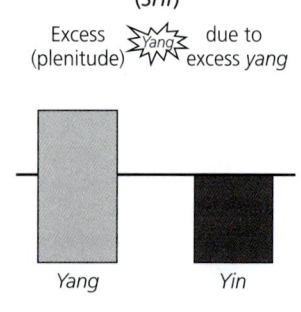

A Pathological state: plenitude (*SHI*)

Excess (plenitude) → *Yang* ← due to excess yang

Yang   Yin

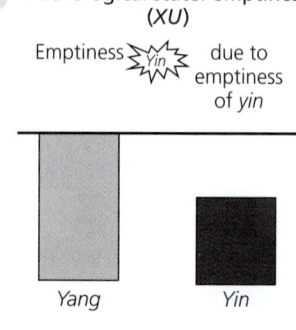

B Pathological state: emptiness (*XU*)

Emptiness → *Yin* ← due to emptiness of *yin*

Yang   Yin

FIGURE 15.5 ■ (A) Pathological state of plenitude or excess (*Shi*) of *yang*. (B) Pathological state of deficiency or emptiness (*Xu*) of *yin*.

TABLE 15.3	Fire element correspondences
Organ	Heart
Viscera	Small intestine
Sense	Tact
Colour	Red
Taste	Sour
Season	Summer
Emotions	Word/joy
Nourishes	Blood vessels/complexion
Climatic factor	Heat

TABLE 15.4	Earth element correspondences
Organ	Spleen
Viscera	Stomach
Sense	Taste
Colour	Yellow
Taste	Sweet
Season	Midsummer heat
Emotions	Reflection/obsession
Nourishes	Connective tissue/lips
Climatic factor	Humidity

TABLE 15.5	Metal element correspondences
Organ	Lung
Viscera	Small intestine
Sense	Smell
Colour	White
Taste	Spicy
Season	Autumn
Emotions	Soul/sadness
Nourishes	Skin/hair
Climatic factor	Dryness

TABLE 15.6	Water element correspondences
Organ	Kidney
Viscera	Bladder
Sense	Hearing
Colour	Black
Taste	Salty
Season	Winter
Emotions	Willpower/fear
Nourishes	Bones/hair
Climatic factor	Cold

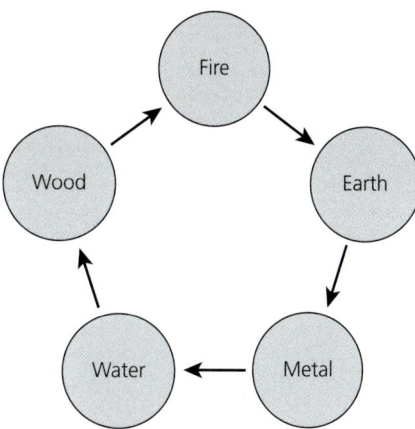

FIGURE 15.6 ■ *Sheng* cycle (generation).

the next but, at the same time, is generated by the previous one (and so on). Each element is considered the 'mother' of the element that follows and the 'son' of the previous. In this manner, wood generates fire, but is also generated by water; fire generates earth and is generated by wood; earth generates metal and is generated by fire; metal generates water and is generated by earth; and water generates wood and is generated by metal. This cycle, whose mission it is to generate, engender and stimulate, could be compared with the sympathetic system of the body (figure 15.6).

• The *Ko* cycle is related to the control that some elements establish over others that, at the same time, are also controlled. In this manner, wood controls earth but is controlled by metal, fire controls metal but is controlled by water, earth controls water but is controlled by wood, metal controls wood but is controlled by fire, and water controls fire but is controlled by earth. This cycle, whose mission it is to control in order to avoid the excess of a stimulus, could be compared with the parasympathetic system (figure 15.7).

Thanks to these two cycles of generation and control (sympathetic and parasympathetic), a system is established which helps to maintain the balance of our organism. When this balance is disrupted, pathological cycles appear.

15.5.2.4 The pathological cycles

When an organ/viscera has an excess of energetic stimulus and if the balance system does not function properly, this may affect the rest of the elements, causing the development of the characteristic symptoms of each system. There are four such cycles, two in relation to the

five elements and which explain the influence that some of these can have over the others.

There are two physiological cycles: generation (*Sheng*) and control (*Ko*).[19,21]

• The *Sheng* cycle is related with generation or creation, so that one element generates

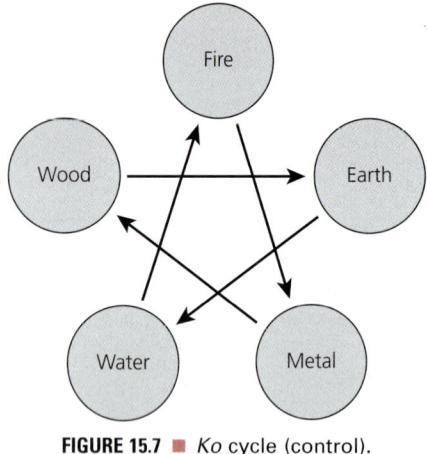

FIGURE 15.7 ■ *Ko* cycle (control).

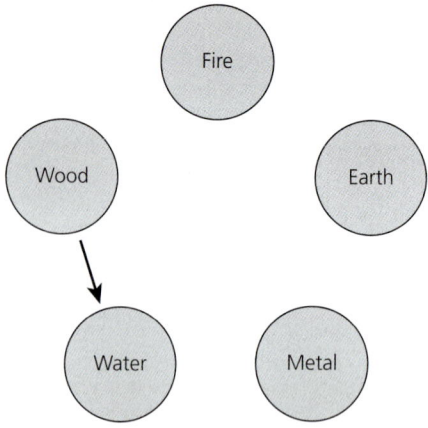

FIGURE 15.9 ■ *Zi-Mu* cycle.

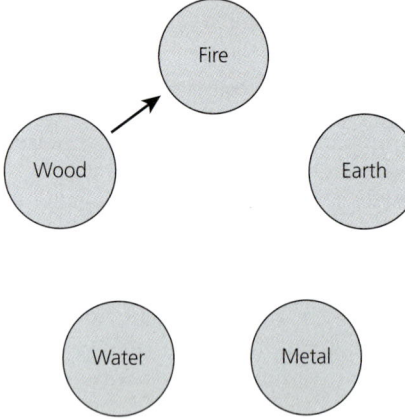

FIGURE 15.8 ■ *Mu-Zi* cycle.

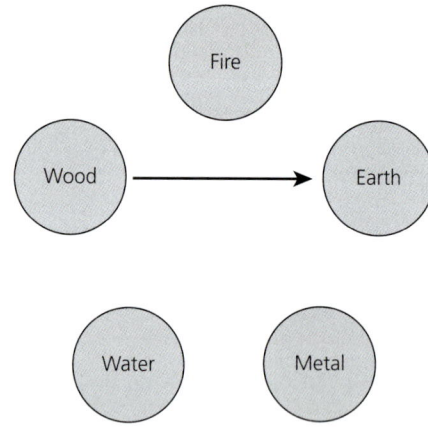

FIGURE 15.10 ■ *T'Cheng* cycle.

generation cycle (*Mu-Zi* and *Zi-Mu*) and two in relation to the control cycle (*T'Cheng* and *Wu* cycle).

- *Mu-Zi* cycle (the mother can tire the son): 'An excess of wood can generate an excess of fire' (figure 15.8). For example: an excess of muscular activity or of stress can over-stimulate the liver (wood). If the systems are not properly balanced, this overstimu-lation will affect the heart (fire), and symp-toms such as palpitations and arrhythmias may appear.
- *Zi-Mu* cycle (the mother can be tired by the son): 'An excess of wood can consume water' (figure 15.9). An excess of energetic stimulus over the liver, if water is not in balance, could be harmful and cause the appearance of symptoms pertaining to that element, such as tinnitus and low-back pain.
- *T'Cheng* cycle (excess of dominance): 'An excess of wood can block earth' (figure 15.10). The excess of energetic stimulus over the liver can produce a blockage of the

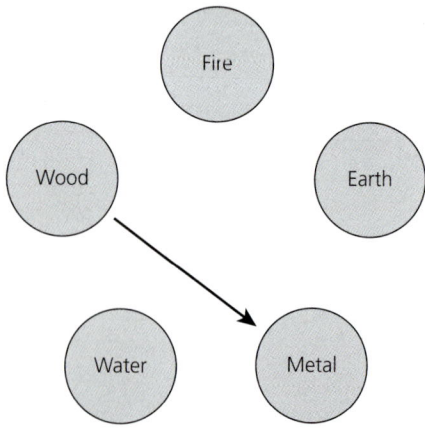

FIGURE 15.11 ■ Insulting *Wu* cycle.

spleen, producing the appearance of diges-tive symptoms.

- Insulting (*Wu*) cycle: 'An excess of wood can break metal' (figure 15.11). An excess of energetic stimulus from the liver, if the movement of water is unbalanced, can affect the lung, producing corresponding symptoms such as coughing, dyspnoea or skin disorders.

15.6 THE ACUPUNCTURE MERIDIANS (*JING MAI*)

15.6.1 Definition

The acupuncture meridians are the channels along which the different types of energy circulate, according to the type of meridian: the *rong* energy circulates along the main meridians, and the *wei* energy circulates along the TMM. As these are pathways that carry energy (*Qi*), they accompany great paths of matter (*Xue*). They have a precise topography, with a beginning, an end and a well-defined circulation sense.

These meridians are bilateral and symmetrical and they flow through the human body forming a network made up of main branches, secondary branches and capillaries. Therefore, they are an instrument of communication between the surface of the body and the organs.

The main meridians conduct the energy to the next meridian by means of an external pathway, which is where the acupuncture points are found (and on which the therapist will focus during treatment). These lead to the corresponding energy unit (organ/viscera) following an internal pathway. An example is the bladder meridian, which accompanies the pathway of the sciatic nerve.

These meridians receive the name of five organs (*yin*) and five viscera (*yang*) together with two meridians that correspond with both functions:

- Six organs: LU: lung; P: pericardium (corresponds with a function); HE: heart; SP: spleen; LIV: liver; and KID: kidney.
- Six viscera: LI: large intestine; TB: triple burner or *sanjiao* (corresponds with a function); SI: small intestine; BL: bladder; GB: gall bladder; and ST: stomach.

These organs/viscera can be grouped into pairs, forming what is called an energetic unit. Thus, LU/LI form an energetic unit, as do ST/SP, HT/SI, UB/KD, PC/TH and GB/LV.

15.6.1.1 Types

Twelve main meridians, 12 secondary TMMs and eight annex meridians are described (marvellous vessels, extraordinary vessels).

- The TMM have the same name as the main corresponding meridian, therefore a TMM

of the LU, PC, HT, LI, TH, SI, UB, GB, ST, SP, LV and KD is described.

- There are eight marvellous vessels: *Ren Mai, Du Mai, Yang Qiao, Yin Qiao, Yang Wei, Yin Wei, Chong Mai* and *Dae Mai*. These meridians fulfil a function of coordination and establish links with the remaining meridians. They do not have their own points, except for *Ren Mai* and *Du Mai*, but they have some master points or points of opening and cross-points that they share with the main meridians.
- The 12 main meridians form the so-called great circulation, whereas the small circulation is formed by the *Ren Mai* and *Du Mai* meridians.

15.6.2 Circulation sense of the meridians

The main meridians have an energy circulation sense (figure 15.12) which is as follows. As occurs in the organs and the viscera, the meridians are grouped into pairs, forming what are known as coupled meridians, due to their proximity and because they are found communicating through a vessel or the secondary meridian, known as transverse *Luo*. Therefore, LU is coupled with LI (and vice versa), ST with SP, etc.

On the other hand, an energy timetable is defined: each organ meridian has a 2-hour period during which energy is at its peak, while 12 hours later is the period of minimal or depleted energy. This timetable has a practical application when performing a diagnosis as it can be used to confirm how the patient's symptoms regarding an organ or a viscera vary within its timetable of peak or depletion of energy.

- *LU*: 3–5 a.m.
- *LI*: 5–7 a.m.
- *ST*: 7–9 a.m.
- *SP*: 9–11 a.m.
- *HE*: 11 a.m. to 13 p.m.

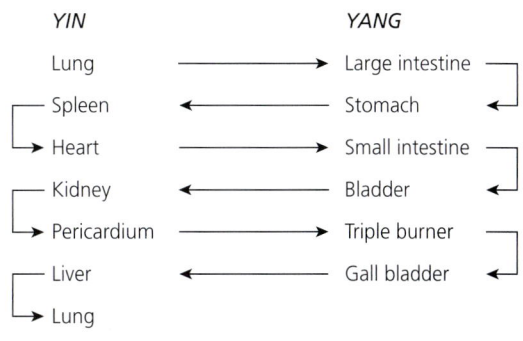

FIGURE 15.12 ■ Sense of energy circulation.

- *SI:* 1–3 p.m.
- *BL:* 3–5 p.m.
- *KID:* 5–7 p.m.
- *P:* 7–9 p.m.
- *TB:* 9–11 p.m.
- *GB:* 11 p.m. to 1 a.m.
- *LIV:* 1–3 a.m.

KEY POINTS

The acupuncture meridians are paths of energy circulation which run through the body similar to a network, and which enable communication from the interior (organs) to the exterior. They maintain the harmony and dynamic balance of all functional activities (homeostasis).

15.7 THE ACUPUNCTURE POINTS

15.7.1 General notions

The acupuncture points are specific, biologically active points, upon which one can act with a needle and/or any other medium (e.g. pressure, moxa) with a therapeutic objective.

Despite the scientific recognition surrounding acupuncture and the points that form the network of channels or meridians within which *Qi* energy circulates, the tendency is to simplify the location of the acupuncture points, locating them sometimes in a random and imprecise manner.

As professionals particularly trained in the fields of anatomy, exploration and the treatment of patients, therapists are urged to be precise in the location of the points.

15.7.2 Characteristics of the acupuncture points

The acupuncture points are mainly distributed along the meridians, in precise anatomical localizations.[23–25]

In the West, they are referred to by the name of the meridian they are located on followed by a number, whereas in the East, their Chinese name is used (which has a concrete meaning). For example, the Western nomenclature uses ST36, representing point 36 of the stomach meridian, whereas in Mandarin Chinese nomenclature (or *pinyin*), this is known as *Zusanli* (three distances below the knee).

Normally, acupuncture points are found located in small depressions or dips[26], close to bony structures, vasculonervous complexes, depressions, processes or bony prominences and musculotendinous junctions, but individual factors are considered, especially as there is individual variation in the location of points and therefore the practitioner must be careful to find the correct location.[27] The situation and depth may vary depending on the age, physical state and anatomy of the point, pathway of the meridian and even the season.

In the current, more modern and contemporary phase, numerous scientific studies have shown that the subcutaneous tissue adjacent to the acupuncture point contains a large amount of nerve terminals, arteriovenous blood vessels, lymphatic vessels, neuromuscular motor points and plexuses.[26,28–30]

It is also important to note some of the electric properties of the acupuncture points (e.g. voltage, resistance, impedance).

A simple definition of electric resistance is the opposition to the passing of electric energy by matter. In contrast, impedance is the sum of several related resistances ($R1 + R2 + R3$ ...), which is less than the adjacent surrounding tissue.

Acupuncture points provide less electric resistance to the passing of a low-voltage electric current compared to the acupuncture meridians. Therefore they can be easily detected using electronic equipment (electronic acupuncture point finders).

The electric resistance (measured in ohms [Ω]) to the reactive acupuncture points is inferior to the rest (or to the non-acupuncture points); that of the acupuncture point is relatively less than that of neighbouring tissue.[31–33] In deteriorated, degenerated or degraded zones, areas with lesions or *ashi* points of local pain, inferior values are shown which display less resistance, as occurs with the acupuncture points. An injured or degraded region is the tissue or area that shows degenerative changes, tendinopathies, fibrosis or tears (with a value of 200–250 Ω). In normal regions, where we find healthy tissue, we can find values of above 800 Ω.

Acupuncture points have a higher local voltage: an acupuncture point has an electric potential higher than that of the neighbouring tegument. An acupuncture point has around 40–80 mV. A healthy surrounding tissue has approximately 10–20 mV.

Skin electric conduction devices exist (that measure the electric resistance in the skin and the voltage) and these can aid in correctly locating the acupuncture points, as well as their electrical stimulus (figure 15.13).

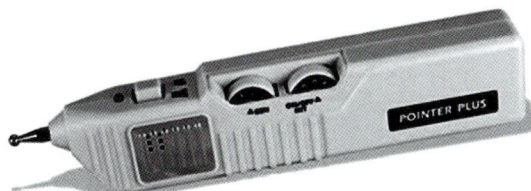

FIGURE 15.13 ■ Pointer Plus device. (Colour version of figure is available online).

15.7.3 Location of acupuncture points

One of the fundamental aspects determining effectiveness of treatment is the precision employed while locating an acupuncture point. Although the vast majority of points are sensitive to palpation, or are located in small anatomic depressions (and thus clearly detectable upon palpation), the location of acupuncture points is based on three fundamental references. These are: measurements using finger lengths, the proportional measure, and the use of anatomical landmarks.[18]

15.7.3.1 The finger-cun measurement method

This is the use of different finger segments for the location of the points. This is considered an approximate measurement system and uses a proportional measurement method, based on the size of the fingers of the person who is to be measured.

The term 'distance' or *cun* (*tsun*) is defined as the length of the middle interphalangeal joint of the third finger (second phalanx of the middle finger). It measures approximately 2.5 cm, which corresponds to the width of the distal phalanx of the thumb.

- width of the thumb: 1 distance (*cun*)
- width of the hand: 3 distances (*cun*)
- width of two triphalangeal fingers: 1.5 distances (*cun*).

15.7.3.2 The proportional measure

These are the measurements of the bony segments which were established in the distant past, and which are used as references of length and width for the location of acupuncture points. These measurements are proportional to each person, and therefore valid for all, whether they are tall or short, children or adults, or fat or thin.

These measurements are called *cun* (*tsun*) and represent the parts in which a bone segment is divided. There are a series of bone measurements that are most commonly used by clinicians. For example:

- 9 *cun* = mastoid process
- 8 *cun* = chondrosternal angle, centre of the umbilicus
- 19 *cun* = greater trochanter, centre of the patella
- 16 *cun* = centre of the patella, lateral malleolus.

15.7.3.3 The use of anatomical landmarks

This involves locating the acupuncture points by using anatomical references or landmarks.

Several types of anatomical references are distinguished:

- fixed: ears, bony processes, nail, nipple, umbilicus, pubis, joints and condyles
- moving: folds, muscle-tendon aponeurosis.

15.7.4 Functions of the acupuncture points

Some points have a diagnostic function, as they represent the superficial reflexes of the activity and state of the internal organs. This can be manifested in different ways, such as spontaneous pain on palpation, skin disorders, changes in skin coloration and/or temperature or scaling of the skin.

For example, deep pressure applied to point LU1 can produce local pain and/or irradiated pain in the path of the meridian and may be indicative of illness in the lung meridian.

Although the points mainly fulfil a therapeutic function, by re-establishing the balance between the superficial system and the internal organs, the balance between the energy (*Qi*) and the blood (*Xue*) is re-established, the immune system is stimulated and the body becomes strengthened.

15.7.5 Action of the points

Acupuncture points can have different actions:

- Local action: they can be used to treat alterations of nearby areas and can act upon tissues or organs close by. For example, the LI4 point can be used for pain in the hand and wrist.
- Distal action: they can treat alterations of distant areas: 'there where the meridian reaches, the treatment reaches'. For example, the LI4 point can be used for disorders

of the head and face (special action point over the head and the face).

- Specific action: some points have a specific action over specific alterations or can regulate alterations of an opposite nature. For example, the ST37 point can be used to treat disorders such as constipation or diarrhoea, as it is a special action point which unblocks the large intestine.
- Empirical action: certain points have properties based on empiricism, which may or may not have a scientific correlation. For example, SP10, apart from having a special action role over the blood or 'the sea of the blood', is used empirically in order to strengthen and tonify the blood. There are descriptions of treatments within the *Ode to the Jade Dragon* (a poem or text based on an old compendium with simple combinations of acupuncture points), which uses the combination of various points for the treatment of the pathology.

15.7.6 Types of acupuncture points

Several different types of acupuncture points exist:
- transporting or command points: 'classical *shu* points'
- *Yuan* source points
- *Luo* connecting points
- *Xi* cleft points
- back *Shu* points and front *Mu* points
- *Hui* meeting points and special-effect points
- extra or non-meridian points.

The first four of these are found within the so-called command group, located between the fingers and the elbows of the upper limb, and the toes and knees of the lower limb. The reason they are so named is that, through these points, one can act upon the energetic flow of each of the meridians and, thus, command the energy of the channel, the energy as a whole and the blood. In order to do so, the cycles of the five elements are taken into consideration.

15.7.6.1 'Classical Shu' points

Each of the 12 main meridians has five transporting or command points within the so-called command pathway. These points are able to control the meridian energetically and are named: *Jing* (well), *Ying* (spring), *Shu* (stream), *Jing* (river) and *He* (sea).
- *Jing* (or *ying*) points: these are points where the energy enters the meridian,

and all, except for one, are located on the border of the nails: LU11, P9, HE9, LI1, TB1, SI1, KID1, LIV1, SP1, GB44, ST45, BL67.
- *Ying* points: in these points the energy is more dynamic. These are found within the interdigital spaces: LU10, P8, HE8, LI2, TB2, SI2, KID2, LIV2, SP2, GB43, ST44, BL66.
- *Shu* points: in these points, the energy is powerful and broad. These points are situated in the intermetacarpal and intermetatarsal spaces: LU9, P7, HE7, LI3, TB3, SI3, KID3, LIV3, SP3, GB41, ST43, BL65.
- *Jing* points are used when the energy is blocked. They are found in the small joints (wrists and ankles): LU8, MC-5, HE4, LI5, TB6, SI5, KID7, LIV4, SP5, GB38, ST41, BL60.
- *He* points are found in the intermediate joints (elbows and knees): LU5, P3, HE3, LI11, TB10, SI8, KID10, LIV8, SP9, GB34, ST36, BL40.

Within these classical *shu* points there are tonifying and sedating points:
- Tonifying points stimulate the organ or corresponding function: LU9, P9, HE9, LI11, TB3, SI3, KID7, LIV8, SP2, GB43, ST41, BL67.
- Sedation or dispersion points inhibit the organ or corresponding function: LU5, P7, HE7, LI2, TB10, SI8, KID1, LIV2, SP5, GB38, ST45, BL65.

15.7.6.2 Yuan *source points*

These are points that absorb energy. They have the capacity to tonify or disperse the corresponding organ when connecting to the *Luo* points through the transverse *Luo* channel: LU9, P7, HE7, LI4, TB4, SI4, KID3, LIV3, SP3, GB40, ST42, BL64.

15.7.6.3 Luo *connecting points*

These are points of energy drainage that are connecting to the main flow: LU7, P6, HE5, SI7, TB5, LI6, KID4, LIV5, SP4, GB37, ST40, BL58.

15.7.6.4 Xi *cleft points*

These are points that unblock the energy unit: LU6, P4, HE6, LI7, TB7, SI6, SP8, LIV6, KID5, ST34, GB36, BL63.

Some of these points are given names of Western drugs, such as 34ST (omeprazole), SP8 (Xanax), LU6 (salbutamol).

15.7.6.5 *Back* Shu *points*

These are found in the back, more exactly, in the first line of the urinary bladder meridian, at 1.5 *cun* from the midline on both sides, at the level of the paraspinal muscles (figure 15.14).

Each meridian has its own *Shu* point, which represents the metameric origin of the organ/viscera. It is important to highlight that, at a segmental level, there is a metameric and segmental correspondence between the back *Shu* points of traditional acupuncture and the related organ. Mainly, there is a segmental correspondence for the dermatomes, myotomes and viscerotomes (table 15.7).

The *Shu* points have been studied by numerous experts, such as Upledger, Sherrington, Head, Bekkering, Van Bussel and Mackencie J, and they have been described as Head zones, Upledger points, etc.

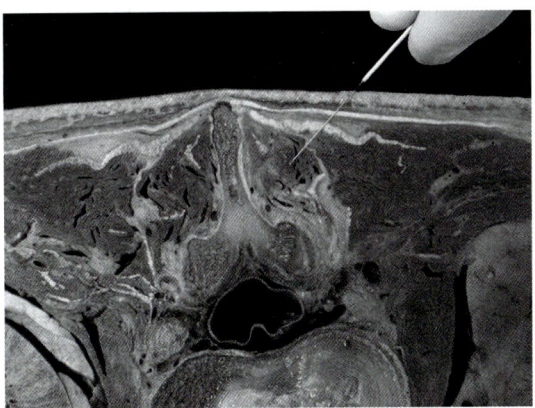

FIGURE 15.14 ■ Puncture of a transverse section at the lumbar level acting upon the *Shu* point at 1.5 *cun* lateral to the midline (*DuMai*). (Colour version of figure is available online).

These are general stimulation points, and are used both for tonification and sedation. They are particularly effective in chronic disorders (figure 15.15).

- lung: BL13 (T3)
- pericardium: BL14 (T4)
- heart: BL5 (T5)
- liver: BL18 (T9)
- gall bladder: BL19 (T10)
- spleen: BL20 (T11)
- stomach: BL21 (T12)
- triple burner: BL22 (L1)
- kidney: BL23 (L2)
- large intestine: BL25 (L4)
- small intestine: BL27 (S1)
- bladder: BL28 (S2).

Apart from this segmental and metameric correspondence (which is not altogether clear, due to the fact that the similarities are not exact), there are other acupuncture points which are used empirically. Depending on the point and its location, an explanation can be found for correspondence, or not. For example, the BL32 point is located in the second sacral foramen at 0.75 *cun* lateral to S2, and is used empirically in genitourinary pathologies of the female lower pelvis in combination with SP6. However, it can be used for disorders of the vasculonervous innervation of the second sacral foramen, such as gynaecological alterations – inflammation of the lower pelvis, irregular menstruation, dysmenorrhoea and infertility. In this case it is important to locate the BL32 point with precision. A direct stimulus with the needle is then performed by introducing the needle into the second sacral hole.

Regarding the complementarity of BL32 with SP6, a formal scientific explanation is not available; however, SP6 is the main point to be used

TABLE 15.7   Correspondence of the *Shu* points (back) with the dermatome and myotome

Meridian	Acupuncture point	Dermatome	Myotome
Lung	BL13	T3 (T4)	C3–C5; T1–T4
Pericardium	BL14	T4 (T5)	C3–C5; T1–T5
Heart	BL15	T5 (T6)	C3–C6; T5–T6
Governing vessel	BL16	T6 (T7)	C3–C4; C6–C8; T6–T7
Diaphragm	BL17	T7 (T8)	C3–C4; C6–C8; T7–T8
Liver	BL18	T9 (T10)	C3–C4; C6–C8; T10–T11
Gall bladder	BL19	T10 (T11)	C3–C4; C6–C8; T9–T10
Spleen	BL20	T11 (T12)	C6–C8; T9–T12
Stomach	BL21	T12 (L1)	C6–C8; T9–L1
Triple burner	BL22	L1 (L2)	C6–C8; T9–L2
Kidney	BL23	L2 (L3)	C6–C8; L2–L3
Large intestine	BL25	L4 (L5)	L4–L5
Small intestine	BL27	S1 (S2)	L5–S2
Bladder	BL28	S2 (S3)	L5; S1–S2

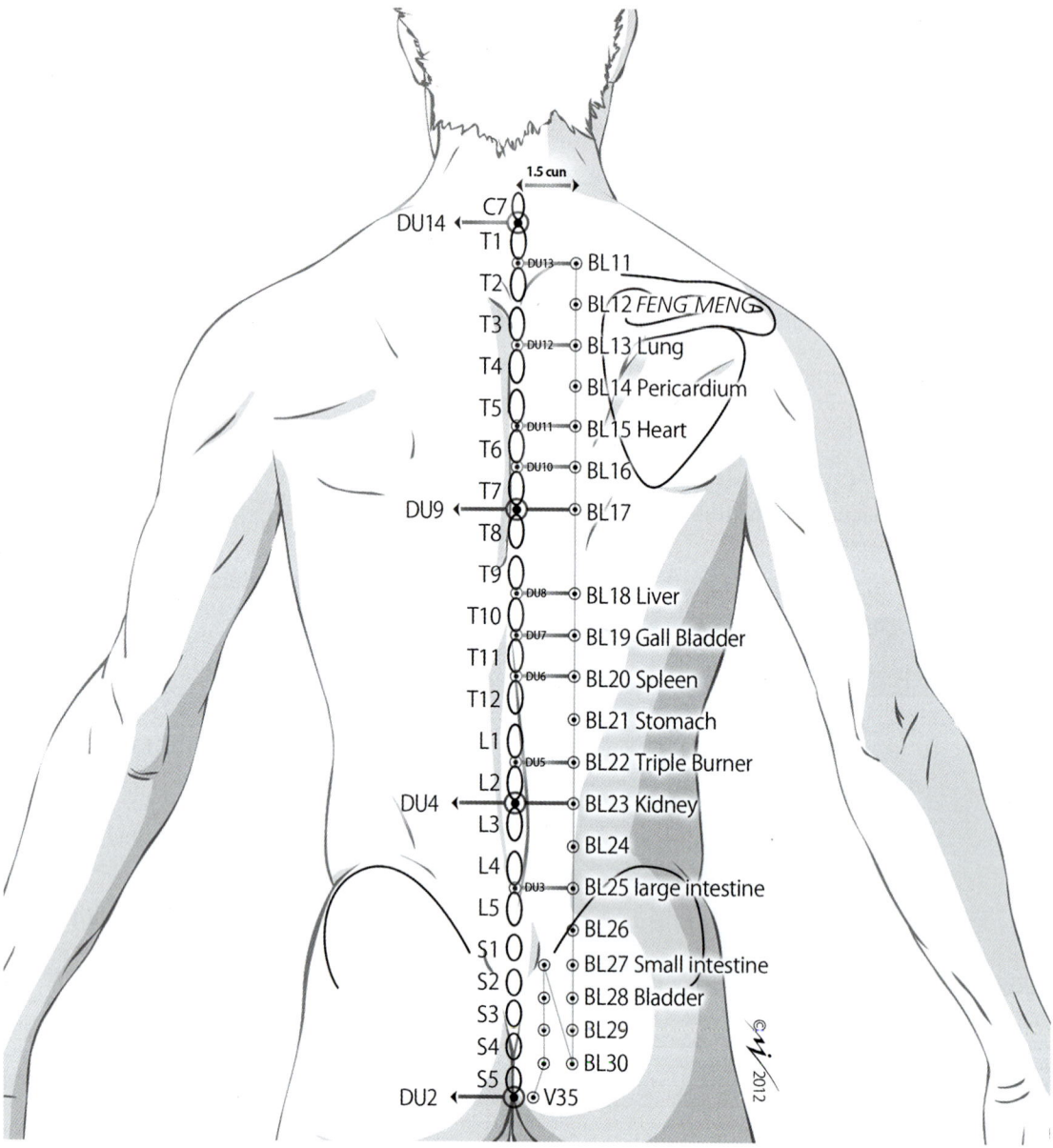

FIGURE 15.15 ■ *Shu* points of the back. (Colour version of figure is available online).

in gynaecological and urinary disorders, especially in women. This SP6 point (known as *San Yin Jiao*) has a powerful effect on pathologies of the inferior *Jiao* and, due to its location, is a cross-point of the three *yin* meridians of the leg (spleen, liver, kidney), as its name indicates.

KEY POINTS

Acupuncture is considered within the scope of practice for physiotherapists.

For general gynaecological and urinary treatment (the latter, mainly for women) the SP6 + BL32 formula is used in order to produce a direct stimulus to the lower pelvis.

SP6 will be used as a bilateral opening point and BL32 is used due to its action over the local sacral openings.

Furthermore, depending on both the pathology and the clinical symptoms, more points will be added, depending on the process.

This procedure is contraindicated in pregnancy, as it can produce uterine contractions, movement of the fetus, bleeding and even abortion.

TABLE 15.8 **Correspondence of the ventral *Mu* points with the dermatome and myotome**

Meridian	Acupuncture point	Dermatome	Myotome
Lung	LU1	T2 (C4)	C5–T1
Pericardium	REN17	T4 (T5)	C5–T1; T4–T5
Heart	REN14	T7	T7–T12
Large intestine	ST25	T10	T10
Triple burner	REN5	T11	T7–T12
Small intestine	REN4	T11 (T12)	T7–T12
Spleen	LIV13	T10	T8–L1
Liver	LIV14	T6–T7	T8–L1
Kidney	GB25	T9 (T11)	T8–L1
Stomach	REN12	T8	T7–T12
Gall bladder	GB24	T7	C3–C5; T7–L1
Urinary bladder	REN3	T12 (L1)	T7–T12

15.7.6.6 Front Mu *points/alarm points*

These are located in the front of the body (table 15.8), and are used for diagnosis and treatment. They are sore when there is a disorder affecting the organ and are used mainly in acute disorders (figure 15.16).

- lung: *LU1*
- pericardium: *REN17*
- heart: *REN14*
- liver: *LIV14*
- gall bladder: *GB24*
- spleen: *LIV13*
- stomach: *REN12*
- triple burner: *REN5*
- kidney: *GB25*
- large intestine: *ST25*
- small intestine: *REN4*
- bladder: *REN3*.

15.7.6.7 Hui *meeting points*

These are special points where the *Jing Qi* of eight types of body structures meet: *Zhang, Fu, Qi* (energy), blood (*Xue*), tendons, bones, medulla and channels. These points are used in the treatment of pathology affecting these structures or substances and, when stimulated, show a multiple and extensive action.

- *LU9:* meeting point of the vessels
- *GB34:* meeting point of muscles and tendons
- *LIV13:* meeting point of organs (*yin*)
- *REN12:* meeting point of the viscera (*yang*)
- *REN17:* meeting point of the vital energy
- *BL17:* meeting point of the blood
- *BL11:* meeting point of the bones
- *GB39:* meeting point of the marrow.

15.7.6.8 Special-effect points

These are empirical points that have an important effect on energy balance.

- *BL10:* acts upon the parasympathetic nervous system. Indicated in states of plethora with cerebral symptoms
- *BL38:* acts upon haematopoiesis. Indicated in pathologies which are accompanied by signs of weakness, e.g. anaemia, amenorrhoea, weight loss
- *BL40:* lumbar column
- *LU7:* head and neck
- *LI4:* head, face and mouth
- *P6:* chest, heart, stomach (problems with an internal aetiology)
- *TB5:* thoracic pains (external problems)
- *SP6:* gynaecological alterations
- *ST32:* meeting point of arteries and veins
- *ST36:* acts upon general energy, indicated in depressive and nervous states
- *SP5:* action upon the connective tissue and upon the venous tone. Indicated in varicose veins and arthropathies
- *BL60:* relaxing action upon the nervous system and an antalgic point, in general.

15.7.6.9 Extra or non-meridian points

These are points that are not found on the pathway of any of the meridians. The number of these points can vary according to different authors. It is worth highlighting the existence of extra points named *huatuo jiaji* (or Ex-B2 'paravertebral' points) due to their metameric correspondences (figure 15.17).

There are 34 *huatuo jiaji* points: 17 extra points located on either side of the midline. Each is located at the height of the inferior depression

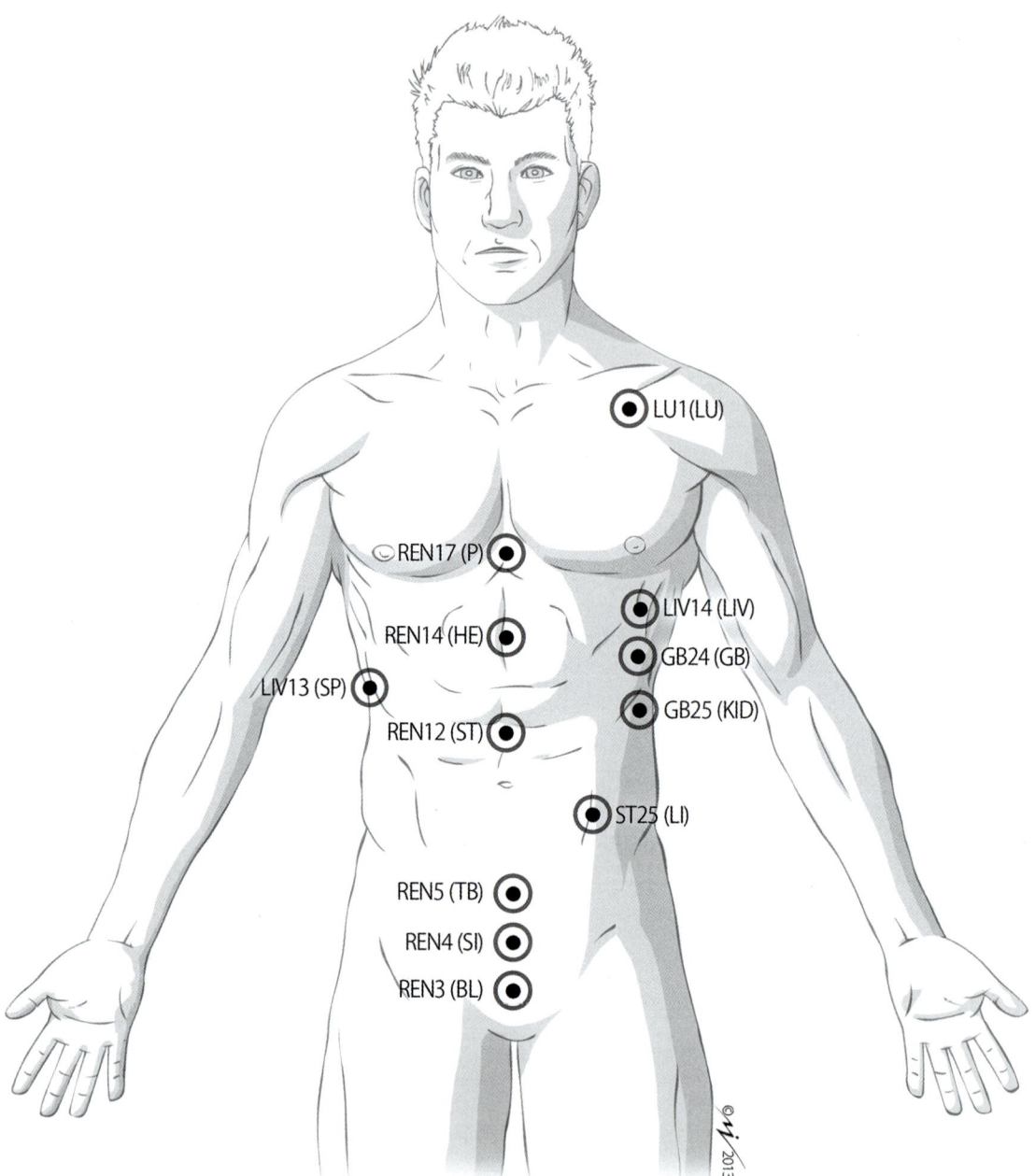

FIGURE 15.16 ■ Ventral *Mu* points. (Colour version of figure is available online).

and lateral to the spinous process (at 0.5 *cun* lateral to the posterior midline), from T1 (which corresponds with DU14) up to L5 (which corresponds with DU3). Therefore, there are 12 pairs of thoracic points (between T1 and T12) and five pairs of lumbar points (between L1 and L5). Depending on the school of thought, the lateral points, corresponding with the cervical column, are described as 'cervical *huatuo jiaji*'.

Regarding the puncture technique for these points, it is important first to consider the correspondence with the organ or viscera associated with the acupuncture point. The insertion is performed at 0.5–1 *cun* perpendicular or oblique at 45° in the direction of the midline. Locally this does not correspond with the facet joints, as these remain slightly lateral, but a translation from *pin-yin* could be: 'facet joint syndrome'. The puncture should never be performed in a lateral direction (due to the possibility of injuring a vital organ at a different level).

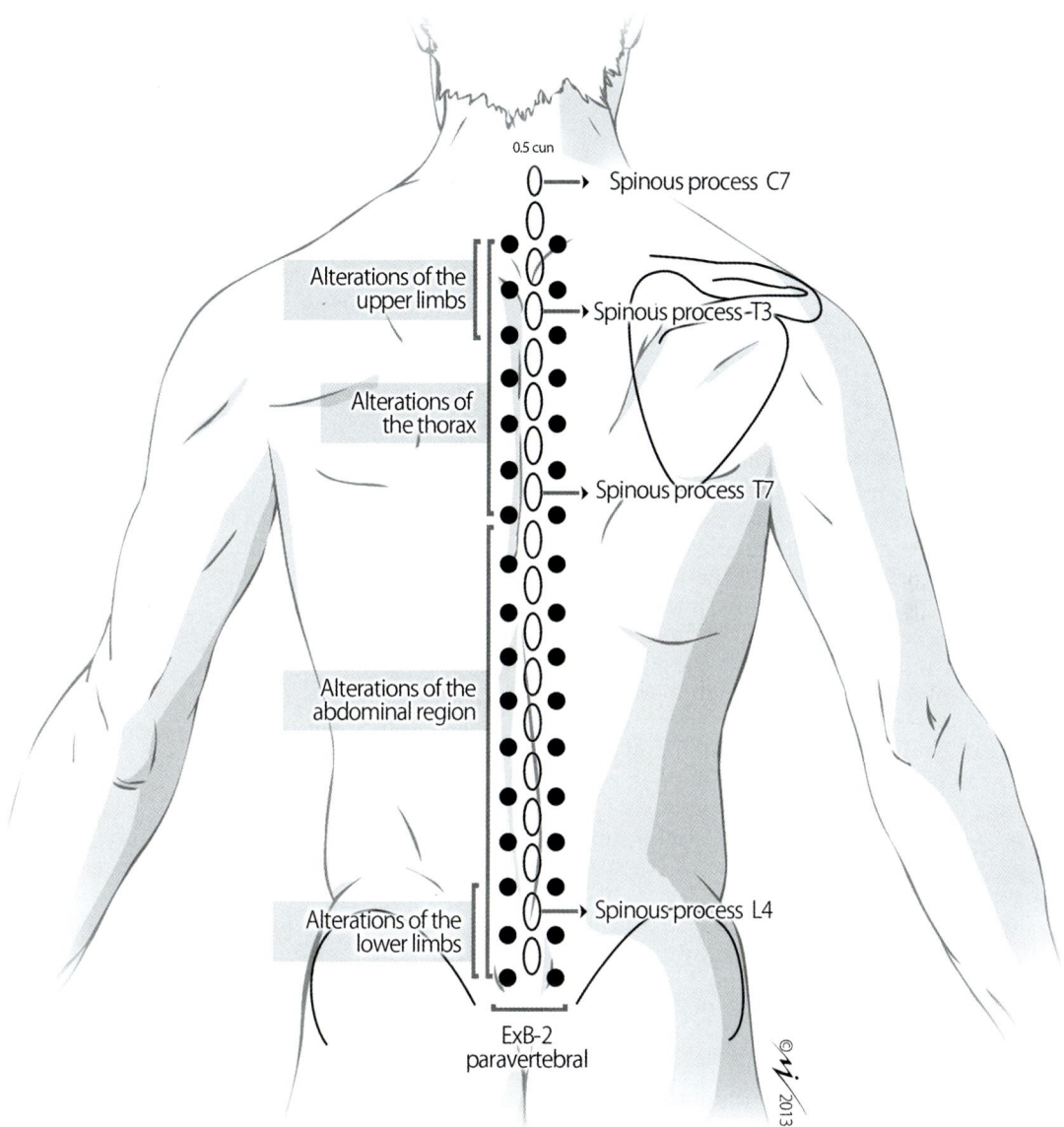

0.5 cun

Spinous process C7

Alterations of the
upper limbs

Spinous process-T3

Alterations of
the thorax

Spinous process T7

Alterations of the
abdominal region

Spinous process L4

Alterations of the
lower limbs

ExB-2
paravertebral

FIGURE 15.17 ■ *Huatuo jiaji* points or paravertebral points. (Colour version of figure is available online).

Once the arrival of *Qi* is obtained, the needle can be either manually or electrically stimulated using electroacupuncture (see chapter 13).

Oblique insertions are also used (45° in a medial direction) in the treatment of the dorsal *Shu* points (back), directing the needle towards the area of the extra points *huatuo jiaji*, and reinforcing the therapeutic action of the latter.

It is important to note that with this type of puncture precaution is advised in treatments during pregnancy, due to the connection with the fetus, especially in the lumbosacral region.

In TCM puncture of these points is indicated in order to regulate and balance the organs and viscera according to the *Zhang-Fu* theory (in China, punctures in segments of the cervical spine were also performed in order to regulate chronic disorders and osteoarthrosis of this cervical segment). In the West, these points are understood to provide segmental regulation for illnesses and disorders by stimulating the local nerve root and local facet disorders.

The approximate metameric correspondences are:

- *T1–T3:* for the treatment of the lung and the upper extremities
- *T–T7:* chest, heart
- *T8–T10:* liver and gall bladder

- *T11–T12:* stomach and spleen
- *L1–L2:* kidney, lower extremities
- *L3–L5:* bladder, intestines and lower extremities.

15.8 THE *DE-QI* PHENOMENON

The *de-Qi* phenomenon is defined as the sensation the patient experiences when the needle stimulates the acupuncture point. It can be translated as the 'needle phenomenon' or 'needle sensation' (see chapter 2). In general, the *de-Qi* is sought for in the exact location of the acupuncture point, while appreciating that this point is individual for each patient, and must be located using the patient's own measures or landmarks. A thorough knowledge of anatomy and a careful visual inspection, as well as previous palpation, are also recommended. In certain applications, the therapist seeks the *de-Qi* in the sense of the energy flow he or she is most interested in. For example, in the stimulation of *Yu-Yiao* ('fish loin' point or the midpoint of the eyebrow), the needle may be oriented either towards the outer edge of the eyebrow (in the case of a temporal headache) or towards the beginning of the eyebrow in order to support the function of the *inn-trang* (third eye) and as an anxiolytic.

De-Qi is found mainly within fascial planes of connective tissue[34], subcutaneous cellular tissue, and sometimes, the *de-Qi* or 'the arrival of *Qi*' phenomenon is sought with needle stimulations in intramuscular, intrabursal or intra-articular planes, or against the periosteum. This depends on the intended application and the location of the acupuncture point.

An important and definitive factor in this process is the diameter of the acupuncture needle used: needles of 0.26–0.30 mm diameter are used mainly for treatment with acupuncture, with a few exceptions in certain points and/or patients.

For the generation of *de-Qi*, many methods exist, such as the use of rotation, thrusting, stimulation of the needle handle (such as by scratching or flicking) and electroacupuncture. The objective is to mobilize the needle in order to attract energy towards it and generate a response in the surrounding tissues (see chapter 2). Also, the therapist will notice a certain tension in the tissues surrounding the needle.

On the other hand, when rotation is applied to the needle, this causes the mechanotransduction phenomenon (mechanical stimulus) of the connective tissue (see chapter 2). This will trigger the main biocellular and physiological mechanisms of acupuncture which, to date, are

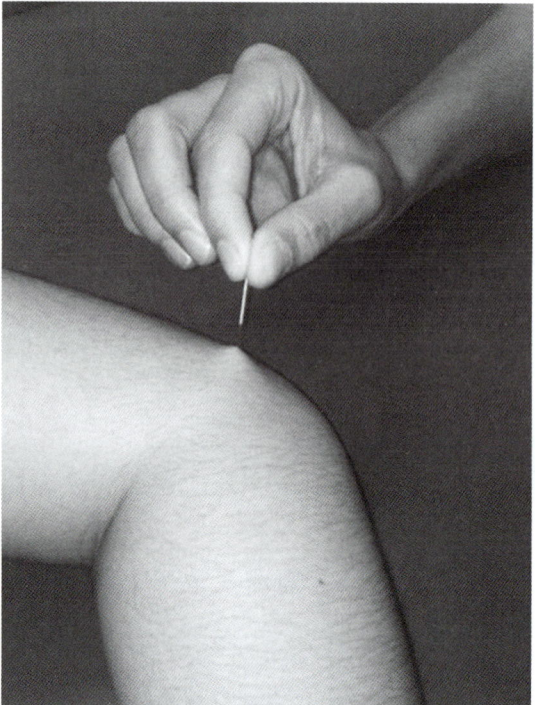

FIGURE 15.18 ■ Needle removal upon point LI11 after several needle rotations have been performed. (Colour version of figure is available online).

still only partially understood. For example, little is known regarding the effects on the tissue when performing needle rotations in order to obtain the *de-Qi* response in the area surrounding the needle. What has been proven, however, is that the resistance offered by the needle upon removal depends on the location of the puncture (or the acupuncture point) and that this increases with the frequency of needle manipulations (figure 15.18).[34–36] Several studies have proved that acupuncture produces multiple effects in the fibrocytes and the surrounding connective tissues. The fibrocytes can divide and participate in the maintenance and metabolic turnover of the matrix by releasing determined enzymes (matrix metalloproteinases). During scarring these can be transformed into contractile myofibroblasts. Together with extracellular phosphorylation kinase, this generates gene expression, synthesis and secretion of proteins, modification of the extracellular medium and muscle contraction.

15.9 ANATOMICAL DESCRIPTION OF THE MERIDIANS

Below, we will describe the pathways of the main acupuncture meridians according to their external pathways, together with the location and

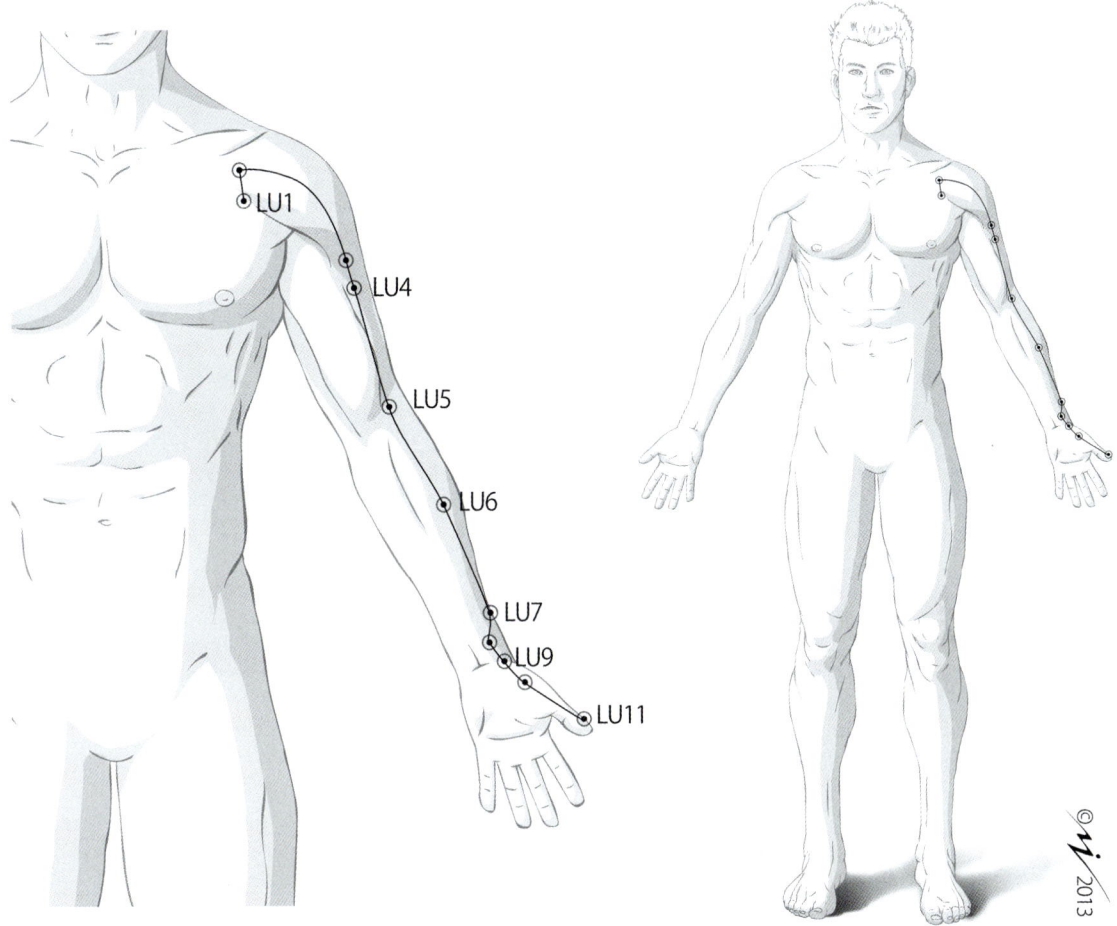

FIGURE 15.19 ■ Lung meridian (*Tsou Tai Yin*). (Colour version of figure is available online).

indications of the most important points, along with the corresponding anatomical relations.[37–40]

15.10 LUNG (*HAND TAI YIN*)

The path of the lung meridian runs from the thorax to the fingertips. There are 11 acupuncture points found along this meridian (figure 15.19).

Its external pathway begins in the deltopectoral groove, at a distance below the clavicle, and it wraps around the anterior aspect of the shoulder (anterior deltoid) and continues along the lateral border of the biceps brachii to the elbow (flexion crease, lateral to the tendon of the biceps brachii). This pathway then continues over the anteroexternal aspect of the arm (brachioradialis muscle), passing by the wrist between the tendon of the abductor hallucis longus and the radial artery, crossing the thenar eminence (radial border) and ending in the external nail border of the thumb.

- Function: this is the master of energy, regulating water passage, as well as governing the health of the skin and the hair. The nose is its superficial opening.
- Most important points: LU11, LU9, LU7, LU6, LU5.

15.10.1 LU11

- Location: 0.1 *cun* proximal and lateral in the radial border of the nail of the thumb.
- Indications: painful inflammation of the larynx and the pharynx, cough, dyspnoea and other illnesses of the respiratory pathways.
- Cerebrovascular accident, hot flushes, disorders of consciousness accompanied by high fever.
- *Jing*-well point.

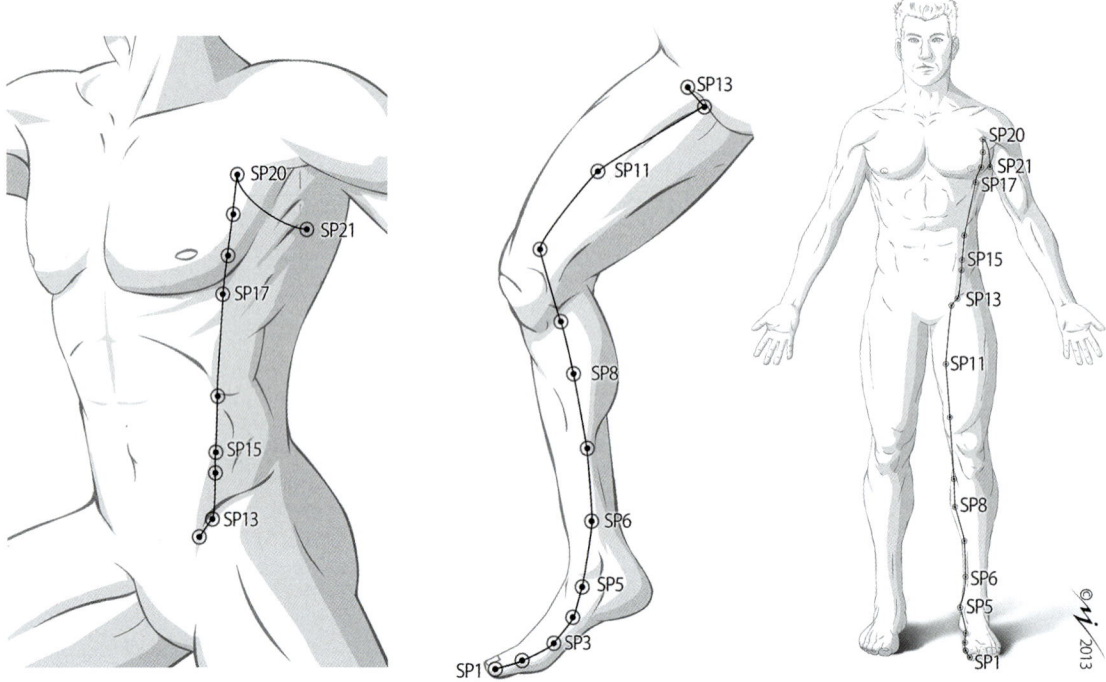

FIGURE 15.20 ■ Spleen meridian (*Zu Tai Yin*). (Colour version of figure is available online).

15.10.2 LU9

- Location: at the radial aspect of the distal volar wrist crease, external to the radial artery, ulnar to the tendon of the abductor hallucis longus muscle.
- Precaution: separate the radial artery towards the ulnar aspect beforehand.
- Indications: chronic lung pathology, dryness of the respiratory pathways, cough, dyspnoea, lack of energy, lack of vitality, not feeling like speaking.
- Neuromuscular joint disorders of the wrist (e.g. disorders of the radial nerve, rhizarthrosis, radial wrist pain, tenosynovitis).
- Point of systemic stimulation of the blood vessels.
- Tonification point of the LU meridian.
- *Jing*-well point. *Ying*-spring point.

15.10.3 LU7

- Location: 1.5 *cun* proximal to the distal flexion crease of the wrist, proximal depression of the styloid process of the radius, between the tendons of the brachioradialis and the abductor hallucis longus muscles.
- Considerations: firstly, lift the skin covering the radial styloid process.
- Indications: cough, dyspnoea and other illnesses of the respiratory tracts (rhinitis).

Radial paralysis, pain in the forearm, stenosing tenosynovitis, neck pain and nuchalgia (experience point). Bell's palsy, migraine, cough, wrist weakness. Also used in tobacco addiction.
- *Lu*-connecting point. *Shu* point.

15.10.4 LU6

- Location: 7 *cun* above the distal flexion crease of the wrist, in the internal radial aspect of the forearm, on the line joining LU5 and LU9.
- Indications: cough, dyspnoea and other diseases of the respiratory system. Pain in the anterior aspect of the forearm (radial aspect).
- *Xi*-cleft point.

15.10.5 LU5

- Location: at the cubital crease, in the radial depression of the biceps brachii tendon (figure 15.20).
- Indications: cough, dyspnoea, infectious illnesses of the superior respiratory tracts. Disorders of the skin and of the lung (mainly due to heat).
- Enthesopathy of the biceps brachii and the brachioradialis muscles, pain in the

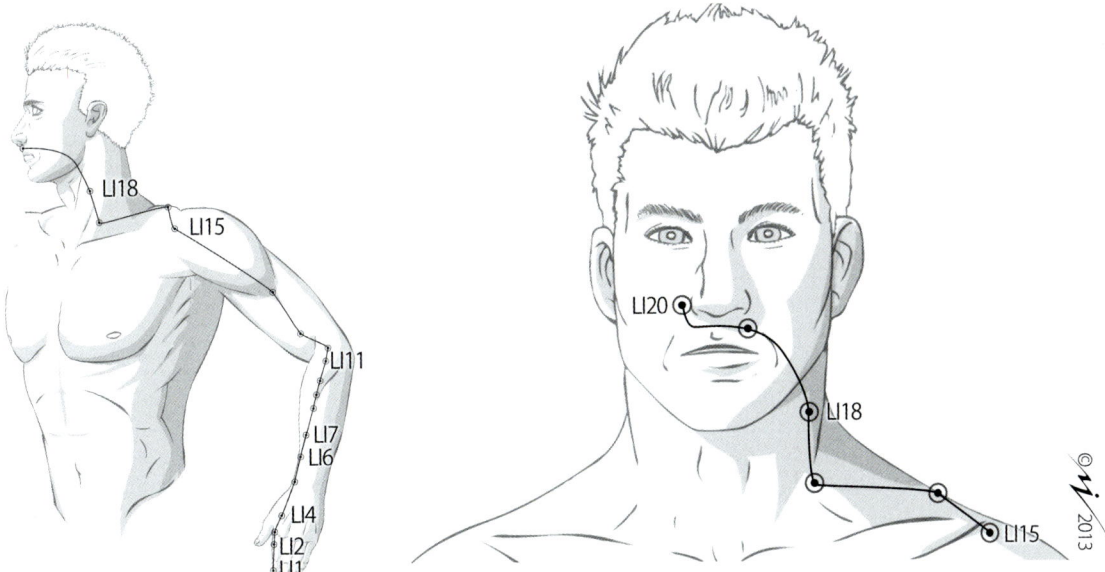

FIGURE 15.21 ■ Large-intestine meridian (*Tsou Yang Ming*). (Colour version of figure is available online).

anterolateral aspect of the elbow, pain irradiated to the upper limb (in the path of the lung meridian).
- Sedation point of the meridian.
- *He*-sea point.

15.11 LARGE INTESTINE (*HAND YANG MING*)

This meridian runs from the tip of the second finger to the face, and is where we can find 20 acupuncture points (figure 15.21).

The external pathway begins in the external nail border of the second finger, and runs along the dorsal radial border of the second metacarpal bone. At the level of the wrist it passes in between the tendons of the abductor hallucis longus and extensor hallucis longus muscles (the anatomical snuffbox), and runs along the radial aspect of the forearm on the dorsal side to the lateral epicondylar region, continuing along the external side of the arm to the acromioclavicular joint. From this point it continues to the seventh cervical and supraclavicular fossa, rising along the posterior border of the sternocleidomastoid muscle to the nasolabial sulcus, crossing above the lip to the nasogenian sulcus on the opposite side.
- Function: this meridian acts upon the large intestine, but it has a very specific action upon the head and the face.
- Most important points: LI1, LI2, LI4, LI15, LI6, LI7 and LI11.

15.11.1 LI1

- Location: 0.1 *cun* proximal and lateral to the corner of the nail on the radial side of the index finger.
- Indications: acute inflammation of the face, mouth and throat (e.g. phyaryngitis, tonsillitis, mumps, periodontitis). Unconsciousness, coma (used as a starter point or a first-aid measure).
- *Jing*-well point.

15.11.2 LI2

- Location: on the radial side of the index finger distal to the metacarpophalangeal joint, in the union of the head and neck of the proximal phalanx (ventral to the second metacarpophalangeal joint).
- Indications: acute inflammation of the head, face, eyes, mouth and otorhinolaringeal system. Motor and sensitive disorders of the second finger, metacarophalangeal arthropathy of the second finger. Distal point for mouth and teeth.
- *Ying*-spring point.

15.11.3 LI4

- Location: on the dorsal aspect of the hand, in the middle of the second metacarpal on the radial side (over the adductor hallucis muscle).
- Indications: acute inflammation of the neck, head and face.

- Motor disorders of the wrist and fingers (thumb). Special-effect point over the head and the face. Effects on the uterus if energetically manipulated (contractions and abortion).
- *Yuan*-source point.

15.11.4 LI6

- Location: with the elbow slightly flexed, 5 *cun* above the dorsal crease of the wrist, on the external aspect of the forearm, on the line that joins LI5 and LI11.
- Indications: acute inflammation at the otorhinolaryngological, ocular and mouth level, such as, for example, laryngitis, pharyngitis, epistomatitis, rhinitis, epistaxis.
- *Xi*-cleft point.

15.11.5 LI11

- Location: with the elbow flexed to 90°, between the lateral end of the articular line of the elbow (flexion crease) and the lateral epicondyle of the humerus. At its depth we find the extensor carpi radialis longus muscle.
- Indications: acute inflammation at the level of the head and neck with fever and headache. Hives (helps calm the itching). Constitutes a symptomatic point in allergies.
- Pain at the level of the elbow, the forearm and all the upper extremity.
- Tonification point of the meridian.
- *He*-sea point.

15.12 STOMACH (*FOOT YANG MING*)

The pathway of the stomach meridian is from the face to the toes. Forty-five points are distinguished (figure 15.22).

Its external pathway begins in the inferior border of the eye orbit, descending vertically towards the mouth commissure, passing by the inferior maxilla and the mandible angle and ascending in front of the ear to the temporal zone (balding area above the forehead). From the inferior border of the mandible, it descends in front of the sternocleidomastoid muscle and the sternoclavicular joint, crossing the supraclavicular fossa and descending vertically along the thorax at the level of the mammillary line (two distances from the midline) to the groin. It continues descending along the anteroexternal part of the thigh (vastus lateralis), the external knee compartment and the anterolateral aspect

of the leg (tibialis anterior) to the neck of the foot, where it continues down the dorsum of the foot, ending in the external nail border of the second toe.

- Function: this is a very important meridian due to its metabolic and energetic function regarding food. It also acts upon the face, mouth and teeth.
- Most important points: ST45, ST42, ST41, ST40, ST39, ST37, ST36 and ST34.

15.12.1 ST45

- Location: 0.1 *cun* lateral to the nail border of the second finger.
- Indications: disorders of the sense organs (ears, eyes, mouth, nose, tongue). Odontology and otorhinolaryngology (odontology, rhinitis, sinusitis, epistaxis, inflammations of the pharynx and the larynx). Insomnia due to heat.
- *Jing*-well point.

15.12.2 ST42

- Location: most elevated point of the dorsum of the foot, between the tendons of the extensor hallucis longus and the extensor digitorum longus muscles, over the dorsalis pedis artery (in the depression lateral to the pedal pulse).
- Indications: gastralgia, flatulence.
- Pain in the dorsum of the foot, loss of strength in the toes and the foot. Paralysis of the external popliteal nerve (drop foot).
- *Yuan*-source point.

15.12.3 ST41

- Location: centre of the anterior transverse fold of the ankle joint, between the tendons of the extensor hallucis longus and the extensor digitorum muscles.
- Indications: distal point important for frontal headaches, vertigo and stupor (of a *yang-ming* or anterior type).
- Important local point for the ankle joint (anterior impingement); residual anterior pain of the ankle.
- Precaution: in deep insertions penetration will become intra-articular (risk of articular contamination).
- *Jing*-river point.

15.12.4 ST40

- Location: 8 *cun* above the maximal prominence of the lateral malleolus, at the level

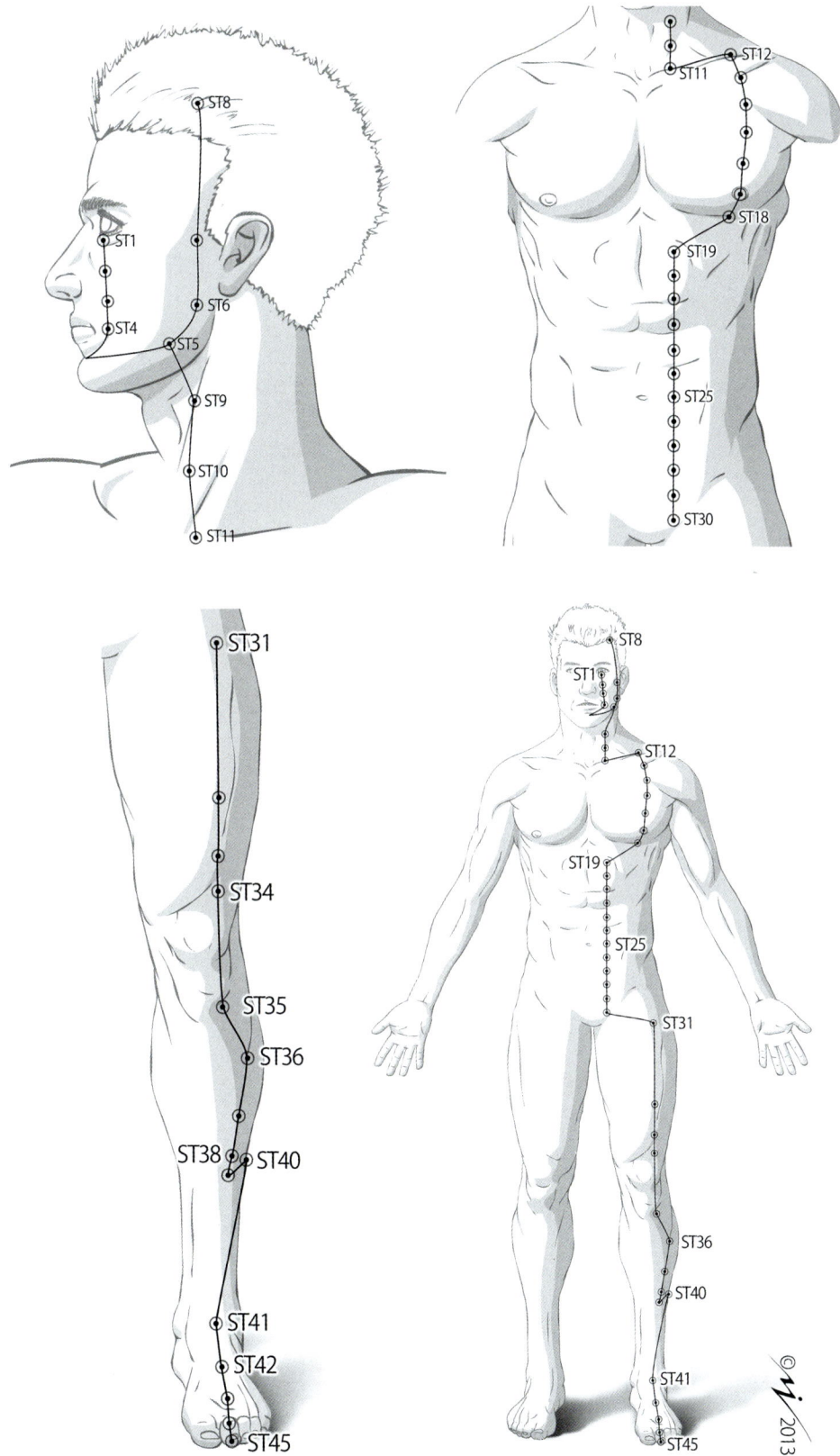

FIGURE 15.22 ■ Stomach meridian (*Zu Yang Ming*). (Colour version of figure is available online).

of ST38 and 1 *cun* lateral (between the extensor digitorum longus and peroneus brevis muscles).
- Indications: bronchial asthma, bronchitis, pneumonia and other illnesses with major mucus production.
- Main point: (mucolytic action) elimination of phlegm or other substances insufficiently metabolized by the body (e.g. digestion, mucus, triglycerides, calculus).
- Mental and psychosomatic disorders, epilepsy (calms the *shen* or spirit).
- Pain, paralysis and swelling of the lower limbs.
- *Luo*-connecting point.

15.12.5 ST39

- Location: 9 *cun* below the ST36 (external eye of the knee) and 1 *cun* below ST28, one finger width lateral to the anterior aspect of the tibia.
- Indications: regulates and balances the small intestine and illnesses of the small intestine. Pain and motor disorders of the lower limb.
- *He*-sea point with special action on the small intestine.

15.12.6 ST37

- Location: 6 *cun* below ST35, one finger width lateral to the anterior border of the tibia.
- Indications: regulates and balances the large intestine, illnesses of the large intestine. Pain and motor disorders of the lower limb.
- *He*-sea point with special action on the large intestine.

15.12.7 ST36

- Location: 3 *cun below ST35*, 1 *cun* lateral to the border of the tibialis anterior muscle, at the height of the distal border of the anterior tuberosity of the tibia (tibialis anterior muscle).
- Indications: strengthening of the whole body, preventive action and reinforces the tonifying immunity of the *Qi* and of the blood, insufficiency syndromes, weakness and convalescence. Disorders of the digestive system.
- Pain, motor disorders and disorders of the lower extremities, stroke, paralysis of the common fibular nerve, hemiplegia.
- *He*-sea point.

15.12.8 ST34

- Location: knee flexed, in the line joining the anterior superior iliac spine and the superolateral border of the knee, 2 *cun* proximal to this border.
- Indications: this is an important local point for the knee.
- Immediate and calming effect on gastrointestinal motility.
- *Xi*-cleft point to unblock stomach energy.

15.13 SPLEEN (*FOOT TAI YIN*)

The pathway for the spleen meridian begins at the toes until the thorax. It contains 21 points (figure 15.20).

The external pathway begins in the internal nail border of the big toe, passing over the internal aspect of the foot and then in front of the medial malleolus and ascending along the internal aspect of the leg, close to the tibial periosteum, until it reaches the internal condyle of the femur. It then continues along the anterointernal aspect of the thigh (vastus medialis) to the groin, before entering the abdomen between the mediocostal line and the stomach meridian. It continues ascending to the second intercostal space and descends to finish at the level of the sixth intercostal space, in the middle axillary line.

- Function: its main action is upon the digestive system, but it also acts on the psyche, in transformation (digestion) and transport (distribution). Its superficial opening is the mouth, emerging through the lips; it regulates the muscles and also nourishes the limbs. The spleen controls both the circulation and distribution of the blood.
- Most important points: SP1, SP2, SP3, SP4, SP5, SP8.

15.13.1 SP1

- Location: on the medial side of the big toe, 0.1 *cun* from the corner of the nail.
- Indications: distension, oedema and sensation of thoracic and abdominal fullness. Acute gastroenteritis.
- Antihaemorrhagic. Regulates the blood.
- *Jing*-well point.

15.13.2 SP2

- Location: distal depression of the metatarsophalangeal joint of the first toe, in the limit between the red and white skin (change of coloration of the skin of the sole as opposed to that of the dorsal part of the foot).

- Indications: acute and chronic gastroenteritis. Diarrhoea in digestive disorders.
- Pathology of the big toe, tendinopathy of the big toe. Sesamoiditis.
- *Ying*-point (spring).

15.13.3 SP3

- Location: proximal and plantar depression of the metatarsophalangeal joint of the big toe, at the limit between the red and white skin.
- Indications: acute and chronic gastroenteritis, acute and chronic dysentery, eliminates humidity. Digestive disorders.
- *Yuan*-source point and *shu*-spring point.

15.13.4 SP4

- Location: distal and plantar depression on the base of the first metatarsal, at the limit between the red and white skin.
- Indications: acute and chronic gastritis, acute and chronic enteritis, acute and chronic dysentery. Flatulence and abdominal pain due to diverse causes.
- Calms the *shen* (eliminates obstruction in the chest).
- Local point for metatarsalgias.
- *Luo*-connecting point.

15.13.5 SP5

- Location: anterior and distal depression of the medial malleolus, at the midpoint between the tuberosity of the navicular bone of the tarsum and the tip of the medial malleolus.
- Indications: articular, tendon and bone disorders of the ankle. Collateral medial ankle sprain, chronic and residual pain of the ankle, limitation of dorsal flexion, osteochondritis.
- Precaution: in deep insertions the penetration is intra-articular (there is a risk of articular contamination).
- Sedation point of the meridian.
- *Jing*-river point.

15.13.6 SP8

- Location: 3 *cun* below the internal tibial condyle (SP9), on the line that joins the tip of the medial malleolus and SP9.
- Indications: chronic diarrhoea, chronic dysentery. Some gynaecological disorders

(irregular periods, dysmenorrhoea, uterine myomas, ovarian cysts).
- *Xi*-cleft point.

15.14 HEART (*HAND SHAO YIN*)

The pathway is from the thorax to the fingertips. Nine points are found along this meridian (figure 15.23).

The external pathway begins in the axillary fossa, passing by the internal border of the humerus, between the biceps brachii and the triceps brachii muscles until it passes in front of the medial epicondyle of the elbow. It continues to descend along the flexor carpi ulnaris muscle to become radial to the pisiform bone (Guyon's canal). It then enters the palm of the hand (hypothenar eminence) and ends in the external nail angle of the little finger.

- Function: it has effects on the physiology and physiopathology of the heart. It controls the blood vessels, and also acts on mental traits (*shen*). The essence of the heart is reflected in the face and tongue and it controls the sense of taste.
- Most important points: HE9, HE7, HE6, HE5, HE3.

15.14.1 HE9

- Location: 0.1 *cun* above and lateral on the radial side of the fifth finger.
- Indications: pain in the cardiac region, cardiac illness (functional). Mental and psychosomatic disorders. Calms the mind.
- Tonification point of the meridian.
- *Jing*-well point.

15.14.2 HE7

- Location: ulnar aspect of the distal flexion crease of the wrist, radial depression of the tendon of flexor carpi ulnaris muscle, close to its insertion in the pisiform bone (Guyon's canal).
- Precaution: bear in mind the ulnar neurovascular bundle.
- Indications: cardiac pain, palpitations and other coronary symptoms (functional). Mental disorders, psychosomatic and anxiodepressive states (calms the *shen*), insomnia, stage fright.
- Disorders of the wrist (ulnar pain and pathology of the triangular fibrocartilage).
- Sedation point of the meridian.
- *Yuan*-source and *shu*-spring point.

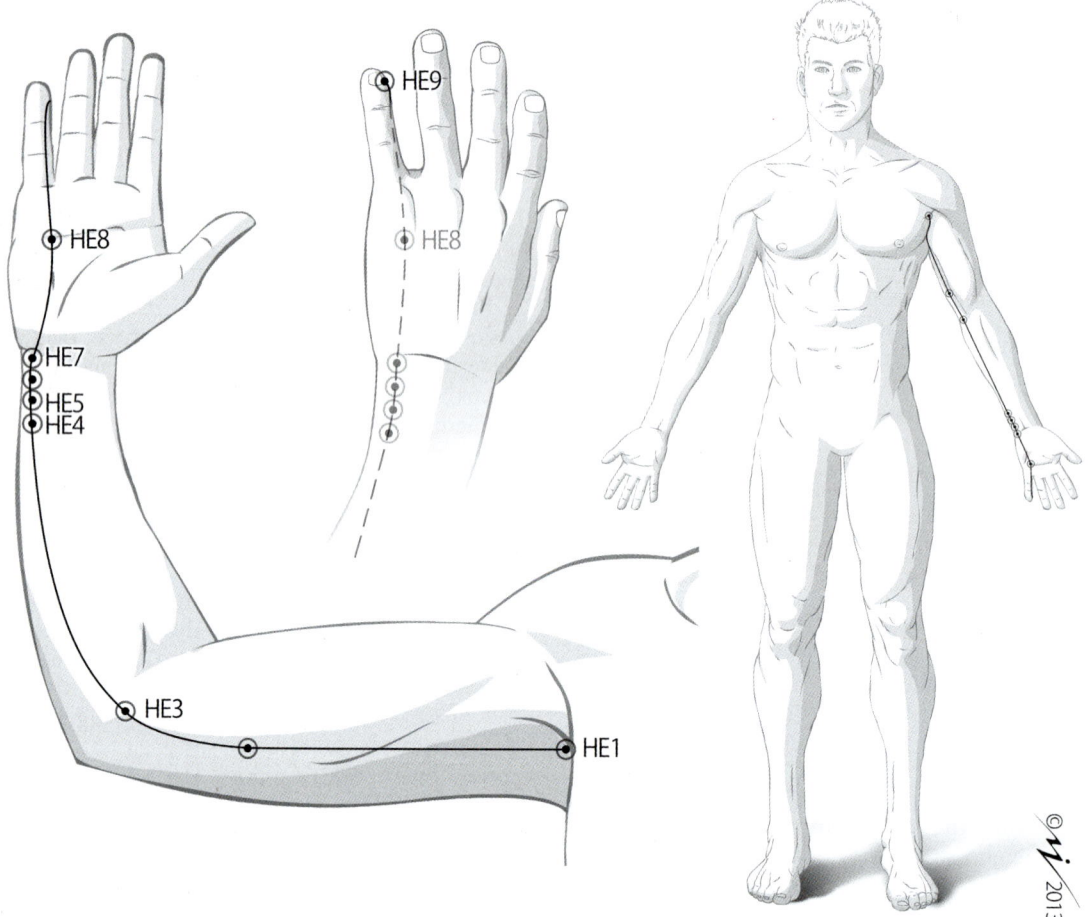

FIGURE 15.23 ■ Heart meridian (*Tsou Shao Yin*). (Colour version of figure is available online).

15.14.3 HE6

- Location: 0.5 *cun* above the distal flexion crease of the wrist, external in relation to the tendon of the flexor carpi ulnaris muscle.
- Precaution: bear in mind the ulnar neurovascular bundle (Guyon's canal).
- Indications: angina pectoris, epistaxis, haemoptysis, haematemesis and other forms of haemorrhage through the orifices of the superior part of the body.
- *Xi*-cleft point.

15.14.4 HE5

- Location: 1 *cun* proximal to the distal flexor wrist crease, external in relation to the tendon of flexor carpi ulnaris muscle.
- Indications: cardiac pain (functional), palpitations. Psychoemotional lability.
- Sudden aphonia, connection with the tongue.
- *Luo*-connecting point.

15.14.5 HE3

- Location: elbow flexed, in the centre between the internal side of the elbow crease and the medial epicondyle of the humerus.
- Indications: pains of cardiac aetiology. Calms the *shen* (important calming point).
- Entrapment syndrome and neuropathy of the ulnar canal. Dysaesthesia and irradiated pain (ulnar territory). Medial epicondyle tendinosis and compartment syndrome of the forearm.
- *He*-sea point.

15.15 SMALL INTESTINE (*HAND TAI YANG*)

Its path goes from the fingers to the head. Nineteen points are found on this meridian (figure 15.24).

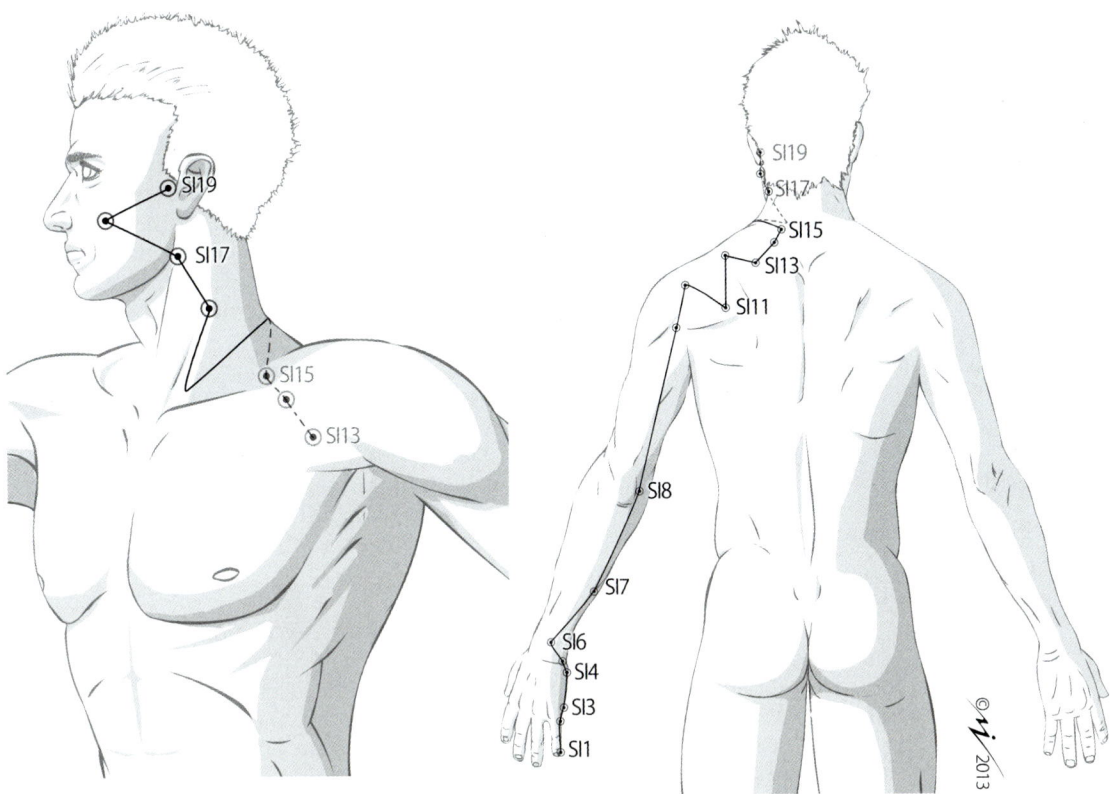

FIGURE 15.24 ■ Small-intestine meridian (*Tsou Tai Yang*). (Colour version of figure is available online).

Its external pathway begins at the internal nail border of the fifth finger, passing along the internal side of the fifth finger and the dorsal aspect of the hand, then continues along the dorsal ulnar border to situate itself in the groove between the medial epicondyle and the olecranon, and then continues upwards along the posterior part of the arm. In the scapular zone it takes a zig-zag path over the supraspinatus and infraspinatus muscles, coinciding with scapular MTrPs. From here it heads towards the seventh vertebra and crosses the suprascapular fossa, ascending along the lateral neck area and crossing the inferior maxilla towards the cheekbone, ending in the anterior depression of the tragus, in front of the external ear.

- Function: its actions are widespread. Apart from its effect on the organ, it acts upon the nape area, neck pain, pain in the scapular area, and mental and fever-related disorders.
- Most important points: SI1, SI3, SI4, SI6, SI7, SI8.

15.15.1 SI1

- Location: 0.1 *cun* in the ulnar nail angle of the fifth finger.

- Indications: illness of the breast (e.g. acute mastitis, low milk supply after birth).
- Fever, lack of sweating, pain in the pharynx and the larynx in the first stage of a cold.
- Loss of consciousness, starter point.
- *Jing*-well point.

15.15.2 SI3

- Location: fist slightly closed, ulnar aspect of the proximal transverse metacarpophalangeal crease of the fifth finger (limit between white and red skin).
- Indications: eye inflammations. Epilepsy, mental and psychosomatic disorders.
- Pain in the forearm, wrist and fingers. Distal point important for pain, rigidity, contracture along all the meridian and disorders of the cervical spine. Cervical syndrome, low-back pain. Tonifying point of the meridian.
- *Shu*-stream point.

15.15.3 SI4

- Location: ulnar border of the hand; depression between the base of the fifth metacarpal

and the pisiform bone (limit between red and white skin) in the wrist crease.
- Indications: pain in the ulnar wrist (triangular fibrocartilage and instability).
- *Yuan*-source point.

15.15.4 SI6

- Location: with the palm on the chest, in the external aspect of the forearm, in the proximal and radial depression of the styloid process of the ulna.
- Indications: pain in the upper extremity. Low-back pain.
- *Xi*-cleft point.

15.15.5 SI7

- Location: external part of the forearm, 5 *cun* proximal to the dorsal wrist crease (line joining SI5 and SI8).
- Indications: mental and psychosomatic disorders, psychoemotional disorders.
- Pain in the forearm. Cervicobrachialgia. Ulnar neuropathy.
- *Luo*-connecting point.

15.15.6 SI8

- Location: groove between the olecranon and the medial epicondyle of the humerus.
- Precaution: when performing a deep puncture, it is recommended to avoid the ulnar nerve.
- Indications: epilepsy, mental and psychosomatic disorders (sedating and antispasmodic).
- Cervicobrachialgia. Irradiated pain along the meridian pathway. Ulnar neuropathy.
- Sedation point of the meridian.
- *He*-sea point.

15.16 BLADDER (*FOOT TAI YANG*)

This path runs from the face to the toes. There are 67 acupuncture points along this meridian (figure 15.25).

The external pathway begins in the internal corner of the eye and continues upwards over the forehead to the occipital bone in a pathway that is parallel to the midline, at a distance of approximately 1 *cun*. From this point it divides into two branches: the first runs across the back, parallel to the midline at a distance of 1.5 *cun*, passing over the sacral foramina and the posterior aspect of the thigh in its midline (where it overlaps with the sciatic nerve), to the popliteal fossa. The second branch descends vertically parallel to the midline at 3 *cun* (at the level of the internal border of the scapula), goes across the gluteal zone and joins with the anterior branch in the popliteal fossa. From this point it continues descending along the midline between the two gastrocnemii, the tip of the lateral gastrocnemius and the external part of the Achilles tendon. It borders the external malleolus and continues along the external border of the fifth metatarsal bone to end up in the external nail border of the fifth toe.

- Function: this meridian acts upon the posterior part of the genital and urinary organs. It also has effects upon the eyes, nose, head, nape region and the dorsal part of the back.
- Most important points: BL67, BL65, BL64, BL63, BL58, BL40.

15.16.1 BL67

- Location: 0.1 *cun* behind the external nail border of the fifth toe.
- Indications: headaches, rhinitis, epistaxis.
- Malpositions of the fetus (moxa). Other disorders during labour (e.g. slow labour, placental abruption).
- Tonification point of the meridian.
- *Jing*-well point.

15.16.2 BL65

- Location: lateral aspect of the foot, in the proximal depression of the metatarsophalangeal joint of the fifth toe (limit between red and white skin).
- Indications: mental and psychosomatic disorders. Tension headache.
- Local pain, pain in the posterior aspect of the leg. Sciatica S1.
- Sedation point of the meridian.
- *Ying*-spring point.

15.16.3 BL64

- Location: below the tuberosity of the fifth metatarsal.
- Indications: epileptic seizures. Ischiolumbalgia. Keratitis.
- *Yuan*-source point.

15.16.4 BL63

- Location: below the anterior border of the lateral malleolus, distal to the cuboid bone.
- Indications: epileptic seizures. Low-back pain. Pain at the level of the lateral malleolus.
- *Xi* cleft point.

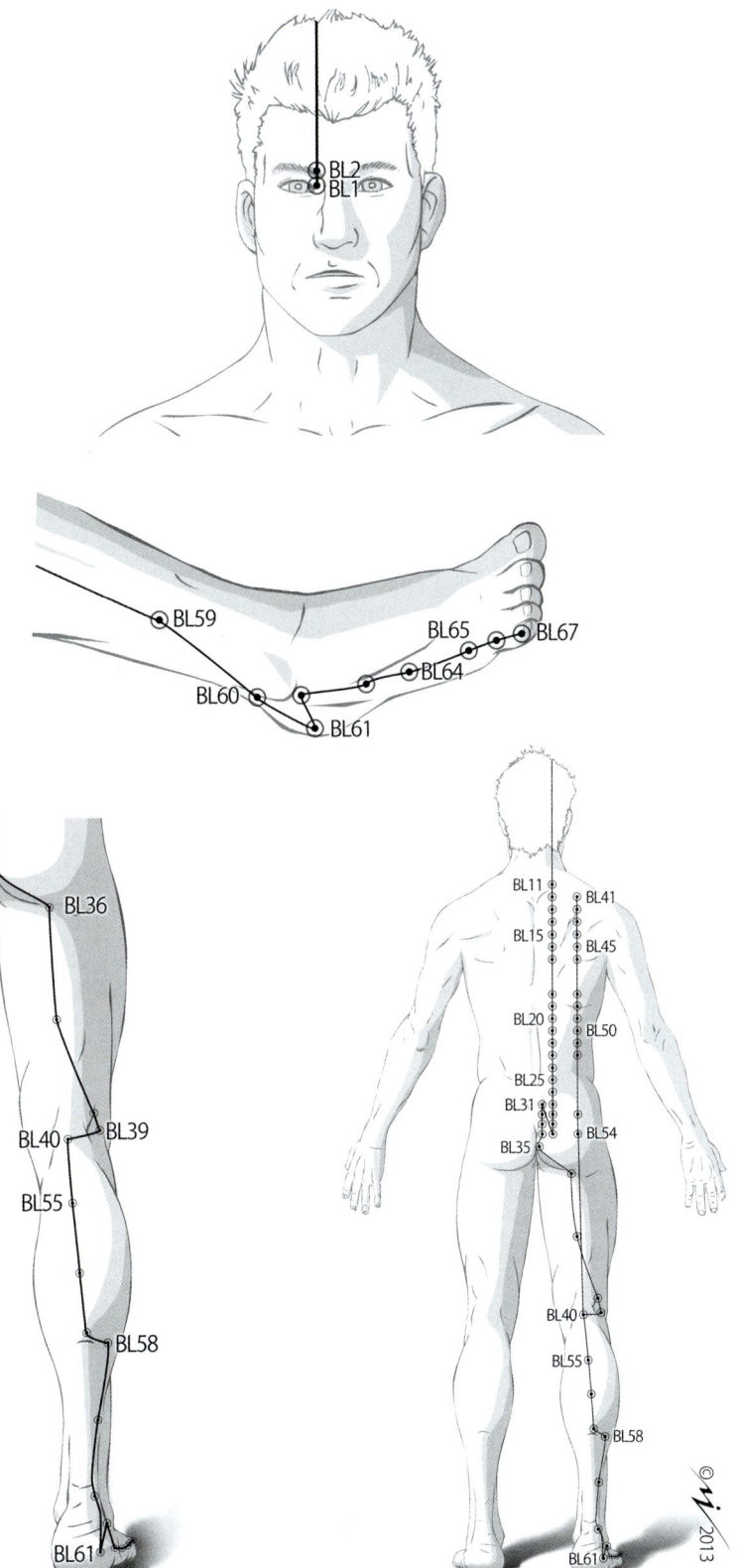

FIGURE 15.25 ■ Bladder meridian (*Zu Tai Yang*). (Colour version of figure is available online).

15.16.5 BL58

- Location: 7 *cun* above BL60 (lateral malleolus), 1 *cun* lateral and inferior to BL57, between the lateral gastrocnemius and the soleus muscle.
- Indications: haemorrhoids, tension headaches, rhinitis, epistaxis.
- *Luo*-connecting point.

15.16.6 BL40

- Location: centre of the knee crease (popliteal fossa).
- Indications: beneficial for the back and the knees. Sudden disorders of consciousness in the brain and cerebrovascular illnesses. Motor disorders, pain and spasms in the lower limbs.
- Low-back pain. Irradiated pain from the lower limbs. Vascular pathology of the lower limbs. Knee pain (popliteal).

- Acute and chronic gastroenteritis.
- Precaution is advised with popliteal cysts (Baker).
- *He*-sea point.

15.17 KIDNEY (*FOOT SHAO YIN*)

The pathway of the kidney meridian runs from the feet to the thorax and contains 27 acupuncture points (figure 15.26).

Its external pathway begins in the sole of the foot, continuing along the arch towards the navicular bone and the posterior part of the medial malleolus, where it loops around the inferior part of the ankle to continue upwards along the medial aspect of the tibia, alongside the anterior border of the Achilles tendon, and continues to the knee in the internal part of the popliteal fossa. It then continues medial in the thigh (gracilis muscle) to the pubic spine. It continues along the abdomen parallel to the

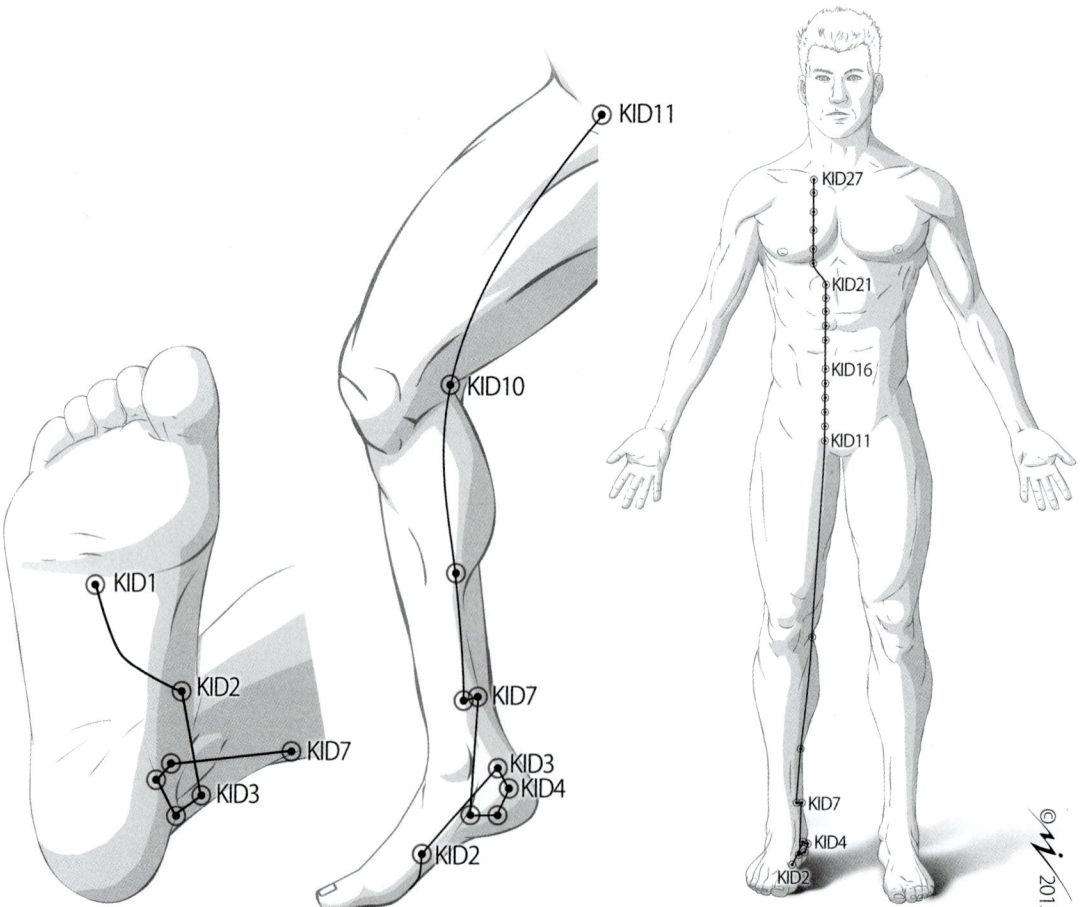

FIGURE 15.26 ■ Kidney meridian (*Zu Tai Yin*). (Colour version of figure is available online).

midline at 0.5 *cun* to the thorax (fifth intercostal space), which is situated at *2 cun* from the midline, ending at the level of the sternoclavicular joint.

- Function: the kidney meridian acts upon the urinary tracts, genital organs, intestines and lungs. Also upon the hearing system, the bones and the follicle system.
- Most important points: KID1, KID3, KID4, KID5, KID7, KID10.

15.17.1 KID1

- Location: in the depression which forms in the anterior part of the sole of the foot (between the second and third metatarsal) when performing plantar flexion, approximately in the transition between the anterior and middle third of the sole of the foot.
- Indications: chronic laryngitis and pharyngitis. Aphonia of a psychosomatic origin. Urine retention. Headaches, vertigo and stupor. Pain in the sole of the foot.
- Sedation point of the meridian.
- *Jing*-well point.

15.17.2 KID3

- Location: the depression formed in the maximal protuberance of the medial malleolus and the Achilles tendon (0.5 *cun* posterior to the medial malleolus).
- Indications: hypertension, vertigo, stupor. Chronic laryngitis, chronic pharyingitis, tinnitus, deafness. Disorders of masculine and feminine sexual function. Motor disorders of the lower limb. Strengthening of the inferior aspect of the back (local point).
- *Yuan*-source point and *ying*-spring).

15.17.3 KID4

- Location: 0.5 *cun* inferior and posterior KID3, medial border of the Achilles tendon.
- Indications: chronic bronchitis. Constipation. Urinary retention. Heel pain. Posterior ankle impingement syndrome.
- *Luo*-connecting point.

15.17.4 KID5

- Location: below and behind the medial malleolus, 1 *cun* below KID3, in the medial depression of the calcaneal tuberosity.
- Indications: some gynaecological disorders (e.g. irregular periods, amenorrhoea, uterine prolapse).
- *Xi*-cleft point.

15.17.5 KID7

- Location: 2 *cun* above KID3, anterior to the Achilles tendon.
- Indications: regulates and balances sweat and body fluids. Scarce or exaggerated sweating (together with LI4). Oedema (water regulation). Strengthens the lumbar region.
- Tonification point of the meridian.
- *Jing* point-river.

15.17.6 KID10

- Location: internal portion of the popliteal fossa, with the leg flexed, between the tendons of the semitendinosus and the semimembranosus muscles. Located at the same level as BL40.
- Indications: disorders of male sexual function (impotence). Anovulatory disorders, dysfunctional uterine haemorrhage. Knee joint pain. Tendinopathy of the pes anserinus, bursitis.
- *He*-sea point.

15.18 PERICARDIUM (*HAND JUE YIN*)

Its pathway goes from the thorax to the fingers. This meridian contains nine points (figure 15.27).

The external pathway begins lateral to the nipple, goes upwards above the axilla and descends along the internal part of the arm, accompanying the vasculonervous bundle to the anterior elbow, where it is situated medial to the tendon of the biceps brachii muscle. It then continues along the medial aspect of the forearm between the radius and the ulna. In the wrist it passes between the tendons of the flexor carpi radialis and the palmaris longus muscles, crossing the palm between the second and third metacarpals and ending at the tip of the third finger.

- Function: the pericardium meridian acts upon the precordial region, the chest, the palms of the hands and the internal aspect of the forearms up to the axilla.
- Most important points: P9, P7, P6, P4, P3.

15.18.1 P9

- Location: in the centre of the tip of the third finger. Some authors locate it on the external nail border of the same finger.
- Indications: cerebrovascular illness, heat stroke, vasovagal syncope and high fever (as an emergency measure).

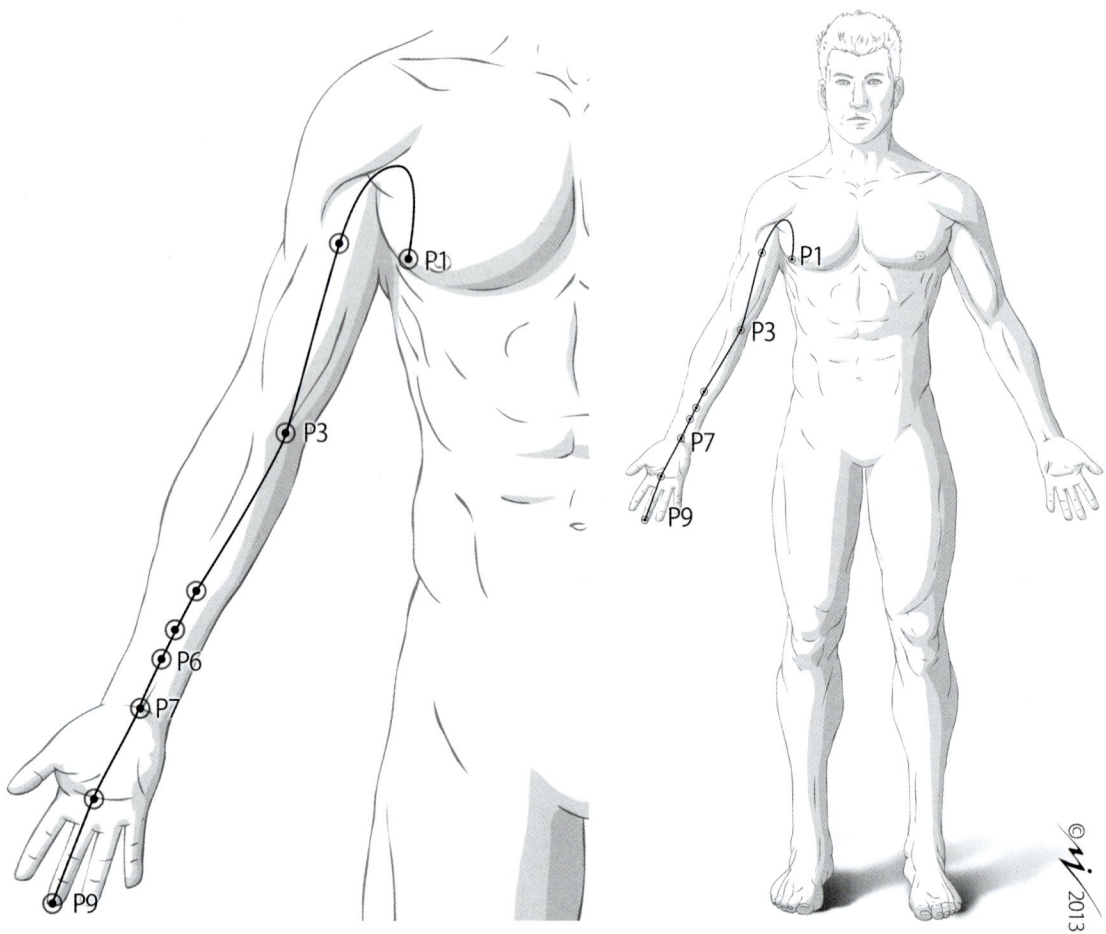

FIGURE 15.27 ■ Pericardium meridian (*Tsou Jue Yin*). (Colour version of figure is available online).

- Tonification point of the meridian.
- *Jing*-well point.

15.18.2 P7

- Location: centre of the distal articular crease of the wrist, between the tendons of the palmaris longus and the flexor carpi radialis muscles.
- Indications: angina pectoris. Mental and psychosomatic disorders, epileptic seizures (sedating and spasmolytic action).
- Carpal tunnel syndrome (take care not to manipulate the needle; there is a direct relation with the median nerve).
- Sedation point of the meridian.
- *Yuan*-source point and *ying*-spring point.

15.18.3 P6

- Location: 2 *cun* proximal to the distal wrist crease, between the tendons of the palmaris longus and the flexor carpi radialis muscles.

- Indications: angina pectoris, palpitations, feelings of thoracic fullness. Disorders of consciousness and hemiplegia in cerebrovascular illness. Factors of internal aetiology (anxiety-depressive disorders).
- Gastralgia, nausea and vomiting.
- An important point for decongestion of the chest and the stomach.
- Pain and motor disorders of the forearm.
- Main point for nausea and vomiting during pregnancy. Prescription: SP4 + P6.
- *Luo*-connecting point.

15.18.4 P4

- Location: internal aspect of the forearm, 5 *cun* proximal to the distal wrist crease, between the tendons of the flexor carpi radialis and the palmaris longus muscles.
- Indications: angina pectoris, palpitations, feelings of thoracic fullness, palpitations in coronary cardiopathies. Antihaemorrhagic action in haematemesis and epistaxis.

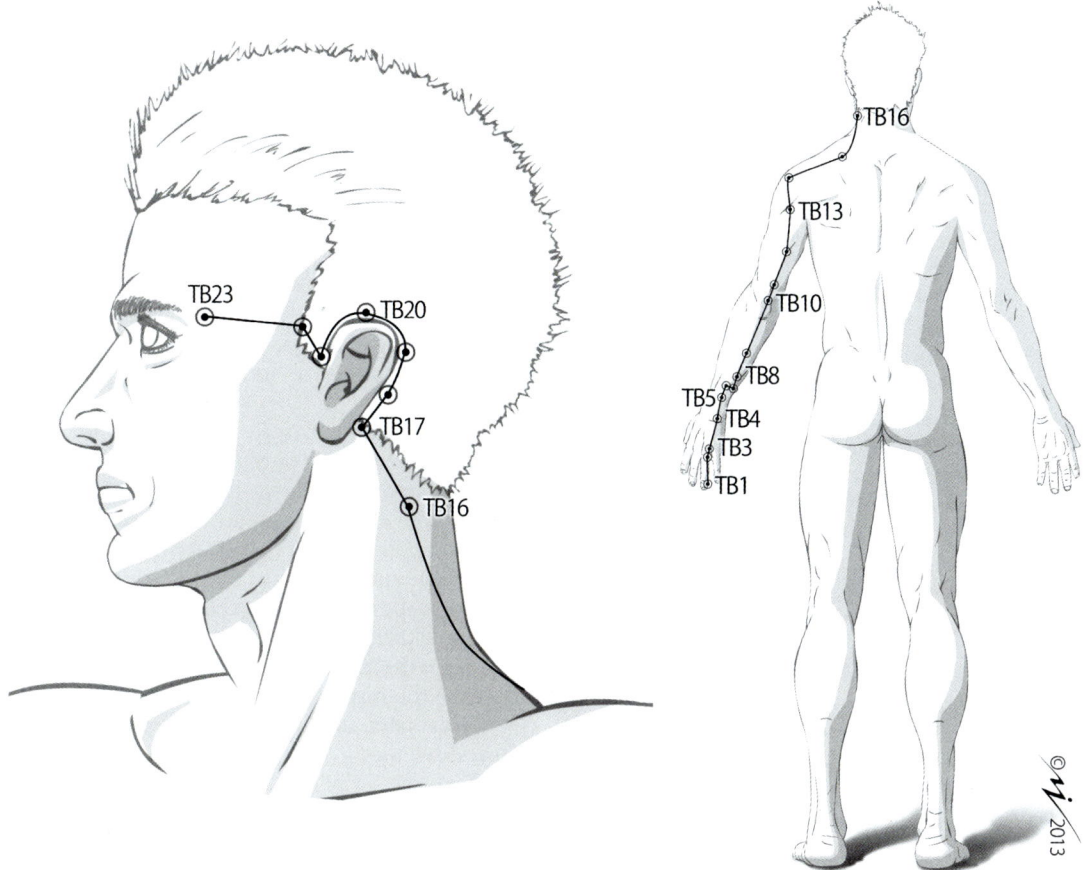

FIGURE 15.28 ■ Triple burner meridian (*Tsou Shao Yang*). (Colour version of figure is available online).

- Unspecific pains of the volar aspect of the forearm. Neuropathies (median nerve) and irradiated pain.
- *Xi*-cleft point.

15.18.5 P3

- Location: centre of the elbow crease, ulnar to the tendon of the biceps brachii muscle (between the tendon and the brachial artery).
- Indications: angina pectoris, feelings of thoracic fullness, palpitations in coronary cardiopathies. Gastralgia, nausea and vomiting in acute gastritis.
- Local important point.
- *He*-sea point.

15.19 TRIPLE BURNER/*SANJIAO* (*HAND SHAO YANG*)

Its pathway runs from the fingers to the face. Twenty-three points are located along this meridian (figure 15.28).

Its external path begins in the internal nail border of the fourth finger. From here it runs along the dorsum of the hand between the fourth and fifth metacarpals, ascending along the dorsal side of the forearm to the radius and ulna. It then passes along the olecranon fossa and continues along the posterior border of the arm and shoulder, reaching the supraclavicular fossa and ascending around the external ear, ending at the outer end of the eyebrow.

- Function: the triple burner meridian acts upon the external portion of the eye, the ear, the periauricular region, and the elbows and shoulders.
- Most important points: TB1, TB3, TB4, TB5, TB7. TB10.

15.19.1 TB1

- Location: 0.1 *cun* from the ulnar nail border to the fourth finger.
- Indications: acute inflammations of the pharynx and larynx, acute amygdalitis.
- Hearing disorders (e.g. deafness, tinnitus).

- Beneficial for ears and tongue.
- *Jing*-well point.

15.19.2 TB3

- Location: dorsum of the hand, proximal to the metacarpophalangeal joint of the fourth finger, angle between the heads of the fourth and fifth metacarpals.
- Indications: hemicranial headache. Acute inflammation of the eyes (e.g. conjunctivitis, keratitis).
- Important distal point for hearing/hearing disorders (e.g. deafness, tinnitus).
- Pain and motor disorders of the upper extremity and the hand. Clears the head and the eyes.
- Radial nerve paralysis (wrist drop).
- Tonification point of the meridian.
- *Ying*-spring point.

15.19.3 TB4

- Location: centre of the dorsal wrist crease, in the ulnar depression of the common extensor tendon and radial to the tendon of the extensor digiti minimi muscle.
- Indications: pain in the shoulder, the back and the wrist.
- *Yuan*-source point.

15.19.4 TB5

- Location: 2 *cun* proximal to the dorsal wrist crease, between the ulna and the radius.
- Indications: fever, eye inflammation, hearing disorders (deafness, tinnitus).
- Pain and motor disorders of the shoulder, back, upper extremity and hand.
- Analgesic point for the upper extremity (e.g. shoulder, elbow).
- Closes the external wind barrier (factors of external aetiology).
- *Luo*-connecting point.

15.19.5 TB7

- Location: 3 *cun* above the dorsal wrist crease, exterior to TB6, in the radial border of the ulna.
- Indications: deafness, epilepsy.
- *Xi*-cleft point.

15.19.6 TB10

- Location: with the elbow flexed, in the depression 1 *cun* above the olecranon distal point.
- Indications: pain at the shoulder, the arm and the elbow joint. Epilepsy.

- Non-specific lymphadenitis and tuberculose lymphadenitis of the neck, the nape and the axilla. Enthesitis of the triceps brachii.
- Sedation point of the meridian.
- *He*-sea point.

15.20 GALL BLADDER (*FOOT SHAO YANG*)

Its pathway goes from the face to the toes. Forty-four points are found on this meridian (figure 15.29).

The external pathway begins in the outer corner of the eye and surrounds the external ear to the mastoid process. From here it forms another arch over the temporal region until the forehead and then moves back with a slight deviation at the nape, passing over a portion of the superior trapezius towards the shoulder and the anterior aspect of the axilla. It continues in a zig-zag path along the lateral border of the thorax to the hip, crossing the piriformis muscle (posterior part of the coxofemoral joint) and descending along the lateral aspect of the leg (iliotibial tract), the head and lateral aspect of the fibula, the anterior border of the lateral malleolus, the dorsum of the foot (between the fourth and fifth metacarpal) and ending in the external nail border of the fourth toe.

- Function: the gall bladder meridian has effects over the outer corner of the eye, the temporal zone, the nape, the lateral portion of the thorax and abdomen, the gluteals and the external aspect of the leg and foot.
- Most important points: GB44, GB43, GB40, GB38, GB37, GB36, GB34.

15.20.1 GB44

- Location: 0.1 *cun* posterior to the corner of the nail on the lateral side of the fourth toe.
- Indications: hemicranial headache, acute eye inflammations (conjunctivitis). Tinnitus.
- *Jing*-well point.

15.20.2 GB43

- Location: between the fourth and fifth metatarsophalangeal joint, the border of the interdigital space between the fourth and fifth toe (limit of red and white skin).
- Indications: hypertension. Hearing disorders (deafness, tinnitus). Illnesses of the gall bladder.
- Tonification point of the meridian.
- *Ying*-spring point.

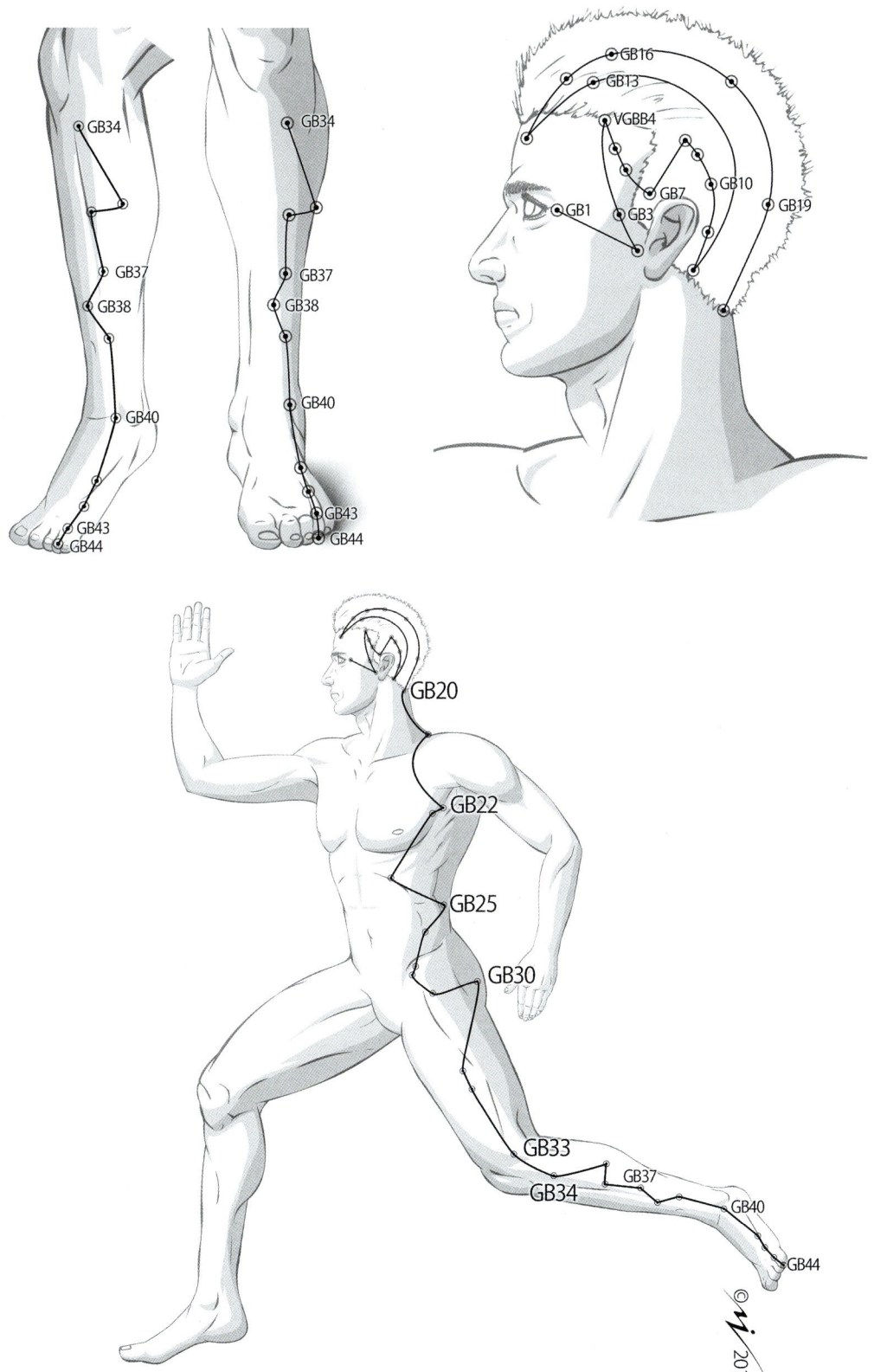

FIGURE 15.29 ■ Gall bladder meridian (*Zu Shao Yang*). (Colour version of figure is available online).

15.20.3 GB40

- Location: anterior and inferior to the external malleolus in a depression on the lateral side of the tendon of extensor digitorum longus muscle.
- Indications: some acute eye inflammations. Illnesses of the gall bladder. Pain in the lateral malleolus, hemiplegic supinated foot. Lateral ankle ligament sprain. Chronic ankle pain.
- Precaution: in deep insertions the penetration is intra-articular (there is a risk of articular contamination).
- *Yuan*-source point.

15.20.4 GB38

- Location: 4 *cun* superior to the maximum elevation of the lateral malleolus, anterior border of the fibula.
- Indications: hemicranial headache (lateral or *shao-yang*). Lateral thoracic pain, the lateral side and the lower extremities. Hemiplegia in cerebrovascular accident.
- Sedation point of the meridian.
- *Jing*-river point.

15.20.5 GB37

- Location: 5 *cun* superior to the maximum elevation of the lateral malleolus, in the anterior border of the fibula.
- Indications: ocular illnesses; keratitis, night-blindness, glaucoma. Sensation of tension and pain in the breast (initial stage of mastitis). Pain and loss of strength in the leg.
- *Luo*-connecting point.

15.20.6 GB36

- Location: 7 *cun* above the maximum elevation of the lateral malleolus, in the anterior border of the fibula.
- Indications: depressive disorders. Intercostal neuralgia.
- *Xi*-cleft point.

15.20.7 GB34

- Location: anterior-inferior and distal depression of the head of the fibula; between the peroneus longus and the extensor digitorum longus. The needle can reach the interosseous membrane and the epineural tissue of the peroneal nerve.
- Indications: gall bladder illnesses and disorders of the bile ducts, such as cholecystitis or cholelithiasis.

- Pain at the knee joint. Hemiplegia, hemiparaesthesias and pain affecting one-half of the body due to cerebrovascular disease.
- Systemic stimulation point for tendons (tendons, muscles and joints).
- *He*-sea point.

15.21 LIVER (*FOOT JUE YIN*)

Its pathway goes from the toes to the thorax. Fourteen points are found along this meridian (figure 15.30).

Its external pathway begins in the external nail border of the big toe, continues along the dorsum of the foot between the first and second metatarsal and then becomes anterior to the internal malleolus, crossing with the meridian of the spleen and ascending along the medial border of the tibia. Under the knee it crosses again with the spleen meridian and continues along the internal aspect of the knee and thigh to the groin. It continues its ascent to the ribcage, ending at the level of the sixth intercostal space on the mammillary line.

- Function: the liver conserves and stores blood. It drains energy and regulates blood circulation. It controls the tendons, muscles and nails. Regulation of the vision.
- Most important points: LIV1, LIV2, LIV3, LIV5, LIV6, LIV8.

15.21.1 LIV1

- Location: 0.1 *cun* from the tip of the external nail of the big toe.
- Indications: external abdominal hernias, dysfunctional uterine haemorrhage. Vesical illnesses (retention and urinary incontinence), infection of the urinary tract (balancing and regulating action).
- *Jing*-well point.

15.21.2 LIV2

- Location: between the first and the second toe, interdigital border for the skin between the limit of the red and white skin.
- Indications: hypertension. Some gynaecological disorders, dysfunctional uterine haemorrhage, dysmenorrhoea, amenorrhoea. Infection of the urinary tract, urinary incontinence.
- Cardiovascular illness, cerebrovascular accident.
- Sedation point of the meridian.
- *Ying*-spring point.

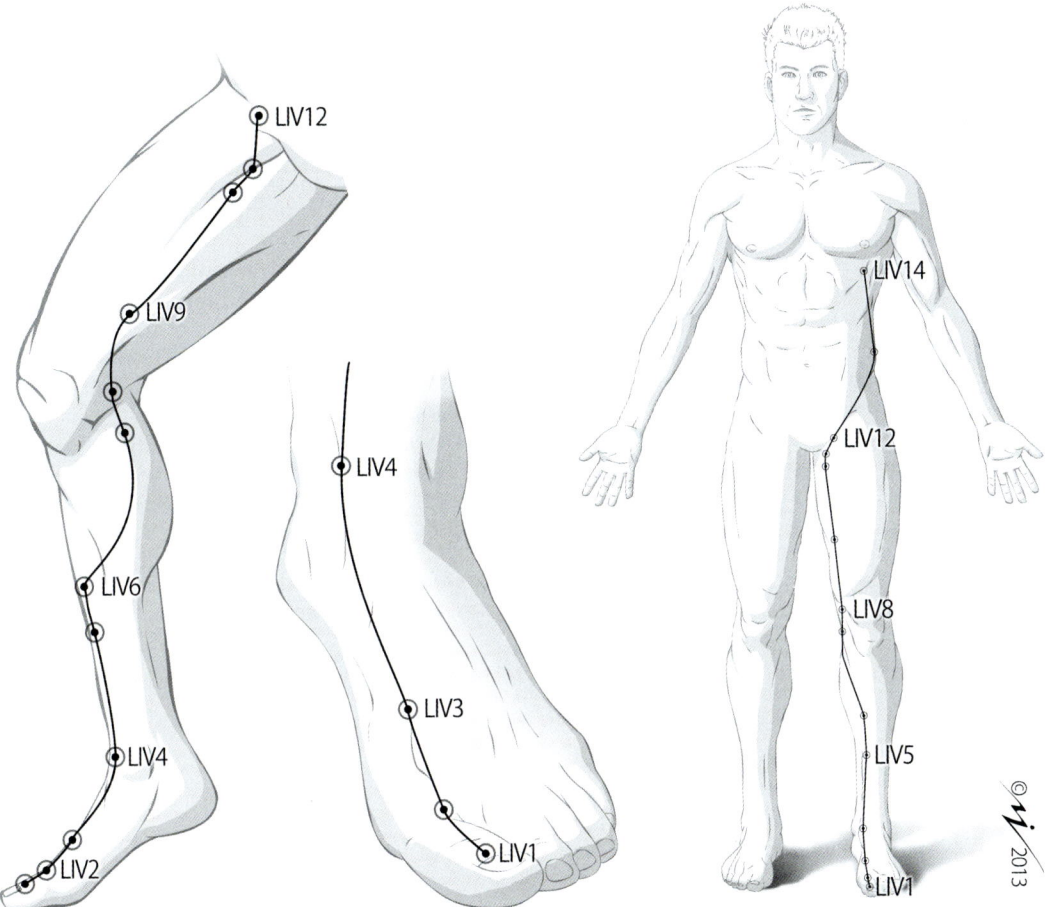

FIGURE 15.30 ■ Liver meridian (*Zu Jue Yin*). (Colour version of figure is available online).

15.21.3 LIV3

- Location: in the angle formed by the first and second metatarsals, in the proximal metatarsophalangeal depression.
- Indications: hypertension. Menstrual disorders. Incontinence and urinary retention. Mental and psychosomatic disorders, epileptic seizures. Clears the head. Acts upon the eyes. Pain and motor disorders of the lower extremity and foot.
- *Yuan*-source point and *shu*-spring point.

15.21.4 LIV5

- Location: 5 *cun* superior to the maximal protuberance of the medial malleolus, centre of the internal aspect of the tibia.
- Indications: gynaecological disorders, such as irregular menstruation, inflammation of the lower pelvis, uterine prolapse. Acute inflammation of the external genitals in the male, scrotal hernia. Thigh pain.
- *Luo*-connecting point.

15.21.5 LIV6

- Location: 7 *cun* above the maximal protuberance of the medial malleolus, in the centre of the internal aspect of the tibia.
- Indications: haemorrhagic uterine anovulatory dysfunction. External abdominal hernias.
- *Xi*-cleft point.

15.21.6 LIV8

- Location: flexed knee, internal border of the knee crease, behind the internal femoral epicondyle, depression of the anterior border of insertions of the semimembranosus and semitendinosus muscles.
- Indications: some gynaecological disorders (genitals, uterus), especially vulvar pruritus. Disorders of male sexual function. Pain and motor disorders of the knee joint and the lower extremities. Medial gonalgia. Enthesitis of the pes anserinus.
- Tonification point of the meridian.
- *He*-sea point.

In this section we will add two of the regulatory vessels that are included with the principal meridians due to the fact that they are the only ones of the eight that present their own points.

15.22 CONCEPTION VESSEL (*REN MAI*)

Its pathway goes from the perineum to the chin. This meridian contains 24 points (figure 15.31).

Its external pathway begins in the perineum, between the genital area and the anus, passing through the body along the anterior midline, abdomen and thorax, ending in the mentolabial sulcus.

- Function: it is considered a general energy reservoir, with regulating action acting upon it. It also has genitourinary, digestive and respiratory effects.

- Most important points: REN4 REN6, REN12, REN17.

15.22.1 REN4

- Location: in the anterior midline, 3 *cun* below the umbilicus, 2 *cun* above REN2 (pubis).
- Indications: all states of weakness (strengthens the body and reinforces health). Illnesses of the urinary tracts, urine retention, urinary incontinence. Disorders of male sexual function, prostatitis. Gynaecological and obstetric disorders.
- *Mu*-alarm point of the small intestine.

15.22.2 REN6

- Location: in the anterior midline, 1.5 *cun* below the umbilicus.

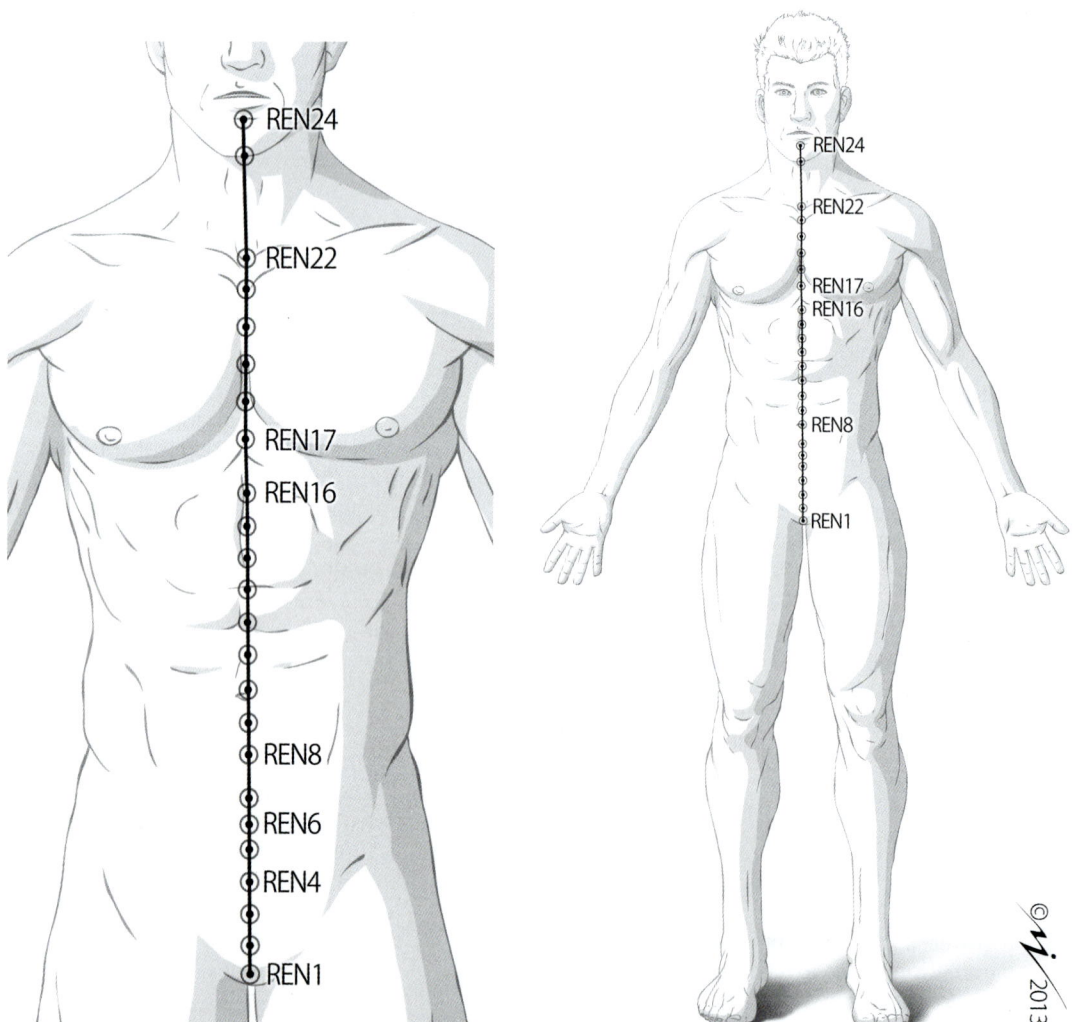

FIGURE 15.31 ■ Conception vessel meridian. (Colour version of figure is available online).

- Indications: all states of weakness (strengthens the body and reinforces immune function. Gynaecological disorders. Disorders of male sexual function.

15.22.3 REN12

- Location: in the anterior midline, 4 *cun* above the umbilicus.
- Indications: acute and chronic gastroenteritis. Gastric ulcer, gastralgia. Acute and chronic cholecystitis. Hiccups.
- *Mu*-alarm point of the stomach and reunion point of the viscera.

15.22.4 REN17

- Location: in the anterior midline, at the level of the fourth intercostal space, in the centre between both nipples.
- Indications: coronary cardiopathy. Bronchial asthma, spastic bronchitis. Low milk supply.
- *Mu*-alarm point of the pericardium and reunion point of vital energy.

15.23 GOVERNING VESSEL (*DU MAI*)

Its pathway runs from the coccyx to the superior maxillary bone. It consists of 28 points (figure 15.32).

Its external pathway begins at the tip of the coccyx and it runs through the whole lumbar, dorsal cervical and nape zones along the posterior midline, continuing along the head, forehead and nose and ending in the upper gum.

- Function: it is considered to be a general energy reservoir, acting upon the physical, mental and otorhinolaryngological spheres. It acts upon rigidity of the vertebral column and heaviness of the head.
- Most important points: DU4, DU14, DU20.

15.23.1 DU4

- Location: in the posterior midline, in the inferior depression of the L2 spinous process.
- Indications: disorders of male sexual function (impotence). Some gynaecological and

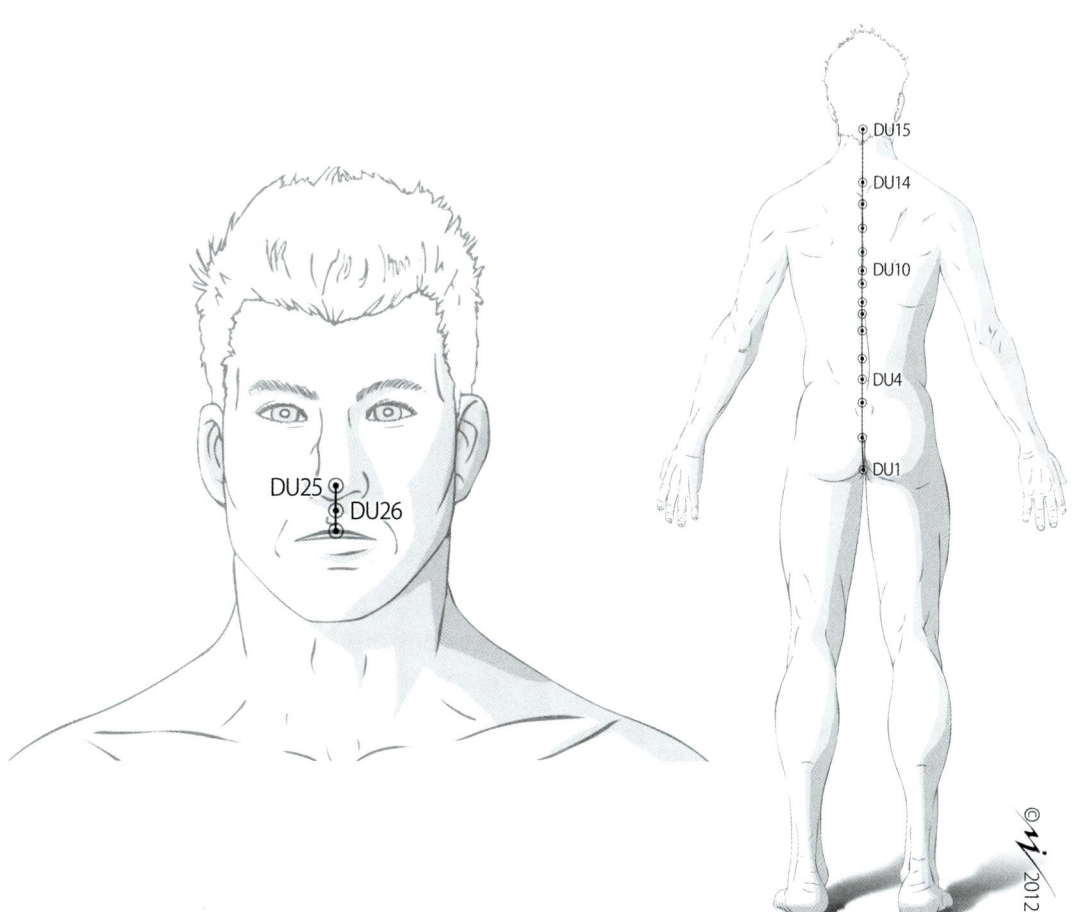

FIGURE 15.32 ■ Governing vessel meridian. (Colour version of figure is available online).

TABLE 15.9   Summary of the main points classified by meridian

Meridian	*Ting*	Tonification	Sedation	*Luo*	*Yuan*	Back *Shu*	Front *Mu*	*Xi* cleft
LU	11LU	LU9	LU5	LU7	LU9	BL13	LU1	LU6
LIV	1LIV	LIV11	LI2	LI6	LI4	BL25	ST25	LI7
ST	45ST	ST41	ST45	ST40	ST42	BL21	REN12	ST34
SP	1SP	SP2	SP5	SP4	SP3	BL20	LIV13	SP8
HE	9HE	HE9	HE7	HE5	HE7	BL15	REN14	HE6
SI	1SI	SI3	SI8	SI7	SI4	BL27	REN4	SI6
BL	67BL	BL67	BL65	BL58	BL64	BL28	REN3	BL63
KID	1KID	KID7	KID1	KID4	KID3	BL23	GB25	KID5
P	9P	P9	P7	P6	P7	BL14	REN17	P4
TB	1TB	TB3	TB10	TB5	TB4	BL22	REN5	TB7
GB	44GB	GB43	GB38	GB37	GB40	BL19	GB24	GB36
LIV	1LIV	LIV8	LIV2	LIV5	LIV3	BL18	LIV14	LIV6

obstetric disorders. Epileptic seizures. Low-back pain.

15.23.2 DU14

- Location: In the posterior midline, in the inferior depression of the C7 spinous process.
- Indications: persistent high fever, colds, flu. Cervical syndrome. Epilepsy.

15.23.3 DU20

- Location: in the midline, 5 *cun* behind the midpoint of the ideal anterior hairline, in the centre, between the ears.
- Indications: acute cerebrovascular accident. Headache; vertigo and stupor. Anal and rectal prolapse. Uterine prolapse.

In table 15.9 the integrations between the main acupuncture points are presented by meridians.

15.24 DESCRIPTION OF THE TECHNIQUE: TREATMENT MODEL USING THE TENDINOMUSCULAR MERIDIANS

15.24.1 Definition

The TMM correspond with the representation of the muscles, tendons and ligaments found along the main meridian pathways, sharing most of the pathway within its external path.

15.24.2 Functions

The main functions of the TMM are the distribution of energy (*wei*) and the blood through the musculoskeletal system and blocking the access of perverse energies to deeper planes with the ensuing worsening of the illness. Thus, this constitutes defensive functions towards illness.[21]

This treatment model is indicated in the approach of any pathology originated in the musculoskeletal system that is found within the area of influence of the meridian. Osteomuscular pain is, according to Chinese medicine, a localized pain in the secondary paths, such as the TMM. Therefore these are the first line of defence in the interior of the body in order to neutralize perverse exogenous energy. A battle is thus established between the biological energy (*wei*) and the pathological energy that produces a stagnation of energies in the meridian, leading to stagnation of blood and causing the appearance of an acute osteomuscular pain. This pain is due to an aggression of perverse external energy to a TMM, which can be caused either by repeated microtraumas or by a more intense trauma, which can produce a pain of *yang*-type characteristics, which are:

- pain: of an acute onset that tends to remit at rest, which worsens with movement, increases with heat and decreases with cold
- flushing: redness and an increase in temperature
- tumour: oedema
- functional impotence: incapable of movement.

15.24.3 Objectives of treatment with tendinomuscular meridians

The main objectives are:
- Extract the perverse energy through the *Jing* points of the affected meridians, which are very analgesic points for emergency treatments, and through the *Ashi* points, which are to be superficially punctured and thread-needled.
- Impede progression of the perverse energies to deeper planes by increasing the

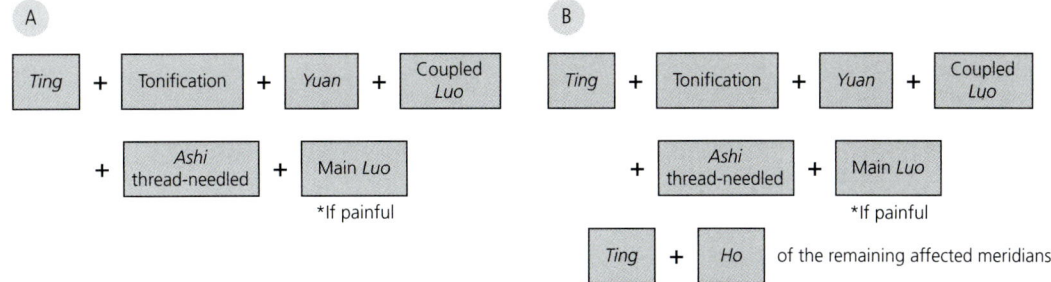

FIGURE 15.33 ■ Treatment protocol with tendinomuscular meridian. (A) In the case of only one affected tendinomuscular meridian. (B) In the case of more than one affected tendinomuscular meridian.

energy flow of the main meridian. For this purpose, puncture of the following points is used:

- tonification and *yuan*-source points of the main meridian
- *Luo*-connecting points of the coupled meridian.

In order to check whether the perverse energy has penetrated to deeper planes, press on the *luo* point of the affected meridian: if it is painful, it means the perverse energy has gone deeper and this point (*luo*) must be punctured perpendicularly.

15.24.4 Working protocol

The working protocol of the TMM treatment model is as follows (figure 15.33):

- localization of the painful points and identification of the most affected meridian (or the one that has the most painful points)
- puncture of the *Jing* point of the most affected meridian
- puncture of the tonification point of the most affected meridian
- puncture of the *yuan* point of the affected meridian and the *luo* of the coupled meridian
- puncture of the *Ashi* points (painful under pressure and spontaneously) and the local painful points
- verification of whether the *luo* point of the affected meridian is painful under palpation.

The *Ashi* points are treated with needles superficially and thread-needled using some of the following techniques:

- surrounding the painful zone with several dispersed needles
- use of an electrodispersion technique: continuous waves, with a pulse width of 200–250 μs, at a high frequency (60 Hz or more) and a tolerable intensity.

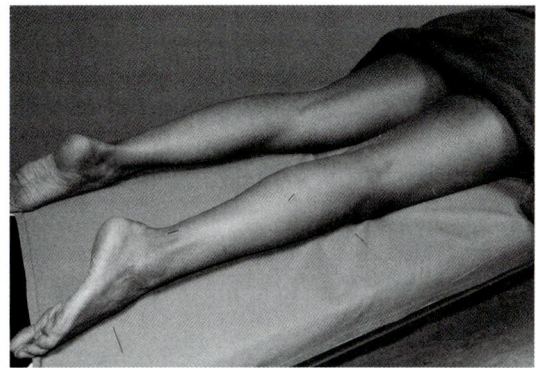

FIGURE 15.34 ■ Acupuncture application over the lumbar region.

15.25 CLINICAL CASE

15.25.1 Herniated disc with L5–S1 irradiation (figure 15.34)

The patient is a 40-year-old woman (a bank clerk), who spends extended periods of the day in a sitting position both at the office and at home.

Personal history and reason for consultation: she has suffered from frequent episodes of low-back pain, with a feeling of weakness in both lower limbs and generalized asthenia which she treats with non-steroidal anti-inflammatory drugs and muscle relaxants on demand. Recently, she suffered from a flare-up, with pain irradiating to the right leg along the L5–S1 region.

When she came for consultation she presented with fluctuating pain of moderate intensity in the lumbopelvic region, pain in both sacroiliac joints, more intense on the left, and pain with paraesthesias in the right lower limb from the gluteus to the lateral ankle.

Physical exam: she presents with pain and hypertonia in response to palpation of the paravertebral lumbar muscles, as well as the piriformis, iliopsoas and quadratus lumborum muscles on the right side. She has positive sclerotome pain in L4–L5–S1 segments, and general hypoaesthesia of the whole limb. The dermatome findings reaffirm greater involvement of the L5–S1 segment.

From the point of view of TCM she presents with pain under palpation of the back *shu* points (BL23–BL32); furthermore, the pain irradiation corresponds with the pathway of the urinary bladder meridian and is tender under palpation of BL56, BL57, BL58 and BL34 points.

She was seen by the traumatology service and a magnetic resonance image scan was performed. It revealed focal protrusion of the posterior and central border of the L5–S1 disc, compatible with a herniated disc.

The patient received pharmacological treatment consisting of Celebrex® and Myolastan®, as well as physiotherapy consisting of magnetotherapy, thermotherapy, analgesic electrotherapy and manual therapy for 2 weeks. During this period she referred to a discrete alleviation of symptoms; however, occasional irradiation into the right lower limb persisted, more intensely towards the sacroiliac joints.

(*Clinical case continued on page 491*)

15.26 REFERENCES

1. Huang di Neijing Suwen. Yellow emperor's inner classic of medicine, common questions. Commercial press edition. Shanghai: Shang-wu yin-shu-kuan; 1955. p. 261.
2. Soulié de Morant G. Compendio de la verdadera acupuntura china. Madrid: Editorial Alhambra, S.A.; 1984.
3. Wancura-Kampik I. Segment-anatomie. München Dtsch Arztebl Int 2009;106:728.
4. Mayor D. The Chinese back shu and front mu points and their segmental innervation. Rev Int Acupuntura 2008;51:26–36.
5. Pomeranz B, Stux GS. Scientific bases of acupuncture. Berlin: Springer-Verlag; 1989. p. 94-9.
6. Mayer DJ. Biological mechanisms of acupuncture. Prog Brain Res 2000;122:457–77.
7. Filshie J, White A. Medical acupuncture. A western scientific approach. Edinburgh: Churchill Livingstone; 1998.
8. Baldry P. Acupuncture, trigger points and musculoskeletal pain. 3rd ed. London: Elsevier, Churchill Livingstone; 2005.
9. Yun-tao Ma, Mila Ma, Zang Hee Cho. Biomedical acupuncture for pain management. London: Churchill Livingstone; 2011.
10. Melzack R, Wall PD. Pain mechanisms: a new theory. Science 1965;150:971–9.
11. Pomeranz B, Stux GS. Scientific bases of acupuncture. Berlin: Springer-Verlag; 1989. p. 94-9.
12. Shen E. Participation of descending inhibition in acupuncture analgesia. In: Zhang XT, editor. Research on acupuncture, moxibustion and acupuncture anesthesia. Beijing: Science Press; 1986. p. 31–8.
13. Dorsher PT, Fleckenstein J. Puntos gatillo y puntos de acupuntura clásica. Tercera parte: relación entre los patrones de dolor miofascial referido y los meridianos de acupuntura. Rev Int Acupuntura 2009;3:108–14.
14. Melzack R. Trigger points and classical acupuncture points, part I: qualitative and quantitative anatomic correspondences. Dt Ztschr f Akup 2008;51:15–24.
15. Travell JG, Simons DG. Myofascial pain and dysfunction. The trigger point manual. 2nd ed. Madrid: Panamericana; 2004.
16. Birch S. Trigger point-acupuncture point correlations revisited. J Altern Complement Med 2003;9:91–103.
17. Chen E. Cross-sectional anatomy of acupoints. Edinburgh: Churchill Livingstone; 1995.
18. Fundamentos de Acupuntura y Moxibustión de China. Beijing: Ediciones en lenguas extranjeras; 2003.
19. Maciocia G. The foundations of Chinese medicine. 2nd ed. London: Aneid-Press Elsevier; 2005.
20. Gómez Hernández F. Acupuntura, Restauración bioenergética. Madrid: Nueva Editorial Dilema; 2004.
21. Nogueira Pérez AC. Fundamentos de Bioenergética. Ediciones CEMETC, S.L.; 1987.
22. Principles of acupuncture within the framework of Traditional Chinese Medicine (TCM). In: Kubiena G, Sommer B, editors. Practice Handbook of Acupuncture. 3rd ed. Churchil Livinstone. Elsevier; 2010.
23. Sussman DJ. Acupuntura Teoría y Práctica. Buenos Aires: Ed. Kier; 2007.
24. Hoopwood V. Acupuncture in physiotherapy. Oxford: Elsevier; 2004.
25. Embid A. Enciclopedia de medicina China. Madrid: Medicinas Complementarias; 1998.
26. Langevin HM, Yandow JA. Relationship of acupuncture points and meridians to connective tissue planes. Anat Rec 2002;269:257–65.
27. Miguel-Pérez M, Ortiz-Sagristà JC, Pérez-Bellmunt A, et al. Descripción anatómica de puntos de acupuntura en la extremidad superior. Revista Internacional de Acupuntura 2008;2:126–31.
28. Académie de médecine traditionnelle chinoise. Précis d'acupuncture chinoise. académie de médecine traditionnelle chinoise. Pekin: Ed. en langues etrangeres; 1977.
29. Bossy JH. Atlas anatómico de los puntos de Acupuntura. Barcelona: Ed. Masson; 1984.
30. Peuker E, Filler T. Guidelines for case reports of adverse events related to acupuncture. Acupunct Med 2004;22:29–33.
31. Van Wijk R, Kwang-Sup S, van Wijk EPA. Anatomic characterization of acupuncture system and ultraweak photon emission. Asian J Phys 2007;16:443–74.
32. Niboyet J. La moindre résistance á l'electricité de surfaces punctiformes et de trajets cutanés concordant avec les points et méridiens bases de l'acupuncture. Gap: Louis Jean; 1963.
33. Reichmanis M, Marino AA, Becker RO. Electrical correlates of acupuncture points skin conductance variation at acupuncture loci. Am J Chin Med 1976;4:69–72.
34. Langevin HM, Churchill DL, Wu J, et al. Evidence of connective tissue involvement in acupuncture. FASEB J 2002;16:872–4.
35. Langevin HM, Churchill DL, Cipolla MJ. Mechanical signaling through connective tissue: A mechanism for the therapeutic effect of acupuncture. FASEB J 2001;15:2275–82.
36. Langevin HM, Churchill DL, Fox JR, et al. Biomechanical response to acupuncture needling in humans. J Appl Physiol 2011b;91:2471–8.
37. Lian Y-L, Chen Ch-Y, Hammes M, et al. Atlas Gráfico de Acupuntura. Representación de los puntos de acupuntura. Konemann; 2005.
38. Deadman P, Al-Khafaji M, Baker K. A manual of acupuncture. 2nd ed. East Sussex: Journal of Chinese Medicine Publications, 2007.
39. Chang-ging G, Hu Bo D, Liu Nai-gang M.A. Anatomical Illustration of acupuncture points. People's medical publishing house; 2008.
40. Focks C. Atlas de acupuntura. 2nd ed. Barcelona: Elsevier; 2009.

CHAPTER 16

ELECTROACUPUNCTURE

Antonio García Godino • Roberto Sebastián Ojero • Francisco Minaya Muñoz

The sceptic is someone who does not believe in science, but who believes in himself; he believes enough in himself to dare to deny science and to affirm that science is not bound by fixed and determined laws. The doubter is the true scientist; he only doubts himself and his interpretations, but he believes in science.

CLAUDE BERNARD

CHAPTER OUTLINE

KEYWORDS

analgesic acupuncture; acupuncture for facial paralysis; intramuscular acupuncture; pulse width; energy blockages; higher nervous centres; cell damage; chronic pain; electroacupuncture; electrolipolysis; traditional Chinese medicine (TCM); microcurrent stimulation; endogenous opioids.

16.1 INTRODUCTION TO ELECTROACUPUNCTURE AND ACU-TENS

According to the World Health Organization, the Western understanding is that the term acupuncture:

is used in its broad sense to include traditional body needling, moxibustion, electric acupuncture (electro-acupuncture), laser acupuncture (photo-acupuncture), microsystem acupuncture such as ear (auricular), face, hand and scalp acupuncture, and acupressure (the application of pressure at selected sites).[1]

Electroacupuncture (EA) is a technique that combines the action of acupuncture with that of electrical stimulation of the points, via needles, with the objective of producing an intense analgesic effect. It consists of the general application of a transcutaneous electrical nerve stimulation (TENS)-type current to the acupuncture needles in order to increase the therapeutic effects. EA generates an increased *Qi* and blood response within the acupuncture points and a greater biological stimulus with polarity changes of those same points, hence the use of the term acu-TENS – the combination of acupuncture and TENS.

EA is mainly indicated for the treatment of pain via the production of analgesia. It is generally used where manual acupuncture is indicated, especially when acupuncture does not achieve the expected results, or when it is necessary to apply a stronger stimulus in order to generate any of the following:

- a greater dispersion or sedation effect
- an enhanced tonifying effect
- to provide relief in processes of *Qi* and blood stagnation
- in order to produce a greater response in acute, subacute, chronic and fibrosis pathologies, where other techniques may have failed.

According to different authors, the alleviation of pain with acupuncture cannot be attributed simply to a placebo effect, as stimulation with acupuncture produces changes within the transmission of pain, blocking it at different levels of the central nervous system.[2,3]

Certain pathologies exist in which one can affirm that the beneficial effects of acupuncture and classic electrotherapy are multiplied when using EA, as long as a good praxis is performed and a series of precautions, indications and contraindications are considered.[3]

The main benefits of EA are:

- improvement of microcirculation
- elimination of local algogenic substances
- production of an anti-inflammatory effect
- in cases of increased tone, it helps decrease the tone of the smooth-muscle fibre.

16.1.1 Characteristics of electroacupuncture: parameters

Most commonly, EA uses TENS-type currents such as rectangular asymmetrical biphasic pulses. However, other types of TENS waveforms are also employed, such as symmetrical biphasic waves, triangular biphasic waves, spike-like biphasic pulses and monophasic pulses (e.g. square, triangular) (figure 16.1).[4]

During the stimulation phase, the surface of the area is equal to the area of the compensation phase. In contrast, the compensation phase is not wide enough to generate an active potential. Consequently, this type of TENS current does not have galvanic effects, as the net galvanic effect of the asymmetrical rectangular impulse is zero (or rather, it produces zero values or values very close to zero). Therefore, it is a type

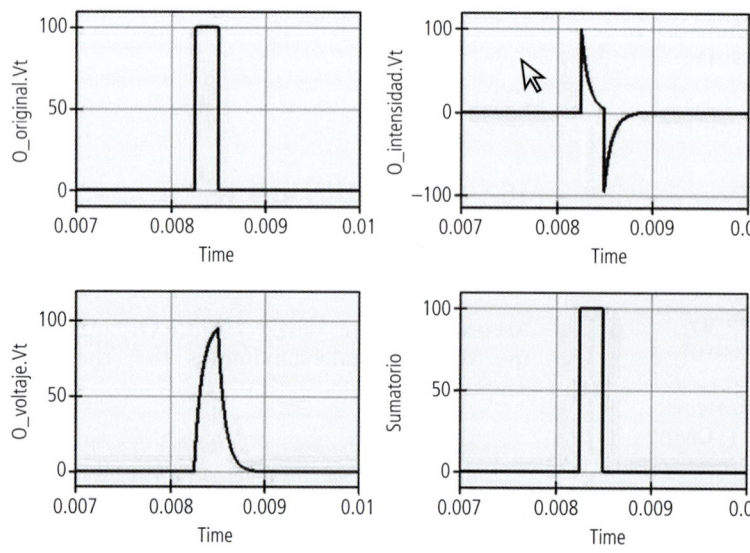

FIGURE 16.1 ■ Pulse waveform of the transcutaneous electrical nerve stimulation-type currents used in electroacupuncture. (Colour version of figure is available online).

of electrotherapy without polarity or without galvanism.

In accordance with the premises of classical electrotherapy, the cathode (negative electrode) is the most stimulating electrode and, therefore, the electrode that provides the greater effect. Hence, this electrode is applied in the area where more effectiveness is sought and where it will be used as a native electrode.[5]

16.1.2 Types of acu-TENS and biological basis

16.1.2.1 Basis

The biological foundation of acu-TENS is based on the following points:

- The physiological purpose of TENS (used in analgesic mode) is to activate different groups of nerve fibres selectively in order to trigger the analgesic mechanisms that produce clinically significant pain relief.[5]
- TENS currents work by inhibiting transmission of nociceptive information to the spinal cord, thus reducing central sensitization.[4]
- The action of the electrical impulses manages to inhibit the painful stimulus, favouring an increase in the production of natural analgesic substances (β-endorphins).[6]
- A current is generated in the area of the lesion that triggers biological repair, ensuring migration of the necessary cells towards the lesion area.[5]
- Several studies point to a relation between direct electrical currents and the process of cell mitosis (or cell growth), as live tissues naturally tend to produce electric potentials which help to control the scarring processes of injuries.[7,8]

16.1.2.2 Types

- Western TENS: this is the conventional device commonly used by physiotherapists (box 16.1).
- Chinese TENS: these are devices that have been used in China since ancient times to stimulate acupuncture points (box 16.2).

The types of Chinese electric waves used (continuous, intermittent and dense-disperse waves) correspond with the continuous or interrupted waveforms, periodically interrupted waves and modulated waves (frequency modulation, amplitude modulation or both) which are commonly used in the West.

BOX 16.1 Characteristics of Western TENS

PARAMETERS

- Waveform: asymmetrical biphasic square (in general)
- Frequency: 1–150 Hz
- Pulse width: 50–250 ms
- Controls: 2 or 4
- Battery: 1.5 V or 220 V
- Can be used in conventional or burst mode
- The devices can be portable (1.5 V or 9 V battery) or fixed (220 AC/DC)
- The intensity is dosed in milliamps (1 mA = 10^{-3} A)

Adaptors can be found (2–4 mm female to male for a variety of outlets).

BOX 16.2 Characteristics of Chinese transcutaneous electrical nerve stimulation

PARAMETERS

- Waveform: asymmetrical biphasic rectangular (in general, although there are many that work with monophasic pulses)
- Frequency: 1–150 Hz
- Pulse width: 50–250 ms
- Controls: 4, 6, 8, 10
- Battery: 9 V (2) or 220 AC/DC
- Wave types: continuous, intermittent and dense-disperse
- Outlets: 4–10 pairs of electrodes with filiform needles (metal handle)
- The intensity is dosed in milliamps (1 mA = 10^{-3} A)

The Chinese devices are usually light, more straightforward to use and cheaper, although they must bear a CE mark or the equivalent (figure 16.2A). Recently, Enraf-Nonius®-Spain and PRIM® have developed the first Western device (Physio Invasiva®) (figure 16.2B) to apply different electrotherapy modalities (TENS, microcurrents (MCRs), galvanic current, high-voltage pulsed current) through the needle.

Figure 16.3 shows the results of an oscilloscope analysis of the waveforms used in these devices.

16.1.3 Clinical application of electroacupuncture in physiotherapy

As a reminder of the premises of classical electrotherapy, it is important to consider that,

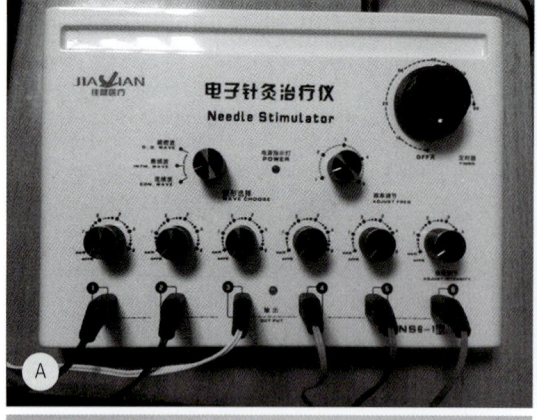
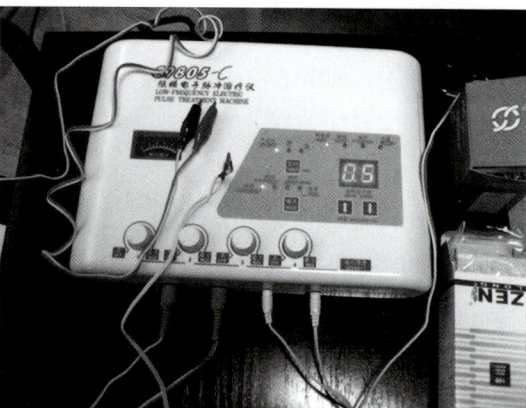
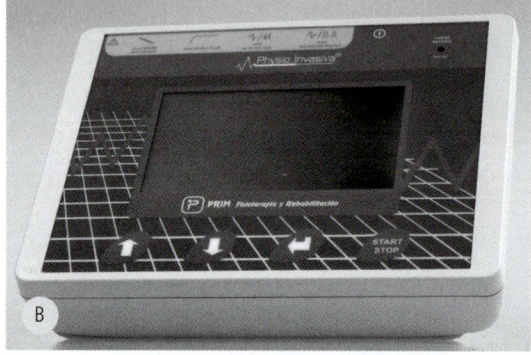

FIGURE 16.2 ■ Electrotherapy equipment. (A) Chinese devices commonly used in treatments with electroacupuncture. (B) Physio Invasiva®: the first Western device to apply different electrotherapy modalities through a needle. (Colour version of figure is available online).

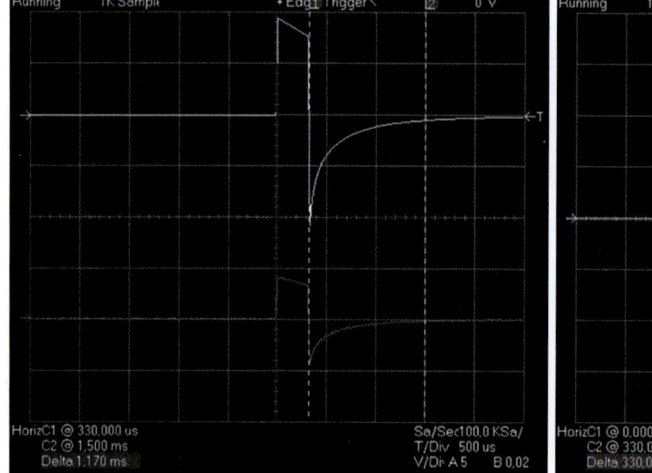
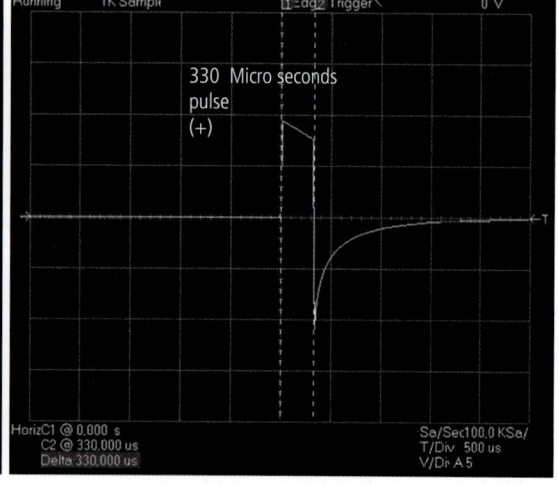

FIGURE 16.3 ■ Oscilloscope analysis of the waveforms of Chinese transcutaneous electrical nerve stimulation. (Colour version of figure is available online).

within a conventional physiotherapy programme, in each outlet provided by a device, two electrodes are used; these are known as the anode (or positive electrode) and the cathode (or negative electrode). The cathode is the most active and stimulating electrode; it acts upon the axon by exciting and depolarizing it (i.e. both the nerve and muscle cells), accompanied by propagation of the action potential. In turn, the anode (or

positive electrode) hyperpolarizes the axon, thus inhibiting the action potential. Nonetheless, the stimulus produced by both electrodes has beneficial effects for the treatment of pain.[8–10]

The form of application is thus bipolar, mainly seeking interpolar effects over the polar effects. The bipolar application can be transverse (leaving the structure to be treated in the centre – commonly used for articular and capsular applications) or longitudinal (for tendons, ligaments, muscles).

16.1.3.1 Most frequent applications

1. Analgesic applications: the electrodes are applied in the region with the most pain, clinically symptomatic areas, points that are tender to palpation, or areas that were confirmed as being positive during exploratory testing. These points are called *Ashi* acupuncture points or points of local pain.
2. Vasotropic applications: the cathode is placed central to the heart as a distal therapeutic mode (in relation to the anode) or proximally (by placing the cathode in the region of more sensitive innervation and the anode distally).
3. Intramuscular applications (motor point): EA is used in the myofascial trigger points (MTrPs) that correspond with acupuncture points. Special consideration with regard to the anatomy, function and innervation of the muscle or muscle group within which we are seeking a response is recommended. The purpose of this application is to activate the motor efferents in the myotomes related to the origin of pain.[5,11]
4. Applications on the *huatuo jiaji* points (paravertebral points): these are stimulated bearing in mind their metameric correspondence and the segmental level implicated. Such applications are indicated for the treatment of painful syndromes, local facet syndromes and rheumatism. For this application we shall consider the correspondence with the organs and viscera (according to the *Zhang-Fu* theory of traditional Chinese medicine [TCM]). This is especially interesting in the autonomic nervous system together with areas that depend on autonomic innervation (sympathetic and parasympathetic systems).

KEY POINTS

The *huatuo jiaji* points (paravertebral points) tend to respond very well to treatment with EA. In this type of treatment there are several points worth bearing in mind:

- The locations of the *huatuo jiaji* are selected according to the level of the rheumatism.
- Electrical stimulation can be performed beginning with low frequencies (2–5 Hz), later increasing to higher frequencies (50–100 Hz), in order to decrease the habituation effect.

5. Clinical applications in the common pathologies seen in physiotherapy clinics include:
   a. pathologies of the musculoskeletal system: periarthropathies, coxalgia, gonalgia, tendinopathies, bursitis, fasciitis, sprains, muscular fibrosis, muscular contractures, nerve paralysis, backache, sciatica (also for the symptomatic treatment and recovery of a range of musculoskeletal pathologies, in situations of chronic pain, neuralgia and recurring pain)
   b. as a form of functional treatment for the remaining body systems, such as the reproductive, cardiovascular, respiratory, gastrointestinal, genitourinary systems
   c. other pathologies: those secondary to the adverse effects of medicine, convalescence, insomnia, stress, additions and states of anxiety, etc.
6. Applications in general acupuncture points: the more generic points are activated via stimulation or tonification of the contributing systems (according to the Chinese methodology)[12,13]:
   a. ST36: ailments of the stomach and the abdomen
   b. BL40: ailments of the dorsolumbar region
   c. LU7: ailments of the head and neck
   d. LI4: ailments of the face and mouth
   e. SP6: female ailments; lower abdomen and lower limbs
   f. P6: ailments of the thoracic cavity.

16.1.4 Precautions and contraindications

We will continue by describing the various precautions and contraindications associated with EA.

16.1.4.1 Precautions

- As a general rule, do not go beyond the midline in the region of the cardiac plexus in order to avoid producing interferences between the sinus rhythm and the cardiac nerves of the sympathetic trunk.
- Be aware of the presence of neurovascular bundles: exercise special precaution when introducing intense needle manipulation techniques and EA directly over these areas.
- Be aware of patients who may be especially sensitive, such as the elderly, patients in convalescent care, malnourished or obese patients.

In the case of a vasovagal response, or cardiovascular depression, hypotension, loss of consciousness or vomiting, proceed by extracting the needle, placing the patient in a secure position and stimulating the so-called 'resuscitation points' for the restoration of *yang*. An effective technique consists of stimulating the GV25 and GV26 points using a light pinch or by stimulating any of the *Jing*-well points (this is a widespread method of resuscitation used in China).

16.1.4.2 Contraindications

- Pregnancy: EA is contraindicated due to the risk of abortion. Mainly this is true for infraumbilical points (due to the connection with the fetus), lumbosacral roots (these depend on abdominal innervation) and points that mobilize the blood of the inferior *Jiao* and the uterus (LI4 and SP6). Some studies mention the possibility of using acupuncture symptomatically as long as risk points are avoided.
- Children during their growth years: metadiaphyseal regions, areas of bone growth and points such as ST36 are contraindicated as these can produce stunted growth (this is an empirical observation, bearing in mind that there is no scientific evidence to support this theory).
- Epilepsy: EA may increase the risk of epileptic attack and seizures.
- Active neoplastic processes: avoid active tumoral zones due to the possible risk of cell multiplication. However, EA can be used to treat the secondary effects of degenerative autoimmune illnesses such as cancer or other immunocompromised situations. The idea is that the energy systems may be improved as well as the gastrointestinal metabolic system.
- Always consider possible cardiac disorders (cardiac decompensation), coagulation illnesses, skin problems, sensory alterations and infections. All of these are considered relative contraindications.
- EA should not be used on the viscera and appendages.

16.2 MECHANISM OF ACTION

16.2.1 The neurophysiology of electroacupuncture

16.2.1.1 Generalities and objectives

One of the objectives sought by EA is to produce an immediate inflammatory response and to initiate the self-defence system of the patient's body in response to pathology and cell damage. In this manner, the body acts by generating anti-inflammatory substances and autologous mechanisms for pain control. Furthermore, an activation of the small-diameter afferents of the muscle (A-δ fibres) occurs, causing a muscular contraction and activity of the receptors of the type 3 group of afferents (GIII).

As a general rule, in the treatment of chronic pain, stimulation and tonification are preferably performed with low frequency and high intensity. However, for the treatment of acute pain, sedation and dispersion are preferred with the contrasting parameters of high frequency and low intensity.[14,15]

KEY POINTS

In the treatment of chronic pain, stimulation with low frequency and high intensity is performed for a maximum of 30 minutes (signs of fatigue may appear due to the visible muscular contraction). The objective is to achieve a stimulation or tonification of the tissue in the presence of numbness and organic states of insufficiency or apoplexies, according to Chinese medical methodologies. In the treatment of acute pain, high-frequency and low-intensity stimulation is preferred for a duration of 15–20 minutes. The aim is to produce sedation or dispersion of the acute process or the excess, in line with Chinese medical practices.

16.2.1.2 Mechanisms

The impulses generated by EA in the small-diameter afferent fibres (A-δ) of the muscles, motor point, myotome and site of pain will trigger the following mechanisms (figure 16.4):

- Extrasegmental analgesia: via the activation of descending pathways that inhibit pain, causing liberation of endogenous opioids in the superior nervous centres: the periaqueductal grey matter, the nucleus raphe magnus, the paragigantocellular nucleus of the raphe and the thalamic elements (caudate nucleus, accumbens nucleus, limbic system).
- Segmental analgesia: similar to the general effects of classical electrotherapy (a similar effect to conventional TENS applied percutaneously). Activation of the A-δ occurs and generates the 'gate-control' phenomenon or the closing of the 'nerve gates', and modulation of neural coding at the level of the spinal cord, thus inhibiting incoming noxious information.[16–18]

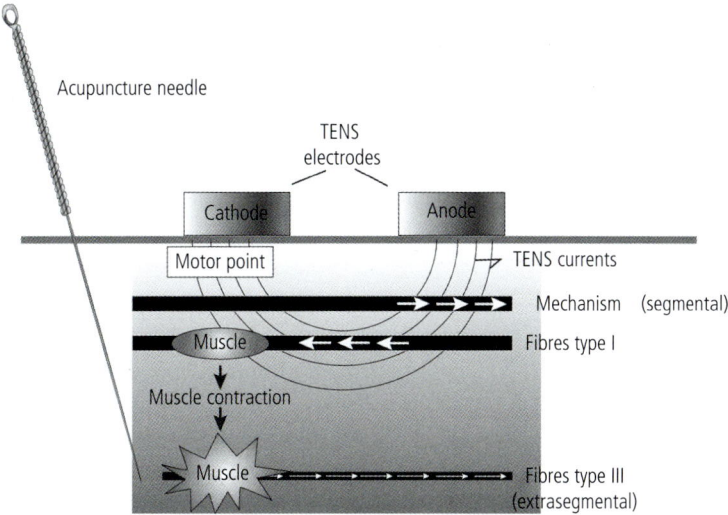

FIGURE 16.4 ■ Effect of electroacupuncture on the motor point in order to trigger neuromuscular responses and stimulation of the higher nervous centres. TENS, transcutaneous electrical nerve stimulation. (Adapted from: Watson T. Electroterapia: Práctica basada en la evidencia. Barcelona: Elsevier; 2009).

KEY POINTS

The phasic muscular contractions that are produced with the application of EA generate activity of the small-diameter muscle afferents, activating the inhibitory paths of descending pain and producing both types of analgesia – segmental and extrasegmental.

On the other hand, EA facilitates the release of different substances in different areas within the nervous system:

- At the spinal level: enkephalins, endorphins, γ-aminobutyric acid system and dynorphins. Pain is blocked presynaptically, inhibiting the system of ascending information along the spinothalamic pathway (anterolateral).
- In the midbrain: enkephalins, 5-hydroxytryptamine, noradrenaline. These neurotransmitters inhibit pain pre- and postsynaptically. They modulate the ascending information along the spinothalamic tract (they activate the centres of nucleus raphe magnus and of periaqueductal grey) and send descending signals along the dorsolateral pathway of the spinal cord.
- Along the hypothalamic–pituitary–adrenal axis: β-endorphins, adrenocorticotrophic hormone and the hormonal system.
- In the central nervous system: EA activates the central cerebral mechanisms and promotes internal homeostasis.

16.2.1.3 Application modalities: forms and methods

Some applications for the use, form and methodology of EA are:

- The 10 Hz frequency (or intermediate frequency) is systematically the most commonly used by contemporary authors (in bioenergetics and cosmetic pathologies).[19,20]
- The most frequently used points for the treatment of lumbar pain with acupuncture are DU4 and BL23, together with EA in local points (*Ashi*) and in extra-articular points (*huatuo jiaji*). The distal points are found in the territory of the bladder (posterior), gall bladder (lateral) and stomach (anterior) meridians.[21]
- Lundeberg performed a randomized controlled trial in chronic lumbar pain and observed that EA at 2 Hz produced better results than manual acupuncture and EA at 80 Hz.[22]
- Eriksson et al.[23] performed studies of the use of EA in bursts; this produced a more tolerable muscular contraction than that of single pulses at low frequency and provoked the liberation of central endorphins. Sjölund[24] also affirmed that a frequency of 80 Hz is more efficient in order to calm pain.
- Treatments with EA are performed at low frequencies (1–4 Hz) in a continuous manner and with a pulse width duration of 200 ms.[25] Omura[26] also uses high intensities

for the sake of producing a muscular contraction and triggering a response in the superior nervous centres.

KEY POINTS

Several clinical studies indicate that elecroacupuncture could offer better results than manual acupuncture and transcutaneous electrotherapy in lumbar and sciatic pain.

16.2.2 Clinical expertise and electroacupuncture

Clinical and professional experience is decisive for the placement of acupuncture needles, as there is no set path to follow in order to perform that 'perfect' treatment.

In the practice of EA, clinical experience has shown that treatment does not consist of blindly following a set of agreed protocols or miraculous formulas, but rather it is the professional who must determine the mode of action and the frequency with regard to the phase of pathology, and depending on the aetiology and symptoms of each individual clinical case.

16.3 DESCRIPTION OF THE TECHNIQUE

16.3.1 Electroacupuncture of the *Ashi* points

16.3.1.1 Concepts and characteristics

The *Ashi* points are points that are painful on palpation and which usually produce clinical symptoms in the patient. These traditionally correspond to the painful palpation points theoretically defined by *Sun Si Miao*, as they do not normally coincide with points within the acupuncture channels (acupuncture points).

In TCM these are known as *āshì* or *āshì-xué*, translated as: 'oh yes'.

KEY POINTS

Where there is pain there is an *Ashi* point, and acupuncture and moxibustion can be applied directly over local areas of pain. In the clinic, the *Ashi* points can produce beneficial therapeutic effects in pain and rheumatism syndromes.

The *Ashi* points are characterized by[27]:
- leukocyte infiltration and inflammatory hyperplasia
- fibroblastic proliferation with serofibrinous exudation
- lipid infiltration
- loss of transverse strands of the skeletal muscle with the formation of fibrous nodules due to local secretion of nociceptive substances.

16.3.1.2 Methodology

The application of EA in the *Ashi* points is based on the use of the technique of thread needling, with the needle inserted at an angle of 30–45° to the skin surface, and searching for the painful region. Several pairs of needles can be used (e.g. two, four, six, eight) according to the intensity of pain, its location and pathology. The pairs must face each other, with the focal point of pain in the centre of the needles (figure 16.5).

The needles to be used for the performance of this method must be 1 inch or 1.5 inch (25 or 40 mm) in length and 0,25 mm, 0,26 mm or 0,30 mm in diameter.

In general (according to the praxis of TCM), high frequencies are used for electrodispersion where there is acute *yang*-type pain and in order to sedate the structure that is found to be in excessive pain. High frequencies can also be combined at the beginning of the treatment, together with low frequencies at the end. An effective and very commonly used method is the alternation of 60 Hz and 4 Hz (15 minutes and 5 minutes).

In any case, the best placement of the electrodes heavily relies on the clinician's clinical and professional experience and should be adjusted according to the pathology, aetiology and symptoms of each individual clinical case.

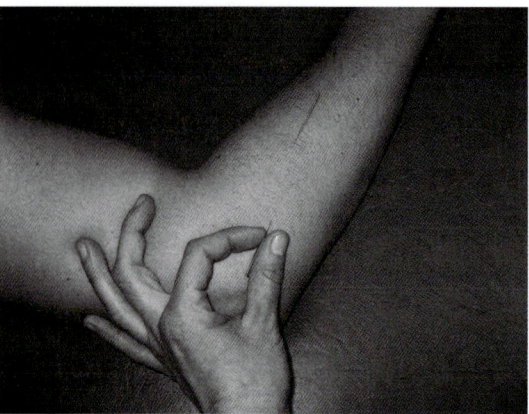

FIGURE 16.5 ■ Thread needling technique applied over local pain sites or *Ashi* points. (Colour version of figure is available online).

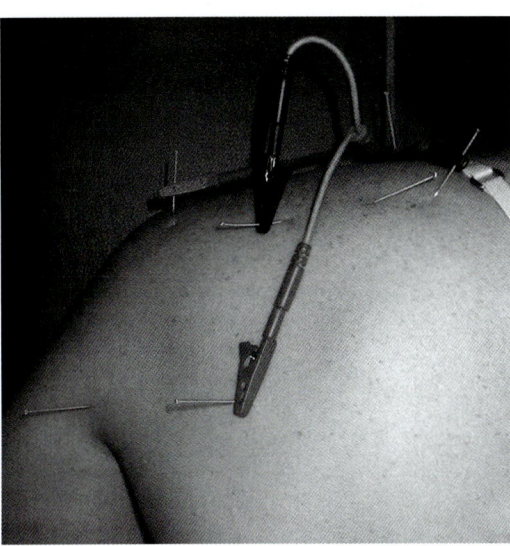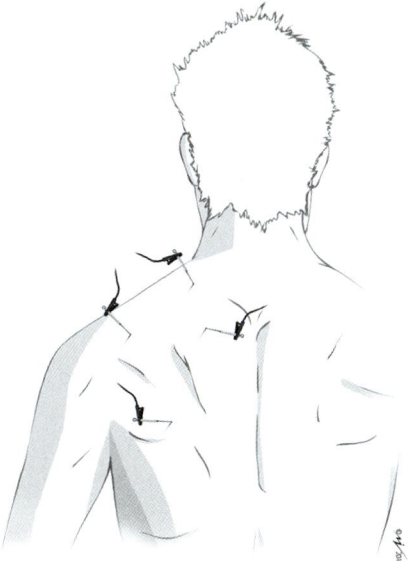

FIGURE 16.6 ■ Electroacupuncture with intramuscular application in scapular acupuncture points, using the 'zigzag points of the scapula' corresponding to the small-intestine meridian for the treatment of local symptoms at this level; the points are SI9–SI13. (Colour version of figure is available online).

16.3.2 Intramuscular electroacupuncture

16.3.2.1 Concept and characteristics

Intramuscular EA consists of the application of needles over the MTrPs that coincide with the acupuncture points. Furthermore, it is in parallel with the *Ashi* points (as they are also points that are sensitive to pain).

Local acupuncture points that coincide with MTrPs are used. The difference of EA applied intramuscularly is that, normally, these intramuscular points are not punctured in an isolated manner but are combined with other classical acupuncture points, such as opening points, special-effect points, row points and master points.

This procedure can be applied in myofascial pain syndrome, mainly within intramuscular points, and related to clinical manifestations of cervicalgia, dorsalgia, low-back pain, pseudo-sciatica syndrome (piriformis syndrome), lateral epicondylalgia and scapular pain. It may also be applied in areas where there are clinically relevant acupuncture points that can clearly be pathognomonic with myofascial pain syndrome.

16.3.2.2 Methodology

The professional will decide which parameters are to be used in EA for the purpose of proper therapeutic practice, thus optimizing the results based on what has been previously described. The intramuscular needles, after correct insertion, should remain in the site for 20 minutes.

The most common clinical application of this technique is within large-muscle regions.[28,29]
- scapular girdle (figure 16.6):
  - superior trapezius: GB21 (apex point of the lung, taking care not to produce a pneumothorax)
  - levator scapulae: SI14, SI15
  - teres major: SI9
  - infraspinatus: SI11
  - supraspinatus: SI12, SI13
- muscle bellies of the forearm: extensor carpi radialis: SI10, SI11, SI12
- lumbopelvic girdle: piriformis: GB30 (a 50 mm needle may be used)
- head and face: masseter: ST6
- lower limb:
  - rectus femoris: ST31, ST32. ST33, ST34
  - triceps surae: BL55, BL56, BL57, BL58.

The technique of intramuscular puncture is applied in clear myofascial pain syndromes, and not used on isolated points but, rather, in combination with other acupuncture points.

16.3.3 Electrolipolysis

16.3.3.1 Concept

Electrolipolysis consists of implanting various pairs of needles in areas of fat accumulation, with

EA taking place via connection of the needles with a device that generates low-frequency currents similar to TENS.

16.3.3.2 Physiopathology of obesity and cellulalgia

The main functions of the hypodermis are thermoregulation, trauma absorption, caloric reservoir and participation in the metabolism of fat and water.

Atrophy of the hypodermic tissue occurs due to a lax connective tissue formed by large lobules of fat tissue and limited by septum formed by fibres of thin collagen tissue and few elastic fibres. Due to this process of atrophy, a decrease in the functions of caloric reservoir and thermoregulation occurs, and this facilitates the appearance of wrinkles, flaccidity and loose-hanging skin.

The flaccidity associated with cellulite occurs due to intrinsic ageing associated with the most severe grades of cellulite, due to vascular involvement and the influence of the effect of gravity of the fat lobules upon the septum of the collagen tissue fibres, the elastic fibres, and over the dermis itself. With the appearance of flaccidity associated with cellulite, an alteration in the amount, width and quality of fibrous bands occurs.

The common zones of fat accumulation are the abdominal and side regions, the thighs, the internal aspect of the knees, the posterior arm region and the double-chin area. In clinical practice it is important to be thorough and really to get to know the tissue upon which we are working in order to avoid producing iatrogenesis.

16.3.3.3 Characteristics and effects

Electrolipolysis allows one to:
- modify the permeability of the adipocytes, eliminate their fat, decrease localized fat deposits and areas of accumulation and thus increase diuretic metabolism

- slim down
- eliminate flaccidity and mould the body.
These generalities depend on the type of patient, the location of the fat, size of fat deposits, etc..

16.3.3.4 Methodology

The region where the treatment is applied is within the hypodermic tissue (subdermis).[30]

For this type of EA technique, long needles are used (at least 1.5 *cun* or 40 mm; the most recommended are 2 *cun* or 50 mm). This technique is described using needles of 30 mm or 32 mm in diameter in order to cover the largest quantity of fat tissue and thus favour the lipolytic effect (table 16.1).

According to TCM, Japanese-type needles without a needle head or guide tube are used.

The needles must be facing each other and must not touch each other in order to prevent producing a short circuit of the system (figure 16.7).

The professional must be able to go through the cellular tissue and orient the needle towards the region of fat on which he or she will be working.

Available on the market are bifurcators and Y-adaptor cables that multiply the outlets, so that the areas of fat accumulation to be treated can be increased.

The EA that is used in this procedure consists of TENS-type currents applied in a specific way over the adipocyte.

The therapeutic procedure consists of selecting a fold of fat upon which to act on the adipose tissue.

The needles are placed facing each other in parallel and without touching.

16.3.4 Electroacupuncture in scars

16.3.4.1 Concept and characteristics

Considering the physiopathology of the system of channels and meridians, one must bear in

---

TABLE 16.1 Electroacupuncture technique in the lipolysis phases

Phase	First phase	Second phase	Third phase	Fourth phase
Effect	Ionizer	Vasodilation (evacuation)	Drainage (stagnation)	Tonification (retraction of the skin and adipose tissues
Intensity	Sensitive	Higher intensity (according to tolerance)	Decrease the intensity, only sensitive	Intensity according to tolerance
Frequency	5 Hz	20 Hz	40 Hz	40 Hz
Type of wave	Dense-disperse	Intermittent	*Tui na*	Continuous
Time	20 minutes	20 minutes	20 minutes	20 minutes

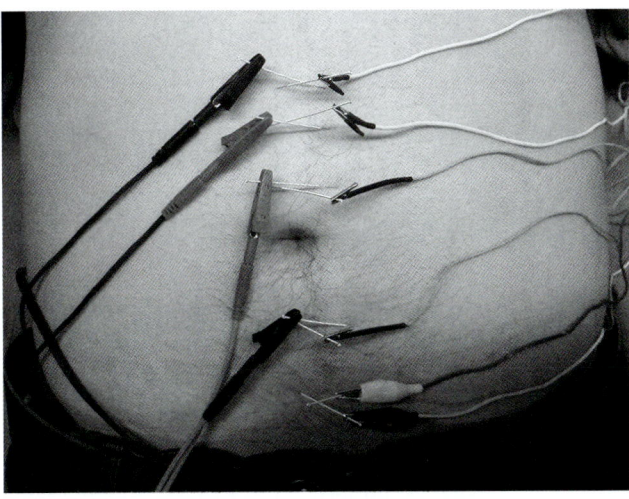
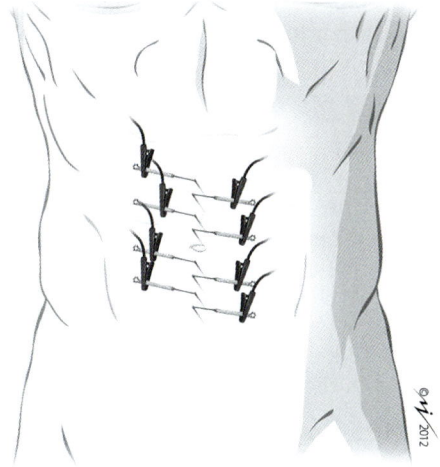

FIGURE 16.7 ■ Electrolipolysis procedure for the area of fat accumulation of the anterior abdomen. Long needles are used with a medial to lateral orientation, pinching the fat region in order to access the subcutaneous tissue. Japanese needles of 0.32 × 40 mm are used. (Colour version of figure is available online).

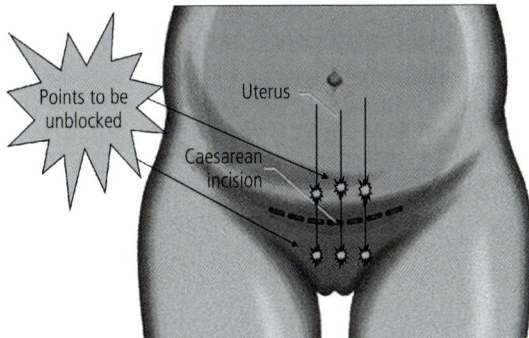

FIGURE 16.8 ■ Caesarean-section scar that cuts across the two meridians of the kidney and the *Ren Mai* meridian. One needle is positioned proximally, and another distally on both sides of the scar, unblocking the energetic channels of *Ren Mai*, and both kidney meridians, as well as providing an additional local effect. (Colour version of figure is available online).

mind the energy blockages caused by scars along the meridian paths.

According to TCM, a scar is an interruption of the circulation of energy (*Qi*) and the blood system (*Xue*) and produces a sensation of pain, emptiness, pins and needles and dysaesthesias and can even trigger more profound illnesses, as well as chronic and/or organic pain.

16.3.4.2 Methodology

For this technique of EA, needles are inserted on both sides of the scar that is interfering with the course of the meridian (these do not necessarily have to exactly coincide with the described acupuncture points) (figures 16.8 and 16.9).[16,31]

FIGURE 16.9 ■ Electroacupuncture applied on a scar in the lumbar spine. (Colour version of figure is available online).

16.3.5 Monopolar stimulation

16.3.5.1 Concepts and characteristics

Monopolar stimulation refers to stimulation of the body's nerves via electric currents using single-electrode TENS.

This modality of EA is applied with the objective of alleviating different types of pain: acute, subacute, chronic and postoperatory.

Any part of the body can be induced in order to produce a signal that allows for the location of a point, depending on the amount of energy used at that location.

16.3.5.2 Methodology

In clinical practice, there are several forms of EA treatment using monopolar stimulation of the acupuncture points.

There are devices of cutaneous electroconductivity (measuring electric resistance of the skin and its voltage) that can help determine the correct location of the acupuncture points (diagnostic function). As well as fulfilling a diagnostic function, these can be used therapeutically, stimulating the acupuncture point with local TENS and thus triggering a therapeutic response (in symptomatic acupuncture, in active zones of the lesion or in the perilesional area).

These systems of monopolar stimulation are also used in the microsystems and in reflex systems, e.g. reflexology, auriculotherapy, acupuncture of the hand, craniopuncture in both modalities – diagnostic as well as therapeutic.

16.3.5.3 Types

- Acu-pen stimulator: this is a portable point stimulator. It is used to test the location of the acupuncture points, as well as for stimulation with percutaneous electrotherapy. The EA stimulus can also be created via the needle for approximately 10 seconds (figure 16.10).
- Pointer Plus stimulator: this is also a portable point stimulator. It locates and stimulates acupuncture points and trigger points of myofascial pain with a high degree of precision. It has a sound and light indicator for pulse detection and two interchangeable probes (for body points and auriculotherapy). It generates continuous pulses of TENS-type waves (asymmetric biphasic) and the intensity ranges from 0 to 22 mA. It also provides stimulation of a fixed and continuous frequency (8–10 Hz) with a pulse width of 240 µs. An EA stimulus can also be performed via the needle for approximately 10 seconds (figure 16.11). Prior to the application of the stimulator, one has to adjust the settings to the threshold and the level of sensitivity of the patient.
- Ryodaraku or electric point detector: the Ryodaraku health monitor is a multipurpose instrument for measuring the Ryodaraku energy of the meridians and for applying EA and electrostimulation treatments. This device has a neurometer of great precision for determining the intensity of the electric current and performing bionergetic measurements. It has an asymmetric biphasic TENS-type square wave, and has outlets for connections with electrode handles, searching electrodes, electrode pads for therapy and commutators of function for diagnosis, measurement and treatment. It exercises a constant pressure on the points or affected areas, providing greater precision during the location of the points to be treated.

All these devices of monopolar EA (acu-pen, Pointer-Plus, Ryodaraku) can be used on any acupuncture point, both for diagnosis (testing function) as well as for treatment of the free nerve terminals of any region.

In the back, correspondence with the *huatuo jiaji* Ex-B2 or paravertebral extra points can be sought (figure 16.12). Their location can serve as a guide to find a response in the proximal

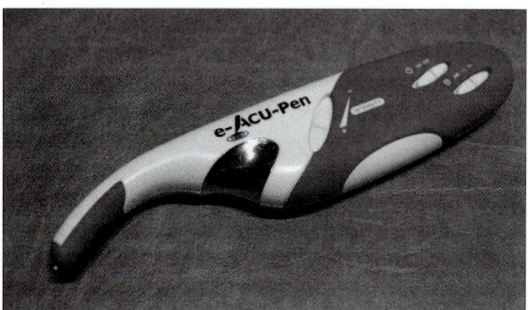

FIGURE 16.10 ■ Acu-pen stimulator. (Colour version of figure is available online).

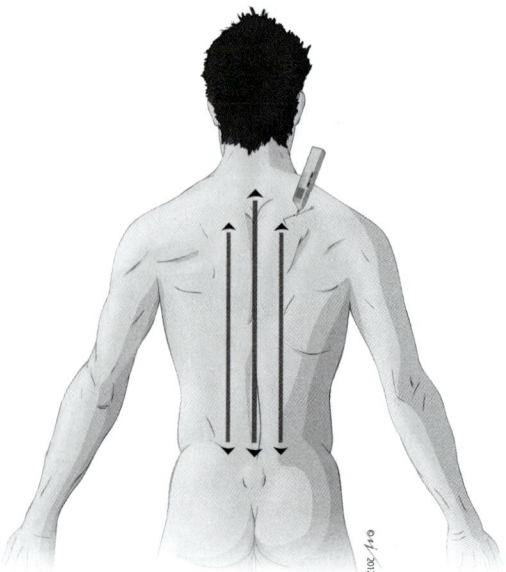

FIGURE 16.11 ■ Application with a pointer stimulator along metameric levels of the spine. (Colour version of figure is available online).

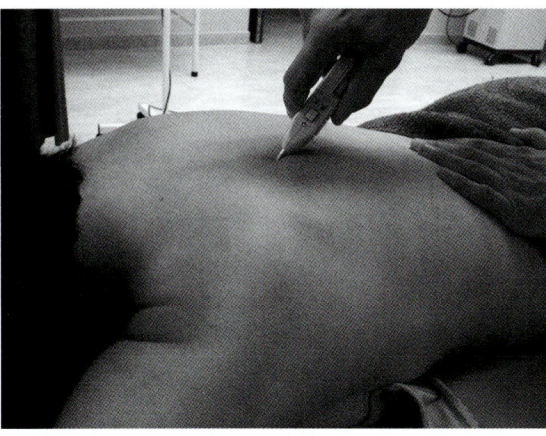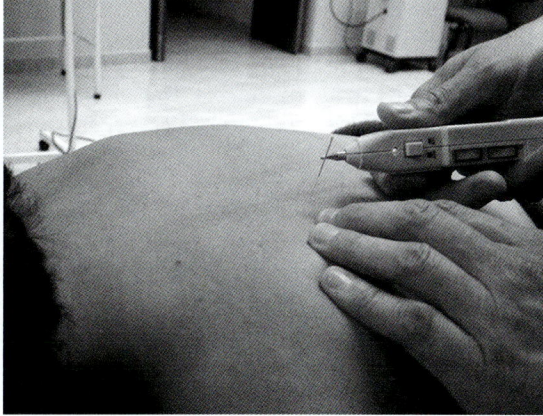

FIGURE 16.12 ■ Evaluation and treatment of the different segmental levels or *huao jiaji* points Ex-B2 or 'paravertebral' points for pathology of the upper limbs and *Zhang-Fu* theory. (Colour version of figure is available online).

nerve root for treatment of a distal pathology. Over these levels, peripheral sensitization techniques can be used (e.g. the skin-rolling technique) while searching for the stimulus at the level of the metamere, the hyperalgic zones and areas with allodynia. This is where the desensitizing treatment can be performed with monopolar EA, reducing the level of nociceptive activity of the cells on the dorsal horn of the spinal cord.

As a clinical example, monopolar EA can be used to locate points along the gall bladder meridian (found at a distance around the ear) and along the triple heater meridian (at two distances). The points to be stimulated would be those that came out positive in diagnostic tests for hearing disorders, tinnitus and lateral headaches.

16.3.6 Acupuncture in peripheral paralysis

Treatment with EA is commonly used in cases of alterations of the peripheral nerves, such as facial paralysis, paralysis of the radial nerve, paralysis of the common peroneal nerve, sensorimotor disorders, dysaesthesias and hypoaesthesias.

It is important always to rely on a medical diagnosis together with the corresponding medical treatment and, better still, to have access to complementary follow-up tests (i.e. neurophysiological studies such as electromyography).

16.3.6.1 Electroacupuncture in peripheral paralysis

- The effects of EA in peripheral paralysis are improvement of speed of neuromuscular conductivity, increase in number of

muscle fibres and increase in muscle, nerve and blood capacity.
- EA acts upon the motor points of the muscle (stimulation) and produces muscle contractions. This stimulus can be directed towards the nerve terminals using TENS-type impulses.
- Strong stimulations tend to sedate, whereas light stimulations tend to excite. It is important to consider that tonification will mainly occur with low frequencies and interrupted pulses.
- Ideally, the muscle group being worked on should be isolated. In order to achieve this successfully, the correct selection of points is important, with regard to the insertion and treatment areas, as this will avoid the phenomenon of aberrant innervations (in cases of facial paralysis).
- EA is applied in the affected meridians with the aforementioned parameters (interrupted waves, low frequencies and low intensity for at most 20 minutes).
- In more chronic stages, stimulation can be applied (as this is an insufficiency and/or state of emptiness) and, in the case of acute and more recent pathologies, sedation may be preferable (as it is a state of excess-plenitude or *yang*-type pain).
- It is important to select the most conflicting points, as well as always to consider the special-effect points.

16.3.6.2 Bell's palsy

Concept. According to the Yale[36] Medical Group, Bell's palsy or facial paralysis is defined as an episode of weakness or paralysis of the facial muscles with no known explanation, and which begins suddenly and tends to worsen considerably within 3–5 days.

This situation results from an injury of the seventh cranial pair of nerves (facial nerve). Usually the pain or discomfort occurs on one side of the face or the head, affecting the muscles innervated by the facial nerve. The facial nerve supplies motor fibres to muscles responsible for expression, lips, nose, cheeks, eyelids and forehead (the frontal region, the cheek and the perioral area are the most commonly affected areas).

This illness progresses with hemifacial weakness, rigidity and inability to frown, lift the eyebrows, move the mouth or blow. Also, tear production, disappearance of expression lines, retroauricular or facial pain, loss of taste in the anterior two-thirds of the tongue, hypoacusia and even some cases of hyperacusia can be found.

The so-called Bell's phenomenon, commonly observed, is characterized by the paralysed eye being displaced upwards when the patient attempts to close the eyelids.

According to TCM, Bell's palsy is thought to be an injury caused by the wind. In TCM, the wind is a perverse climatic factor that attacks the meridians of the craniofacial system and the upper parts of the body, producing damage due to obstruction of the *Qi* and the blood, which affects the collateral meridians. It appears suddenly and with variable or erratic symptoms and is usually associated with other perverse climatic factors that attack the superficial defence system, such as the cold and humidity.[31]

Methodology. The main acupuncture points used for the treatment of Bell's palsy are:
- Local points: ST2, ST3, ST4, ST6, ST7, SI18, LI20, BL2, TB23, *yu-yao* (Ex-HN-4), *yin-tang* (Ex-HN-3) and *tai-yang* (Ex-HN-5). Clearly, not all these points should be selected during the same session as that would be excessive; rather, they must be alternated throughout successive treatment sessions. It is important to differentiate the meridian and the most affected region of the face – the eye, the nose, the mouth – with the purpose of selecting the most involved meridian (this is usually the stomach, which passes along the anterior region of the face) in order to begin treatment. Consider that 'where the meridian reaches, the treatment reaches':
  - ST2 and ST3 (the infraorbital foramen and the border of nasolabial groove)
  - BL2 (the beginning of the eyebrow, action of lifting the eyebrow)
  - SI18 (trigeminal), ST8 (superior branches of the temporal muscle)
  - GB8 and GB14 (action on the eye and the ear)
  - TB21, SI19, GB2 (outer-ear trumpet, extraosseous portion of the facial nerve)
  - DU24 or DU20: points for ending the session
- Extraordinary points: these reinforce the action of the main points and have a local effect: *Inn-tang, shao-yang, yu-yao*.

All these described points can be subjected to light EA of tolerable intensity.

The recommended duration is 15–20 minutes and an exhaustive knowledge of the location of the points and the facial anatomy is necessary, as well as considerable dexterity and skill.

In EA treatment, the main points to be considered are ST4 and ST6. The puncture method consists of puncturing ST4 subcutaneously in the direction of ST6, and vice versa, for the treatment of the mouth and nose. These points are reinforced with ST7 (which corresponds with the exit of the facial nerve and the lateral pterygoid muscle). In the case of a greater denervation or paralysis, longer needles may be introduced (ideally 1.5 inch or 40 mm).
- Points for commencing treatment:
  - If the most involved meridian is the stomach (*yang-ming* of the leg), which circulates along the anterior head and neck region, the treatment can be initiated with a distal point of the stomach, ST44, ST43, ST42, ST41 (choose any of these), as they are used empirically due to correspondence with the five elements: *jing*-well point, *ying*-spring point, *shu*-stream point and the *yuan*-source point (from the five elements of nature: metal, water, wood, fire and earth). The most used command point of all is ST44 (*ying*-spring point of the stomach, which corresponds with the water element in the theory of the five elements), used for treatment of feverish illnesses or those that course with wind-heat in the head, plus for treatment of the musculoskeletal system.
  - Use the LI4 opening point (bilaterally and for tonification), seeing as it is a point of special action for the head and the face, as well as one of the circulating meridians (ending in the nasolabial sulcus of the opposite side).
  - If the most affected region is the lateral part or *shao yang* of the head and the face, we would begin with distal points from both *shao yang* meridians (triple burner

and gall bladder); for example, GB41, GB42, GB43 or TB2, TB3.
- Other points:
  - GB20 is the point to remove the wind from the head and the face.
  - Other points of special action: on the bones, tendons, medulla, blood, energy, and as support points for the local points and the circulating meridian (BL11, GB34, GB39, BL17, SP10, ST36, REN17).[31,32]

16.3.6.3 Radial nerve palsy

Concept. Paralysis of the radial nerve is a common peripheral paralysis seen in the therapist's daily clinical practice, and produces sensorimotor problems in the muscles supplied along the pathway of the radial nerve. In its pathological state it produces functional incapacity for wrist and finger extension, and a clinical picture of wrist drop.

Methodology. To start treatment, it is advisable to begin at the initiation points selected by the professional, and continue with manual acupuncture along the following meridians and surrounding points:
- the large intestine due to its parallelism with the radial nerve: LI2, LI3, LI4, LI6, LI10, LI11, LI12
- the triple burner due to its pathway with collaterals dependent on the radial nerve: TB4, TB5, TB6, TB10.

16.3.6.4 Paralysis of the common peroneal nerve

Concept. Paralysis of the common peroneal nerve is another common peripheral paralysis seen in the therapist's daily clinical practice. It produces sensorimotor problems in the muscles depending on the pathway of the nerve and causes considerable functional inability as regards gait, as well as affecting the muscles responsible for dorsiflexion and eversion of the ankle (tibialis anterior, extensor hallucis longus, extensor digitorum and peroneus brevis and longus muscles).

Methodology. With this technique, treatment begins with the so-called initiation points (as chosen by the professional), and continues with manual acupuncture in the following meridians and surrounding points:
- the stomach: ST36, ST37, ST38, ST39, ST40, ST41, ST42, etc. (as seen in chapter 15, these points are dependent on the common peroneal nerve)

- the gall bladder: for treatment of the branches of the common peroneal nerve (such as the superficial peroneal nerve): GB34, GB37, GB38, GB39.

KEY POINTS

It has been demonstrated that EA is very useful for this pathology, especially if it is used at a low frequency with weak and brief stimulation, and with intermittent electrical waves for 20 minutes. Shorter rest periods are used in relation to manual acupuncture.

16.3.7 Other electroacupuncture modalities: microcurrents or MENS

16.3.7.1 Concepts and characteristics

MCRs or microcurrent electrical neuromuscular stimulator (MENS) are based on the application of EA at very low intensities (µA), at a subsensory level (the patient hardly perceives the passing of the current).

In general, the maximum intensity (depending on the make) is around 2 or 3 mA.

When treatment is applied with MCR percutaneously, the patient hardly perceives the passing of the current or has very little sensation of it. However, in the application of MCR combined with EA, the patient perceives the passing of electricity below the acupuncture needles very clearly (figure 16.13).

This method of applying EA stimulates cell growth, produces an increased cellular energy metabolism (adenosine triphosphate) of up to 500% and can introduce transporter amino acids in the synthesis of proteins, which, in turn, produces important results for healing and regenerating purposes. Treatment with MCR produces energy in the same scale as that which the body produces at the cell level. For this reason, it is said that treatment with MCR provides a physiological contribution at the cellular level.[33,34]

In the event of a traumatic mechanism, tissue damage takes place, with involvement of the electric potentials (voltage). In the lesional area, a greater electrical potential is found compared to that of the surrounding tissues.[35] As a result, this decreases electrical conductivity and cellular capacitance, and subsequently impedes progression of the repair mechanisms.

16.3.7.2 Methodology

The use of EA with MCR is similar to that used in the anterior sections of EA with TENS.

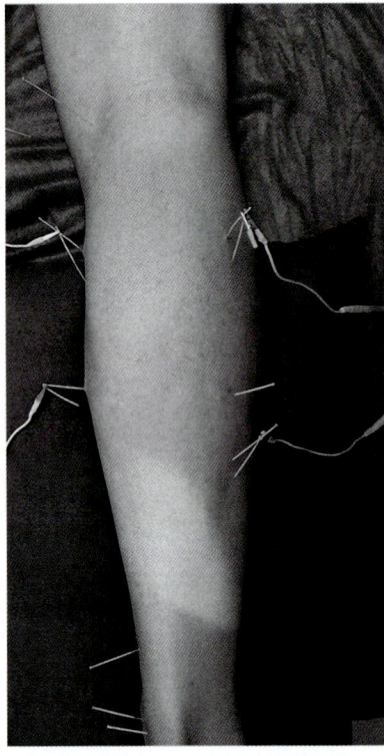

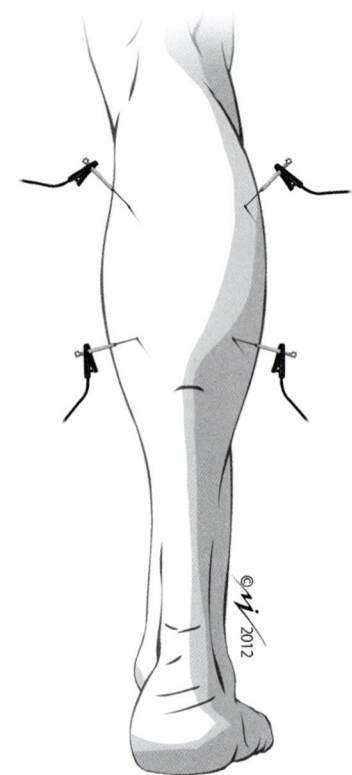

FIGURE 16.13 ■ Application of microcurrents in a patient with a gastrocnemius muscle injury. (Colour version of figure is available online).

This form of EA is used to stimulate the acupuncture points or for use in local zones where one wishes to achieve an extraordinary energetic input, as well as producing the general effects described: anti-inflammatory, antioedema, muscle relaxant, accelerator of the repair process of wounds and scars and improvement of joint range.

Regarding the particular characteristics of this special type of EA, it offers a series of advantages, effects, indications, contraindications and special precautions with regard to conventional EA with TENS:

- Advantages:
  - greater safety (dosed in µA)
  - comfort (the sensations it produces are less unpleasant for the patient, as they are subsensory)
  - decreased acute and chronic pain (clinically, this method is extensively used for the treatment of painful illnesses and in acupuncture anaesthesia)
  - rapid recovery of the tissues and improvement of wounds, scars and even bony lesions
  - production of collagen tissue fibres, improving tissue elasticity
  - allows for application in more delicate regions, such as the face, the inferior *jiao*

(low abdomen) and in craniopuncture, in the following pathologies:
  eye: neuralgia, conjunctivitis, tics, tear production
  ear: tinnitus, hypoacusia
  temporomandibular joint: trismus, contracture of the muscles of mastication, dental pain
  nose: rhinitis, anosmia, sinusitis
  head: headaches, migraines, vertigo
  - other pathologies: entrapment syndromes (carpal tunnel, tarsal tunnel, ulnar neuropathies) tendinopathies, oedema, fractures
  - almost total absence of side effects and complications.
- Effects:
  - reduction of pain
  - increase in the repair index of the tissue and the wounds
  - increased protein synthesis
  - stimulation of regeneration of the damaged fine tissue
  - stimulation of the autonomic nervous system: used for the treatment of insomnia
  - stimulation of the lymphatic flow
  - inhibition of MTrPs.
- Indications:
  - treatment of trigger points within myofascial pain syndromes and fibromyalgia

- treatment of the nerves (neuralgias and neuropathies)
- regeneration of contractile tissues
- liberation of adherences and retractile scars
- tendinopathies and enthesopathies, joint impingement, fasciitis/fasciosis, periostitis, postsprain residual pain, luxation
- muscular atrophy: stimulates the metabolic processes of the muscle and motor end-plate
- aesthetic treatments: increases microcirculation; the production of collagen has a lymph-draining effect and strengthens the skin and the connective tissue
- other pathologies: epilepsy, flaccid syndrome, neurasthenia, hypertension, insomnia.
- Contraindications:
  - pregnancy
  - cardiac pacemakers
  - alterations of cardiac rhythm
  - direct application over the eyes, viscera, plexus
  - tumours
  - haemophilia.
- Precautions:
  - In patients with a weak physical constitution or nervousness, an excessive intensity of current is not advisable as it can cause fainting.
  - In the case of a vasovagal response, cardiovascular depression, hypotension, loss of consciousness, vomiting, the needles are withdrawn, the patient is positioned in a stable position and the so-called resuscitation points are stimulated, in order to restore the *yang*. An effective technique is to stimulate with a slight pinch on the DU25 and DU26 points or on any of the *Jing*-well points (this is a commonly used method in China).

16.4 CLINICAL CASE

16.4.1 Cervical spine and craniocervical symptoms

The patient is a 34-year-old business owner who sells electrical supplies, and also works on a sports team. She spends a lot of time travelling by plane with the team due to her work.

Personal background and reason for consultation: she has suffered from a number of previous pathologies related to cervicalgia (pain in the cervical spine and in the muscles of the shoulder girdle), and has received many previous treatments directed at alleviating the symptoms experienced in these areas.

She suffers from episodes of irradiated pain along the right upper limb, as well as from dizziness, vertigo, loss of balance, tinnitus and other related craniocervical symptoms. She has consulted an ear, nose and throat specialist as well as a neurologist and both have told her that she has a lesion due to a structural alteration affecting the bones of the inner ear, which have suffered from an early deterioration process.

Medical treatment: sulpiride (Dogmatil®), antihistamines (Ebastel®).

Physiotherapy: treatment of the cervical spine and vestibular physiotherapy programme.

16.4.2 Acupuncture

Physical exam: pain on palpation of the muscles of the shoulder girdle and the suboccipital muscles. Rigidity of the cervical spine; cervical rotation produces and increases craniocervical symptoms. Dysaesthesia and pain in the C6–C7 territory. The myotomes of the right biceps brachii and triceps brachii muscles show alterations. Positive sclerotome in segments C6 and C7.

X-ray findings: cervical osteoarthrosis.

She receives physical therapy and acupuncture treatments once a week.

(*Clinical case continued on page 492*)

16.5 REFERENCES

1. WHO. Acupuncture: review and analysis of reports on controlled clinical trials. Geneva: WHO; 2003.
2. Kerr FW, Wilson PR, Nijensohn DE. Acupuncture reduces the trigeminal evoked response. Exp Neurol 1978;61:84–95.
3. Mayor D. Scientific and clinical foundations. Edinburgh: Elsevier; 2007. p. 3333.
4. Maya Martín J, Albornoz Cabello M. Estimulación eléctrica y transcutánea neuromuscular. Barcelona: Elsevier; 2010.
5. Watson T. Electroterapia: Práctica basada en la evidencia. Barcelona: Elsevier; 2009.
6. Cheng RS, Pomeranz B. Electroacupuncture analgesia could be mediated by at least two pain-relieving mechanisms: endorphin and non-endorphin systems. Life Sci 1979;25:1957–62.
7. Sluka KA, Walsh D. Transcutaneous electrical nerve stimulation: basic science mechanisms and clinical effectiveness. J Pain 2003;4:109–21.
8. Low J, Reed A. Electrotherapy explained: principles and practice. 2nd ed. London: Butterworth-Heinemann; 1994.
9. Savage B. Practical electrotherapy for physiotherapists. London: Faber & Faber; 1960.

10. Eriksson M, Sjölund B. Acupuncture-like electroanalgesia in TNS resistant chronic pain. In: Zotterman Y, editor. Sensory functions of the skin. Oxford/New York: Pergamon; 1976.

11. Baldry P. Acupuncture, trigger points and musculoskeletal pain. 3rd ed. London: Elsevier; 2005.

12. Embrid A. Enciclopedia de Medicina China. Madrid: Ed. Medicinas complementarias; 1998.

13. Sussman DJ. Acupuntura Teoría y Práctica. Buenos Aires: Ed. Kier; 2007.

14. Chao AS, Chao A, Wang TH, et al. Pain relief by applying transcutaneous electrical nerve stimulation (TENS) on acupuncture points during the first stage of labor: a randomized double-blind placebo-controlled trial. Pain 2007;127:214–20.

15. Mayor DF. Electroacupuncture: a practical manual and resource. London: Churchill Livingstone Elsevier; 2007.

16. Yun-Tao M. Biomedical acupuncture for sports and trauma rehabilitation. Dry needling techniques. London: Churchill Livingstone, Elsevier; 2011.

17. Yun-tao M, Mila M, Zang Hee CH. Biomedical acupuncture for pain management. London: Elsevier; 2011.

18. Filshie J, White A. Medical acupuncture: a western scientific approach. Edinburgh: Churchill Livingstone; 1998.

19. Thambirajah R. Acupuntura energética. Madrid: Elsevier; 2008.

20. Thambirajah R. Acupuntura cosmética. Tratamiento de los trastornos y las patologías de la piel. Madrid: Elsevier; 2008.

21. Mayor DF. Electroacupuntura para la ciática. Un recorrido por la literatura a través de la base de datos de estudios clínicos disponible en www.electroacupunctureknowledge.com. Rev Int Acupuntura 2009;03:72–7.

22. Lundeberg T. Electrical stimulation techniques. Lancet 1996;348:1672–3.

23. Eriksson MB, Sjölund BH, Nielzén S. Long term results of peripheral conditioning stimulation as an analgesic measure in chronic pain. Pain 1979;6:335–47.

24. Sjölund BH. Peripheral nerve stimulation suppression of C-fiber-evoked flexion reflex in rats. Part 1: parameters of continuous stimulation. J Neurosurg 1985;63: 612–16.

25. Melzack R, Wall PD. Acupuncture and transcutaneous electrical nerve stimulation. Postgrad Med J 1984;60: 893–6.

26. Omura Y. Basic electrical parameters for safe and effective electro-therapeutics [electro-acupuncture, TES, TENMS (or TEMS), TENS and electro-magnetic field stimulation with or without drug field] for pain, neuromuscular skeletal problems, and circulatory disturbances. Acupunct Electrother Res 1987;12:201–25.

27. Villaverde JR. Los puntos ah-shi. Tratamiento de los síndromes dolorosos del aparato locomotor mediante los puntos ah-shi. Madrid: Ed. Las Cuatro Fuentes; 1996.

28. Dreadman P, Al-Khafagi M. A manual of acupuncture. London: Journal of Chinese Medicine Publications; 2007.

29. Chang-ging G, Bo H, Nai-gang L. Anatomical illustration of acupuncture points. Beijing: People's medical publishing house; 2008.

30. Chunsheng L. Modern Obesity [M]. Beijing: Science, Literature and Technology Publishing House; 2004.

31. Maciocia G. The Foundations of Chinese Medicine. 2nd ed. London: Aeneid-Press Elsevier; 2005.

32. Wang SM, Kain ZN, White PF. Acupuncture analgesia: II. Clinical considerations. Anesth Analg 2008;106(2): 611–21.

33. Mercola JM, Kirsch ML. The basis of microcurrent electrical therapy in conventional medical practice. J Adv Med 1995;8:107–20.

34. Smith RB. Microcurrent therapies. Emerging theories of physiological information processing. Neurorehabilitation 2002;17:3–7.

35. Pearson S, Colbert AP, McNames J, et al. Electrical skin impedance at acupuncture points. J Altern Complement Med 2007;13:409–18.

36. Yale Medical Group (YMG). Available at: <http://yalemedicalgroup.org/info/health.aspx?ContentTypeId=85&ContentId=P00774>; [Accessed 20 July 2014].

PART **VIII**

MESOTHERAPY

MESOTHERAPY IN THE MUSCULOSKELETAL SYSTEM

Juan Ruiz Alconero

The physician's high and only mission is to restore the sick to health, to cure, as it is termed.
SAMUEL HAHNEMANN

CHAPTER OUTLINE

KEYWORDS

mesotherapy; dermis; homeopathy; homotoxicology; platelet-rich plasma; growth factors; allopathy; non-steroidal anti-inflammatory drugs (NSAIDs); fibroblasts; collagen; angiogenesis; wound.

17.1 INTRODUCTION

Mesotherapy is the introduction of therapeutic substances into the dermis. This structure (the dermis), as will be subsequently discussed, has certain pharmacokinetic and pharmacodynamic qualities that differentiate it from other routes of administration, such as intramuscular, intravenous or oral.[1] It is important to bear in mind the above definition as, unfortunately, due to the use of mesotherapy for cosmetic medicine, this name has been used to associate it together with other techniques that have nothing to do with the principles of this therapeutic technique, such as electroporation, virtual mesotherapy (via the opening of ionic channels in the epidermis), or even, in a much more misleading and deceptive manner, 'oral mesotherapy'.

KEY POINTS

Mesotherapy is the introduction (injection) of therapeutic substances into the dermis.

17.1.1 Brief historical overview

Although mesotherapy was developed in 1952 by the rural French doctor M. Pistor, since the beginning of humanity there has always been an interest in introducing medicine to the interior of the body. Examples are acupuncture and the application of punctures and lesions with plant thorns and insect bites as well as the use of scarification, to break up the skin layer and be able to apply medicine to injuries.

However, it was not until the medical advances of the nineteenth century (sadly due to the great number of wars that occurred during this period) that the need for rapid mechanisms for pain relief emerged. This is how, in 1841, Pravaz and Wood almost simultaneously developed the modern syringe and hypodermic needle; later on Rynd began the administration of subcutaneous morphine to treat chronic pain.

Once these tools were made available, the search was centred on finding the correct medication. The American civil war and the Franco-Prussian war left a great number of morphine addicts. Cocaine was demonstrated to have a great number of toxins and heroin (the word is the feminine of hero, as it was going to be the 'heroine' in the battle against pain), demonstrated addiction habits that were even greater than those produced by morphine.

This situation was resolved with the discovery of procaine by Eihnor in 1905, as it had superior analgesic effects and fewer toxins. Procaine (known as novocaine in the USA) began to be systemically used within the medical field as an anaesthetic and bronchodilator.

In a French rural village, a humble doctor, Dr Pistor, made a haphazard discovery. A shoemaker with asthma consulted him and, typical of that time, Pistor treated him with procaine injections. A few days later, in consultation, the patient commented that, although the asthma was the same, he had begun to hear the bells of the village church, which is something that had not happened in a long time due to his deafness, although the improvement to his hearing acuteness had gradually faded since the time of the injection. Pistor, seeing that the only thing that had changed in the treatment of his patient was the application of procaine injections, began to inject around the ear area with surprising results, and thereafter he gradually began to apply it in all fields of practice. This was the birth of mesotherapy (1958), based on two fundamental pillars: the injection site and the amount of product to be administered ('a little, a few times, and in the right place').

17.2 OBJECTIVES OF MESOTHERAPY

Mesotherapy is useful in multiple areas of health. It is a technique that can be added to our therapeutic arsenal as it offers a certain flexibility in the planning of a therapeutic programme, whatever our speciality. Mesotherapy has these main aims:

- stimulation of natural healing
- regulation of inflammatory processes
- regeneration of damaged tissue
- stimulation of blood circulation
- regulation of neural reflexes
- stimulation of the endocrine-immunological pathways
- stimulation of detoxification mechanisms.

Over the years, several models have been developed that attempt to explain how this technique works. The first were mere hypotheses that were totally empirical. Currently, however, with the

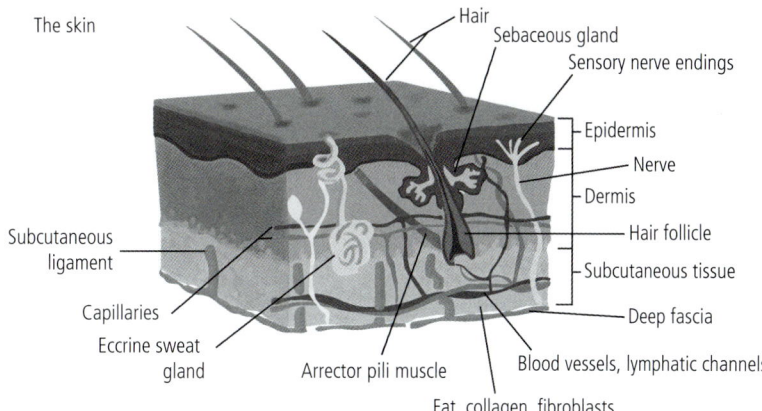

FIGURE 17.1 ■ Structure of the skin. (Colour version of figure is available online).

advent of new discoveries regarding the structure and physiology of the dermis, it is possible to develop new theories, coming to the one which today better explains the functioning of this therapy: the so-called revisionist theory.

17.3 STRUCTURE OF THE SKIN

It is necessary to make an indepth study of the mesotherapy site of application before explaining the mechanisms of action, seeing as, in contrast to other techniques, application within the correct anatomical structure is as important as the medication used. This type of treatment is site-dependent.

The skin is divided into three main structures[2,3] (figure 17.1):

1. The epidermis: this is an epithelial structure formed of cells and which, therefore, is nourished by the dermis. Some of these cells are epithelial themselves, such as keratinocytes. Others are of a neuroectodermal and mesenchymal origin, which is why, in some cases, the epidermis can be a site for mesotherapy application.
2. The hypodermis: this structure contains the cutaneous annexes, namely the sweat glands and the hair follicles.
3. The dermis: this is the application site of mesotherapy.[4] It has a width that varies between 1 and 9 mm, and it is made up of connective tissue and a series of vessels and nerves that cross this layer, together with the resident population of immunological cells. This creates a perfect site for stimulating the nervous, vascular and immunoendocrine networks.

As far as mesotherapy is concerned, there are two main components in the dermis: vascular and cellular.

KEY POINTS

The dermis is the site of mesotherapy application.

17.3.1 Cellular composition of the dermis

The cellular composition of the dermis is as follows:

- the immune system: Langerhans cells, macrophages and receptors for neuromediators and neurotrophics (interleukin-6, nerve growth factor, fibroblast growth factor-beta, substance P, calcitonin gene-related peptide)
- the nervous system: Merkel cells, in connection with the neurons that go through the dermis, and which transmit the information via neuromediators
- the endocrine system: in the dermis paracrine signalling (local cell with local cell) takes place between the nerve cells and the immune cells – this is very rare in the rest of the body.

17.3.2 Microcirculation of the dermis

Within the dermis[5], there are three types of circulation:

1. blood microcirculation
2. lymphatic microcirculation
3. interstitial microcirculation.

Microcirculation of the dermis is distributed in five differentiated compartments:

1. arterial: responsible for blood distribution depending on pH
2. venous: evacuation of excess CO_2

3. capillary: blood diffusion mechanisms
4. lymphatic: drainage system
5. interstitial: collagen localization, fibroblasts and haematic cells.

The interstitial circulation and its compartment are the site of action of mesotherapy, as, although in the past this was thought to be a static area, it is now known that the interstitial compartment presents two phases, sol and gel, and that it passes from one phase to the other according to pH, circadian rhythm, stress and manual manipulation.

Interstitial circulation is essential for two important factors:

1. This is the union between the blood circulation and the local cellular population. It separates the cellular membrane from the capillary endothelia.
2. It has a buffering and regulating effect.

17.4 MECHANISM OF ACTION

The mechanism of action is shown in figure 17.2.

17.4.1 First theories

The first theories about how mesotherapy works were slaves of their time; in other words, they reduced the explanation to what was known at the time, usually with simple empirical processes, and without scientific evidence supporting these theories.

Naturally, the first theory was proposed by Pistor, who tried to provide an explanation using nervous stimulation, arguing that the treatment effect provoked a reflex effect that interrupted the visceral–medullar–cerebral pathway, provoking a temporary medullar shock in the lateromedullary sympathetic centre.[6,7] Shortly after, based on the Melzack and Wall's gate-control theory, it was possible to explain the analgesic and profound effect that local stimulation has on nervous pathways.[8]

However, Bicheron[9] found that the neurological explanation in itself was not enough and, on realizing that all pathologies produce microcirculatory vascular suffering, he discovered that the locoregional action of the medication produced above all local stimulation of this microcirculation.

Thanks to the electronic microscope and the use of radiotracers, both the theory of the three units by Dalloz-Bourguinon[10] and the unified theory of Kaplan[11,12] led to consideration of neurological and immune receptors, besides vascular receptors, as the following three structures are found in the dermis:

• dermal terminals of the capillary loops
• afferent neurons
• immunohaematogenic cells, such as plasma cells and mast cells.

Kaplan went further and was able to observe that the action of mesotherapy produces three different types of pharmacokinetics in the dermis: a localized short-range action, another long-range action and a mixed action.

17.4.2 Ordiz's[13] revisionist or integrated theory

Three main agents responsible for the effects of mesotherapy can be distinguished: the immune, nervous and endocrine systems.

Each one is responsible for the treatment response that we encounter:

1. an immediate, rapid and unspecific action triggered by the needle pricks themselves, stimulating the neuro-immunoendocrine pathway both mechanically and locally
2. a sustained action, mediated by T and B lymphocytes, with an immunoinflammatory character
3. a local action of the medication itself.

This mechanism, that integrates the immune, vascular and neuroendocrine systems, is what makes the pharmacokinetic behaviour of the intradermal pathway so special, and explains the positive effects.

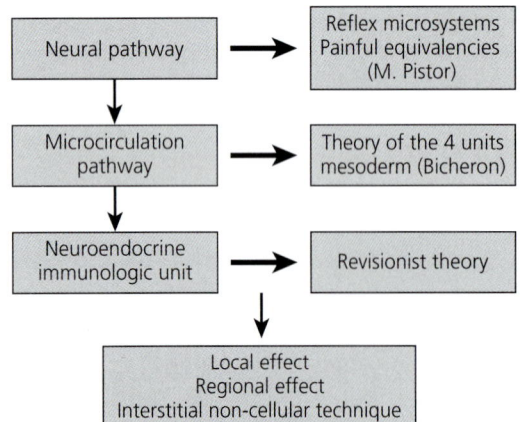

FIGURE 17.2 ■ Evolution of models regarding the mechanism of action of mesotherapy.

KEY POINTS

Mesotherapy is not a therapy that acts upon the cell level in the same way as traditional medication, but rather it acts upon the interstitial level.

17.4.3 Growth factors

Growth factors have gained a great deal of importance in recent years due to their regenerative and healing capacity in all fields of medicine and physiotherapy.[14] Their activation within the frame of mesotherapy can be key to understanding complex intercellular communication systems and the relation between the local effects of therapy, which do not have anything to do with medication *per se*, but rather with local cellular stimulation (box 17.1).

These are a group of molecules with a protein origin and the capacity to exercise external control over the cell cycle. They act by joining with specific receptors and in very reduced quantities. They have a local action and are produced by a large number of cells, such as fibroblasts, osteoblasts, endothelial cells, macrophages and monocytes.

It is the capacity of stimulation of the cell cycle that makes these essential in repair processes, such as the proliferation of fibroblasts and keratinocytes, the angiogenesis phenomenon, the remodelling of the extracellular matrix and debridement and elimination of the injured tissue.[15]

Furthermore, as will be explained, this capacity for modification can be used as a therapy in itself and not only as a theoretical basis for mesotherapy functioning. Growth factors can be easily extracted and isolated during ambulatory consultation and can be applied via mesotherapy or intralesional administration methods, thus increasing their concentration in injured areas up to four times with regard to the basal concentration.[16]

BOX 17.1 Growth factors in the different stages of wound repair

- Antimicrobial activity: nitric acid, reactive oxygen species
- Chemotaxis and proliferation of fibroblasts and keratinocytes: platelet-derived growth factor (PDGF); transforming growth factor-beta (TGF-β); interleukin-1 (IL-1); recombinant human growth factor (KGF-7)
- Angiogenesis: vascular endothelial growth factor (VEGF); fibroblast growth factor (FGF-2); PDGF
- Remodelling of the extracellular matrix: PDGF; TGF-β; tumour necrosis factor (TNF); osteopontin (OPN); IL-1; collagenase; matrix metalloproteinases (MMPs)

Adapted from Kuma et al.[53]

17.4.4 'Virtual' mesotherapy or electroporation

As previously explained, mesotherapy is the introduction of substances into the dermal layer. Until now this had only been performed using inoculation with needles. Given that many people are scared of needles, there has always been the need to find a way of introducing medication without causing discomfort and pain such as that which occurs with punctures. In 2003, Agre and MacKinnon received the Nobel prize, after discovering hydropores – a series of channels within transmembrane proteins that could communicate with the dermis without the need for puncture.[17] With the generation of a simple transmembrane potential of 0.5–1.5 V, these pores could be opened, allowing for the passage of substances.[18,19]

The problem has always been the size of the molecules (as there are molecules that are much larger than the diameter of the pores) and their erratic passage to the dermal plane.[20]

However, most importantly, electroporation only consists of the administration of substances without the capacity for stimulation of the mesotherapy technique.[4]

Therefore, it is erroneous to describe electroporation as a form of mesotherapy as, although it is a useful technique in many cases, it does not have the effects or mechanisms of action previously described.

17.5 MATERIALS

Many physiotherapists may not be altogether familiar with the characteristics of the needles and syringes available on the market. For those interested in the field of invasive physiotherapy this is considered essential knowledge.

17.5.1 Syringes

Although syringes of 10 mL and 5 mL can be used in mesotherapy, for physiotherapy purposes, and due to the smaller quantities of medication used, 5 mL is sufficient. There are even smaller sizes available, 2 mL and 3 mL, but these require a play of pressures and considerable dexterity and, in the author's opinion, a 5 mL syringe is better.

Syringes with two and three bodies are available. Ideally, three bodies should be used, as these give a greater control of the medication contained.

17.5.2 Needles

A great variety of needles are available and, for this reason, it is important to consider two factors:

1. The calibre: this is the diameter of the needles and is measured with a number followed by the letter 'G' (gauge). The greater the number associated with 'G', the smaller the needle diameter. Therefore, a 30G needle is smaller than a 27G one. These diameters are coded with a single colour; therefore the calibre can also be identified just by recognizing the colour.
2. The length: this is measured in either inches or millimetres.

In mesotherapy, needles of 27G and 32G are used, with the classic needle being 30G. Regarding length, there are specific mesotherapy needles that are actually very short, 4 mm, whereas generic 30G needles measure 12 mm. Although these generic 30G needles require a greater control of needle insertion depth by the professional, they are more versatile in seeking the appropriate depths.

Remember that a much thicker needle is needed to extract medication from the vials. The extraction of medication with a 27G or 30G needle is almost impossible, as the needle diameter is so small that only minimal flow is able to pass through it. For this reason, it is necessary to have a thicker needle available, 18G or 19G. Given that this is a needle that is clearly visible, it is important to explain to the patient that the needle is only going to be used to import the liquid or perform an aspiration out of the patient's sight.

It is essential to be familiar with the different types of needles and syringes, as what can be useful for one professional may be a worse choice for another, and this also depends on the size of the operator's hand and its steadiness. The author has always used 12 mm 30G needles, but it is important to know how to use and control the pressures and depths of each type of needle.

KEY POINTS

In mesotherapy needles of between 27G and 32G are used, with 30G being the classic size.

17.5.3 Mesotherapy guns

After a stagnant period of research on mesotherapy guns, there has recently been an increase in availability and modernization of the classic systems. This has seen the weight of the mechanism reduced and made more compatible with various syringes, as well as the introduction of pneumatic motors, thus controlling the depth, the repetition of the punctures and the amount of product administered with each injection.

These are useful but expensive systems, which do not offer the versatility that can be achieved by the manual system.

Ordiz offers the following key considerations when selecting the perfect gun[13]:

- The parts in contact with the patient must be disposable.
- The medication must not go through hidden paths.
- The depth of the puncture, dosage and frequency must be calibrated by the professional.
- It must be ergonomic.
- It must be of low economic cost.

Finally, it is important to have gauze and a good antiseptic to hand. Alcohol is not advisable, as it is a vasodilator and may increase the little bleeding experienced, as well as irritate the area. Clorhexidine is more useful, as it does not irritate the nostrils or the application area and it does not soil the skin or clothing. The author does not recommend povidone-iodine, as, due to the multiple punctures that can be made during a session, one can run the minimal, but real, risk of marking these punctures and essentially 'tattooing' them.

Seeing as the main threat is secondary microbial infection of the administration site (as will be discussed later), ideally, one must have the correct antiseptic to hand which will help provide protection from these pathogens. Given that there is no commercial product with these properties, a pharmaceutical preparation is used (box 17.2).

Finally, the room to be used must meet minimal health requirements. It must be well lit and ventilated and the furniture must be disinfected and meet the relevant CE regulations. All the material must be at hand and patients should be positioned so that they can be easily accessed from all angles.

BOX 17.2	Ideal antiseptic preparation for mesotherapy

Benzilic acid 10 mL
Benzalkonium chloride 0.65 g
Chlorhexidine 5 mL
Distilled water q.s. to 500 mL

17.6 CONTRAINDICATIONS AND SIDE EFFECTS

17.6.1 Contraindications

The contraindications depend on the medication to be injected. In general, the absolute contraindications are as follows:

- cancer sufferers undergoing treatment
- patients taking autoimmune treatment
- allergy to one of the products to be used
- ongoing treatment with anticoagulants
- pregnancy.

There are also several relative contraindications depending on the state of the patient at the time of treatment which oblige the therapist to postpone the procedure for a few days. Among these are the need to do exercise immediately after the session (which may cause an increase in haematomas) and unavoidable sun exposure to the treated area (causing postinflammatory hyperpigmentation due to sun exposure).

It is important to consider that mesotherapy is one more tool within the range of techniques available to physiotherapists and, until the legal position of this speciality is resolved, especially regarding the competency of physiotherapists to prescribe medication, in many places around the world it is preferable to choose other therapeutic methods in complicated or ambiguous cases.

17.6.2 Side effects

The side effects of mesotherapy are generally few and minor. If the safety protocols are followed and well-known medication from well-known laboratories is used, this technique can be applied without placing patients in any danger.[21]

Nonetheless, to say that this is a painfree treatment without any consequences would be misleading patients, however mild the reactions may be. As in all invasive treatments, the information provided must be complete and exact.

17.6.2.1 Pain

Obviously, when puncturing patients' skin, they will feel pain, although the extent of this is subjective. It is important never to deny to the patient that there will be pain, but it is appropriate to avoid the word 'pain' itself. It is better to speak of discomfort or a needle prick than of pain, as the term used will very much condition what the patient feels.

Nonetheless, pain is limited to the session, and once the punctures have finished, there should be no discomfort.

Currently, there are topical anaesthetic products (see chapter 2) that can be very useful for patients who are very sensitive to punctures.[22]

17.6.2.2 Erythema

This refers to redness in the injection point. Most frequently this is normal and relatively unimportant, but it is always necessary to perform a differential diagnosis between an allergic reaction and an infection, especially when more than 2 hours have passed.

If the erythema arises quite soon (2 hours or more after the session), most probably it is an allergic reaction. If it appears later on (1 week or more), it is most likely an infection.

There is medication that is more susceptible to producing erythema (vasodilators). Furthermore, people with atopical skin can see a completely normal erythema worsen, although in these cases, without any negative consequences.

17.6.2.3 Haematomas

Haematomas are common and can be caused both by poor technique, as well as by chance. Some people are more predisposed to suffer haematomas than others.

Although per se, haematomas do not entail any problem, it is important to control them, as they can cause both complications and infections.

Ideally, compress the area immediately, and with predisposed people, use homeopathic prevention (arnica 9CH 1 day beforehand in granules).

17.6.2.4 Vagal reactions

Vasovagal reactions (otherwise known as fainting) are frequent in patients who are sensitive and susceptible. They are also encouraged by excessively warm and stuffy treatment rooms.

These reactions usually begin with major sweating and tachycardia. Patients usually experience what is known as a sensation of anticipation, where they realize that they will lose consciousness. Then the patient turns pale and there is a drop in tension, which can lead to the loss of consciousness if nothing is done to prevent it.

Loss of consciousness is usually brief, lasting only a few seconds, and the patient recovers, although may be pale, cold and suffering from tremors. This is not accompanied by relaxation of the sphincter or myoclonus contractions.

Place the patient in a supine position with the legs elevated, or if this is not possible, have the person sitting and leaning forwards and place the head between the knees. The patient should be covered with a light blanket, with the clothing loosened if it is tight and the room should be ventilated. The key is patience, because an attempt to raise the patient too soon can make the vasovagal reaction reappear.

The best way to avoid this is simply to prevent it, by informing the patient of the whole process, avoiding punctures while the patient is standing, having a well-ventilated and calm room, with soothing music and, if possible, ensuring patients have had sufficient sustenance (i.e. have not fasted) at the time of their visit. It is important to be able to recognize the reaction, and anticipate and control the situation without displaying any agitation.

17.6.2.5 Mechanical injuries in nerves or vessels

Although the needles used are very thin, this does not exempt the professional from a perfect knowledge of the regional anatomy of the area to be punctured in order to avoid lacerating neighbouring structures. Do not forget that the side of the needle is sharp and may cut.

17.6.2.6 Postinflammatory hyperpigmentation

In infiltrated regions that are exposed to the sun immediately after treatment, a reactive pigmentation may arise. This is more frequent in tanned people or those with dark skin, and is associated with a poor treatment prognosis. Therefore it is very important to avoid sun exposure in the treated area for at least 48 hours after the session.

17.6.2.7 Skin necrosis

This is the loss of irrigation and finally the death of a section of skin. This is extremely rare and usually occurs in the distal regions where vaso-constrictors are used.

17.6.2.8 Tuberculoid granuloma

This is an inflammatory reaction surrounding the area and depends on the type of medication, the depth of the injection and, often, it just happens by chance.

17.6.2.9 Skin infections

These are probably the most serious complication of mesotherapy, although luckily they are extremely rare.

There are three mechanisms of contamination:

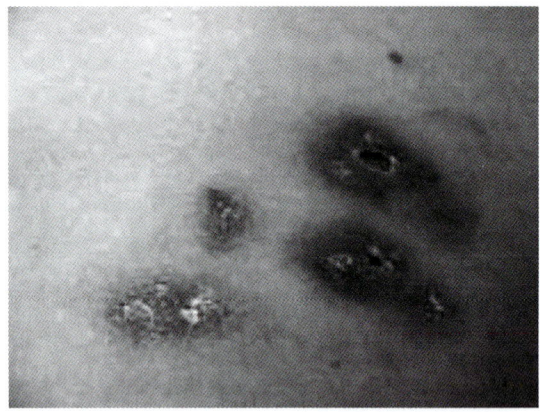

FIGURE 17.3 ■ Wounds caused by a microbial infection after mesotherapy treatment. (Colour version of figure is available online).

1. direct inoculation due to product contamination. Buy medication from laboratories that offer a guarantee and always note down the serial number of the product. Also, one vial must be used per patient and treatment; vials must never be shared or left open for any period of time. Ensure that the vial that is about to be used is permitted for parenteral administration
2. contamination via non-protected punctures
3. contamination via pathogen agents found in the skin.

Skin asepsis and disinfection of the material are essential to avoid infection. Disposable material must be used and written protocols for asepsis and disinfection must be maintained.

Infections due to atypical microbacteria are more frequent and also more serious[23] (figure 17.3). They usually appear due to product contamination and are highly resistant to antiseptics and disinfectants. They have an incubation period of between 3 weeks and 3 months and, therefore, if they appear, it is a long time after the treatment sessions.

Although 20% of these cases resolve spontaneously, they can leave after effects.[24]

The diagnosis is made on biopsy and, as these cases are very resistant to antibiotics, it is necessary to perform an antibiogram in order to select the correct medication, which generally is taken for up to 6 months, in order to treat the problem correctly.[25]

KEY POINTS

The infections caused by atypical mycobacteria are the most frequent, and also cause the most serious possible side effects.

17.6.2.10 Allergic reactions

The most serious is anaphylactic shock, although this is extremely rare. Most commonly allergic reactions are local and rapidly established and are accompanied by hives and wheal (swelling) reactions located at and limited to the injection area.

17.7 THE MESOTHERAPY TECHNIQUE

As in every manual technique, professionals must use what best suits them, considering the size of their hands, their manual dexterity and the size of the material to be used.

Familiarize yourself with the different syringes and try the different guns but, essentially, you must be comfortable and have various support points to control the depth of the puncture and perform the procedure safely.

Regarding the sessions, it is imperative to follow Pistor's principle – 'a little, many times and in the correct site'.

It is also crucial to respect the principle of therapeutic response whereby, in the measure that we have a response, the sessions must be spaced between them. The author does not recommend more than one session per week, as it is important to bear in mind that, apart from the pharmacological effect of the product administered, the local stimulation effect inherent to the technique itself is also sought.

17.7.1 Manual techniques

There are three techniques recognised as orthodox, although professionals will use the one that is best suited to their own hand (figure 17.4).

When injecting, and in relation to depth, the following techniques are described.

17.7.1.1 The epidermal injection

This is very superficial, does not cause bleeding and is applied with the bevel pointing upwards and visible underneath the skin. This stimulates the epidermal receptors and actually has little use except in specific areas (such as the elbow and the bony edges). It is always used in combination with other techniques.[13]

17.7.1.2 Intradermal injection

This is the mesotherapy technique par excellence. This type of injection usually has a depth of 2–4 mm at 45° with respect to the skin surface, leaving little micropapules (elevations) in the skin. It is useful in painful and reflex points and in the insertion points.

KEY POINTS

The intradermal injection is the mesotherapic technique par excellence.

17.7.1.3 Intradermal nappage

This technique consists of multiple repeated injections at 2 mm, which requires extraordinary coordination of the hand movements. It is useful for tracing muscular and tendinous paths, especially when muscle relaxants are used.

17.7.1.4 Intradermal papule

This consists of leaving a great papule, requiring a greater injected volume than usual. It is useful mainly in corporal cosmetic mesotherapy applications, and not very useful in clinical mesotherapy.

17.7.1.5 Coup par coup injection or mesotherapy

This is a deeper injection, 4–10 mm, with an injection of major volumes. It is useful as the antalgic treatment of chronic pain. The application of this technique is also described in acupuncture points.

17.7.1.6 Mesoperfusion

Also known as small mesotherapy, this consists in using intravenous perfusion material and placing it into the dermal route, letting it perfuse slowly upon the area. This technique may be continuous or sequential and has the inconvenience of more easily causing haematomas.

17.8 MEDICATION USED IN MESOTHERAPY

In mesotherapy, both allopathic as well as homeopathic medicine can be used and, therefore, it is important to know the difference between the two.

Allopathy is a therapeutic modality that combats disease by using medication that produces effects in a healthy individual that are different from those produced by the disease to be treated. A clear example of this are the vasodilators used in arterial hypertension which, independently of the cause (whether this is renal, cardiac or unknown) work by decreasing arterial

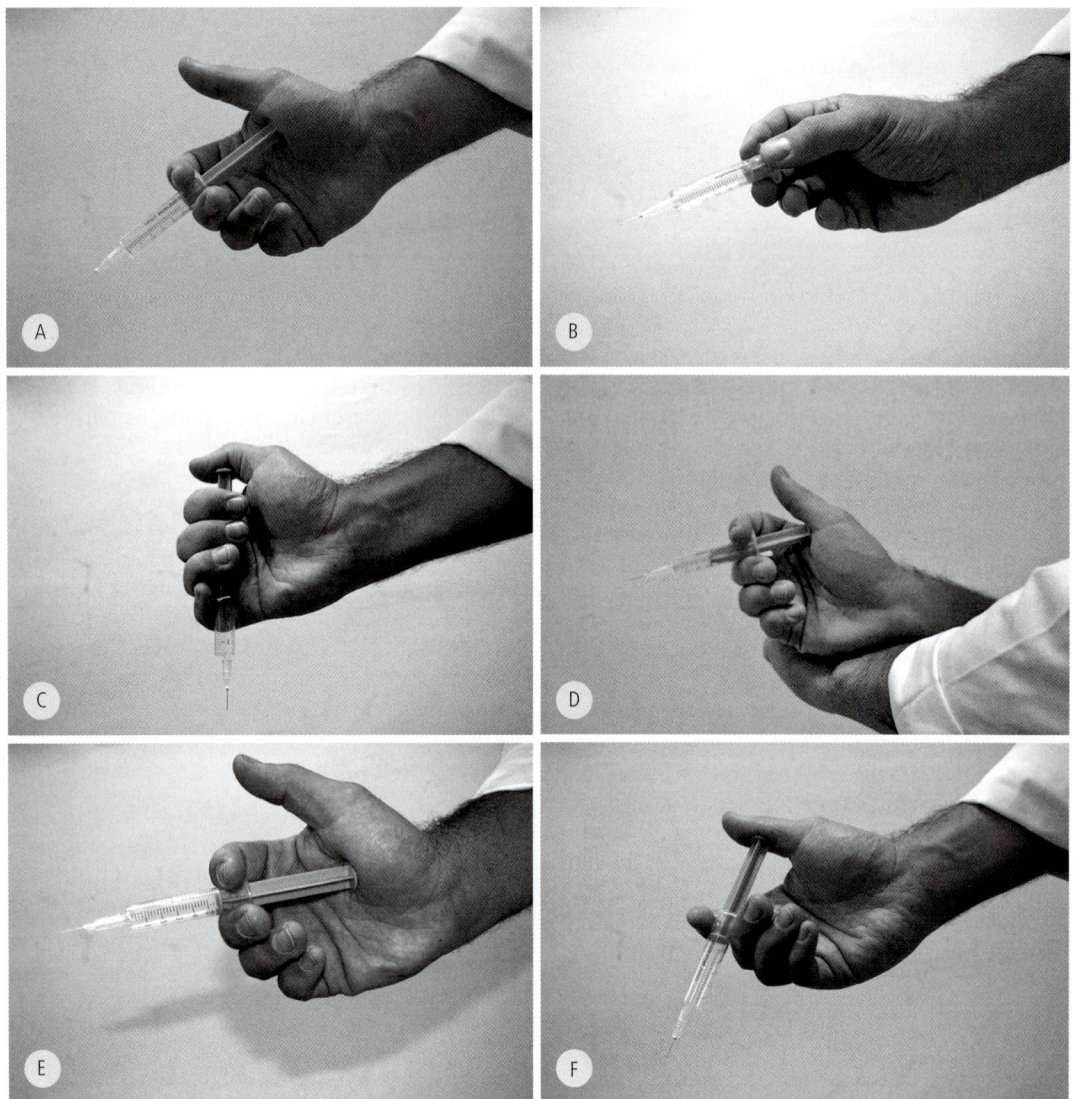

FIGURE 17.4 ■ (A–F) Different manual techniques for mesotherapy. (Colour version of figure is available online).

tension or increasing blood and kidney flow, which has nothing to do with the pathogenic mechanism of the illness. Normally high concentrations are used. This is classic pharmacology.

Homeopathy is a system for healing that applies minimal treatment doses to illnesses. These are the same substances that, in greater quantities, would produce in a healthy human being the same or similar symptoms to those that the person is fighting. A typical example of this is the use of *Apis mellifica*, which is a diluted version of a bee sting, indicated in red oedema with throbbing pain that decreases with the use of cold water. It causes the same symptoms in the human body as bee stings.

Phytotherapy is the treatment of illnesses using plants or herbal substances. For this reason,

it is important to stress that not all homeopathy is natural and that phytotherapy and allopathy are not opposites. In fact, medicine derived from plants is still being used in classic pharmacology, just as it was hundreds of years ago.

KEY POINTS

Homeopathic medicines are 'drugs' according to the Spanish Ministry of Health, and therefore are only sold in pharmacies. They bear a national medicine code and are approved by the Spanish Agency of Medicines and Medical Devices (Agemed). These medicines are never sold in health food shops or parapharmacies, at least in Spain.

In general, the main difference between homeopathy and allopathy is the amount of the product to be used. In homeopathy this is minimal and, thus, it is almost impossible to incur side effects. However, the allopathic effect is faster.

Several advantages of homeopathy include the fact that it does not come up positive in antidoping testing and it can be used safely during pregnancy.

Although an exhaustive explanation of homeopathy is beyond the scope of this book, it is commonly used with great success by a number of mesotherapy professionals. Although its mechanism of action cannot be explained at present,[26] because of the positive results when compared to placebo, it is important to consider the use of homeopathy in the treatment of musculoskeletal pathology.[27]

At present in mesotherapy, an evolution of classical homeopathy is used, called homotoxicology.[28] It was developed by Dr Reckeweg, and is the nexus between allopathy on the one hand and the more classical homeopathy on the other.

When performing mesotherapy, the following points must be clear[4,13]:
- Do not inject any substance.
- Do not inject haphazardly.
- Do not inject a patient undiscerningly.
- Use selection criteria according to the indications.
- The medication used must be water-soluble.
- Use well-known and safe medications.
- Do not mix homeopathic and allopathic medicine within the same syringe, as the pH changes can deactivate the effect of the homeopathic medication.
- Do not combine more than three medications within the same syringe, especially with allopathy.
- Do not use more than 3 mL per syringe; in general, use 1 mL per medication.
- Use certain medication with caution and always with prior knowledge, especially as regards the use of vasoconstrictors, due to the risk of necrosis and degenerative fibrosis.

17.8.1 Allopathic medication

17.8.1.1 Local anaesthetics

The most frequently used local anaesthetics are procaine and lidocaine. Procaine, as discussed previously, is the first type of medicine used in mesotherapy. Although both are local anaesthetics, they belong to completely different pharmacological families and, increasingly, lidocaine is taking the place of procaine, as it is generally used more often and has a lower risk of producing allergic reactions. If patients who have never received mesotherapy are asked whether they have ever gone to the dentist and they give a positive response, they will certainly have been anaesthetized with lidocaine or one of its derived medicines, and therefore one can be almost sure of not provoking an allergic reaction. This is not the case with procaine, as it is not used in general medicine.

The use of these substances, apart from producing anaesthesia, is as a vector for medication, as they will allow better passage of the therapeutic agents to the dermis.[29]

17.8.1.2 Calcitonin

This has three well-defined actions in mesotherapy, apart from its own general actions as a hormone in the metabolism of calcium[30]:
- vasodilator action
- analgesic action (this is not well known; although it was originally thought that it was mediated by neurotransmitters on a central level, it also acts at a peripheral level)[31]
- anti-inflammatory action via the reduction of vascular permeability and partial inhibition of cyclooxygenase, an enzyme that enables synthesis of prostaglandins and, therefore, moderates the inflammatory phenomenon).

17.8.1.3 Non-steroidal anti-inflammatory drugs (NSAIDs)

In standard texts,[13,32] piroxicam is cited; however, since it has been included within the group of drugs that need special approval it is preferable to use ketoprofen or diclofenac.

17.8.1.4 Vasodilators

Buflomedil. This drug is particularly useful in venous-lymphatic insufficiencies. Its mechanism of action is less understood.

Monoethanolamine nicotinate. This is a potent vasodilator, so much so that it may cause a facial flush (sudden redness of the face and upper limb) which can cause a hypotensive syncope, and therefore it is only recommended in select cases, such as circulation pathologies

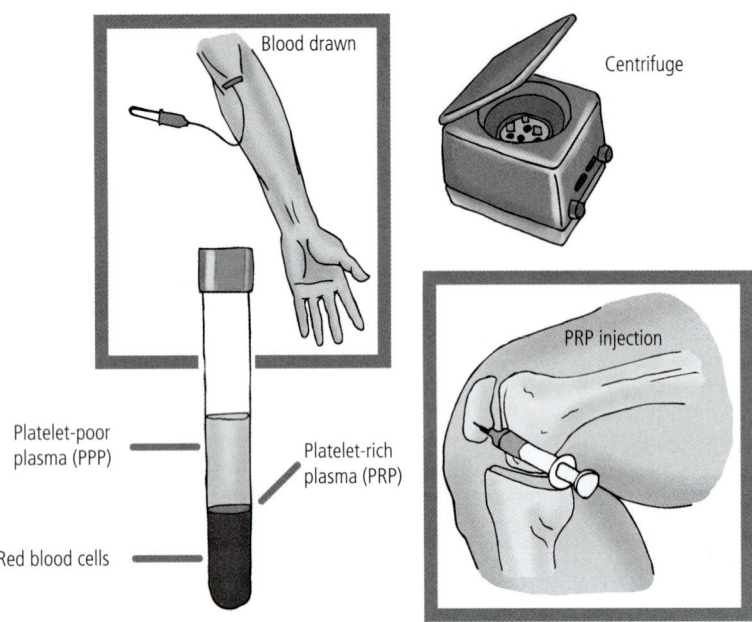

FIGURE 17.5 ■ Treatment using plasma-rich growth factors. (Colour version of figure is available online).

and always with a prior warning of this possibility. It is important for the professional to be trained to handle these situations.[13]

Pentoxifylline. Its analgesic activity is summated to vasodilation. This is probably the vasodilator of choice in processes in which there is vascular compromise.

17.8.1.5 Muscle relaxants

Both thiocolchicoside and, particularly, diazepam are useful in cases of muscle compromise.

17.8.1.6 Group B vitamins

In particular, vitamins B_1, B_6 and B_{12} are highlighted, as these are neurotrophic vitamins. These may be used in chronic and degenerative processes, with nervous compromise.

17.8.1.7 Ethylenediaminetetraacetic acid (EDTA)

EDTA is a chelating agent of metallic ions, especially calcium, and therefore is indicated for use with mesotherapy in the treatment of calcifications, in 5% concentration.[32]

17.8.2 Growth factors

The mechanisms of action of growth factors as well as their capacity for cell modulation and regeneration on many levels (e.g. vasodilation, angiogenesis, chemotaxis, cellular remodelling) have been described in section 17.4.3.[14,15]

By intervening in all body repair processes, growth factors are useful if they can be artificially transported to the lesioned site (via an injection or direct application in surgery).

The best access is via platelet growth factors (figure 17.5), as, with a mere blood extraction, and processing that includes centrifugation at 1800 rpm for 7 minutes, the separation of the platelet-rich plasma phase from the rest of the plasma occurs and, with the addition of 0.05 cm^3 calcium chloride, a concentration of growth factors is obtained which has, on average, a concentration of up to four times more growth factors than physiologically normal. This can then be used in both mesotherapy[33] and intralesional injection.[34] Although the American school advocates a second centrifugation in order to obtain a greater concentration, there are studies that demonstrate that, with a larger concentration, cellular rupture increases and, ultimately, the final number and effectiveness are very similar.[35]

The advantages of this treatment are that there are no side effects, such as allergies (it is 100% autologous) or infections (platelet-rich plasma is bactericidal) and it allows for combination with any other therapy.[36]

An important consideration, however, is that its use will depend very much on the number of platelets and, therefore, the total number of growth factors varies from one person to another depending on the patient's overall health. Its use is under debate in people with autoimmune illnesses (e.g. rheumatoid arthritis, lupus) and whether in theory its capacity for cellular cycle modulation could influence cancer cell changes.[35–38]

At present, and with several million treatments in the world based on growth factors, adverse cases have not been reported among those previously cited, and therefore it is considered to be a safe and effective treatment.[36,38]

17.8.3 Homotoxicological medication in mesotherapy

Homeopathic drugs for use via injection are only authorized in two Spanish laboratories. As homeotoxic preparations are used, which are combinations of several unitary homeopathic medications, the commercial preparations will be cited (see conflict of interests declaration, below).

Homotoxicological medications can be mixed together without any problem, but they should never be mixed within the same syringe together with allopathic medicine (the pH of allopathic medicine can deactivate the homotoxic medication). Furthermore, if necessary, more than three homtoxicological medications can be combined.

As previously mentioned, remember that homeopathy, and therefore homotoxicology, is overseen by the Spanish Ministry of Health and Agemed, and therefore can only be bought in pharmacies or directly from the laboratory, but never in herbal medicine shops or parapharmacies.

Due to the near-inexistence of side effects, it is recommended that professionals who are beginning their treatment with mesotherapy start with homotoxicology administration for the sake of safety. The clinical effects have been published[39–43] and there are enough in many cases to satisfy even the most demanding clinician and, in many cases, the use of allopathy in mesotherapy will not be necessary.

It is also true that, as has been previously mentioned, at present the mechanism of action is not completely understood.[26,27]

Once the basic techniques are mastered, the professional will be confident of knowing what, where and why one punctures, and can start with allopathy.

17.8.3.1 Heel Laboratories

- Traumeel®: inflammatory processes.
- Zeel®: degenerative processes.
- Discus®: vertebral spine

- Spascupreel®: muscle spasm
- Lymphomyosot®: oedema
- Kalium Compositum®: periarthritis, periostitis
- Belladona Homacord®: localized inflammation
- Neuralgo-Rheum-Injeel®: rheumatism of soft tissues
- Colocintis Homacord®: neuralgic and throbbing pain, paraesthesias.

17.8.3.2 Reckeweg Laboratories

- Anginacid® (R1): inflammation
- Lumbagin® (R11): low-back pain
- Calcossin® (R34): alterations of calcium metabolism
- Manurheum® (R46): shoulder and upper-limb pathologies
- Rutavine® (R55): traumas
- Spondarthrin® (R73): arthrosis

In general, although it is not strictly the case, Anginacid® and Traumeel® can be compared to NSAIDs; Spascupreel® to a muscle relaxant, both for smooth muscle as well as striated muscle; Spondarthrin® and Zeel® are used as agents for treating arthrosis and all degenerative pathologies; Discus® or Lumbalgin® are used as remedies for vertebral pathologies and Lymphomyosot®, Rutavine® and Anginacid® are used as regulators of oedematous processes, whether acute or chronic.

For this reason, it is necessary to assess the state and clinical presentation of the patient, as well as the localization and evolution of the pathological process at all times in order to select the correct medication.

17.9 MESOTHERAPY PROTOCOLS IN MUSCULOSKELETAL PATHOLOGY

Before listing the various protocols, both allopathic and homeopathic, it is important to understand that mesotherapy can be one of the treatments available, and, therefore, any reader of this work can use several techniques integrated within clinical protocols.

It is necessary always to follow the basic rules of precaution and information. Commonly, in musculoskeletal pathology, in addition to the classic contraindications, we have to add the precaution of not performing mesotherapy on fracture sites and acute muscle ruptures.

Have patients complete a health questionnaire in which they must declare any allergies and current pharmacological treatments. The patient is to sign an informed consent statement which has previously been explained, indicating the pros and cons of the treatment, possible side effects and possible therapeutic alternatives, in accordance with the requirements of the Spanish law of patient autonomy (Law 41/2002, 14 November).

A mesotherapy session should never be performed without having the patient first sign an informed consent and being adequately informed of the treatment.

KEY POINTS

Patients must fill in a health status questionnaire in which they declare any allergies or current pharmacological treatments. An informed consent is to be signed.

The sessions are planned according to the character of the lesion, the therapeutic relation and the response to treatment.

The goals are based on alleviating pain, reducing oedema and improving blood perfusion, as well as facilitating functional recovery.

As far as the puncture site is concerned, although it is very tempting to show images with fixed locations for the purpose of mapping out the punctures, it is preferable to assess the patient clinically and, depending on the structures involved, puncture as follows:
- *coup par coup* technique, performed deeply in reflex points that are painful to palpation
- micropapule technique, in points of anatomical reference of the affected structures, insertions, tendinous channels
- *nappage* in extensive muscular territories.

Lumbar pathologies are an exception to this, as the points noted by Ordiz[13] are truly useful in the treatment of painful pathologies affecting the lumbar spine.

Patients may experience pain related to their pathology and site of involvement, and it is important to adapt treatment accordingly.

17.9.1 Acute pathology: acute trauma

Syringe 1: lidocaine 1% 1 cm^3 + calcitonin 100 IU 1 cm^3 + diclophenac 50 mg/2 cm^3.

In homeopathy:
Syringe 1: Traumeel® or Anginacid® + Rutavine® or Lymphomiost® + Kalium® or Belladonna® if bone structures are affected or if it is localized.

17.9.2 Pathology of the soft tissues: protocol

Syringe 1: lidocaine 1% 1 cm^3 + pentoxifylline 2 cm^3 + diclofenac 50 mg/1 cm^3.

Syringe 2: lidocaine 2 cm^3 + EDTA 2 cm^3 or diazepam® 5 mg/1 cm^3.

Always assess the muscular involvement or calcification in order to select between EDTA or diazepam. When using homotoxicology, and if it is possible to complement treatment with syringe 2, with calcifications (but always using separate syringes), the protocol would be:

Syringe 1: Traumeel® + Zeel® or Calcossin® + Manurheum® (adding Spascupreel® if there is important muscular involvement).

17.9.3 Pathologies of the tendon

Syringe 1: lidocaine 1% 1 cm^3 + calcitonin 100 IU 2 cm^3 + diclofenac 50 mg/1 cm^3.

Syringe 2: lidocaine 1% 1 cm^3 + diazepam 5 mg/2 cm^3.

In homeopathy:
Syringe 1: Traumeel® or Angiacid® + Spascupreel® + Rutavine® and Belladonna® if acute.

17.9.4 Degenerative pathologies

Syringe 1: pentoxifylline 2 cm^3 + B complex (B$_1$–B$_6$–B$_{12}$) 1 cm^3 + calcitonin 100 IU/1 cm^3.

In homeopathy:
Traumeel® or Angionacid® + Zeel® or Calcossin® + Spondarthin®.

17.9.5 Carpal tunnel syndrome

Mesotherapy can be useful in carpal tunnel syndrome. In such cases, mucopolysaccharidoses, which modulate the inflammatory effect are used; where there is significant chronic pain, a tricyclic antidepressant can be useful, such as amitriptyline and, in cases of chronic fibrosis, use low-molecular-weight heparin.

In homeopathy cases, use Traumeel® + Angionacid® + Phosphor® + Lymphomiosot®.

17.9.6 Pathology of the hand

There are three hand pathologies for which classical treatment protocols are described: Dupuytren's disease, trigger finger and Raynaud's syndrome.

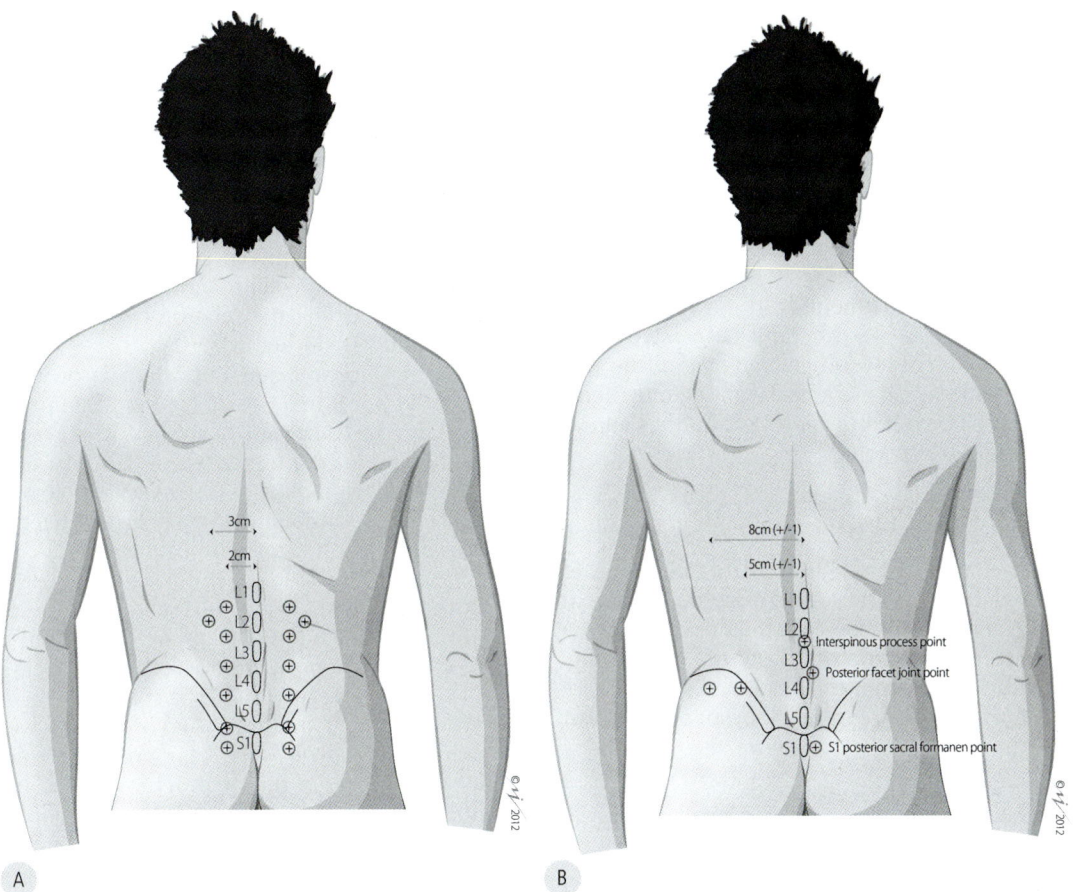

A   B

FIGURE 17.6 ■ (A, B) Summary of the puncture points for lumbar spine pathology. (Adapted from Ordiz and Gomis Devesa.[46]). (Colour version of figure is available online).

17.9.6.1 Dupuytren's disease

Syringe 1: lidocaine 1% 1 cm^3 + coumarin/1 cm^3 + salicylate/1 cm^3 + mucopolysaccharidoses/ 1 cm^3.

17.9.6.2 Trigger finger

Syringe 1: pentoxifylline/1 cm^3 + vitamin B complex/1 cm^3 + calcitonin 100 IU/1 cm^3.

Syringe 2: lidocaine 1% 1 cm^3 + diazepam 5 mg/1 cm^3.

17.9.6.3 Raynaud's phenomenon

Syringe 1: nicardipine 2 mg/1 cm^3 + lidocaine 1% 1 cm^3 + pentoxifylline 1 cm^3.

17.9.7 Pathology of the spine

In addition to the general contraindications in mesotherapy treatments of spinal pathologies, the following specific contraindications apply:

- fractures of the vertebrae
- active infections
- neurological compressions of surgical solution.

Because of the common neurological component to these pathologies, add B-complex vitamins routinely to any preparation administered.[44,45]

As commented at the beginning of this section, it is especially helpful to follow a strict series of points in lumbar pathology (figure 17.6). Recent studies have demonstrated a great effectiveness of the mesotherapy route in the treatment of this pathology and with fewer side effects.[47,48]

17.10 MESOTHERAPY IN OTHER BRANCHES OF MEDICINE

It is important to note that mesotherapy can be used in any branch of medicine.[49] After all, its creator, Dr Pistor, was a rural doctor who used it for any treatment he saw fit.

17.10.1 Cosmetic medicine

Perhaps the best-known application of mesotherapy is in the field of cosmetic medicine. For many years, corporal mesotherapy has been the only far-reaching treatment for cellulite or adiposis oedematosa. Although, at first, allopathic and homeopathic medicine were used interchangeably, at present only homotoxicology can be used, as well as other products such as organic silicium, for its treatment.

Furthermore, mesotherapy associated with growth factors or low reticulated hyaluronic acid has had widespread use in facial antiageing medicine, in order to help conceal small lines and as a refirming treatment.

17.10.2 Hair disorders

Mesotherapy is widely used in this field due to its good results. These range from the use of corticosteroids in the treatment of alopecia areata to the injection of finasteride and biotine for androgenetic alopecia, as well as the use of growth factors to strengthen the hair and support hair transplant surgery.

17.10.3 Acne

Both mesovaccination as well as antibiotics and corticosteroids have been used for the treatment of acne, with varying results. Commonly the *nappage* technique is used and combined with oligoelements.

17.10.4 Angiology

All sorts of vascular pathologies can be treated using mesotherapy, subject to having a good array of vasodilator, venotonic and lymphotonic medication, both allopathic and homeopathic.

17.10.5 Neurology

Headaches, facial neuralgias and chronic pain can be treated with amitriptyline, muscle relaxants or even botulinum toxin, which is usually known as mesobotox.

17.11 SCIENTIFIC EVIDENCE

If you search for mesotherapy on the web page of the National Center for Biotechnology Information (http://www.ncbi.nlm.nih.gov/) based in the USA (the reference web page when searching for scientific articles), up to 166 articles are referenced, 134 published in the last 10 years and 107 in the last 5 years. Furthermore, in the last

2 years the number is 52; therefore, one-third of articles concerning this treatment were published very recently. This means that mesotherapy is attracting interest in the scientific community and the goal of realizing larger scientific reviews is being fulfilled.

Most of these studies are centred on cosmetic medicine applications (facial, corporal and capillary) and on the side effects of mesotherapy. More recently, important studies have also been published regarding the relation between mesotherapy and physiotherapy.

The most recent and important is probably the study published in 2012 by Mammucari et al.,[50] in which a review of studies on the use of mesotherapy for the treatment of pain of a musculoskeletal origin was performed. The conclusions were that, although more studies are needed, the results so far indicate clinical benefits.

One of these studies compared the use of mesotherapy with traditional allopathy in the treatment of acute low-back pain.[51] A total of 84 randomized patients were treated with a cocktail of NSAIDs, lidocaine and corticosteroids using mesotherapy, and another group of patients were treated orally with NSAIDs and corticosteroids. The effectiveness of the treatment was similar in both groups, with the advantage of using a lower amount of medication in the patients treated with mesotherapy and having a lower potential of side effects compared to the oral administration group.

Another study was published by Cachio et al.,[32] in which 80 patients with calcified tendonitis were treated with EDTA using mesotherapy together with ultrasound, compared to placebo. The results were total disappearance of calcifications in 62.5% and partial disappearance in 22.5%, as opposed to only 15% in the control group.

Finally, the University of Oviedo in Spain published a study by Ordiz et al.[52] in which 138 patients belonging to federated sports teams of the University of Oviedo were treated for 158 pathologies: exclusively homotoxicological medications were used (Traumeel®, Zeel® and Spascupreel®). Healing occurred in 71% of patients, and a great improvement in symptoms occurred in 16.4%, while only 3.4% reported no change.

17.12 CLINICAL CASE

17.12.1 Mesotherapy in lumbar pain
(figure 17.7)

The patient is a 28-year-old-male, an elite fencer, diagnosed with disc protrusion of L4/L5, who

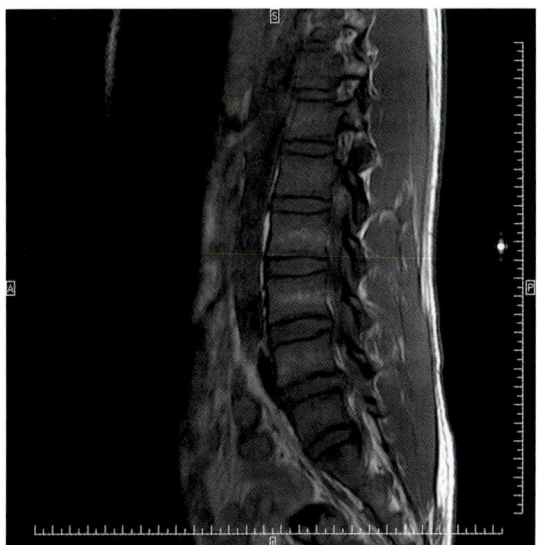

FIGURE 17.7 ■ Magnetic resonance image: sagittal section of the lumbar region.

has seen a gradual reduction in capacity for training and an increase in pain at rest. He is awaiting assessment for possible surgery. Meanwhile, the lesion incapacitates him for everyday work, and makes training and competition impossible. He has tried several physiotherapy sessions which have not been able to reduce the amount of discomfort or pain, which he only manages to control with oral NSAIDs (ibuprofen 600 mg).

(Clinical case continued on page 492)

Conflict of interest declaration

The author reports no financial relationships or conflicts of interest.

17.13 REFERENCES

1. Wepierre J. Theorie et pratique therapeutique, 5. Paris: Editions Guy le Part; 1980. p. 13.
2. Lázaro Ochaita P. Dermatología. texto y atlas. 2nd ed. Madrid: Editorial Luzán; 1994.
3. Freedberg IM, Eisen AZ, Wolff K, et al. Fitzpatrick's dermatology in general medicine. 9th ed. New York: McGraw Hill; 2004.
4. CHOS. Analyse des différentes conceptions du mode d'action de la mesotherapie. BSFM 1983;58:22–5.
5. Merlen JF. Microcirculation cutaneé sanguine, interstitialle et lymphatique. Journal de Medicine Estetique et de Chirurgie Dermatologique 1982;9:219–29.
6. Pistor M. Actas del Boletín de la Sociedad Francesa de Mesoterapia 1970;20:12–16.
7. Pistor M. Actas del Boletín de la Sociedad Francesa de Mesoterapia 1975;36:5–7.
8. Melzack R, Wall PD. Pain mechanisms: A New Theory Science 1965;150:971–9.
9. Einholtz B, Maudet D, Bicheron M. Use of nhai via mesotherapy in oral surgery. Actualites Odonto-Stomatologiques 1990;44(170):285–98.
10. Dalloz-Bourguignon A. A new therapy against pain: mesotherapy. J Belge de Medecine Physique et de Rehabilitation 1979;2(3):230–4.
11. Kaplan A. Mésoscintigraphie: contribution de la techniqueméso à la scintigraphie diagnostique. Implications pharmacocinétiques. In: Libro de resúmenes del V Congreso Internacional de Mesoterapia. Paris: 1988. p. 48–50.
12. Kaplan A. Mésoscintigraphie et proposition d'une théorie unifiée de la Mésothérapie. In: Libro de resumenes del VI Congreso Internacional de Mesoterapia. Bruxelles: 1992. p. 42–9.
13. Ordiz I. Tratado de Mesoterapia. Edición digital 2008.
14. Lacci K, Dardik A. Platelet-rich plasma: support for its use in wound healing. Yale J Biol Med 2010;83:1–9.
15. Rozman P, Bolta Z. Use of platelet growth factors in treating wounds and soft-tissue injuries. Acta Dermatovenerol Alp Panonica Adriat 200;16:156–65.
16. Marx RE, Carlson ER, Eichstaedt RM, et al. Platelet-rich plasma: growth factor enhancement for bone grafts. Oral Surg Oral Med Oral Pathol Oral Radiol Endod 1998;85:638–46.
17. Dutzler R, Campbell EB, MacKinnon R. Gating the selectivity filter in ClC chloride channels. Science 2003;300:108–12.
18. Finkelstein A. Water movement through lipid bilayers, pores, and plasma membranes. New York: Wiley Interscience; 1987.
19. Potts RO, Bommannan D, Wong O, et al. Transdermal peptide delivery using electroporation. In: Sanders LM, Hendren RW, editors. Protein delivery – physical systems. New York: Plenum; 1997. p. 213–38.
20. Santoianni P. Intradermal delivery of active principles. G Ital Dermatol Venereol 2005;140:549–55.
21. Le Coz J. Effets secondaires et incidents en mésothérapie. BSFM 1983;57:4–7.
22. Eidelman A. Topical anesthetics for dermal instrumentation: a systematic review of randomized, controlled trials. Ann Emerg Med 2005;46:343–51.
23. Ruiz Manzano J, Manterola JM, Ausina V, et al. Nomenclatura y clasificación de las micobacterias. Arch Bronconeumol 1998;34:154–7.
24. Medina MV, Sauret J, Valet JA, et al. Enfermedades producidas por micobacterias ambientales. Med Clin (Barc) 1999;113:621–30.
25. Esteban J. Current treatment of nontuberculous mycobacteriosis: an update. Expert Opin Pharmacother 2012; 13:967–86.
26. Vickers AJ. Clinical trials of homeopathy and placebo: analysis of a scientific debate. J Altern Complement Med 2000;6:49–56.
27. Linde K. Are the clinical effects of homeopathy placebo effects? A meta-analysis of placebo-controlled trials. Lancet 1997;350:834–43.
28. Ernst E, Schmidt K. Homotoxicology: a review of randomised clinical trials. Eur J Clin Pharmacol 2004;60(5): 299–306.
29. Huteau Y. Les anesthésiques locaux employés en Mésothérapie. In: Libro de resúmenes del V Congreso Internacional de Mesoterapia. Paris: SFM; 1988. p. 29–37.
30. Munson PL. Physiology and pharmacology of thyrocalcitoninum. In: Handbook of physiology. 7th ed. Washington, DC: American Physiological Society; 1976. p. 443–64.
31. Ito A. Anti-hyperalgesic effects of calcitonin on neuropathic pain interacting with its peripheral receptors. Mol Pain 2012;8:42.
32. Cachio A, De Blasis E, Desiati P, et al. Effectiveness of treatment of calcific tendinitis of the shoulder by disodium EDTA. Arthritis Rheum 2009;61:84–91.

33. Bulam H, Ayhan S, Sezgin B, et al. The Inhibitory Effect of Platelet-Rich Plasma on Botulinum Toxin Type-A: An Experimental Study in Rabbits. Aesthetic Plast Surg 2014.

34. Dallaudière B, Pesquer L, Meyer P, et al. Intratendinous injection of platelet-rich plasma under US guidance to treat tendinopathy: a long-term pilot study. J Vasc Interv Radiol 2014;25(5):717–23.

35. Martínez González JM. ¿Existen riesgos al utilizar los concentrados de Plasma Rico en Plaquetas (PRP) de uso ambulatorio? Medicina Oral 2002;7:375–90.

36. Carter MJ. Use of platelet rich plasma gel on wound dealing: a systematic review and metaanalysis. Eplasty 2011;11:e38.

37. Wan Hl, Avila G. Platelet rich plasma. Myth or reality. Eur J Dent Editorial 2007;1:192–4.

38. Sampson S, Gerhardt M. Mendelbaum B. Platelet rich plasma injection grafts for musculoskeletal injuries: a review. Curr Rev Musculoskelet Med 2008;1:165–74.

39. Zenner S, Metelmann H. Posibilidades de utilización de Traumeel solución inyectable. Resultados de un estudio de aplicación multicéntrico en 3241 pacientes. Med Biol 1996;1:132–40.

40. Weiser M, Zenner S. Terapia oral de afecciones traumáticas, inflamatorias y degenerativas con un medicamento homeopático. Med Biol 1997;1:4–9.

41. Potrafki B. Terapia biológica de contusiones, distorsiones y tendopatías. Med Biol 1998;2:186–7.

42. Riedel I. Estudio comparativo del empleo de los medicamentos bioterapéuticos Zeel y Traumeel en la práctica médica. Med Biol 1989;2:171–3.

43. Molino M. Revisión de experiencias clínica con Traumeel. Med Biol 1991;3-4:411–13.

44. Perrin JJ. Cervico-dorso-lombalgies: approchedynamiquemesotherapique. BSFM 2006;127.

45. Bigorra E. Lombalgies chroniques, place de la Mésothérapie. BSFM 2004;120.

46. Ordiz I, Gomis Devesa AJ. Mesoterapia en aplicaciones reumato traumatológicas. Available online at:: <http://www.ordizmesoterapia.com>; [accessed 15 December 2013].

47. Cosimo C. Mesotherapy versus systemic therapy in the treatment of acute low back pain: a randomized trial. Evid Based Complement Alternat Med 2011;Article ID 317183.

48. Bonnet C, Laurens D, Perrin JJ. Guía Práctica de Mesoterapia. Paris: Ed. Masson; 2008.

49. Le Coz J. Mesoterapia en medicina general. Edición Española. Barcelona: Ed. Masson; 1994. p. 100.

50. Mammucari M, Gatti A, Maggiori S, et al. Role of mesotherapy in musculoskeletal pain: opinions from the Italian Society of Mesotherapy. Evid Based Complement Alternat Med 2012;2012:436959.

51. Costantino C, Marangio E, Coruzzi G. Mesotherapy versus systemic therapy in the treatment of acute low back pain: a randomized trial. Evid Based Complement Alternat Med 2011;2011:pii. 317183.

52. Ordiz I, Egocheaga J, Del Valle M. Mesoterapia Homotoxicológica en Lesiones Deportivas en Partes Blandas. Escuela de Medicina Deportiva. Universidad de Oviedo 2004.

53. Kuma V, Abbas AK, Fausto N, et al. Robbins basic pathology. London: Saunders. Elsevier; 2007.

INJECTION THERAPY

CHAPTER 18

INJECTION THERAPY FOR PHYSIOTHERAPISTS

Stephanie Saunders

For every complex problem, there is an answer that is neat, plausible – and wrong.

HL. MENCKEN

CHAPTER OUTLINE

KEYWORDS

injection technique; corticosteroid; local anaesthetic; inflammatory damage cycle; dosages; injection protocol.

18.1 INTRODUCTION

I was trained in London by Dr. James Cyriax and was responsible for running and teaching on his courses in Orthopaedic Medicine both in Britain and overseas. This involved teaching doctors how to do injections into joints and soft tissue, but I was always uncomfortable about teaching a skill that I had never used personally.

Enquiries to my medical colleagues about the evidence regarding choice and action of injectable drugs, dose, volume, placement and possible outcomes or side effects showed that very little was known and that most approaches were empirically based.

Eventually I started giving injections myself and was surprised to find that, using the excellent training given by Dr. Cyriax, usually patients responded very well to the intervention. I came to the conclusion that injection therapy is a valid extra tool that should be available to all physiotherapists working with musculoskeletal conditions. The ability to relieve pain rapidly enables the clinician to reduce morbidity and initiate early rehabilitation.

I therefore designed the first course in injection therapy for physiotherapists in 1995, which was given in Birmingham, England. Since then we have run many courses and now over 2000 have completed their training and are using this additional skill in the UK.

All research on injection therapy shows that it works, but only in the short term. After varying periods of time there is no evidence of superiority over other physical or chemical treatments, or doing nothing. Few studies are performed that examine a combination of injection followed by appropriate regimes that address the cause of the lesion. Experienced physiotherapists are placed in an ideal situation: they have good knowledge of anatomy, excellent diagnostic and handling skills and are able to apply the additional treatments that almost always are required after any injection. These may include manual treatments as well as preventive advice on posture, rest and exercise.

The following is a brief outline of the theory and practice of injection therapy. Further detailed information can be found in *Injection Techniques in Musculoskeletal Medicine*.[1]

18.2 THE DRUGS

18.2.1 Corticosteroids

The commonly used injectable corticosteroids are synthetic analogues of the adrenal glucocorticoid hormone cortisol (hydrocortisone), which is secreted by the innermost layer (zona reticularis) of the adrenal cortex. Cortisol has many important actions, including anti-inflammatory activity. Corticosteroids influence the cells involved in the immune and inflammatory responses primarily by modulating the transcription of a large number of genes. They act directly on nuclear steroid receptors to control the rate of synthesis of mRNA. However, they also reduce the production of a wide range of proinflammatory mediators, including cytokines and other important enzymes.[2-9]

18.2.1.1 Rationale for using corticosteroids

We know surprisingly little about the precise pharmacological effects of corticosteroids when they are injected directly into joints and soft tissues.[10-12] Local steroid injections are thought to work by:

- Suppressing inflammation in inflammatory systemic diseases, such as rheumatoid or psoriatic arthritis and gout. Synovial cell infiltration and proinflammatory cytokine expression are reduced in a multifaceted manner by intra-articular corticosteroid injection.[3,5,13-16]
- Suppressing inflammatory flares in degenerative joint disease. However, the pathophysiology of osteoarthritis is poorly understood, and there are no reliable clinical features that predict which osteoarthritic joints will respond to injection. Often, the only way to find out is with an empirical trial of injection therapy.[4,15-18]
- Breaking up the inflammatory damage–repair–damage cycle which is postulated to set up a continuous low-grade inflammatory response, inhibiting tissue repair and sound scar formation, while forming adverse adhesions. There is little direct evidence to support this, however.[11,19,20]
- Protecting cartilage: there may be a direct chondroprotective effect on cartilage metabolism or other effects not related to anti-inflammatory activity of the steroids, e.g. promotion of articular surfactant production.[4,7,21-29]
- Direct analgesic effect: Inflammation is a complex cascade of molecular and cellular events. The precise role of inflammation in 'tendinitis' is the subject of considerable debate, and many authors prefer the terms 'tendinosis' or 'tendinopathy' to describe the pathological changes. Tendon pain may not be due to inflammation (tendinitis) or structural disruption of the tendon fibres (tendinosis), but might instead be caused by the stimulation of nociceptors by chemicals such as glutamate, substance P and chondroitin sulphate released from the damaged tendon. Corticosteroids (and possibly local anaesthetics) may inhibit release of noxious chemicals and/or the long-term behaviour of local nociceptors. *In vitro*, corticosteroids have also been shown to inhibit the transmission of pain along unmyelinated C-fibres by direct membrane action.[3-34]

18.2.1.2 Commonly used corticosteroids

Triamcinolone acetonide
- Adcortyl® (10 mg/mL – dilute)
- Kenalog® (40 mg/mL – concentrated)

Kenalog® is recommended for ease of administration. This drug can be used in very small quantities so is ideal for small joints and tendons where distension may increase pain. Adcortyl®, however, is useful where larger volume is required, as in larger joints and bursae. The duration of action of the drug is approximately 2–3 weeks.

Methylprednisolone acetate
- Depo-Medrone® (40 mg/mL – concentrated)

This drug may give more postinjection pain than triamcinalone acetonide. It is available also premixed with local anaesthetic as Depo-Medrone® (40 mg/1 mL) with lidocaine (10 mg/mL) in 1 mL and 2 mL vials, which we do not recommend as it is a fixed-dose combination and therefore difficult to adjust.

Hydrocortisone
Hydrocortistab® (25 mg/mL – very dilute) Very soluble – this has the shortest duration of action of the steroids mentioned here, perhaps as little as 6 days. It may be particularly useful for superficial injections in thin, dark-skinned patients, where depigmentation or local fat atrophy may be more noticeable. Hydrocortistab® 20 mg is equal to 4 mg triamcinolone or methylprednisolone[35–37] (table 18.1).

18.2.2 Local anaesthetics

These membrane-stabilizing drugs act by causing a reversible block to conduction along nerve fibres. The smaller nerve fibres are more sensitive, so that a differential block may occur where the small fibres carrying pain and autonomic impulses are blocked, sparing coarse touch and movement. Uptake into the systemic circulation is important for terminating their action and also for producing toxicity. Following most regional anaesthetic procedures, maximum arterial plasma concentrations of anaesthetic develop within 10–25 minutes, so careful surveillance for toxic effects is recommended for 30 minutes after injection if significant volumes are used.[38]

18.2.2.1 Rationale for using local anaesthetics

- Analgesic: although the effect is temporary, it may make the overall procedure less unpleasant for the patient, break the pain cycle (by reducing nociceptive input to the 'gate' in the dorsal horn) and increase the confidence of the patient in the clinician, diagnosis and treatment. In one study, pain inhibition was better with bupivacaine than lidocaine during the first 6 hours, presumably because of its longer half-life; in later evaluations no differences in outcomes were observed. In another study, bupivacaine was superior to lidocaine at 2 weeks, but not at 3 and 12 months. Some practitioners inject a mixture of short- and long-acting local anaesthetic in order to obtain both the immediate diagnostic effect plus more prolonged pain relief.[39,40]
- Diagnostic: pain relief following an injection confirms the diagnosis and the correct placement of the solution. Sometimes even the most experienced practitioner will be unsure exactly which tissue is at fault; in this situation a small amount of local anaesthetic may be injected into the most likely tissue and the patient re-examined after a few minutes. If the pain is relieved then the source of the problem has been identified, and further treatment can be accurately directed.[11]

TABLE 18.1 Commonly used corticosteroids

Drug	Dose	Potency	Manufacturer
Short-acting		+	
Hydrocortisone acetate	25 mg/mL		Sovereign
Hydrocortistab®	1 mL ampoules	++++	
Intermediate-acting			
Methylprednisolone acetate	40 mg/mL		Pharmacia
Depo-Medrone®	1 mL, 2 mL, 3 mL vials		
Depo-Medrone® + lidocaine	1 mL, 2 mL vials		
Triamcinolone acetonide			Squibb
Adcortyl®	10 mg/mL		
	1 mL ampoules, 5 mL vials		
Kenalog®	40 mg/mL		
	1 mL vials		

- Dilution: the internal surface area of joints and bursae is surprisingly large, due to the highly convoluted synovial lining with its many villae, so an increased volume of the injected solution helps to spread the steroid around this surface.[11]
- Distension: a beneficial volume effect in joints and bursae may be the physical stretching of the capsule or bursa with disruption of adhesions. Distension is not advised at entheses, so the smallest practicable volume should be used; distension in tendons by bolus injection of a relatively large volume of solution may physically disrupt the fibres and compress the relatively poor arterial supply, and also give rise to distension pain.[41–44]

18.2.2.2 Commonly used local anaesthetics

Local anaesthetics vary widely in their potency, duration of action and toxicity.[38] The most commonly used for joint and soft-tissue injection are as follows.

- Lidocaine hydrochloride (previously lignocaine hydrochloride): the most widely used local anaesthetic, it acts more rapidly and is more stable than others. The effects occur within seconds and duration of block is about 30 minutes; this is the local anaesthetic recommended in this book.
- Marcain® (bupivacaine) has a slow onset of action (about 30 minutes for full effect) but the duration of block is up to 8 hours. It is the principal drug for spinal anaesthesia in the UK. We do not use it for routine outpatient injections because the delayed onset of action precludes the immediate diagnostic effect available with lidocaine, and if there is an adverse effect this will take a long time to dissipate. There is no evidence of any long-term benefit from using bupivacaine instead of lidocaine. Compared to placebo, the effect of intra-articular bupivacaine wears off in less than 24 hours.[40,45]

Lidocaine (under the brand name Xylocaine®) and Marcain® are also manufactured with added adrenaline (which causes vasoconstriction when used for skin anaesthesia, and so prolongs the local anaesthetic effect). These preparations are not recommended for procedures involving the appendages because of the risk of ischaemic necrosis. Xylocaine® with adrenaline added is clearly marked in red. We recommend that clinicians who administer injection therapy avoid these combination products altogether.

18.3 POTENTIAL SIDE EFFECTS

Side effects from injection therapy with corticosteroids and/or local anaesthetics are uncommon and when they do occur are usually mild and transient. Nonetheless it is incumbent upon the clinician practising injection therapy to be aware of the presentation and management of all the potential minor and more serious side effects associated with this treatment.[46–49]

Injection of the wrong drug is a potentially serious and totally avoidable problem with severe consequences for all concerned. Strict attention to the preparation protocol should prevent this.

Consider carefully before giving corticosteroid injections to pregnant or breastfeeding women; this therapy has been recommended for carpal tunnel syndrome and de Quervain's tendovaginitis in these patients, but these conditions usually resolve following delivery. If used, a detailed discussion of the pros and cons of injection therapy should be carefully documented.[50–53]

KEY POINTS

Side effects from injection therapy with corticosteroids and/or local anaesthetics are uncommon.

18.3.1 Local side effects

Local side effects may occur when an injection is misdirected or too large a dose in too large a volume is injected too often. Subcutaneous placement of the steroid and the injection of a drug bolus at entheses must both be avoided. Serious local side effects are rare.[46]

- Postinjection flare of pain. The quoted figures are about 2–10% but this is well in excess of our own experience. When it does happen it is usually after a soft-tissue injection, and rarely follows a joint injection. When corticosteroid is mixed with local anaesthetic the solution should be inspected carefully for flocculation/precipitation before injecting, as this may be related to postinjection flare of pain, which may also be caused by rapid intracellular ingestion of the microcrystalline steroid ester and must always be distinguished from sepsis. There may be more frequent postinjection flares with methylprednisolone, but this may have more to do with the preservative in the drug than with the steroid itself. An early increase in joint stiffness following intra-articular corticosteroids is consistent with a transient synovitis.[12,48,54–56]

- Multidose bottles of lidocaine contain parabens as a preservative. Many steroids will precipitate when added to it and this precipitate may be responsible for some cases of postinjection flare of pain and 'steroid chalk'. Parabens may also be responsible for some allergic reactions to local injections. The use of multidose bottles increases the risk of cross-infection and should be avoided. Single-dose vials of lidocaine do not contain parabens.
- Subcutaneous atrophy and/or skin depigmentation. In one meta-analysis of shoulder and elbow injections, 'skin modification' had a frequency of 4%. Skin changes may be more likely to occur when superficial lesions are injected, especially in dark-skinned patients. The injected drugs should not be allowed to reflux back through the needle tract – pressure applied around the needle with cotton wool when withdrawing may help. In thin, dark-skinned patients especially, it may be preferable to use hydrocortisone for superficial lesions. Patients must always be advised of the possibility of this side effect, and the fact recorded. Local atrophy appears within 1–4 months after injection and characteristically proceeds to resolution 6–24 months later, but may take longer.[57–60]
- Bleeding or bruising may occur at the injection site, possibly more frequently in patients taking warfarin, aspirin, or oral non-steroidal anti-inflammatory drugs (NSAIDs) with significant antiplatelet activity, e.g. naproxen. It is important to apply firm pressure to the injection site immediately following needle withdrawal.
- Steroid 'chalk' or 'paste' may be found on the surface of previously injected tendons and joints during surgery. Suspension flocculation, resulting from the mixture of steroid with a local anaesthetic containing preservative, may be responsible. The clinical significance of these deposits is uncertain.[61]
- Soft-tissue calcification. Corticosteroid injections into osteoarthritic interphalangeal joints of the hand may result in calcification or joint fusion, possibly because of pericapsular leakage of steroids due to raised intra-articular pressure. No deleterious effects have been ascribed to this calcification.[62]
- Steroid arthropathy is a well-known and much feared complication of local injection treatment – it is also largely a myth. In many instances injected steroid can be chondroprotective rather than destructive. There is good evidence linking prolonged high-dose oral steroid usage with osteonecrosis, but almost all the reports linking injected steroids with accelerated non-septic joint destruction are anecdotal, and mainly relate to joints receiving huge numbers of injections. A reasonable guide is to give injections into the major joints in the lower limbs at no less than 3–4-month intervals, although this advice is based on consensus rather than evidence. Reports of Charcot-like accelerated joint destruction after steroid injection in human hip osteoarthritis may reflect the disease itself rather than the treatment. Currently no evidence supports the promotion of disease progression by steroid injections. Repeat injections into the knee every 3 months seem to be safe over 2 years.[10,21–29,62–66]
- One study determined the relationship between frequent intra-articular steroid injection and subsequent joint replacement surgery in patients with rheumatoid arthritis who had received four or more injections in an asymmetric pattern in a single year. A subset of 13 patients with an average of 7.4 years of follow-up was established as the cohort of a 5-year prospective study. This highly selected cohort received 1622 injections; joint replacement surgery was not significantly more common in the injected joints. The authors concluded that frequent intra-articular steroid injection does not greatly increase the risk inherent in continued disease activity for these patients and may offer some chondroprotection.[67]
- Tendon rupture and atrophy. The literature does not provide precise estimates for complication rates following the therapeutic use of injected or systemic steroids in the treatment of athletic injuries but tendon and fascial ruptures are reported complications of injection. This is probably minimized by withdrawing the needle slightly if an unusual amount of resistance is encountered, and using a peppering technique at entheses with the smallest effective dose and volume of steroid. The whole issue of steroid-associated tendon rupture is controversial, disputed, anecdotal, and in humans not well supported in the literature, although it is widely accepted that repeated injection of steroids into load-bearing tendons carries the risk of rupture.[68–78]
- The current climate of opinion is antithetical towards steroid injection into and around the Achilles tendon. If this is being

contemplated it is advisable to image the tendon first to confirm that it is a peritendinitis with no degenerative change (with or without tears) in the body of the tendon. Low-dose peritendinous steroid injections appear to be safe and it might be safer to infiltrate with local anaesthetic alone. The patient should rest from provocative activity for 6–8 weeks. In rabbits, injections of steroid, both within the tendon substance and into the retrocalcaneal bursa, adversely affect the biomechanical properties of Achilles tendons. Additionally, rabbit tendons that received bilateral injections demonstrated significantly worse biomechanical properties compared with unilaterally injected tendons. Bilateral injections should be avoided as they may have a systemic effect in conjunction with the local effect, further weakening the tendon. Surgery for chronic Achilles tendinopathy has a complication rate of around 10% and should not be assumed to be a trouble-free treatment option.[79–82]

- Delayed soft-tissue healing may be associated with local steroid injection. In a study of rabbit ligaments the tensile strength of the injected specimens returned to a value that was equal to that of the non-injected controls; however, the peak load of the injected specimens remained inferior, with a lag in histological maturation. This has implications for the timing of return to activity following injection therapy.[82]

- Sepsis. Joint sepsis is the most feared complication of steroid injection treatment; it may be lethal, but it is a rarity. Local infection occurs in only 1 in 17,000–162,000 patients when joint and soft-tissue injections are performed as an 'office' procedure. In one study local sepsis following injection of a pre-packaged corticosteroid in a sterile syringe was 1 in 162,000 injections compared with 1 in 21,000 using a non-prepackaged syringe. Soft-tissue infections and osteomyelitis can also occur after local soft-tissue injection.[46,49,62,83–89]

- Prompt recognition of infection is essential to prevent joint and soft-tissue destruction, although diagnosis may be delayed if symptoms are mistaken for a postinjection flare or exacerbation of the underlying arthropathy. Following an injection, swelling at the site, increased pain, fever, systemic upset (e.g. sweating, headaches) and severe pain on all attempted active and passive movements should raise clinical suspicion of infection.[83,89–91]

- Fragments of skin may be carried into a joint on the tip of a needle and may be a source of infection. Joint infections may also possibly occur by haematogenous spread, rather than by direct inoculation of organisms into the joint. Steroid injection may create a local focus of reduced immunity in a joint, thus rendering it more vulnerable to blood-borne spread. Rarely, injection of contaminated drugs or hormonal activation of a quiescent infection may be to blame.[83,87]

- All cases of suspected infection following injection must be promptly admitted to hospital for diagnosis and treatment. Blood tests (erythrocyte sedimentation rate [ESR], C-reactive protein [CRP], plasma viscosity, white blood cell differential count, blood cultures) should be taken along with diagnostic aspiration of the affected joint or any other localized swelling. The needle used for attempted aspiration may be sent for culture if no aspirate is obtained. X-ray changes may be absent in the early stages of joint infection and more sophisticated imaging techniques such as magnetic resonance imaging and isotope bone scans may be helpful.[83,87]

- To avoid injecting an already infected joint, have a high index of suspicion in rheumatoid patients, elderly osteoarthritic patients with an acute monarthritic flare (especially hip) and patients with coexistent infection elsewhere, e.g. chest, urinary tract and skin, especially the legs. Joint infection has been reported as occurring between 4 days and 3 weeks after injection. Exotic infections may occur in immunocompromised patients following joint injection.[92,93]

- Aggressive therapy, including powerful immunosuppressive and cytotoxic drugs, is increasingly used in the treatment of rheumatoid arthritis, and may confer increased susceptibility to infections. The high frequency of delayed septic arthritis in rheumatoid patients after intra-articular steroid administration should alert clinicians to this complication.[94,95]

- Concern has been raised that prior steroid injection of the knee and hip may increase the risk of a subsequent joint infection following joint replacement, although this has been disputed. Some surgeons deprecate the routine use of intra-articular steroids following knee surgery because of a perceived increased risk of infection, while others advocate this for postprocedural pain relief.[96–101]

- If infection occurs following an injection, vigorous attempts must be made to isolate the causative organism. If this is *Staphylococcus aureus* the clinician should have nasal swabs taken and, if positive, appropriate antibiotic treatment should be instituted and no more injections given until further swabs confirm clearance. A review of aseptic technique used should also be undertaken.[87,102]
- Intra-articular corticosteroids may be effective following septic arthritis where pain and synovitis persist despite intravenous antibiotic treatment, and where lavage and repeat synovial fluid and blood cultures are sterile. Multidose bottles and vials should be avoided as they may become contaminated and act as a source of infection. Drugs for injection must be stored in accordance with the manufacturer's instructions.[103]
- Rare local side-effects include nerve damage (severe pain and 'electric shocks' if you needle a nerve), transient paresis of an extremity (from an inadvertent motor nerve block), and needle fracture.[49,52]

KEY POINTS

The most important local side effects that occur with an injection are postinjection flare of pain, subcutaneous atrophy and/or skin depigmentation, bleeding or bruising, steroid 'chalk' or 'paste', soft-tissue calcification, steroid arthropathy, tendon rupture and atrophy, joint sepsis and, rarely, nerve damage, transient paresis and needle fracture.

18.3.2 Systemic side effects

Systemic complications are rare[12]:
- Facial flushing is probably the most common systemic side effect, occurring in less than 1% of patients to 5%. It may appear within 24–48 hours after the injection and may last 1–2 days.[61,64,104]
- Deterioration of diabetic glycaemic control. Diabetic patients must be warned about this possible temporary side effect. A common observation is that blood sugar levels undergo a modest rise for up to a week, rarely longer. Where larger doses of corticosteroid than recommended here for single-site injection are given (or multiple sites are injected at one time, or over a few days), this may lead to a more prolonged (up to 3 weeks) elevation of blood sugar.

This may require a short-term increase in diabetic drug dosage, so the patient should be informed about the steroid drug and dosage given.[105–107]
- Uterine bleeding (pre- and postmenopausal) may occur. The exact mechanism is unknown but intra-articular steroid treatment causes a temporary, but considerable, suppression of sex steroid hormone secretion in women. In a postmenopausal woman postinjection uterine bleeding creates a difficult dilemma – is the bleeding related to the injection, or should she be investigated to exclude other, potentially serious, causes? If this complication occurs it must always be taken seriously.[108,109]
- Suppression of the hypothalamic–pituitary axis occurs following intra-articular and intramuscular injection of corticosteroids but at the low doses and frequencies described later this usually appears to be of no significant clinical consequence and we do not issue patients with a steroid card after injection. Rarely, however, systemic absorption of corticosteroid may evoke a secondary hypercortisolism similar to Cushing's syndrome.[110–114]
- Clinical improvement of distant joints in polyarthritis is an early clinical feature suggestive of significant systemic absorption of locally administered corticosteroid. This may account for the common observation of symptomatic improvement in joints other than the one injected (box 18.1).
- Significant falls in ESR and CRP levels (mean fall of about 50%). Intra-articular corticosteroid injections can cause this in patients with inflammatory arthritis and

BOX 18.1	**Suppression of the hypothalamic–pituitary axis by corticosteroid therapy**

Probably underrecognized
May occur with single or multiple injections within minimum of 5 weeks
Onset 10–14 days after injection

CLINICAL FEATURES

Moon face/buffalo hump
Acne-like eruptions/flushing
Palpitations/tremors
Dyspnoea/weight gain 5–8 kg
Disturbed menstruation

OUTCOME

Spontaneous resolution at 3 months (1 injection) and 6 months (2 injections)

TABLE 18.2	**Potential side effects of corticosteroid/local anaesthetic injection therapy**
Systemic side effects	**Local side effects**
Facial flushing	Postinjection flare of pain
Impaired diabetic control	Skin depigmentation, fat atrophy
Menstrual irregularity	Bleeding/bruising
Hypothalamic–pituitary axis suppression	Steroid 'chalk', calcification
Fall in erythrocyte sedimentation rate/C-reactive protein	Steroid arthropathy
Anaphylaxis (very rare)	Tendon rupture/atrophy Joint/soft-tissue infection

TABLE 18.3	**Numbers needed to harm patients > 60 prescribed oral non-steroidal anti-inflammatory drugs > 2 months**[53]
Number	**Harm caused**
1 in 5	Endoscopic ulcer
1 in 70	Symptomatic ulcer
1 in 150	Bleeding ulcer
1 in 1200	Die from bleeding ulcer

Reproduced from Tramer et al.[53]

this effect can last for up to 6 months. This needs to be taken into account when using these blood tests to assess the response of patients to disease-modifying drugs.[115]

- Anaphylaxis. Severe anaphylactic reactions to local anaesthetic injections are rare, but can be fatal. Anaphylactic reactions to corticosteroid injections are extremely rare and are probably a reaction to the stabilizers that the drug is mixed with, rather than the drug itself.[55,116,117]
- Other rare systemic side effects from local steroid injection include pancreatitis (patient presents with abdominal pain and the serum amylase is raised), nausea, dysphoria (emotional upset), acute psychosis, myopathy and posterior subcapsular cataracts. In patients with sickle-cell disease a crisis may be precipitated by intra-articular injection of corticosteroids; the mechanism is not clear, but it is suggested that this treatment be used with caution in these patients. Tibial stress fractures and multifocal osteonecrosis have been reported with systemic but not locally injected corticosteroids used for athletic injuries[47,49,110] (table 18.2).

Despite all the above, injection therapy for joints and soft tissues is a relatively safe form of treatment. Adverse events can be minimized by ensuring that well-trained practitioners follow appropriate procedures.

In a large prospective study of 1147 injections, complications of injection therapy were recorded in just under 12% of patients (7% of injections), but almost all of these were transient. Only four patients (with tennis elbow) had subcutaneous atrophy but the steroid dose was four times the one we recommend. The most common

side effect was postinjection pain, but methylprednisolone was used, which we believe can cause more pain than triamcinolone. Twelve per cent of periarticular injections caused postinjection pain, but only 2% of intra-articular injections were painful. Other side effects were bleeding and fainting or dizziness.[48]

It is safe to mix corticosteroids with local anaesthetics prior to injection. High-performance liquid chromatographic analysis to assess the stability of combinations of triamcinolone and hydrocortisone when mixed with combinations of lidocaine and bupivacaine shows that the combinations are stable when mixed together, supporting the continued use of these products in combination.

Compared with the safety profile of oral NSAIDs, the justification for using the minimum effective dose of injectable drugs in the correct place with appropriate preparation and aftercare becomes evident (table 18.3).

18.4 SAFETY

Adverse reactions to corticosteroid are extremely rare: the drug more likely to provoke serious reaction is local anaesthetic. Simple precautions should always be undertaken, such as checking whether the patient has suffered any previous adverse reactions to the drug and ensuring that a strict aseptic no-touch technique is employed every time an infiltration is carried out.

18.4.1 Immediate adverse reactions

The most important immediate adverse reactions to injection therapy are:
- acute anaphylaxis
- toxicity from local anaesthetic
- syncope.

18.4.1.1 Acute anaphylaxis

Patients who have an anaphylactic reaction have life-threatening airway and/or breathing and/or circulation problems usually associated with skin and mucosal changes.[124]

Acute systemic anaphylaxis results from widespread mast cell degranulation triggered by a specific allergen. Clinically, it is characterized by laryngeal oedema, bronchospasm and hypotension. The true incidence of anaphylaxis is unknown; fatal anaphylaxis is rare but probably underestimated. A register established in 1992 recording fatal reactions gave an incidence of only 20 cases a year in the UK, of which half were iatrogenic, mainly occurring in hospital; a quarter were related to food allergy, and a quarter were related to venom allergy.[119,120]

True allergic reactions to local anaesthetic occur very rarely and mainly with the ester-types, e.g. procaine, and less frequently with the amide types, e.g. lidocaine and bupivacaine. The pathomechanism of immediate hypersensitivity reactions to local anaesthetic is largely unknown and is commonly regarded as 'pseudo-allergic' or 'non-immune-type' anaphylaxis. Immunologically mediated reactions have rarely been observed with positive skin prick tests. A patient may be allergic to local anaesthetic and be unaware of it. Previous uneventful injection is not a guarantee the patient will not be allergic this time, though it does provide some reassurance.[121–123]

18.4.1.2 Recognition of an anaphylactic reaction

A diagnosis of anaphylactic reaction is likely if a patient who is exposed to a trigger (allergen) develops a sudden illness (usually within minutes of exposure) with rapidly progressing skin changes and life-threatening airway and/or breathing and/or circulation problems. The reaction is usually unexpected.[118]

Anaphylactic reactions begin rapidly. The time taken for a full reaction to evolve varies. In a fatal reaction following an intravenous drug injection or insect sting the interval between exposure and collapse from cardiovascular shock is usually 5–15 minutes. There are no data specifically relating to injection therapy.

The lack of any consistent clinical manifestation and a range of possible presentations cause diagnostic difficulty. Many patients with a genuine anaphylactic reaction are not given the correct treatment. Patients have been given injections of adrenaline inappropriately for allergic reactions just involving the skin, or for vasovagal reactions or panic attacks. Guidelines for the treatment of an anaphylactic reaction must therefore take into account some inevitable diagnostic errors, with an emphasis on the need for safety.[118]

TABLE 18.4   Features of anaphylaxis

Symptoms	Signs
Nervousness	Skin: blotches, urticaria, decreased capillary filling, clammy (cyanosis – late sign)
Feeling of impending catastrophe	Eyes: puffy, watering, red, sore
Feeling 'drunk' or confused	Nose: runny, sneezing
Metallic taste, difficulty swallowing	Lips/tongue/throat (angio-oedema) noisy breathing
Abdominal or back pain	Voice: stridor, difficulty talking, hoarse voice
Nausea, vomiting, incontinence	Chest: tachypnoea, wheezing, coughing
Itching	Pulse: tachycardia
Chest tightness	Blood pressure: profound hypotension
Difficulty breathing	Neurological: loss of consciousness, convulsions

A single set of criteria will not identify all anaphylactic reactions. There is a range of signs and symptoms, none of which are entirely specific; however, certain combinations of signs make the diagnosis more likely. Skin or mucosal changes alone are not a sign of an anaphylactic reaction; skin and mucosal changes may be subtle or absent in up to 20% of reactions.

The features of an allergic reaction may be any of those shown in table 18.4. Onset is usually abrupt; the patient feels and looks ill.

Circulatory collapse, cardiac arrest and death may follow.

18.4.1.3 Treatment of severe allergic reactions

Patients having an anaphylactic reaction should be recognized and treated using the airway, breathing, circulation, disability, exposure (ABCDE) approach and life-threatening problems treated as they are recognized.

The exact treatment will depend on the patient's location, the equipment and drugs available, and the skills of those treating the reaction. Clinicians give injection therapy in a variety of settings including hospitals with and without 'crash' teams, and various community premises, including primary care and private facilities. Every clinician must prepare for the 'worst-case scenario' in their setting and have a well-thought-out plan of action that is regularly reviewed in the light of current guidelines and individual experience. Basic life support skills

BOX 18.2 **Immediate action in the presence of severe anaphylaxis**

- Stop injecting
- Summon help
- Maintain airway
- Administer adrenaline intramuscularly
- Administer oxygen if necessary
- Give cardiopulmonary resuscitation if necessary
- Transfer the patient to hospital as quickly as possible if in the community

TABLE 18.5 **Features of local anaesthetic toxicity**

Symptoms	Signs
Lightheadedness	Sedation
Feeling drunk	Circumoral paraesthesia
	Twitching
	Convulsions in severe reactions

TABLE 18.6 **Features of Syncope**

Symptoms	Signs
Anxiety prior to the procedure	Apprehension
Lightheadedness, dizziness	Pallor
Tell you they are going to faint	Sweating
Nausea	Slight swaying
Ringing in the ears	Pulse: bradycardia
Vision 'going grey'	Blood pressure: hypotension

should be acquired and maintained. Written protocols may be laminated and mounted in consulting rooms[118] (box 18.2).

18.4.1.4 Adrenaline (epinephrine)

Adrenaline reverses the immediate symptoms of anaphylaxis by its effects on alpha and beta adrenoceptors. It reverses peripheral vasodilatation, reduces oedema, induces bronchodilatation, has positive inotropic and chronotropic effects on the myocardium and suppresses further mediator release. It may be harmful if given outside the context of life-threatening anaphylaxis.[124]

Death can occur after adrenaline overdose in the absence of anaphylaxis. Administering the doses recommended in our guidelines via the intramuscular route should avoid serious problems.[124]

18.4.1.5 Toxicity from local anaesthetic

Toxic effects from local anaesthetic are usually a result of excessive plasma concentrations. Care must be taken to avoid accidental intravascular injection. The main toxic effects are excitation of the central nervous system (CNS) followed by CNS depression[123] (table 18.5).

With intravenous injection, convulsions and cardiovascular collapse may occur rapidly.

Significant toxic reaction to local anaesthetic is very unlikely with dosages given here.

18.4.1.6 Syncope

A few people may faint, not as a reaction to what was injected, but to being injected – the result of pain or needle phobia. Patients who express apprehension before having an injection should lie down for the procedure; the clinician may be so intent upon placing the needle correctly that the warning features are missed. Unlike an anaphylactic reaction, which appears abruptly following the procedure, there are usually warning features before or during the procedure. There may be a history of fainting with previous invasive procedures, so do ask (table 18.6).

Syncope must be distinguished from an adverse drug reaction, and is treated by:

- reassuring patients that they will recover shortly
- lying them down in the recovery position
- protecting the airway and giving 35% oxygen if loss of consciousness occurs.

Syncope may be accompanied by brief jerking or stiffening of the limbs, and may be mistaken for a convulsion by the inexperienced. Distinguishing a simple faint from a fit is helped by the presence of precipitating factors (painful stimuli, fear), and other features described above. Incontinence is rare, and recovery of consciousness usually occurs within a minute.[123]

18.4.2 Prevention of adverse reactions

The clinician must be prepared for any adverse reaction. Take the following precautions:

- Ask the patient about any known allergies to drugs, especially local anaesthetic.
- If in doubt, use steroid alone or diluted with normal saline.
- Lie the patient on a treatment table for the procedure.

- Control the amount of local anaesthetic given (see guidelines).
- Always aspirate before injecting, to check that the needle is not in a blood vessel.
- Ask the patient to wait for 30 minutes after the injection.
- Anyone with a suspected anaphylactic reaction should be referred to an allergy specialist.

Adverse reactions to corticosteroid are extremely rare: the drug more likely to provoke serious reaction is local anaesthetic. Simple precautions should always be undertaken, such as checking whether the patient has suffered any previous adverse reactions to the drug and ensuring that a strict aseptic no-touch technique is employed every time an infiltration is carried out.[124,125]

18.5 INJECTION PROTOCOL

Giving injections is easy; it is selection of the suitable patient that is difficult. It is possible to learn how to administer injections in a weekend; diagnosis, however, takes a lifetime.

It is necessary to understand fully the information the patient is imparting in the history, to interpret clearly the signs and symptoms elicited in the examination and to eliminate the various differential diagnoses to arrive at a definitive diagnosis. Only in this way can one successfully achieve the desired result of selecting the patient who might respond to injection therapy. This, combined with an in-depth knowledge of functional anatomy, should enable the clinician to help relieve the many patients with pain from musculoskeletal lesions (box 18.3 and figure 18.1).

We suggest the use of Kenalog-40® (triamcinolone acetonide 40 mg/mL) throughout. This is a remarkably safe drug but any appropriate corticosteroid can be used. In our experience, Kenalog® gives less postinjection flare than Depo-Medrone®, particularly in soft tissues,

and is equally effective. Another advantage is that Kenalog® can be used in both small and large areas. Adcortyl® (triamcinolone acetonide 10 mg/mL) is useful where the total volume to be injected is over 5 mL; this allows greater volume for the same dose and avoids the need to dilute the local anaesthetic further with normal saline – useful when injecting hip or knee joints. Depo-Medrone® premixed with lidocaine is commonly used but it is more difficult to adjust doses for the individual lesion.

The effect of the corticosteroid does not usually kick in until about 48 hours after the injection, so patients should be warned that they may not see any relief of pain until then. There is great variation in this time lag, with some experiencing almost immediate improvement, others taking several days. The drug action continues for about 3–6 weeks.

In thin, dark-skinned patients hydrocortisone may be used, especially when injecting superficial soft-tissue lesions in order to avoid the potential risk of fat atrophy or depigmentation.

18.6 LOCAL ANAESTHETICS

We suggest the use of lidocaine hydrochloride but any suitable local anaesthetic can be used. Because of the risk of severe allergic reaction, the patient should be checked carefully for possible allergy to the drug before using any anaesthetic – previous dental work or skin stitches. Where any doubt exists, do not use it. Normal saline can be used to dilute the corticosteroid if necessary.

Lidocaine with adreanaline, which comes in ampoules or vials clearly marked in red, should not be used because of risk of ischaemic necrosis in appendages. Because of its potential half-life of 8 hours or more, we do not recommend the routine use of Marcain® but occasionally it can be used when a longer anaesthetic effect is needed. Some practitioners like to mix short- and long-acting anaesthetics to gain both the immediate diagnostic effect and the longer therapeutic effect.

18.7 DOSAGES

The corticosteroid doses suggested are what we use for the average-sized adult and are governed by the individual patient's age, size, general health and clinical history. These are guidelines only and none are 'cast in stone'; it is up to the clinician to decide on variants depending on individual preference and patient presentation.

BOX 18.3	Indications for corticosteroid injections, with or without local anaesthetic

- Acute and chronic bursitis
- Acute capsulitis
- Chronic tendinopathy
- Inflammatory arthritis
- Acute and chronic back pain and sciatica
- Nerve root entrapment

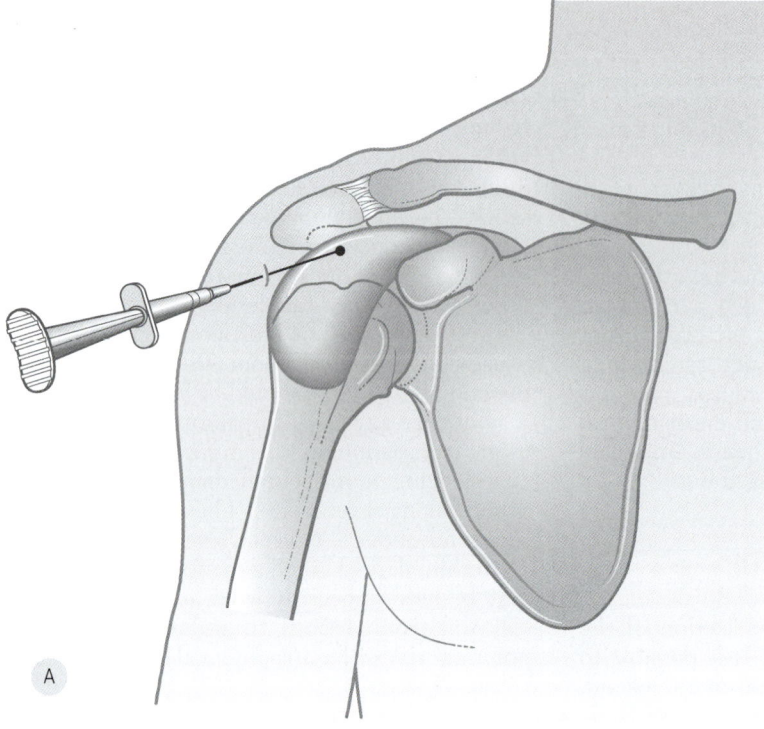

A

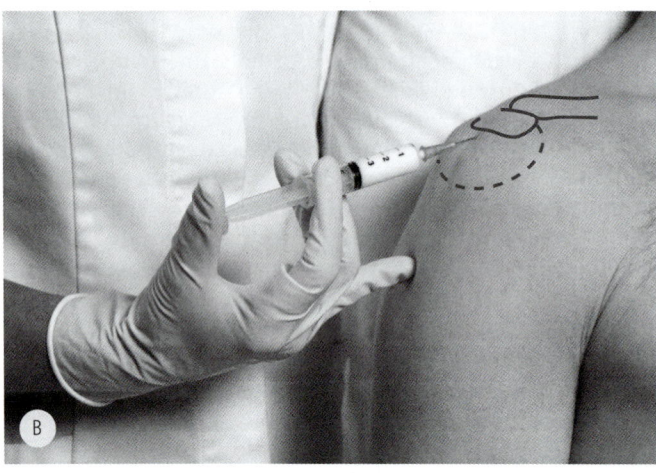

B

FIGURE 18.1 ◼ (A, B) Subacromial bursa injection. (Reproduced from: Saunders S, Longworth S. Injection Techniques in Musculoskeletal Medicine: A Practical Manual for Clinicians in Primary and Secondary Care, 4th edn. Edinburgh: Churchill Livingstone; 2011, with permission). (Colour version of figure is available online).

At all times, the minimum effective dose should be given; this will help prevent the appearance of adverse side effects such as facial flushing, intermenstrual bleeding, hyperglycaemia, skin atrophy and depigmentation.

It is important to keep within the recommended maximum doses of local anaesthetic in order to avoid toxicity. The maximum doses we suggest are half those published in pharmacological texts, so are well within safety limits (table 18.7).

In practice, this translates to the following:
- 2% lidocaine up to a maximum volume of 5 mL
- 1% lidocaine up to a maximum volume of 10 mL

- dilute 1% with normal saline (0.9%) for volumes larger than 5 mL.

KEY POINTS

It is important to keep within the recommended maximum doses of local anaesthetic in order to avoid toxicity.

18.8 VOLUMES

Joints and bursae appear to respond best when a sufficient volume of fluid to bathe the inflamed internal surfaces is introduced. Possibly the

TABLE 18.7 Local Anaesthetics: Suggested Maximum Doses

Drug	Strength	Maximum dose (1)	Suggested maximum
Lidocaine	0.5% 5 mg/mL	200 mg 40 mL	100 mg 20 mL
	1.0% 10 mg/mL	200 mg 20 mL	100 mg 10 mL
	2.0% 20 mg/mL	200 mg 10 mL	100 mg 5 mL
Bupivacaine	0.25% 2.5 mg/mL	150 mg 60 mL	
	0.5% 5 mg/mL	150 mg 30 mL	

TABLE 18.8 Joint injections: suggested average and total volumes

Joint	Dose	Volume
Shoulder	40 mg	5 mL
Elbow	30 mg	4 mL
Wrist	20 mg	2 mL
Thumb	10 mg	1 mL
Fingers	5 mg	0.5 mL
Hip	40 mg	5 mL
Knee	40 mg	5–10 mL
Ankle	30 mg	4 mL
Foot	20 mg	2 mL
Toes	10 mg	1 mL

slight distension 'splints' the structure, or maybe it breaks down or stretches out adhesions. In a small patient the amounts are decreased and in a large patient they may be increased. Greater volume can be obtained by using normal saline, and, especially in the case of the knee joint, where the synovial folds encompass a large total area, greater volume is always recommended in order to bathe all the inflamed surface.

The volumes suggested in table 18.8 are well within safety limits and will not cause the joint capsule to rupture; for instance, it is not unusual to aspirate over 100 mL of blood from an injured knee joint. In any case, the back pressure created by too large a volume would blow the syringe off the fine needle recommended, long before the capsule was compromised (table 18.8 and figure 18.2).

Conversely, tendons should have small volumes injected. This avoids painful distension of the structure and minimizes risk of rupture. An average 'recipe' for tendons is shown in box 18.4.

18.9 CONTRAINDICATIONS TO INJECTION

18.9.1 Absolute contraindications

On no account should an injection be performed in the following:
- hypersensitivity or allergy to any of the drugs used: risk of anaphylaxis
- sepsis: local or systemic: creates focus for microbes
- reluctant patient or no informed consent given: medicolegal factors
- children under 18 (except juvenile arthritis): children usually heal well
- recent fracture site: delays bone formation
- prosthetic joint: risk of infection
- gut feeling: when in doubt, do not inject.

18.9.2 Relative contraindications

Injections should be undertaken only if the extra risk is merited with:
- bleeding risks: anticoagulant therapy: but no good evidence of increased bleeding risk
- haemarthrosis: but this is disputed. Pain relief from aspiration can be dramatic
- diabetes: greater risk of sepsis; blood sugar levels may rise for a few days
- immunosuppressed: by disease, e.g. leukaemia, or drugs, e.g. systemic steroids
- large tendinopathies: e.g. Achilles, infrapatellar tendon (image first)
- pregnancy: medicolegal factors
- psychogenic pain: pain may be perceived to be aggravated.

18.10 PREPARATION PROTOCOL

18.10.1 Prepare patient

- Take history and examine patient.
- Check for absolute or relative contraindications.
- Discuss all treatment options, injection procedure and possible side effects.
- Obtain informed consent and record this.
- Place in comfortable supported position with injection site accessible.

18.10.2 Select drugs

- Decide on total volume based on size of structure.
- Choose dose of drug/s; use minimal effective amount.

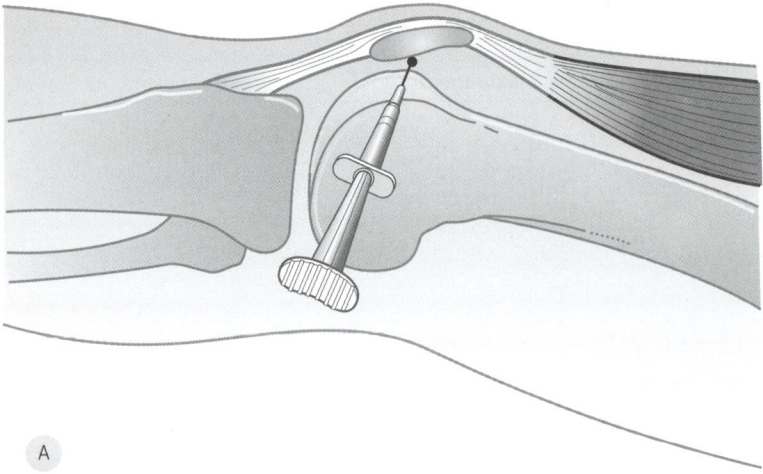

A

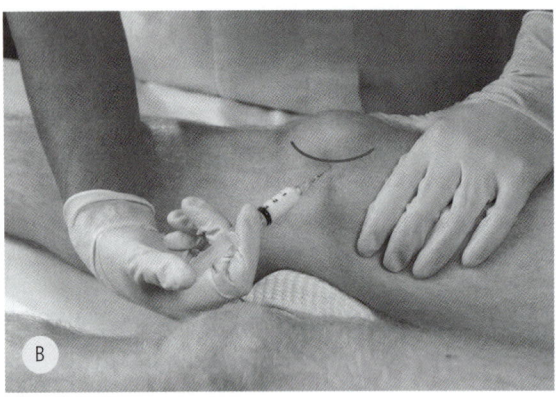

B

FIGURE 18.2 ■ (A, B) Knee joint injection. (Reproduced from Saunders S, Longworth S. Injection Techniques in Musculoskeletal Medicine: A Practical Manual for Clinicians in Primary and Secondary Care, 4th edn. Edinburgh: Churchill Livingstone; 2011, with permission). (Colour version of figure is available online).

> **BOX 18.4** **Tendon injections: suggested average doses and volumes**
>
> - Small tendons: 10 mg of steroid plus local in a total volume of 1 mL
> - Large tendons: 20 mg of steroid plus local in a total volume of 2 mL

- Select corticosteroid and/or single-use local anaesthetic ampoules.
- Check names, strengths and expiry dates.

18.10.3 Assemble equipment

- Appropriate-size in-date sterile syringe.
- Sterile in-date green 21G needle for drawing up.
- Sterile in-date needle of correct length for infiltrating.
- Alcohol swab or iodine skin preparation.
- Cotton wool/gauze and skin plaster – check for allergy.

- Waste bin and sharps box.
- Spare syringe and sterile container if aspiration likely.

18.10.4 Prepare site

- Identify structure and stretch skin strongly between finger and thumb.
- Mark injection site with end of fresh needle cap, then discard.
- Clean skin with suitable preparation in an outward spiral motion.

18.10.5 Prepare injection

- Wash hands with cleanser for 1 minute and dry well with paper towel. Open vial/s and ampoule/s.
- Attach green 21G needle to appropriate-sized syringe.
- Draw up accurate dose of steroid.
- Draw up accurate dose of local anaesthetic if used.
- Discard needle in sharps box.

- Attach needle of correct length firmly to syringe.
- Take loaded syringe and fresh swab to patient.

18.11 INJECTION TECHNIQUE FLOWCHART

Use no-touch technique throughout.

KEY POINTS

Stretch skin strongly both sides of cleansed site

↓

Stabilize injecting hand with needle perpendicular just above skin

↓

Rapidly insert needle short distance through skin

↓

Angle needle slowly and gently towards lesion – do not hit bone

↓

Attempt to aspirate

↓

Inject solution as bolus for joints/bursae; pepper injection for entheses

↓

Withdraw needle rapidly while pressing skin around needle with swab

↓

Get patient to press on swab

↓

Immediately discard syringe and needle into sharps box

↓

Apply plaster unless the patient is allergic

↓

Record drug names, doses, batch numbers and expiry dates, advice and warnings given

↓

Reassess patient and record results

↓

Ensure patient waits for 30 minutes after injection

18.12 FOLLOW-UP

Most injection studies show that injections give demonstrable relief in the short term but there is not much difference from other treatments or no treatment at all in the long term. It is essential, therefore, to address the causes of the pain once the symptoms of pain or paraesthesia have been relieved by the injection. Recurrence of symptoms is common in bursitis and tendinopathy, so appropriate advice on prevention is a vital part of the care package.

The ideal outcome is total relief of pain with normal power and full range of motion. This does not always occur but when local anaesthetic is used there should be significant immediate improvement to encourage both patient and clinician that the correct diagnosis has been made, and the injection accurately placed.

The patient should be told that the relief of pain might be temporary, depending on the strength and type of anaesthetic used, and the pain may return when this effect wears off. Some patients describe this pain as greater than their original pain. This might be due to the flare effect of the cortisone, which is thought to be caused by microcrystal deposition, or because of poor injection technique where the needle has been rammed into bone, but it is also possible that pain that comes back after some relief might appear to be worse. Any afterpain is usually transient and can be eased by application of ice or taking simple analgesia.

The anti-inflammatory effect of the corticosteroid is not usually apparent until about 48 hours after the infiltration and can continue for 3 weeks to 2 months, depending on the drug used, so patients should maximize the drug action during this period by avoiding aggravating activities.

Arrange to review the patient about a week or 10 days later. If the pain is severe or begins to return, as occurs commonly in acute capsulitis of the shoulder, see that patients know that they can return for a further injection if necessary within this period.

KEY POINTS

The anti-inflammatory effect of the corticosteroid is not usually apparent until about 48 hours after the infiltration.

Advise the patient on what to do and what to avoid in the intervening period. Joint conditions usually benefit from a programme of early gentle movement within the pain-free range; studies have shown that 24 hours' complete bed rest after a knee injection for inflammatory arthritis is beneficial but in the case of the wrist immobilization does not appear to improve outcome and might even worsen it. Overuse conditions in tendons and bursae require relative rest; this means that normal activities of daily living can be followed, provided they are not too painful, but return to sport or strenuous repetitive activity should be postponed until the patient is as painfree as possible.

When the symptoms have been relieved, most patients will need a few sessions of treatment for rehabilitation and prevention of recurrence. This is particularly relevant in overuse conditions and might involve correction of posture, ergonomic advice, adaptation of movement patterns, mobilization or manipulation, deep friction massage, stretching and/or strengthening regimes. The advice of a professional sports coach or of an expert in orthotics might also be required.

18.13 CLINICAL CASE

18.13.1 Patient with shoulder pain

A 65-year-old active woman, keen on gardening, decided to prune a 5-metre tree at the end of her garden; she climbed up as high as possible and, using a long cutting pole, spent over 2 hours cutting back long branches above her head.

Two days later she noticed an ache in her left deltoid area. Although she is right-handed, she was holding the pole aloft with her left arm and using her right hand for the cutting action for the duration of the exercise. She expected the ache to go away, but it gradually increased, and after about a week was interfering with her daily activities. There was no pain at rest; she would wake if she slept on her left side, and reaching above her head, out sideways, and behind her back caused the shoulder to hurt at about 6–8 out of 10 on a visual analogue scale.

Three weeks after the pruning episode she decided to seek professional help and consulted a chartered physiotherapist skilled in performing injections for musculoskeletal pain.

18.13.1.1 Examination

The patient presented with pain on active elevation and abduction with a small painful arc, and with some pain on passive lateral rotation but more on passive medial rotation. The painful resisted tests were abduction with weakness, lateral rotation and also slight pain on resisted extension of the elbow.

18.13.1.2 Differential diagnosis

Local causes
- Capsulitis of the glenohumeral joint, as she is female and there was pain on active and passive flexion and passive lateral rotation.

There will of course be some osteoarthritis present due to the patient's age.
- However, the history was not consistent with an acute flare of the joint, there was more pain on passive medial rotation than lateral, and also some resisted tests hurt which did not fit in with the relatively low level of pain.
- Overuse tendinopathy or cuff tear, as the history could indicate this and she presented with pain on three resisted tests – abduction, lateral rotation and elbow extension. This could imply a lesion in the supraspinatus, infraspinatus or triceps – or, indeed, all three tendons.
- However, there was no sudden pain indicating a cuff tear and the triceps is rarely affected, especially at its origin.
- Bursitis of any of the many bursae around the shoulder, particularly the subacromial bursa, as the position of holding the left arm in an elevated position for this length of time could cause impingement of this structure.
- However, there was a complex picture arising from both the history and the examination, so other causes should be considered.
- Haemorrhagic bursitis, but there was no history of trauma and no heat or swelling around the acromion.
- Infection, such as tuberculosis, which is on the increase in the UK, but there was no sign of pyrexia or local heat around the joint.

Referred causes
- Cervical pathology – such as disc lesion, thoracic outlet syndrome, cervical zygaphophyseal joint degeneration or serious bone or lung disease. However, there was no acute neck or arm pain and no paraesthesia and cervical examination was painless with range, which was consistent with the patient's age. There were no red flags indicating serious pathology.

Systemic causes
- Rheumatoid arthritis, gout or pseudogout can all cause shoulder pain, but there was no familial history of these diseases and no other joints were affected. Blood tests for ESR, CRP and uric acid could prove the absence of these potential diagnoses.

Psychosocial causes
- The patient appeared relaxed and there were no inappropriate verbal or physical

reactions to questioning and physical examination.

After considering the above differential diagnoses, it was concluded that the most likely cause of pain was impingement of the subabcromial bursa. The 'muddle' of signs – some passive and some resisted causing symptoms, and the history of overuse – indicated that impingement of the bursa under the acromial arch had occurred. The positive triceps test was not caused by irritation of the tendon but was because of pressure on the bursa by the upward shift of the humerus.

18.13.1.3 Treatment

The diagnosis of subacromial bursitis was explained to the patient using anatomical aids, and various ways of treating it were discussed. The options were to try rest, physiotherapeutic methods such as mobilization, stretching and postural correction, oral anti-inflammatory medication (NSAIDs) or injection of a corticosteroid into the inflamed space.

The patient had tried rest and was anxious to get back to her normal very active life. The evidence for physiotherapeutic intervention for this lesion in the acute stage is poor, and certainly exercise routines would most probably further inflame the bursa. Due to the patient's age, long-term use of NSAIDs was inadvisable because of the established risk of gastric bleeding. She therefore decided that she would undergo subacromial injection into the bursa.

Absolute contraindications – known allergy to the drugs or any infection present – were eliminated and the potential risks of infection or flare were clarified. The patient gave her consent.

The injection consisted of 40 mg triamcinolone acetonide and 4 mL of 1% lidocaine given under sterile conditions. The patient reported minimal discomfort during the injection. Repeat testing of passive flexion and medial rotation, plus resisted testing of abduction and lateral rotation of the shoulder, showed pain was reduced from 7/10 to 2/10 with no evidence of weakness.

Advice on erect posture was given and the patient was instructed to refrain from lifting her left arm above shoulder level for 10 days. The shoulder was taped into a depressed and laterally rotated position with recommendation to keep this on for about 4 days (using clingfilm to cover the tape when showering). She was advised that the effect of the anaesthetic would last about an hour, but the cortisone would probably take about 2–3 days to kick in.

The patient returned for follow-up 10 days later and reported no pain on sleeping or movement after a couple of days. She was then given retraction exercises to encourage more space under the subacromial arch and the importance of good posture, especially when sitting at the computer, was reinforced. She was also told to moderate her gardening activities!

(Clinical case continued on page 493)

18.14 REFERENCES

1. Saunders S, Longworth S. Injection techniques in musculoskeletal medicine. 4th ed. London: Elsevier; 2011.
2. Goulding NJ. Corticosteroids – a case of mistaken identity? Br J Rheumatol 1998;37(5):477–80.
3. Coombes GM, Bax DE. The use and abuse of steroids in rheumatology. Reports on the Rheumatic Diseases (Series 3). Practical Problems (No. 8) 1996.
4. Creamer P. Intra-articular corticosteroid injections in osteoarthritis: do they work, and if so, how? Ann Rheum Dis 1997;56(11):634–6.
5. af Klint E, Grundtman C, Engström M, et al. Intraarticular glucocorticoid treatment reduces inflammation in synovial cell infiltrations more efficiently than in synovial blood vessels. Arthritis Rheum 2005;52(12):3880–9.
6. Goulding NJ. Anti-inflammatory corticosteroids. Reports on the Rheumatic Diseases (Series 3). Topical Reviews (No. 18) 1999.
7. Cutolo M. The roles of steroid hormones in arthritis. Br J Rheumatol 1998;37(6):597–9.
8. Kirwan JR, Balint G, Szebenyi B. Anniversary: 50 years of glucocorticoid treatment in rheumatoid arthritis. Rheumatology (Oxford) 1999;38(2):100–2.
9. Hollander JL, Brown EM, Jester RA, et al. Hydrocortisone and cortisone injected into arthritic joints; comparative effects of a use of hydrocortisone as a local anti-arthritis agent. J Am Med Assoc 1951;147(17):1629–35.
10. Speed CA. Injection therapies for soft-tissue lesions. Best Pract Res Clin Rheumatol 2007;21(2):333–47.
11. Ines LPBS, da Silva JAP. Soft tissue injections. Best Pract Res Clin Rheumatol 2005 Jun;19(3):503–27.
12. Cole BJ, Schumacher HR. Injectable corticosteroids in modern practice. J Am Acad Orthop Surg 2005;139(1):37–46.
13. Anon. Gout in primary care. Drugs and Therapeutics Bulletin 2004;42(5):39.
14. Gossec L, Dougados M. Intra-articular treatments in osteoarthritis: from the symptomatic to the structure modifying. Ann Rheum Dis 2004;63(5):478–82.
15. Kirwan JR, Rankin E. Intraarticular therapy in osteoarthritis. Baillieres Clin Rheumatol 1997;11(4):769–94.
16. Franz JK, Burmester G-R. Antirheumatic treatment: The needle and the damage done. Ann Rheum Dis 2005;64(6):798–800.
17. Jones A, Doherty M. Intra-articular corticosteroid injections are effective in OA but there are no clinical predictors of response. Ann Rheum Dis 1996;55(11):829–32.
18. Brandt KD, Radin EL, Dieppe PA, et al. Yet more evidence that osteoarthritis is not a cartilage disease. Ann Rheum Dis 2006;65(10):1261–4.
19. Dorman T, Ravin T. Diagnosis and injection techniques in orthopaedic medicine. Baltimore, Maryland: Williams and Wilkins; 1991. p. 33–4.

20. Daley CT, Stanish WD. Soft tissue injuries: overuse syndromes. In: Bull RC, editor. Handbook of sports injuries. New York: McGraw Hill; 1998. p. 185.
21. Weitoft T, Larsson A, Ronnblom L. Serum levels of sex steroid hormones and matrix metalloproteinases after intra-articular glucocorticoid treatment in female patients with rheumatoid arthritis. Ann Rheum Dis 2008;67(3):422–4.
22. Verbruggen G. Chondroprotective drugs in degenerative joint diseases. Rheumatology 2006;45(2):129–38.
23. Weitoft T, Larsson A, Saxne T, et al. Changes of cartilage and bone markers after intra-articular glucocorticoid treatment with and without post-injection rest in patients with rheumatoid arthritis. Ann Rheum Dis 2005;64(12):1750–3.
24. Larsson E, Harris HE, Larsson A. Corticosteroid treatment of experimental arthritis retards cartilage destruction as determined by histology and serum COMP. Rheumatology 2004;43(4):428–34.
25. Raynauld JP. Clinical trials: impact of intra-articular steroid injections on the progression of knee osteoarthritis. Osteoarthritis Cartilage 1999;7(3):348–9.
26. Hills BA, Ethell MT, Hodgson DR. Release of lubricating synovial surfactant by intra-articular steroid. Br J Rheumatol 1998;37(6):649–52.
27. Pelletier JP, Mineau F, Raynauld JP, et al. Intraarticular injections with methylprednisolone acetate reduce osteoarthritic lesions in parallel with chondrocyte stromelysin synthesis in experimental osteoarthritis. Arthritis Rheum 1994;37(3):414–23.
28. Jubb RW. Anti-rheumatic drugs and articular cartilage. Reports on the Rheumatic Diseases (Series 2). Topical Reviews (No. 20) 1992.
29. Pelletier JP, Pelletier JM. Proteoglycan degrading metalloprotease activity in human osteoarthritis cartilage and the effect of intraarticular steroid injections. Arthritis Rheum 1987;30(5):541–8.
30. Scott A, Khan KM, Cook JL, et al. What is 'inflammation'? Are we ready to move beyond Celsus? Br J Sports Med 2004;38(3):248–9.
31. Khan KM, Cook JL, Kannus P, et al. Time to abandon the 'tendinitis' myth. BMJ 2002;324(7338):626–7.
32. Khan KM, Cook JL, Maffulli N, et al. Where is the pain coming from in tendinopathy? It may be biochemical, not structural in origin. Br J Sports Med 2000;34(2):81–3.
33. Gotoh M, Hamada K, Yamakawa H, et al. Increased substance P in subacromial bursa and shoulder pain in rotator cuff disease. J Orthop Res 1998;16(5):618–21.
34. Johansson A, Hao J, Sjölund B. Local corticosteroid application blocks transmission in normal nociceptive C-fibres. Acta Anaesthesiol Scand 1990;34(5):335–8.
35. Derendorf H, Mollmann H, Gruner A, et al. Pharmacokinetics and pharmacodynamics of glucocorticoid suspensions after intra-articular administration. Clin Pharmacol Ther 1986;39(3):313–17.
36. Caldwell JR. Intra-articular corticosteroids: guide to selection and indications for use. Drugs 1996;52:507–14.
37. Piotrowski M, Szczepanski I, Dmoszynska M. Treatment of rheumatic conditions with local instillation of betamethasone and methylprednisolone: comparison of efficacy and frequency of irritative pain reaction. Rheumatologia 1998;36:78–84.
38. British National Formulary No 59. Section 15.2 BMA/RPSGB, London 2010.
39. Kannus P, Jarvinen M, Niittymaki S. Long- or short-acting anesthetic with corticosteroid in local injections of overuse injuries? A prospective, randomized, double-blind study. Int J Sports Med 1990;11(5):397–400.
40. Solvebörn S, Buch F, Mallmin H, et al. Cortisone injection with anaesthetic additives for radial epicondylalgia. Clin Orthop Relat Res 1995;316:99–105.
41. Buchbinder R, Green S, Forbes A, et al. Arthrographic joint distension with saline and steroid improves function and reduces pain in patients with painful stiff shoulder: results of a randomised, double blind, placebo controlled trial. Ann Rheum Dis 2004;63(3):302–9.
42. Gam A, Schydlowsky P, Rossel I, et al. Treatment of 'frozen shoulder' with distension and glucorticoid compared with glucorticoid alone: a randomised controlled trial. Scand J Rheumatol 1998;27(6):425–30.
43. Mulcahy KA, Baxter AD, Oni OOA, et al. The value of shoulder distension arthrography with intra-articular injection of steroid and local anaesthetic: a follow-up study. Br J Radiol 1994;67(795):263–6.
44. Jacobs LGH, Barton MAJ, Wallace WA, et al. Intra-articular distension and steroids in the management of capsulitis of the shoulder. BMJ 1991;302(6791):1498–501.
45. Creamer P, Hunt M, Dieppe P. Pain mechanisms in osteoarthritis of the knee: effect of intra-articular anesthetic. J Rheumatol 1996;23(6):1031–6.
46. Habib GS, Saliba W, Nashashibi M. Local effects of intra-articular corticosteroids. Clin Rheumatol 2010;29(4):347–56.
47. Nichols AW. Complications associated with the use of corticosteroids in the treatment of athletic injuries. Clin J Sport Med 2005;15(5):370–5.
48. Kumar N, Newman R. Complications of intra- and peri-articular steroid injections. Br J Gen Pract 1999;49(443):465–6.
49. Dando P, Green S, Price J. Problems in general practice – minor surgery. London: The Medical Defence Union; 1997.
50. Avci S, Yilmaz C, Sayli U. Comparison of nonsurgical treatment measures for de Quervain's disease of pregnancy and lactation. J Hand Surg Am 2002;27(2):322–4.
51. Wallace WA. (letter). Br Med J 2000;320.
52. Lanyon P, Regan M, Jones A, et al. Inadvertent intra-articular injection of the wrong substance. Br J Rheumatol 1997;36(7):812–13.
53. Tramer MR, Moore RA, Reynolds JM, et al. Quantitative estimation of rare adverse events which follow a biological progression: a new model applied to chronic NSAID use. Pain 2000;85:169–82.
54. Berger RG, Yount WJ. Immediate 'steroid flare' from intra-articular triamcinolone hexacetonide injection: case report and review of the literature. Arthritis Rheum 1990;33(8):1284–6.
55. Pullar T. Routes of drug administration: intra-articular route. Prescr J 1998;38:123–6.
56. Helliwell PS. Use of an objective measure of articular stiffness to record changes in finger joints after intra-articular injection of corticosteroid. Ann Rheum Dis 1997;56(1):71–3.
57. Gaujoux-Viala C, Dougados M, Gossec L. Efficacy and safety of steroid injections for shoulder and elbow tendonitis: a meta-analysis of randomised controlled trials. Ann Rheum Dis 2009;68(12):1843–9.
58. Cassidy JT, Bole GG. Cutaneous atrophy secondary to intra-articular corticosteroid administration. Ann Intern Med 1966;65(5):1008–18.
59. Basadonna PT, Rucco V, Gasparini D, et al. Plantar fat pad atrophy after corticosteroid injection for an interdigital neuroma: a case report. Am J Phys Med Rehabil 1999;78(3):283–5.
60. Reddy PD, Zelicof SB, Ruotolo C, et al. Interdigital neuroma. Local cutaneous changes after corticosteroid injection. Clin Orthop Relat Res 1995;317:185–7.

61. Gray RG, Gottlieb NL. Basic science and pathology: intra-articular corticosteroids, an updated assessment. Clin Orthop Relat Res 1983;177:235–63.

62. Gray RG, Tenenbaum J, Gottlieb NL. Local corticosteroid injection therapy in rheumatic disorders. Semin Arthritis Rheum 1981;10(4):231–54.

63. Cameron G. Steroid arthropathy: myth or reality? J Orth Med 1995;17(2):51–5.

64. British National Formulary No 59 Section 10.1.2.2. London: BMA/RPSGB; 2010.

65. Cooper C, Kirwan JR. The risks of local and systemic corticosteroid administration. Baillieres Clin Rheumatol 1990;4(2):305–32.

66. Raynauld J, Buckland-Wright C, Ward R, et al. Safety and efficacy of long term intraarticular steroid injections in osteoarthritis of the knee. Arthritis Rheum 2003;48(2):370–7.

67. Roberts WN, Babcock EA, Breitbach SA, et al. Corticosteroid injection in rheumatoid arthritis does not increase rate of total joint arthroplasty. J Rheumatol 1996;23(6):1001–4.

68. Smith AG, Kosygan K, Williams H, et al. Common extensor tendon rupture following corticosteroid injection for lateral tendinosis of the elbow. Br J Sports Med 1999;33(6):423–5.

69. Shrier I, Gordon O. Achilles tendon: are corticosteroid injections useful or harmful? Clin J Sport Med 1996; 6(4):245–50.

70. Mahler F, Fritsch YD. Partial and complete ruptures of the Achilles tendon and local corticosteroid injections. Br J Sports Med 1992;26(1):7–14.

71. Saxena A, Fullem B. Plantar Fascia Ruptures in Athletes. Am J Sports Med 2004;32(3):662–5.

72. Acevedo JI, Beskin JL. Complications of plantar fascia rupture associated with corticosteroid injection. Foot Ankle Int 1998;19(2):91–7.

73. Fredberg U. Local corticosteroid injection in sport: review of literature and guidelines for treatment. Scand J Med Sci Sports 1997;7(3):131–9.

74. Cyriax JH, Cyriax PJ. Principles of treatment. In: Illustrated manual of orthopaedic medicine. Oxford: Butterworths; 1983. p. 22.

75. McWhorter JW, Francis RS, Heckmann RA. Influence of local steroid injections on traumatized tendon properties; a biomechanical and histological study. Am J Sports Med 1991;19(5):435–9.

76. Read MTF. Safe relief of rest pain that eases with activity in achillodynia by intrabursal or peritendinous steroid injection: the rupture rate was not increased by these steroid injections. Sports Med 1999;33(2):134–5.

77. Mair SD, Isbell WM, Gill TJ, et al. Triceps tendon ruptures in professional football players. Am J Sports Med 2004;32(2):431–4.

78. Mottram DR, editor. Drugs in sport. 2nd ed. London: E & FN Spon; 1996.

79. Gill SS, Gelbke MK, Matson SL, et al. Fluoroscopically guided low-volume peritendinous corticosteroid injection for Achilles tendinopathy; a safety study. J Bone Joint Surg Am 2004;86-A(4):802–6.

80. Hugate R, Pennypacker J, Saunders M, et al. The effects of intratendinous and retrocalcaneal intrabursal injections of corticosteroid on the biomechanical properties of rabbit Achilles tendons. J Bone Joint Surg Am 2004;86-A(4):794–801.

81. Paavola M, Orava S, Leppilahti J, et al. Chronic Achilles tendon overuse injury: complications after surgical treatment. An analysis of 432 consecutive patients. Am J Sports Med 2000;28(1):77–82.

82. Wiggins ME, Fadale PD, Ehrlich MG, et al. Effects of local injection of corticosteroids on the healing of ligaments; a follow-up report (A). J Bone Joint Surg Am 1995;77(11):1682–91.

83. Hughes RA. Septic arthritis. Reports on the Rheumatic Diseases (Series 3). Practical Problems (No. 7) 1996;1.

84. Yangco BG, Germain BF, Deresinski SC. Case report: Fatal gas gangrene following intra-articular steroid injection. Am J Med Sci 1982;283(2):94–8.

85. Charalambous CP, Tryfonidis M, Sadiq S, et al. Septic arthritis following intra-articular glucocorticoid injection of the knee – a survey of current practice regarding antiseptic technique used during intra-articular glucocorticoid injection of the knee. Clin Rheumatol 2003; 22(6):386–90.

86. Seror P, Pluvinage P, Lecoq F, et al. Frequency of sepsis after local corticosteroid injection (an inquiry on 1,160,000 injections in rheumatological private practice in France). Rheumatology 1999;38:1272–4.

87. Grayson M. Three infected injections from the same organism. Br J Rheumatol 1998;37(5):592–3.

88. Jawed S, Allard SA. Osteomyelitis of the humerus following steroid injections for tennis elbow. Rheumatology 2000;39:923–4 (Letter).

89. von Essen R, Savolainen HA. Bacterial infection following intra-articular injection. Scand J Rheumatol 1989;18(1):7–12.

90. Kirschke DL, Jones TF, Stratton CW, et al. Outbreak of joint and soft-tissue infections associated with injections from a multiple-dose medication vial. Clin Infect Dis 2003;36(11):1369–73.

91. Chustecka Z. Intra-articular injections may introduce skin into affected joint. Rheumawire; Available online at: <www.jointandbone.org>; 2001.

92. Gardner GC, Weisman MH. Pyarthrosis in patient with rheumatoid arthritis; a report of 13 cases and a review of the literature from the past 40 years. Am J Med 1990;88(5):503–11.

93. Knight DJ, Gilbert FJ, Hutchison JD. Lesson of the week: septic arthritis in osteoarthritic hips. BMJ 1996; 313(7048):40–1.

94. Ryan MJ, Kavanagh R, Wall PG, et al. Bacterial joint infections in England and Wales: analysis of bacterial isolates over a four year period. Br J Rheumatol 1997; 36(3):370–3.

95. Ostensson A, Geborek P. Septic arthritis as a nonsurgical complication in rheumatoid arthritis: relation to disease severity and therapy. Br J Rheumatol 1991; 30(1):35–8.

96. Gosal HS, Jackson AM, Bickerstaff DR. Intra-articular steroids after arthroscopy for osteoarthritis of the knee. J Bone Joint Surg Br 1999;81(6):952–4.

97. Papavasiliou AV, Isaac DL, Marimuthu R, et al. Infection in knee replacements after previous injection of intra-articular steroid. J Bone Joint Surg Br 2006;88(3):321–3.

98. Kaspar S, de Beer JV. Infection in hip arthroplasty after previous injection of steroid. J Bone Joint Surg Br 2005;87(4):454–7.

99. Chitre AR, Fehily MJ, Bamford DJ. Total hip replacement after intra-articular injection of local anaesthetic and steroid. J Bone Joint Surg Br 2007;89(2):166–8.

100. Pang H-N, Lo N-N, Yang K-Y, et al. Peri-articular steroid injection improves the outcome after unicondylar knee replacement. J Bone Joint Surg Br 2008;90(6):738–44.

101. Wang J-J, Ho S-T, Lee S-C, et al. Intra-articular triamcinolone acetonide for pain control after arthroscopic knee surgery. Anesth Analg 1998;87:1113–16.

102. Lane SE, Merry P. Intra-articular corticosteroids in septic arthritis: beneficial or barmy? Ann Rheum Dis 2000;59(3):240.

103. Pal B, Morris J. Perceived risks of joint infection following intra-articular corticosteroid injections: a survey of rheumatologists. Clin Rheumatol 1999;18(3):264–5.

104. Anon. Articular and periarticular corticosteroid injection. Drug Ther Bull 1995;33(9):67–70.

105. Black DM, Filak AT. Hyperglycemia with non-insulin-dependent diabetes following intra-articular steroid injection. J Fam Pract 1989;28(4):462–3.

106. Younis M, Neffati F, Touzi M, et al. Systemic effects of epidural and intra-articular glucocorticoid injections in diabetic and non-diabetic patients. Joint Bone Spine 2007;74(5):472–6.

107. Wang AA, Hutchinson DT. The effect of corticosteroid injection for trigger finger on blood glucose level in diabetic patients. J Hand Surg [Am] 2006;31(6):979–81.

108. Mens JMA, De Wolf AN, Berkhout BJ, et al. Disturbance of the menstrual pattern after local injection with triamcinolone acetonide. Ann Rheum Dis 1998;57(11):700.

109. Weitoft T, Larsson A, Ronnblom L. Serum levels of sex steroid hormones and matrix metalloproteinases after intra-articular glucocorticoid treatment in female patients with rheumatoid arthritis. Ann Rheum Dis 2008;67(3):422–4.

110. van Tuyl SAC, Slee PH. Are the effects of local glucocorticoid treatment only local? Neth J Med 2002;60(3):130–2.

111. Lazarevic MB, Skosey JL, Djordjevic-Denic G. Reduction of cortisol levels after single intra-articular and intramuscular steroid injection. Am J Med 1995;99(4):370–3.

112. British National Formulary No 59 Section 6.3.2. London: BMA/RPSGB; 2010.

113. Weitoft T, Rönnblom L. Glucocorticoid resorption and influence on the hypothalamic-pituitary-adrenal axis after intra-articular treatment of the knee in resting and mobile patients. Ann Rheum Dis 2006;65(7):955–7.

114. Kumar S, Singh RJ, Reed AM, et al. Cushing's syndrome after intra-articular and intradermal administration of triamcinolone acetonide in three pediatric patients. Pediatrics 2004;113(6):1820–4.

115. Taylor HG, Fowler PD, David MJ, et al. Intra-articular steroids: confounder of clinical trials. Clin Rheumatol 1991;10(1):38–42.

116. Ewan PW. Anaphylaxis (ABC of allergies). BMJ 1998;316(7142):1442–5.

117. Beaudouin E, Kanny G, Gueant JL, et al. Anaphylaxis caused by carboxymethylcellulose: report of 2 cases of shock from injectable corticoids. Allerg Immunol (Paris) 1992;24(9):333–5.

118. Working Group of the Resuscitation Council (UK). Emergency treatment of anaphylactic reactions. Guidelines for healthcare providers. Available online at: <www.resus.org.uk/pages/reaction.pdf>; 2008 [Accessed 16 Jan 2014].

119. Johnston SL, Unsworth J. Clinical review; Lesson of the week. Adrenaline given outside the context of life threatening allergic reactions. BMJ 2003;326(7389):589–90.

120. Pumphrey RSH. Lessons for management of anaphylaxis from a study of fatal reactions. Clin Exp Allergy 2000;30:1144–50.

121. Gall H, Kaufmann R, Kalveram CM. Adverse reactions to local anesthetics: analysis of 197 cases. J Allergy Clin Immunol 1996;97(4):933–7.

122. British National Formulary No 59. London: BMA/RPSGB; 2012. p. 766.

123. Ring J, Franz R, Brockow K. Anaphylactic reactions to local anesthetics. Chem Immunol Allergy 2010;95:190–200.

124. Sander JWAS, O'Donaghue MF. Epilepsy: getting the diagnosis right. BMJ 1997;314(7075):158–9.

125. Snashall D. ABC of work related disorders. Occupational infections. BMJ 1996;313(7056):551–4.

PART X

HIGH-VOLUME IMAGE-GUIDED INJECTIONS

CHAPTER 19

HIGH-VOLUME IMAGE-GUIDED INJECTIONS

Henning Langberg • Peter Malliaras • Dylan Morrissey • Otto Chan • Morten Boesen • Anders Boesen

All truths are easy to understand once they are discovered; the point is to discover them.

GALILEO GALILEI

KEYWORDS

high-volume injection; Achilles tendinopathy; hydrodilatation; image ultrasound guidance; high-volume image-guided injection procedure.

19.1 INTRODUCTION

Despite research into eccentric loading, other rehabilitation and injection therapy, Achilles tendinopathy (AT) often becomes chronic and proves resistant to these interventions for many patients. To deal with chronic AT, a treatment method using high-volume injection under image guidance has been developed. A large volume of saline is injected under ultrasound (US) guidance in the tissue around the tendon to remove adhesions between the tendon and the surrounding tissue and to disrupt ingrown vessels and nerve endings to the tendon.[1,2]

The method of using high volumes of saline in the treatment of soft-tissue injuries is not new, and has previously shown good long-term results in patients with 'frozen' shoulder, where distension of the glenohumeral joint resulted in symptom relief.[3] This hydrodilatation, sometimes referred to as distension arthrography, has been proposed and widely tested as a therapeutic procedure for glenohumeral joint contracture.[4] It is proposed that its benefits are derived from a combination of the anti-inflammatory effect of cortisone with the mechanical effect of joint distension (reflected by radiological distension of the capsule and subacromial bursa), thereby reducing the nociogenic effect of capsular stretch on the glenohumeral joint capsule and its periosteal attachments.[4] Hydrodilatation was first used by Andren and Lundberg in 1965.[5] High-volume image-guided injection (HVIGI) for the treatment of chronic AT was first performed in 2002 and initial data were published in 2008.[1] Since then there have been five further studies from four different centres on HVIGI,[2,6] all reporting similar results, with a decrease in the pain perceived by patients on visual analogue score, a reduction in size and vascularity post-HVIGI, high patient satisfaction and improved functional Victorian Institute of Sports Assessment – Achilles (VISA-A) scores in both the short and medium term, with the critical benefit of rapidly returning many patients to sport.

HVIGI has been most commonly used in AT. AT is a common overuse disorder among recreational and professional athletes, accounting for 6–18% of all running injuries in athletes,[7–9] and with a lifetime risk of 52% in elite distance runners.[10] The non-athletic population is not exempt from AT, with at least 33% of AT patients being sedentary.[11–14] The condition affects both sexes irrespective of age, but with a higher incidence in middle-aged men (35–45 years).[7,15] The overall incidence of AT is about 2.35 per 1000 in the general population.[16]

19.2 AETIOLOGY OF ACHILLES TENDINOPATHY

The aetiology of AT is not well understood, but is considered to be multifactorial.[17–20] The list of potential risk factors for AT is long, including age, obesity, diabetes mellitus, hypertension, dyslipidaemia, systemic inflammatory disorders such as rheumatoid arthritis, fluoroquinolone antibiotics, trauma, abnormal lower-limb anatomy, high-intensity or poor training technique, poor equipment or extreme environmental conditions such as heat, cold and humidity.[16,21–24] In addition, there is growing evidence of genetic predisposition.[25] Many terms have been used to describe AT, such as tendinitis (indicating inflammation), tendinosis (indicating degeneration) and tendinopathy. The general term tendinopathy is most widely used, indicating a failed healing response with characteristic changes in tenocytes (proliferation or apoptosis in more advanced presentations), disruption of collagen fibres, increase in non-collagen matrix and neovascularization.[26] Recent evidence suggests that hypervascularization and neovascularization combined with neoneural ingrowth may play a significant role.[27–31] However, neovascularization is only part of the picture in AT, as it has been reported in athletes without symptoms,[8,32] contradicting earlier findings that it only occurs in symptomatic patients.[31] The combination of both the intratendinous changes and neovessel and neoneural ingrowth leads to thickening and adhesions, in particular around the paratenon and the fascia cruri.[33]

In contrast to failed healing, the severed or ruptured tendon typically undergoes three healing phases: (1) an acute inflammatory phase (lasting days); (2) a proliferative phase (lasting around 3 weeks), during which fibroblasts produce new collagen and endothelial growth factor that facilitates neovascularization; and (3) a collagen remodelling phase, lasting up to a year, accompanied by decreased cellularity and vascularity.[34]

19.3 DIAGNOSIS OF ACHILLES TENDINOPATHY

There is no specific test for the diagnosis of AT, so diagnosis is based on history, pain, localized tendon swelling, morning stiffness and impaired performance with a decrease in calf muscle strength and endurance.[35–37] The development of musculoskeletal US has been helpful to confirm and quantify tendon pathology, but some pathology lesions are asymptomatic and some people with pain do not have pathology, so imaging alone is not diagnostic and it is not possible to confirm pain with imaging.[38] US can be used to measure the size of the tendon, visualize AT shape and location, evaluate tendon echogenicity and assess paratenon change, while also detecting calcification, bony spurs, cystic changes, bursal pathology and partial or complete tears.[39,40] In addition to the grey-scale changes, power and colour Doppler can be used to detect and grade neovascularization within and around the tendon.[31]

19.4 TREATMENT OF ACHILLES TENDINOPATHY

The initial management of AT is typically conservative treatment. Specifically, the mainstay of AT management is rehabilitation and graduated tendon loading. For the last decade a more active approach to AT rehabilitation has become popular.[7,11] Although eccentric exercises are widely practised, scientific data supporting the eccentric rehabilitation regime are sparse.[37,41,42] Most studies[43–46] and systematic reviews,[47,48] however, support the continued use of eccentric exercises. Adjuncts that are useful to manage symptoms include load modification (reducing activities that load the tendon heavily), analgesia with paracetamol or non-steroidal anti-inflammatory drugs (NSAIDs), icing, manual therapy (e.g. frictions) and correction of biomechanics issues (including orthotics) and training errors. If these initial interventions fail, shockwave therapy, injection and surgery may be considered.[7] There are only a few randomized controlled studies published for most treatments of AT.[48] Early intervention is often advised, as the management of manifest AT is complicated and often the condition becomes chronic.[36]

Several substances can be injected to treat AT, including corticosteroids, polidocanol or autologous blood in and around the tendon, with mixed results.[49–51] Corticosteroids have not shown any significant long-term benefit[50] and are anecdotally suspected to result in increased risk of tendon atrophy and rupture.[50] Multiple polidocanol injections under US guidance around the neovascularization were found to reduce pain after activity,[49] but the original results have not been confirmed and the procedure is now rarely practised.[51] Autologous blood injections and other blood products have been used, with no good controlled randomized studies to support their use in AT.[52,53] UK National Institute for Health and Care Excellence (NICE) guidelines state that current evidence on safety and efficacy of autologous blood injections is inadequate in quantity and quality (NICE[54] intervention procedure guidance, January 2013) and they are presently only recommended after special arrangements for clinical governance, consent and audit or research. Platelet-rich plasma applications have not been shown to have any beneficial effects acutely[53] or at long-term follow-up.[55] Similarly, prolotherapy, the injection of hypertonic glucose with local anaesthetic injected alongside the site of maximum pain or neovessels, has not been shown to be more effective than eccentric exercises or a combination of both,[50] although US-guided injections have shown favourable results.[56] Electrocoagulation of the neovascularization has also shown good short-term results.[57] There are numerous other approaches which offer some promise, including tissue engineering, biomaterials[58] and genetics,[59] but none is currently used in routine clinical practice and more research is needed.

19.5 HIGH-VOLUME IMAGE-GUIDED INJECTIONS

The aim of HVIGI is to reduce the pain and stiffness suffered by AT patients, therefore allowing patients an early return to progressive loading and 'normal' activity, with the recommendation to implement an ongoing rehabilitation programme to avoid future relapses.

The theory behind HVIGI is in many ways similar to the theory behind surgical tenolysis. A physical stripping of the tendon and stretching will potentially result in compression or disruption of the neurovascular and neural ingrowth from Kager's fat pad. The distension with saline is thought to physically break down peritendinous adhesions, but injected drugs may potentially also have a positive chemical effect on the AT. Direct neurotoxicity of Marcain® 0.5% on pain fibres may affect the pain sensation. Low-dose cortisone (i.e. 25 mg of hydrocortisone acetate) is used primarily to prevent an acute mechanical inflammatory reaction produced by the large amount of fluid injected and to suppress the local healing response (and therefore reduce the formation of more adhesions). However, the steroid may have effects on tendon pathology and pain, for example, reducing tenocyte proliferation and influencing potential biochemical pain such as substance P.[60]

19.5.1 High-volume image-guided injection procedure (box 19.1, figures 19.1–19.3 and video 19.1)

See box 19.1.

19.6 REHABILITATION FOLLOWING HIGH-VOLUME INJECTION

Rehabilitation following any injection should progress tendon loading, address functional deficits (e.g. strength, power, flexibility) as well as adhere to postinjection guidelines and precautions. Following high-volume injection in the Achilles tendon, the key local consideration is calf muscle function, carefully considered in the context of kinetic chain function. This section provides a brief theoretical rationale and practical rehabilitation outline following HVIGI.

19.6.1 Rationale for rehabilitation post high-volume image-guided injection

The goal of rehabilitation post HVIGI is to treat pain, maximize tendon remodelling and healing

<table>
<tr><td>**BOX 19.1**</td><td>**High-volume image-guided injection (HVIGI) procedure**</td></tr>
</table>

- Clinical diagnosis
- Diagnostic ultrasound to confirm the diagnosis and document the echogenicity, size and site of tendon bulge and other characteristics such as the presence of calcification, cysts, bursa, bony spurs, paratenon changes and exclusion of intratendinous tears, fascia cruris tears and myofascial scars between the gastrocnemius and soleus muscle in the upper and mid-calf
- Assessment and grading of extent of neovascularization using power or colour Doppler (using a semiquantitative scoring system for neovascularization) (Figure 19.1A)
- Explanation of the procedure and obtaining verbal or written consent
- Supine procedure, with hip and knee flexed and hips externally rotated
- 21G green needle insertion transversely from a medial approach using real-time ultrasound guidance and an aseptic technique
- Needle inserted at the level of maximum pain, maximum tenderness, maximum vascularization and maximum anteroposterior diameter (usually same site), touching the ventral surface of the Achilles tendon throughout its course (Figure 19.1B)

- 21G needle is connected to a high-pressure Luer lock connector
- A mixture of 10 mL of Marcain® 0.5% and 25 mg of hydrocortisone acetate) is injected via a 10 mL Luer lock syringe.
- Static and video images are obtained throughout the procedure with extended field of view images taken before and after the HVIGI
- A further 40 mL of normal saline (4 × 10 mL Luer lock syringes) is then injected using high pressure (firm push) (Figure 19.1D; video 19.1)
- At the end of the injection, the power/colour Doppler is turned on to check that there are no residual vascularization. Any residual vessels are treated with a further 50 mL of normal saline injection (figures 19.2 and 19.3)
- Static and video images are taken of the vascularization at the start and end of the procedure using power Doppler

Most of the studies have used a mixture of Marcain® 0.5% with 25 mg of hydrocortisone acetate followed by 40 mL of normal saline. One study used aprotonin (which has now been withdrawn for safety reasons) with similar results.[6] However, there does not appear to be any significant difference in the results with or without steroid.

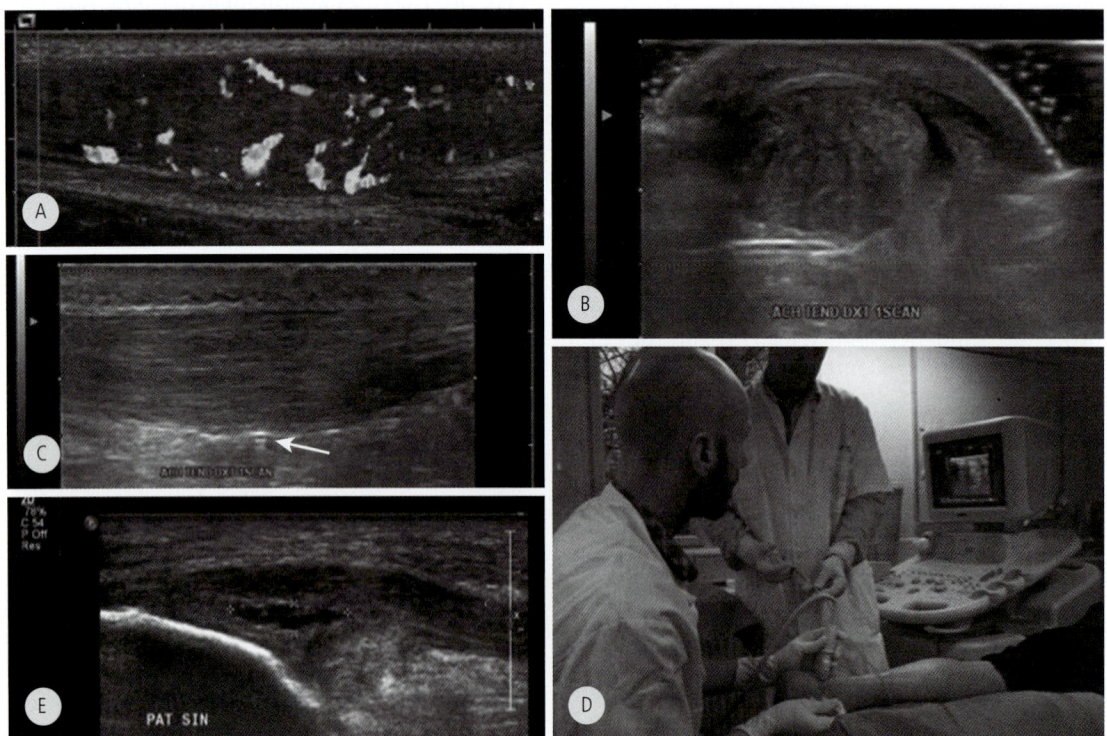

FIGURE 19.1 ■ (A) Achilles tendon with grade 3 Doppler activity. (B) Placement of high-volume image-guided injection (HVIGI) needle in transverse view. (C) Placement of HVIGI needle in longitudinal view. (D) Example of HVIGI set-up. (E) Example of a patellar tendon patient who was rejected from treatment with HVIGI, for obvious reasons. (Colour version of figure is available online).

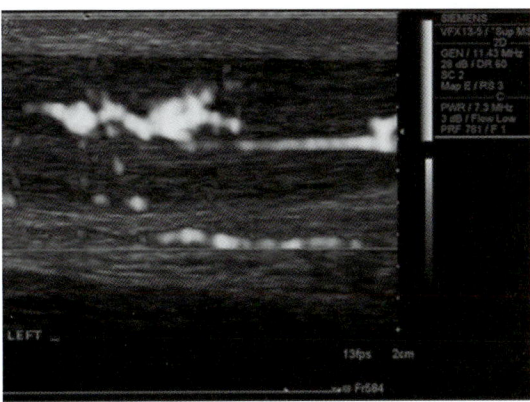

FIGURE 19.2 ■ Doppler ultrasound imaging prior to high-volume image-guided injection. (Colour version of figure is available online).

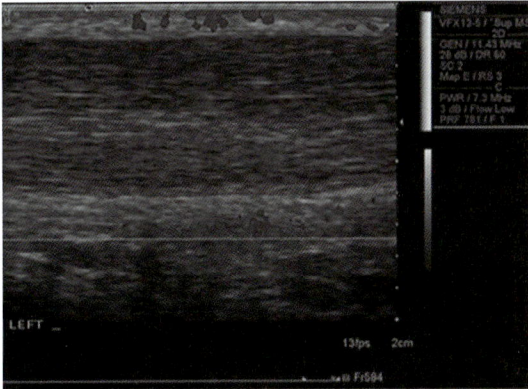

FIGURE 19.3 ■ Doppler ultrasound imaging after high-volume image-guided injection. (Colour version of figure is available online).

and restore function. As discussed, there is an extensive evidence base for the use of eccentric exercise for treating Achilles tendon pain, and this intervention should be considered. Some patients may have poor calf concentric function (e.g. inability to perform a calf raise through full range) so concentric–eccentric training may be a more suitable initial intervention.

Progressive loading is important for tendon adaptation. Tendon response is strain-dependent, and high load and time under tension are important to maximize tendon adaptation. Isometric, concentric–eccentric and eccentric loading that is high-load and slow (allowing high time under tension) has been shown to adapt the tendon, and increase tendon stiffness.[61] Whether abnormal tendons respond in the same way is not known. Kongsgaard et al.[62] found that tendon stiffness reduced following heavy, slow resistance training, the opposite effect to that in normal tendons. Two recent systematic reviews have found no evidence for improved tendon structure or thickness on imaging following

loading.[63,64] Clearly, the adaptation response of abnormal tendons is unclear, but progressive heavy load is likely to be important.

KEY POINTS

After HVIGI, a progressive loading is important for tendon adaptation.

19.6.2 Progressing to impact loading

Commencing high-impact rehabilitation to prepare for activities such as running and jumping is dictated by four criteria: (1) symptoms are stable with tendon-loading exercise and activities of daily living, that is, the patient is not having a flare-up of symptoms that lasts for more than 24 hours following Achilles tendon loading; (2) movement patterns during impact loading are not grossly abnormal; (3) the patient requires this for function and would habitually require such capacity; and (4) other aspects of the kinetic chain are suitably conditioned, or potentially conditionable, for high-impact loading to be safe. The second and fourth points necessitate a sufficient level of underlying neuromuscular function and minimal pain. Gradual progression is the key to commencing impact loading without provoking symptoms. Initially, speed may be introduced to slow rehabilitation exercises (e.g. calf raises) as a bridge towards impact loading and stretch–shorten cycle (SSC)-biased exercise such as jumping. Volume should be progressed prior to intensity, as intense SSC activity involves greater tendon load and is poorly tolerated symptomatically by tendinopathic tendons. Frequency of fast rehabilitation is also important. Initially there should be 2–3 days between loading episodes to allow adequate monitoring of symptom response.

19.6.3 Kinetic chain

It is critical to address kinetic chain dysfunctions. These can be very individual and may be risk factors for injury or dysfunction from past surgery or injury. Dysfunction in the antigravity muscles, including gluteals and quadriceps, is common among AT patients. Functional restriction of movement may also be associated with AT. For example, reduced ankle dorsiflexion with the knee extended, a measure of gastrocnemius flexibility, is associated with AT.[65] Previous injury, such as anterior cruciate ligament reconstruction or meniscal injury, is often associated with contralateral lower-limb overload and AT.

Addressing these kinetic chain factors in rehabilitation wherever possible will facilitate successful return to function and minimize the risk of recurrence.

19.6.4 Acceptable symptoms during rehabilitation

There seems to be clinical benefit from exercise into pain,[7,11,37] but it is not clear whether pain during rehabilitation is necessary (e.g. to produce habituation) or an acceptable byproduct of loading. It is important to educate patients that some symptoms during rehabilitation are acceptable, provided they are transient and non-progressive, as this will minimize fear avoidance. Patients are also best placed to monitor symptoms to ensure that they are remaining stable, and this is practically achieved by monitoring one or two consistent functional aggravating factors over time. As a guide, exercise provocation of up to 5/10 on a visual analogue scale that settles within 24 hours is acceptable. What needs to be conveyed in patient education is the subtle but important distinction between exercising into pain and exercising into irritability. Patients should also expect some symptom provocation when progressing load (e.g. commencing fast loading), but following the gradual progression guidelines outlined above can minimize this. Too fast progression may lead to higher risk of recurrence of the symptoms.

19.6.5 Outline rehabilitation programme post Achilles high-volume image-guided injection

Table 19.1 outlines when functional and rehabilitation activities can be commenced following HVIGI. Immediately after the injection, patients are given a booklet, clearly explaining the strict rehabilitation programme (table 19.2). A dedicated specialist sports physiotherapist goes through the early step-by-step rehabilitation programme immediately after the injection. The suggested timeframe of the outlined rehabilitation has to be adjusted depending on the reduction in symptoms. Return to sports may take 2–6 weeks depending on the age and fitness of the patient and the length of the condition. If patients have been away from sport for an extended period prior to the HVIGI, this increases rehabilitation time post-HVIGI. Typically, athletes multiply by half the time they have been away from sports as a minimum time for rehabilitation. For example, if a football player has not played for 6 months prior to the HVIGI, then s/he will need an additional 3 months of rehabilitation and conditioning before returning to competitive football after the HVIGI (tables 19.1 and 19.2).

19.7 ADVANTAGES OF HIGH-VOLUME IMAGE-GUIDED INJECTION

See box 19.2.

19.8 COMPLICATIONS OF HIGH-VOLUME IMAGE-GUIDED INJECTION

So far only very few major complications (tendon rupture) have been reported. Rupture of the Achilles tendon may be more likely when a patient is rendered asymptomatic or pain free, as 80% of patients who rupture have AT but no symptoms. Similarly, if patients improve clinically, then they are likely to increase their activity and that is likely to increase the risk of

Day	1	2–3	4–6	7–9	10–12	12–
Rest	✓	✓	✗	✗	✗	✗
Drive	✗	✓	✓	✓	✓	✓
Work	✓	✓	✓	✓	✓	✓
Walk	✓	✓	✓	✓	✓	✓
Initial tendon-loading exercise	✗	✗	✓	✓	✓	✓
Swim	✗	✗	✗	✓	✓	✓
Lifting	✗	✗	✗	✓	✓	✓
Aerobic exercise	✗	✗	✗	✓	✓	✓
Strengthening	✗	✗	✗	✗	✓	✓
Sports-specific tendon loading	✗	✗	✗	✗	✗	✓

TABLE 19.1 **Commencement of functional and rehabilitation activity following high-volume image-guided injection**

TABLE 19.2 Outline rehabilitation protocol post high-volume image-guided injection

Time frame	
	Phase one – slow loading
Day 4	Initial tendon loading
	• Double-leg heel raises on flat ground:
	• Start with 3 × 5, knee straight, once daily, slowly
	• Increase as able to 3 × 10
	• Then do single-leg heel raises on flat ground:
	• Start with 3 × 5, knee straight. once daily, slowly
	• Increase until able to do 3 × 10
	Commence Alfredson eccentric training (twice daily) (stop previous exercises)
	• Starting on toes, perform single-leg heel drops over edge of step with knee bent; lift on to toes with other leg and arms
	• Up to 3 × 15, 1-minute rest between sets
	• If bilateral, perform on opposite side between sets
	• May start with 3 × 5 if not able to complete 15
	• Slowly: 6-second downward phase per repetition
	• Repeat 3 × 15 with knee straight
No sooner than day 10	Add weight in backpack if exercise is painfree and able: start with 10 kg and increase by 5–10 kg to maximum of 50% body weight
Day 7	Non-impact fitness work (3–4 × 40-minute sessions/week)
	• Swimming, cycling or rowing
	Phase two – fast/power
Commence when meet criteria	Non-athletic patients:
	• Start when can perform 15 calf raises
	• Progressively increase walking endurance by 5–10 minutes/week
	• Only progress if symptoms are stable
	Athletes:
	• Start when can perform 15 calf raises, ≤3/10 pain with single-leg hop
	• Start running 5 minutes, flat ground, slow/steady pace
	• Increase by 5–10 minutes per week
	• No more than every second to third day
	• Only progress if symptoms are stable
	• When running 30 minutes, progressively commence sport

BOX 19.2	Advantages of high-volume image-guided injection in Achilles tendinopathy patients

• Simple concept
• Simple procedure
• Safe
• Cheap
• No intratendon disruption
• Immediate results
• Rapid results
• Rapid resolution of symptoms
• Early return to activity
• Few complications

rupture. In a 12-year period, the authors report that, to their knowledge, there were two complete ruptures, one 2 years after the HVIGI, one after a month. In both cases there were significant comorbidities, including rheumatoid arthritis and long-term steroid use in one case.

The most frequent complication is pain or discomfort during the procedure or immediately after. The fluid may cause a sensation of distension of the ankle, which can be very uncomfortable. Numbness can be reported after HVIGI and is usually localized around the injection, but occasionally patients report a completely numb foot, which can last for several days. A 'flare response' to the steroid in the treated area is occasionally reported: this is a stinging sensation and is reported in up to 25% of patients for a few days. However, giving NSAIDs in the 2 days after injection seems to reduce the frequency and intensity of the reaction.

KEY POINTS

So far only very few major complications (tendon rupture) have been reported.

Localized muscle acute tears are common in the ipsilateral or contralateral calf or hamstring, as patients often try to return to sport before finishing their conditioning programme. Therefore we recommend that a sports physiotherapist prescribes the rehabilitation in the first period after injection, and monitors late-stage rehabilitation. Patients must be aware of potential time-consuming lifelong eccentric rehabilitation and maintenance exercises. Infection is extremely rare and in a 12-year period two patients presented with localized cellulitis and one patient had a small focal abscess that needed draining.

19.9 CLINICAL CASE

This brief case study focuses on a 46-year-old recreational runner with right midportion AT treated with HVIGI. Symptoms had an insidious onset 5 months prior, following an increase in training volume (20–40 km/week, four runs per week) in preparation for a half-marathon event. Pain was localized in the right Achilles midportion and aggravated and associated with morning stiffness and stiffness after prolonged sitting. Running more than 3 km would result in aggravation in symptoms for 2–3 days, including increase in morning stiffness duration and intensity and more awareness of Achilles pain and stiffness when arising after periods of sitting. He had only run sporadically, a maximum of once per week, over the last 4 months.

Prior to HVIGI he had trialled Alfredson eccentric training exercises for 10 weeks and had also been advised by a physiotherapist to wear heel wedges in his shoes when walking and running. He had tried dry needling and massage around the Achilles and calf. He reported minimal improvement in morning stiffness with exercise but no change in symptoms following running.

There was a relevant history of recurrent ankle sprains on the right side. Potential risk factors, such as lipid imbalance, hypertension, diabetes and inflammatory arthritis, were absent. The patient was a non-smoker and did not take any medication.

The patient was assessed by a sports physician in order to confirm the diagnosis of AT and determine suitability for HVIGI. Tenderness on palpation was isolated to the Achilles midportion, and absent from the retrocalcaneal bursa. There was no diffuse pain around the paratenon or bursa that could indicate pain from these tissues. US imaging excluded bursa and paratenon changes as well as fascia cruris and intratendinous tears.

The patient was suitable for HVIGI as pain from the surrounding tissues (e.g. bursa) was excluded and there was no general health issues that would increase the risk of tendon rupture (e.g. inflammatory arthritis, steroid use). HVIGI was administered as per the injection protocol outlined above. There were no adverse reactions or complications following injection. The patient consulted a sports physiotherapist immediately after the injection for initial guidance regarding the postinjection protocol (table 19.2). Three days postinjection there was a repeat consultation with the sports physiotherapist, including a thorough assessment of musculoskeletal deficits. Main musculoskeletal issues contributing to the presentation included restricted right-ankle weight-bearing dorsiflexion and reduced single-leg calf raise endurance and quality (right = 11, left = 26). As the patient had a deficit in execution of a concentric task, that is, single-leg calf raises, a concentric–eccentric strengthening programme was commenced initially. This was progressed to an Alfredson eccentric programme as per the postinjection protocol (see table 19.2). Sixteen days postinjection he was able to commence a graduated running programme and 5 weeks later he had successfully progressed this running to 30 minutes, three times per week. He then gradually commenced speed work (intervals) as part of his running training; hills and full half-marathon training were gradually introduced at 10 weeks. He continued to have minimal morning stiffness on some mornings after he had run but the 2–3-day reaction of his symptoms after running was absent. At this time he continued his Alfredson eccentric training as a maintenance programme only two to three times a week.

(Clinical case continued on page 493)

19.10 CONCLUSION

HVIGI is a cheap, safe and effective treatment for chronic AT. It reduces stiffness and pain with good short- and long-term function recovery and is effective in returning patients early to sport. Further research with randomized prospective blinded controlled trials is necessary to confirm these early promising results, and to explore HVIGI efficacy in other tendinopathies.

19.11 REFERENCES

1. Chan O, O'Dowd D, Padhiar N, et al. High volume image guided injections in chronic Achilles tendinopathy. Disabil Rehabil 2008;30:1697–708.
2. Humphrey J, Chan O, Crisp T, et al. The short-term effects of high volume image guided injections in resistant non-insertional Achilles tendinopathy. J Sci Med Sport 2010;13:295–8.
3. Watson L, Bialocerkowski A, Dalziel R, et al. Hydrodilatation (distension arthrography): a long-term clinical outcome series. Br J Sports Med 2007;41:167–73.
4. Bell S, Coghlan J, Richardson M. Hydrodilatation in the management of shoulder capsulitis. Australas Radiol 2003;47:247–51.

5. Andren I, Lundberg BJ. Treatment of rigid shoulders by joint distension during arthrography. Acta Orthop Scand 1965;36:45–53.
6. Maffulli N, Spiezia F, Longo UG, et al. High volume image guided injections for the management of chronic tendinopathy of the main body of the Achilles tendon. Phys Ther Sport 2013;14:163–7.
7. Alfredson H, Lorentzon R. Chronic Achilles tendinosis: recommendations for treatment and prevention. Sports Med 2000;29:135–46.
8. Longo UG, Rittweger J, Garau G, et al. No influence of age, gender, weight, height, and impact profile in Achilles tendinopathy in masters track and field athletes. Am J Sports Med 2009;37:1400–5.
9. Schepsis AA, Jones H, Haas AL. Achilles tendon disorders in athletes. Am J Sports Med 2002;30:287–305.
10. Kujala UM, Sarna S, Kaprio J. Cumulative incidence of achilles tendon rupture and tendinopathy in male former elite athletes. Clin J Sport Med 2005;15:133–5.
11. Alfredson H. Chronic midportion Achilles tendinopathy: an update on research and treatment. Clin Sports Med 2003;22:727–41.
12. Astrom M. Partial rupture in chronic Achilles tendinopathy. A retrospective analysis of 342 cases. Acta Orthop Scand 1998;69:404–7.
13. Maffulli N, Sharma P, Luscombe KL. Achilles tendinopathy: aetiology and management. J R Soc Med 2004; 97:472–6.
14. Rolf C, Movin T. Etiology, histopathology, and outcome of surgery in achillodynia. Foot Ankle Int 1997;18: 565–9.
15. Cook JL, Khan KM, Purdam C. Achilles tendinopathy. Man Ther 2002;7:121–30.
16. de Jonge S, van den Berg C, de Vos RJ, et al. Incidence of midportion Achilles tendinopathy in the general population. Br J Sports Med 2011;45:1026–8.
17. Ames PR, Longo UG, Denaro V, et al. Achilles tendon problems: not just an orthopaedic issue. Disabil Rehabil 2008;30:1646–50.
18. Kvist M. Achilles tendon injuries in athletes. Ann Chir Gynaecol 1991;80:188–201.
19. Longo UG, Oliva F, Denaro V, et al. Oxygen species and overuse tendinopathy in athletes. Disabil Rehabil 2008; 30:1563–71.
20. Mahieu NN, Witvrouw E, Stevens V, et al. Intrinsic risk factors for the development of achilles tendon overuse injury: a prospective study. Am J Sports Med 2006;34: 226–35.
21. Carcia CR, Martin RL, Houck J, et al. Achilles pain, stiffness, and muscle power deficits: achilles tendinitis. J Orthop Sports Phys Ther 2010;40:A1–26.
22. Holmes GB, Lin J. Etiologic factors associated with symptomatic Achilles tendinopathy. Foot Ankle Int 2006;27:952–9.
23. Jarvinen TA, Kannus P, Maffulli N, et al. Achilles tendon disorders: etiology and epidemiology. Foot Ankle Clin 2005;10:255–66.
24. Klemp P, Halland AM, Majoos FL, et al. Musculoskeletal manifestations in hyperlipidaemia: a controlled study. Ann Rheum Dis 1993;52:44–8.
25. Magra M, Maffulli N. Genetic aspects of tendinopathy. J Sci Med Sport 2008;11:243–7.
26. Maffulli N, Longo UG, Loppini M, et al. Current treatment options for tendinopathy. Expert Opin Pharmacother 2010;11:2177–86.
27. Alfredson H, Ohberg L, Forsgren S. Is vasculo-neural ingrowth the cause of pain in chronic Achilles tendinosis? An investigation using ultrasonography and colour Doppler, immunohistochemistry, and diagnostic injections. Knee Surg Sports Traumatol Arthrosc 2003;11: 334–8.
28. Knobloch K, Kraemer R, Lichtenberg A, et al. Achilles tendon and paratendon microcirculation in midportion and insertional tendinopathy in athletes. Am J Sports Med 2006;34:92–7.
29. Kristoffersen M, Ohberg L, Johnston C, et al. Neovascularisation in chronic tendon injuries detected with colour Doppler ultrasound in horse and man: implications for research and treatment. Knee Surg Sports Traumatol Arthrosc 2005;13:505–8.
30. Longo UG, Ronga M, Maffulli N. Achilles tendinopathy. Sports Med Arthrosc 2009;17:112–26.
31. Ohberg L, Lorentzon R, Alfredson H. Neovascularisation in Achilles tendons with painful tendinosis but not in normal tendons: an ultrasonographic investigation. Knee Surg Sports Traumatol Arthrosc 2001;9:233–8.
32. Boesen MI, Koenig MJ, Torp-Pedersen S, et al. Tendinopathy and Doppler activity: the vascular response of the Achilles tendon to exercise. Scand J Med Sci Sports 2006;16:463–9.
33. Astrom M, Rausing A. Chronic Achilles tendinopathy. A survey of surgical and histopathologic findings. Clin Orthop Relat Res 1995;151–64.
34. Battery L, Maffulli N. Inflammation in overuse tendon injuries. Sports Med Arthrosc 2011;19:213–17.
35. Magnussen RA, Dunn WR, Thomson AB. Nonoperative treatment of midportion Achilles tendinopathy: a systematic review. Clin J Sport Med 2009;19:54–64.
36. Scott A, Huisman E, Khan K. Conservative treatment of chronic Achilles tendinopathy. CMAJ 2011;183: 1159–65.
37. Silbernagel KG, Thomee R, Thomee P, et al. Eccentric overload training for patients with chronic Achilles tendon pain – a randomised controlled study with reliability testing of the evaluation methods. Scand J Med Sci Sports 2001;11:197–206.
38. Khan KM, Forster BB, Robinson J, et al. Are ultrasound and magnetic resonance imaging of value in assessment of Achilles tendon disorders? A two year prospective study. Br J Sports Med 2003;37:149–53.
39. Archambault JM, Wiley JP, Bray RC, et al. Can sonography predict the outcome in patients with achillodynia? J Clin Ultrasound 1998;26:335–9.
40. Hartgerink P, Fessell DP, Jacobson JA, et al. Full- versus partial-thickness Achilles tendon tears: sonographic accuracy and characterization in 26 cases with surgical correlation. Radiology 2001;220:406–12.
41. Rees JD, Wolman RL, Wilson A. Eccentric exercises; why do they work, what are the problems and how can we improve them? Br J Sports Med 2009;43:242–6.
42. Stanish WD, Rubinovich RM, Curwin S. Eccentric exercise in chronic tendinitis. Clin Orthop Relat Res 1986;65–8.
43. Mafi N, Lorentzon R, Alfredson H. Superior short-term results with eccentric calf muscle training compared to concentric training in a randomized prospective multicenter study on patients with chronic Achilles tendinosis. Knee Surg Sports Traumatol Arthrosc 2001;9: 42–7.
44. Mayer F, Hirschmuller A, Muller S, et al. Effects of short-term treatment strategies over 4 weeks in Achilles tendinopathy. Br J Sports Med 2007;41:e6.
45. Rompe JD, Nafe B, Furia JP, et al. Eccentric loading, shock-wave treatment, or a wait-and-see policy for tendinopathy of the main body of tendo Achillis: a randomized controlled trial. Am J Sports Med 2007;35: 374–83.
46. Roos EM, Engstrom M, Lagerquist A, et al. Clinical improvement after 6 weeks of eccentric exercise in patients with mid-portion Achilles tendinopathy – a randomized trial with 1-year follow-up. Scand J Med Sci Sports 2004;14:286–95.

47. Kingma JJ, de Knikker R, Wittink HM, et al. Eccentric overload training in patients with chronic Achilles tendinopathy: a systematic review. Br J Sports Med 2007;41:e3.

48. Rowe V, Hemmings S, Barton C, et al. Conservative management of midportion Achilles tendinopathy: a mixed methods study, integrating systematic review and clinical reasoning. Sports Med 2012;42:941–67.

49. Alfredson H, Ohberg L. Sclerosing injections to areas of neo-vascularisation reduce pain in chronic Achilles tendinopathy: a double-blind randomised controlled trial. Knee Surg Sports Traumatol Arthrosc 2005;13: 338–44.

50. Coombes BK, Bisset L, Vicenzino B. Efficacy and safety of corticosteroid injections and other injections for management of tendinopathy: a systematic review of randomised controlled trials. Lancet 2010;376:1751–67.

51. van Sterkenburg MN, de Jonge MC, Sierevelt IN, et al. Less promising results with sclerosing ethoxysclerol injections for midportion achilles tendinopathy: a retrospective study. Am J Sports Med 2010;38:2226–32.

52. Bell KJ, Fulcher ML, Rowlands DS, et al. Impact of autologous blood injections in treatment of mid-portion Achilles tendinopathy: double blind randomised controlled trial. BMJ 2014;48:1334.

53. de Vos RJ, Weir A, van Schie HT, et al. Platelet-rich plasma injection for chronic Achilles tendinopathy: a randomized controlled trial. JAMA 2010;303:144–9.

54. National Institute for Health and Care Excellence (NICE). Autologous blood injection for tendinopathy. Available at: https://www.nice.org.uk/guidance/ipg438/chapter/1-guidance (Accessed 10 June 2014).

55. de Jonge S, de Vos RJ, Weir A, et al. One-year follow-up of platelet-rich plasma treatment in chronic Achilles tendinopathy: a double-blind randomized placebo-controlled trial. Am J Sports Med 2011;39:1623–9.

56. Ryan M, Wong A, Taunton J. Favorable outcomes after sonographically guided intratendinous injection of hyperosmolar dextrose for chronic insertional and midportion achilles tendinosis. AJR Am J Roentgenol 2010;194:1047–53.

57. Boesen MI, Torp-Pedersen S, Koenig MJ, et al. Ultrasound guided electrocoagulation in patients with chronic non-insertional Achilles tendinopathy: a pilot study. Br J Sports Med 2006;40:761–6.

58. Longo UG, Lamberti A, Maffulli N, et al. Tissue engineered biological augmentation for tendon healing: a systematic review. Br Med Bull 2011;98:31–59.

59. Lippi G, Longo UG, Maffulli N. Genetics and sports. Br Med Bull 2010;93:27–47.

60. Fredberg U, Stengaard-Pedersen K. Chronic tendinopathy tissue pathology, pain mechanisms, and etiology with a special focus on inflammation. Scand J Med Sci Sports 2008;18:3–15.

61. Malliaras P, Barton CJ, Reeves ND, et al. Achilles and patellar tendinopathy loading programmes: a systematic review comparing clinical outcomes and identifying potential mechanisms for effectiveness. Sports Med 2013;43:267–86.

62. Kongsgaard M, Qvortrup K, Larsen J, et al. Fibril morphology and tendon mechanical properties in patellar tendinopathy: effects of heavy slow resistance training. Am J Sports Med 2010;38:749–56.

63. Drew BT, Smith TO, Littlewood C, et al. Do structural changes (e.g. collagen/matrix) explain the response to therapeutic exercises in tendinopathy: a systematic review. Br J Sports Med 2014;48:966–72.

64. Malliaras P, Kamal B, Nowell A, et al. Patellar tendon adaptation in relation to load-intensity and contraction type. J Biomech 2013;46:1893–9.

65. Kaufman KR, Brodine SK, Shaffer RA, et al. The effect of foot structure and range of motion on musculoskeletal overuse injuries. Am J Sports Med 1999;27:585–93.

PART XI

OUTCOMES: EVIDENCE-BASED PHYSIOTHERAPY

CHAPTER 20

OUTCOME MEASUREMENT IN CLINICAL PRACTICE

Francesc Medina Mirapeix • Pilar Escolar Reina

Measure what can be measured, and make measurable what cannot be measured.
GALILEO GALILEI

KEYWORDS

disability; functioning; measurement; outcome measures; outcomes.

20.1 INTRODUCTION

A result is defined as a characteristic which is expected to change due to an intervention.[1] For example:

The improvement of pain, strength, walking resistance, movement speed or participation in sports after a treatment intervention for a patient with patellar tendinitis and with a limited ability to run short distances.

'Outcome measurement' is a generic term used to describe the process of data collection and to report on the observed effect.[2] In the case of a patient with patellar tendinopathies, this would encompass, for example, the process of using a questionnaire such as the VISA score (Victorian Institute of Sports Assessment – Patella: VISA-P)[3] or others, measured at baseline and after a temporary interval, as well as reporting on the changes observed.

Outcome measurements may be applied to a group of patients or to individual patients. At a group level, measures are usually used for the purpose of assessing the impact of an intervention or any other research question. For example, they may be used to assess the effectiveness of a treatment with percutaneous needle electrolysis on a group with a determined tendinopathy. In this case, the outcome measurements include the same tools and temporal assessment intervals for each member of the group. At an individual level, outcome measurements include a selection of tools and temporal intervals that are relevant to the patient and which, in turn, may differ between patients. This chapter will focus on individual outcome measurements, which are more oriented to clinical practice than to research, and we shall use tendinopathies as an example.

Traditionally, physiotherapists have used individual patient results in the form of goals or 'expected results', which are used at different stages during the course of care:

- during initial assessment, while documenting the aims of treatment
- during reassessments, while evaluating whether or not the goals are being accomplished and while establishing new goals, depending on the new situation as treatment unfolds
- at the end of the episode, to reflect the goals met on a discharge document.

Goals and outcome measures are intimately related, as emphasized in the form shown in table 20.1, proposed by the Canadian Physiotherapy Association.[4] However, the use of outcome measurements in daily clinical practice has been less systematically practised than results measurement per se, despite their relevance for the purpose of establishing treatment goals, monitoring the progress of the patient's health problems and evaluating treatment effectiveness.

TABLE 20.1 **Treatment goal progression and outcome assessment sheet in a patient with low-back pain**

Client: Mr Brown Age: 40

Outcome measures and goals	First visit	1st week	2nd week	3rd week	4th week
Outcome measures					
Pain intensity					
0–10 visual analogue scale	4	3	2	1	0
Activity and participation measures					
Roland-Morris questionnaire (/24)	10		5		1
Impairment measures					
Extension (cm)	0.9	1.4	1.7		1.6
Flexion (modified Shöeber) (cm)	3.1	5.2	6.2		6.3
Initial goals and time frame					
↑ Extension at 1.6 cm in 1 week			Here		
↑ Flexion at 4.5 cm in 1 week		OK			
↓ Pain to 1 in week 1				Here	
↓ Roland-Morris at 5 in 2 weeks			OK		
New goals (established in week 2) and time frame					
↑ Flexion >6 cm (normal) at week 3					Here
↓ Roland-Morris at <2 at week 4					OK

OK, goal acheived at the estimated week; here, goal achieved on the date indicated.
Adapted from: the Canadian Physiotherapy Association.[4]

20.2 SELECTION OF RELEVANT RESULTS

There are many results that may be relevant to clinical practice, as illustrated in the case example cited in the first paragraph of this chapter. In this case, a measurement of all the possible results (e.g. pain, strength) may not be viable in daily clinical practice. Therefore, it is always important to prioritize the most relevant results. In order to make an appropriate selection it is necessary to:

- be knowledgeable about some of the conceptual frameworks on relevant results in physiotherapy
- consider applicable criteria in order to prioritize selected results.

20.2.1 A framework for relevant results in physiotherapy

Traditionally, individuals with health problems have been classified according to their illnesses or health condition. This tendency has emphasized the need to describe the characteristics of the illness (aetiology, pathology and clinical manifestations), whereby the problems of a patient are reduced to a certain label (for example, a paraplegic, a tendinitis). In this healthcare model, known as the biomedical model, the main results are aimed at the pathology and the clinical manifestations. Historically, this model has ignored the many other health dimensions which accompany an illness or condition, such as functioning and disability.

The World Health Organization (WHO) has proposed an expanded model in order to understand the concept of health and its relationship to function and disability.[5] According to this model, shown in figure 20.1, functioning is seen as a generic concept which refers to the performance or the capacity for performance in relation to three factors (in the grey area and in the centre of the figure): body structure and function, activity (or the tasks and actions carried out by the person) and participation (or involvement in a life situation).

This model provides a more indepth description of an individual's health. For example, when applied to the case of the patient with patellar tendinopathy presented at the beginning of the chapter, it describes whether or not the functioning is normal at the level of body function (e.g. muscle strength, pain) and at the level of activity (ability to run). In parallel, it underlines the fact that functioning is understood as a result of a complex interaction between the health condition and the contextual factors (environmental and personal) that surround the person in question.

This model has been the base upon which the *International Classification of Functioning, Disability, and Health* (ICF) was created. This classification is available in print[5,6] and online on the web page http://apps.who.int/classifications/icfbrowser/Default.aspx. It is structured into the components of functioning, and includes a classification of environmental factors. Each component contains a series of domains (or chapters), which are listed in table 20.2.

Each domain (or chapter) is structured into hierarchal categories, which are classification units that help describe the health status of a person in that domain.

For example, in the domain of mobility activities there are certain descriptive categories (for example, changing body position, transferring oneself, walking, lifting up an object), whereas in the self-care domain there are others (such as washing oneself, dressing).

Disability is a generic term which is used to indicate that the functioning of one of the categories in the classification is abnormal or

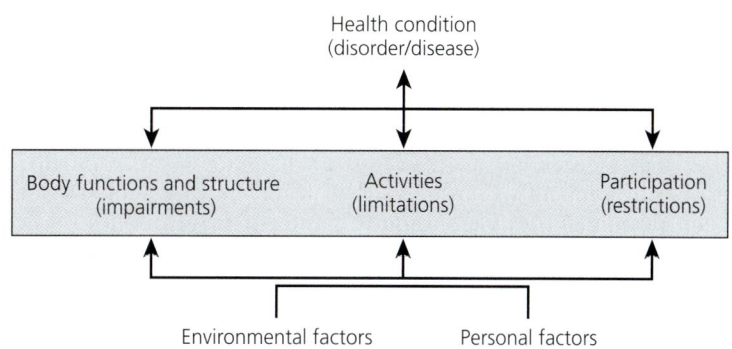

FIGURE 20.1 ■ Model of functioning and disability.[5,6]

TABLE 20.2   **Components and domains (or chapters) of the *International Classification of Functioning, Disability, and Health***

Body component

Structures	Functions
s1 Structure of the nervous system	b1 Mental functions
s2 The eye, ear and related structures	b2 Sensory functions and pain
s3 Structures involved in voice and speech	b3 Voice and speech functions
s4 Structure of the cardiovascular, immunological and respiratory systems	b4 Functions of the cardiovascular, haematological, immunological and respiratory systems
s5 Structures related to the digestive, metabolic and endocrine systems	b5 Functions of the digestive, metabolic and endocrine systems
s6 Structure related to genitourinary and reproductive systems	b6 Genitourinary and reproductive functions
s7 Structures related to movement	b7 Neuromusculoskeletal and movement-related functions
s8 Skin and related structures	b8 Functions of the skin and related structures

Activities and participation	Environmental factors
d1 Learning and applying knowledge	e1 Products and technology
d2 General tasks and demands	e2 Natural environment and human-made changes to environment
d3 Communication	e3 Support and relationships
d4 Mobility	e4 Attitudes
d5 Self-care	e5 Services, systems and policies
d6 Domestic life	
d7 Interpersonal interactions and relationships	
d8 Major life areas	
d9 Community, social and civic life	

negative. It also corresponds to the central part of the model represented in figure 20.1, using the following concepts:

- Impairments: these are problems in function or structure, such as a loss of articular range, strength and muscular resistance or an alteration in the scarring of a tissue.
- Activity limitations: these are difficulties an individual may have while executing an activity such as opening a can, jumping, lifting an object above the head, transporting something heavy.
- Participation restrictions: these are problems an individual may experience while taking part in life situations, such as going for a walk around the neighbourhood, working continuously for several hours, buying groceries.

Traditionally, physiotherapists have based their goals or anticipated results on the improvement of impairments in several systems and even sometimes in the re-education of mobility activities such as walking, maintaining or changing posture. Frequently, however, they have not been aware that they were using ICF categories. The novelty of the WHO model is that it explicitly defines the concepts of functioning and disability, using unified and standardized language, thus allowing the user to use the framework in order to consciously select the most relevant results while, at the same time, describing and assessing the health status of a person.

20.2.2 Criteria needed in order to prioritize the selection of outcomes

Initially, it seems that the ideal is to select an outcome that may be affected by the treatment applied. Thus, when a treatment includes a technique that supposedly impacts on the tissue or on a determined system, the outcome should be selected at the level of the impairment.

Increasingly often, physiotherapy treatments not only seek an impact on an impairment component, but they also take into consideration the outcomes of both activity and participation. Treatments frequently employ a combination of techniques aimed at improving the tissues or deficiencies (for example, laser therapy, strengthening exercises, percutaneous needle electrolysis, flexibility) and interventions aimed at normalizing the performance of activities (such as gait) by means of body-centred techniques (biofeedback, balance, proprioceptive re-education, repetition) or by training the person in the performance of the activity.

When it is just not practical to assess the patient for all the results at different levels, in many cases a good option is to select results at the level of activity due to its mediator role and central relation to other components of functioning. This, in turn, generates a result that is associated with other additional benefits.

Therefore, changes at the level of activity can be associated with changes at the level of participation restrictions (for example, to be able to run must lead to being able to participate once more in sports training) or with benefits at the level of impairments (to be able to do squats again may reflect an improvement in joint range.

For decades, physiotherapists have measured results based on the level of impairment (e.g. strength, range of motion). Far more recent is the interest in combining impairment measures with activities and participation. Nonetheless, some clinicians are still reluctant to apply these more recent measures. The main barrier in these cases has been to assume that measuring the improvement at the impairment level is sufficient because it entails an improvement at the activity level. However this is not necessarily true in all cases.[7,8]

20.3 ASSESSMENT TOOLS

There are many tools available for the measurement of results in physiotherapy for patients with tendinopathies. To measure results of the body function component alone, there are many mechanical instruments (e.g. goniometer, dynamometer), electrical instruments (e.g. electromyography, video, accelerometers) or others.

Because of space limitations, and considering that the activity component is the main result that should be prioritized, this chapter will focus on the available instruments for assessments at the activity level.

20.3.1 Types of assessment tools (at the level of activity)

There are many tests that have been used to measure patient function. These mainly consist of questionnaires with multiple items (see appendices). The existing tools can be classified according to two criteria: the specificity of the items' content and the way in which they are administered.

20.3.1.1 Types of tools according to the specificity of the items' content

These may be:
- Specific: they contain activities that are relevant or become affected when there is a specific problem in an area (for example, the patella) or for a type of patient or aspect. However, such activities are irrelevant for problems in other areas (such as neck pain), patients or aspects. The VISA-P[3] represents a good example of this type of tool.
- Generic: these contain activities that are not specific to any single pathology or diagnosis, e.g. the physical function of the SF-36.[9]

Among the specific tools used to measure results in tendinopathies, there are four types, according to the area in which the items are focused:

1. With a focus on body areas: examples include the Disabilities of the Arm, Shoulder and Hand (DASH)[10] questionnaire or the index of foot function.[11]
2. Patient-centred: the most representative tool is the Patient Specific Functional Scale,[12] which asks patients to identify three activities in which they have difficulty as a consequence of their health condition. Additionally, they are asked to evaluate their capacity to perform each activity on a scale of 11 points, ranging from 0 (unable to perform the activity) to 10 (able to perform the activity with no problem whatsoever). What sets this test apart from other tools is that it does not have a preset list of activities; rather it offers patients the opportunity of creating their own list.
3. Centred on pathology: for example, the VISA-P[3] questionnaire or the VISA index for Achilles tendinopathy (VISA-A).[13]
4. Centred on an ICF domain: a fitting example is the Mobility Activities Measurement for Outpatient Rehabilitation settings (MOBAM).[14]

It is worth highlighting that most of the specific tools available do not contain representative items from a single component or ICF domain. For example:

- The VISA questionnaires use concepts associated with the component of limited activities (items 1–6), as well as restrictions in participation (items 7 and 8).
- The DASH questionnaire includes, among others, activities from both domains of mobility activities and self-care.

This tendency to combine items belonging to different components or domains was the norm before the existence of a conceptual framework with defined domains provided by the ICF. Currently, the tendency for new assessment tools is to centre these on the components and domains defined by the WHO. An example of this is the

MOBAM.[14] However, at present, instruments that use this approach are still scarce.

20.3.1.2 Types of tools according to mode of administration

Following this criterion, measurements are based on observation of the patient's performance or self-reporting by the patient.

- Assessment tools based on patient's self-reporting employ direct questions in order to ask individuals what their level of function is for different activities, e.g. the ability to walk a certain distance or the use of aids. An example is the DASH or the VISA-A. Although most of these activities allow for observation and judgement by the interviewer, the value of this type of tool is that it provides perceptual information from the patient's perspective. Some of these tools are self-administered by the patient, and others have been designed for use by an interviewer, but almost all include multiple items.
- The instruments based on observation of performance are based on the physiotherapist observing the patient while he or she performs an activity. An example of this type of test, as used in tendinopathies, is the assessment scale of ankle lesions (ELT).[15] There are others which are better known, although they have not been applied in tendinopathies: the 6-minute walking test,[16] the functional reach test,[17] the Get-Up and Go Test[18] and the Functional Independence Measure (FIM).[19]

Some of these instruments contain a single test (such as the Get-Up and Go) and others use a battery of multiple items (ELT or FIM). In all cases, the final goal when using them should be to describe the real level of performance or execution of the individual ('reach this position and stop'), to identify the maximal level possible ('reach this position as fast as possible and stop'), or both. The instruction given to the patient determines the sought-after goal.

20.3.2 Format of the items

Most of the existing tools, both those based on performance and self-report measures, contain multiple items. This section is focused on describing the characteristics of two basic structural elements of the instruments containing multiple items (such as the DASH or ELT).

20.3.3 Wording of the items

The item headings contain information that the person who reads or observes must assess.

In the tools that assess the activities domain, the headings usually have two parts: one in which the activity that may be limited is described, and another one that provides contextual information in order to describe it. For example:

- In the DASH, the list of specific tasks is preceded and put into context with the following prompt: 'Rate your ability to do the following activities in the last week'.
- In the VISA-P the 'sitting' task is contextualized by the question: 'For how many minutes can you sit painfree?'

In both of the above examples, for the purpose of contextualizing a given situation, qualifiers may be used (for example, degree of difficulty) or quantifiers (such as the length of time). The most common qualifiers are:

- Difficulty: the degree of extra burden that the activity has due to the presence of slowness, increased effort, pain or changes in the way it is performed.
- Pain: the degree of pain that appears when the patient performs the activity.
- Dependence: the need for human or mechanical assistance in order to perform an activity, and to what degree.

The most common quantifiers are the time it takes to complete an activity and the number of repetitions.

20.3.4 Response formats

The response format represents the context for registering the answers. The most common format is a closed question with a binary answer in a nominal scale, or on a gradual ordinal scale:

- binary answers (able/unable to perform; independent/dependent)
- gradual ordinal scales (no difficulty, mild, moderate, severe, complete). Normally there are three to five response options, although sometimes scales that offer more alternatives are used, especially when qualifying pain, such as numerical scales (from 0 to 10).

20.3.5 Score calculation-summary

Summary scores provide a certain grade of functional capacity that the individual has in the assessed domain. The most common calculation system in this type of scoring is the sum of the codes of the answers provided on all the items. This can be expressed as a proportion of the sum of the total raw score (85/170 in the case of the Five Factor Inventory) or as a percentage (50%).

Assessment tools may provide one or two summary scores: some provide a single summary score, such as the VISA-P. Others provide partial scores by groups of interrelated items (subscales), such as the DASH. This test is composed of a subscale of up to 30 items, in which the scores are summed and transformed, by subtracting 30 from the raw summary score and dividing this by 1.2:

$$Score = (raw\ score - 30)/1.2$$

This transformation allows measurement of a range from 0 to 100, with the high scores indicating larger disabilities. Additionally, there are two optional modules (one for athletes, and another for workers), which are scored separately from the 30 items. The scoring for the module is also transformed to vary between 0 and 100 via the following algorithm:

$$Score = (raw\ score - 4)/1.6$$

Finally, other tests provide a scoring system for their subscales, as well as scores or more global indexes from the ensemble of items, as occurs in the SF-36. This instrument has eight scales, with scores ranging from 0 to 100, with the higher scores indicating a better state of health, and two subcomponents (mental and physical) gathering the items of various scales.

When interpreting a summary score it is important to exercise caution, especially when comparing scores between patients. For example, two patients with a similar score could have different limitations on the ensemble of tasks covered by the tool, as they may have lost (or gained) points in different activities. Therefore, although the summary scores provide a 'gross number' which is commonly considered a measure in an interval scale, this practice ought to be reconsidered.[20]

20.4 SELECTION OF ASSESSMENT TOOLS

The selection of an assessment tool on behalf of the clinician requires a thorough review of the tests and arguments used by the authors who developed the tools or by the researchers who have tested them. The many concepts and technical adjectives used (for example, test–retest reliability, concurrent validity and others) should not disconcert a clinician as, in the end, behind these terms what we have are simply tests and arguments to support the tool, having established measurements on a certain population, without excessive errors (random or systematic) and with an assumable cost.

20.4.1 Assessment tool selection

This section will introduce the clinician to the description and interpretation of the attributes that one hopes to find in an assessment tool and, therefore, help to avoid choosing an inadequate tool. These desirable attributes can be grouped into three big conceptual areas, within which more detailed categories can be established: appropriateness according to the patient's characteristics, adequacy of the metric properties and feasibility.

20.4.2 Appropriateness according to the patient's characteristics

20.4.2.1 Tested on the target population

Ideally, an assessment tool will have been previously tested on the clinical population on which it will be used (such as, for example, patients with patellar tendinopathy). This will provide us with relevant information both on how the metric properties of the tool work out on that specific population group (as it can vary between groups), as well as information on the acceptance of the tool on their behalf.

Additionally, it would be desirable to have normative measures obtained from the tested group, as they will be very useful in the interpretation of the measures gathered in the clinic.

20.4.2.2 Measures which allow for change

Usually, a measurement provides summary scores that allow for patients to demonstrate improvement or deterioration. It is undesirable for a test to provide a measure of the highest levels of function (99 over a maximum score of 100), as very little further improvement will be detected in that patient. This phenomenon is called the ceiling effect. In the opposite circumstance, if the test provides a measure of the lowest levels, this is called a floor effect, and in this case, such a tool would be unable to detect a possible deterioration.

20.4.3 Adequate metric properties

20.4.3.1 Reliability

Reliability is the degree to which, by administering an assessment tool, one obtains scores free from random error – in other words, errors due to undetermined causes that may vary between measurements. The authors or researchers of the assessment tool can basically measure reliability in two distinct ways: repeatability (or reproducibility) and internal consistency.

- The measurement of reliability through repetition requires the tool to be administered at least twice to a group of patients, either by two examiners (interexaminer reliability) or by the same examiner on two different occasions (intraexaminer or test–retest reliability). If the same conditions are met when the measurements are repeated, the existence of discrepancies between both measurements suggests that some type of error or random measurement is taking place. In order to measure the percentage of agreement, coefficients are used (e.g. intraclass correlation coefficient, the kappa index). These coefficients measure the degree of agreement or consistency between two measurements in the group of patients, and may assume values between 0 and 1, with 0 being indicative of null reliability (or that the variations among measurements can be attributed to random measurement errors) and 1 indicative of high reliability (or that the measurement has no error).

- The measurement of internal consistency reliability requires the tool to be administered only once to a group of patients. Internal consistency reliability is desirable, especially in questionnaires with multiple items that seek to measure the same content domain. For the measurement of internal consistency, other coefficients are also used (e.g. Cronbach's alpha coefficient, coefficient KR-20). Unlike the coefficients used to examine reproducibility, these coefficients measure the degree of homogeneity among item scores, but their value also varies between 0 and 1. The interpretation is similar, but follows a different reasoning: if a multi-item questionnaire has a high coefficient of internal consistency, this indicates that someone consistently selects low or high answers in the group of the scale tems (which, in theory, measures nuances of a same result), and therefore that random error is not present in the item response, whether due to aspects such as incorrect reading of the headings, distraction, misunderstanding or other reasons.

Reliability coefficients, estimated use of any of the two procedures (reproducibility or internal consistency), are useful in order to:

- estimate the credibility that can be given to measures established with the given tool. Ideally, the coefficients have a value of between 0.90 and 0.95 in intraindividual comparisons that take place regularly in daily clinical practice, and higher than 0.7 in comparisons between groups

- calculate the standard (or typical) error of measurement (SEM). This measure provides an estimate of the measurement error that could be obtained if the test were repeated on the same patient. The common formula for calculation in the case of tools in which the objective is the measurement of change is as follows (note that the higher the reliability coefficient, the lower the SEM):

$$SEM = \text{Standard deviation} \times \sqrt{1 - \text{reliability coefficient}}$$
(from the test–retest)

For example, imagine a tool that was tested on two occasions (test–retest) on 80 patients, for which the value of the reliability coefficient was 0.85 and the SEM was 5. This latter value means that the application of this tool normally (or typically) entails an error of 5 points.

This value is very useful for interpreting the results of a one-off assessment or to determine whether there is a change between repeated measurements.

20.4.3.2 Validity

The validity of a questionnaire, in which the goal is to measure the results in order to assess changes, refers to the available arguments which support the tool. This, in turn, convinces those who are going to use it that the measures can be used for a stated purpose.

The authors or researchers usually perform what is called a validation process, the objective being to accumulate proof and scientific arguments that support the use of the tool. There are many ways to support claims to validity, e.g. tests based on comparisons with other tools, tests based on content.

For example, validation of the Spanish version of the VISA-P[3] provides proof of the existence of a positive moderate correlation between scores and those offered by the dimensions of the physical function component of the SF-36. This helps the author to reason in favour of the use of the scores provided by the tool. Why? Because if the scoring of the VISA-P is valid and it is useful for the measurement of function associated with tendinopathy, it is expected that it will be empirically related to another accepted measure of function, such as the SF-36.

The decision on behalf of the author or researcher regarding which and what degree of evidence is needed in order for a new questionnaire to be considered as valid depends on what is thought to be convincing. In any case, several tests are usually used. Traditionally, according to the type of evidence used, different adjectives are used to accompany the validity term, e.g. convergent validity (for evidence based on comparison with measures of similar concepts which result in a positive correlation, such as the previous example), content validity. However it is important to emphasize that the cited adjectives must not disconcert the clinician regarding the selection of a measurement tool, because behind these terms, all there is are tests and arguments used by the authors to indicate that errors are not produced when the tool is used.

20.4.4 Feasibility

The feasibility of a tool is determined by availability aspects (availability of the instrument, of the associated material, time) and the burden associated with the use of this tool for the clinician and the patient. For the patient, the burden is related to the amount of time needed to complete the tool, the difficulty derived from comprehension problems and acceptability of the item content. For the clinician, the burden must be considered especially for the tools administered via interview or observation. The time needed for training in the use of the tool and the time it takes to administer the tool are the main areas for consideration. The authors of the tools usually provide information on these aspects.

20.5 INTERPRETATION OF THE RESULTS

The interpretation of the results should be, on the one hand, for the measurements obtained at a determined moment in time, as well as for the changes in scores that occur over time.

20.5.1 Interpretation of a one-time measurement in time

See the following example.

Tom is a 36-year-old man who attends a physiotherapy clinic due to a disabling pain located in his upper limb. On the first visit, the physiotherapist measures, among others, the range of shoulder abduction (120°) and administers the DASH (score = 74).

In order for a score to be of use for a physiotherapist and a patient it must be interpreted and make sense. How are both measures interpreted? The professional will have a clinical image which will provide the measure of the 120° and will

reveal any abnormality for a patient of that age. However, it is probable that the professional will not be able to answer the following questions: what meaning do the 74 points have? What is the measurement error associated with administration of the DASH? And, consequently, what is the interval in which Tom's true score lies?

What follows are several of the methods used to aid in the interpretation of these measures. For a one-off measure to have a meaning, the commonly used method is to interpret the score in terms relative to the normal scores – in other words, the scores previously obtained by the instrument by an interest group, known as the normative group.

The normative scores most commonly used are the percentile values, which represent a percentage of people from the normative sample with scores inferior to a determined score. Table 20.3 presents the percentiles that have been determined by applying a measurement tool of mobility activities on a group of patients who were treated in several centres during the month they started physiotherapy.[21]

TABLE 20.3	Percentiles and basic mobility scores at 1 month of treatment		
Score	Percentile (%)	Score	Percentile (%)
29.17	0	60.75	64
35.50	1	61.28	65
37.73	1	61.64	67
39.61	2	62.18	70
41.21	3	62.53	72
42.11	4	62.98	75
42.64	4	63.43	75
43.98	5	63.87	76
45.23	7	64.41	78
46.39	10	64.76	78
47.46	13	65.30	80
48.53	15	65.66	82
49.51	18	66.28	83
50.49	23	66.64	84
51.38	28	67.26	86
52.27	33	67.62	87
53.08	35	68.33	89
53.97	37	68.60	89
54.24	38	69.49	90
54.77	41	69.76	91
55.58	46	70.83	92
56.20	48	71.01	93
56.38	50	72.26	95
57.18	53	72.52	95
57.98	54	74.04	96
58.79	56	74.22	97
58.97	57	76.45	98
59.68	60	79.13	98
59.86	61	83.05	100
60.48	63	100.00	100

Adapted from: Jette et al.[21]

For example (using table 20.3), if a new patient scores 47.5, this corresponds with the 13th percentile, and could be interpreted as follows: only 13% of patients from the normative group have scores lower than 47.5 on this tool.

For a one-off measure to have any significance, another additional requirement when comparing it with normative data is that the clinician has an idea of what the most common measurement error is. This error is the SEM, already cited in section 2.4.3.1. The authors or researchers usually provide it after testing the tool on a group of participants. The SEM reports on the precision with which a summary score can be offered, as it provides an interval, within which the true measure can be found with a confidence of 95%, according to the following formula:

$$\text{Score} \pm 1.96 \times \text{SEM} = 74 \pm 1.96 \times 7.1 = 74 \pm 14$$

For example, if Tom scored 74 at baseline and the SEM of the instrument is 7.1,[22] it is possible to say that the real score is in the interval of 60–84 points, with a 95% confidence interval (CI).

This last method can be used if the SEM or 95% CI are available. The method based on ordering the percentiles has the inconvenience of being highly dependent on the existence and quality of normative data for the tool.

20.5.2 Interpretation of the measure of change in time

Tom attends a physiotherapy centre for 3 weeks. He progresses and is now able to do more activities with his upper limb. The physiotherapist administers the DASH test at the end of the 3rd week and he scores 24.

Can we affirm without any doubt that the measurement of change $(74 - 24 = 50)$ is not due in any way to the measurement error of the tool? Is the amount of change enough to be representative of truly relevant clinical changes? Or, even though there is a numerical improvement, does this not necessarily constitute one that is clinically relevant?

The interpretation of any change between two measurements taken at different times is usually the result of the comparison between the amount of change registered (50 in the case of Tom) and some of the following reference measures:

- Minimal detectable change (MDC): the MDC represents the smallest difference above which one can consider that actual change beyond measurement error has occurred between assesments. The MDC is usually provided by the authors of the tools. For example, the MDC of the DASH is 12.7.[22]

For example, in the case of Tom, as his measurement of change (50) exceeds the value of the MDC, one can affirm that it is unlikely that the change is due to measurement error.

- Minimal clinically important difference (MCID): The MCID is so called because it represents the smallest difference in score which patients perceive as being beneficial. The MCID is usually provided by the authors of the tools. For example, the MCID of the DASH is approximately 15.[22]

For example, in the case of Tom, as his measurement of change (50) exceeds the value of the MCID, one can affirm that it is probable that the change of score is accompanied by a significant clinical change for the patient and therefore this should probably be accompanied by an update in the therapeutic plan.

The procedure for calculating the MDC and the MCID is beyond the scope of this chapter. What is most relevant on this topic is the interpretation of these measures.

20.6 THE USEFULNESS OF OUTCOME MEASURES

The use of outcome measures in clinical practice can be useful, at least in fulfilling the purposes cited below. Note that group measures are required for all of these, except for the first in the list. Although, up to this point, this chapter has focused on individual measures (or the comparison of measures from the same patient), this section offers an additional vision into the opportunities that are made possible by considering outcomes at a group level.

20.6.1 Decision making in the process of care

The use of outcome measures, especially when applied to activities, provides information that can be used with several goals:

- as a baseline from which to establish the goals of the intervention
- as reference measurements that indicate both the patient's initial capacity and that stimulate a progression towards improvement from the initial episode
- as reference measurements regarding the security and confidence of the patient when performing specific tasks
- as evidence of the effectiveness of the intervention which may be used to change or end the therapeutic plan.

20.6.2 Research

The goal of research is to develop or produce new knowledge which can be, ultimately, generalized to the larger population. This new-found knowledge could be related to the identification of factors associated with a result; the impact of a specific intervention or programme; the understanding of the best result predictors; the metric properties of the applied instruments, or other factors.

Such knowledge can be acquired, for example, via highly controlled experimental studies (clinical trials) or the well-organized analysis of the results that occur in a centre or a network of centres. This last option is called outcomes research, and is accessible to centres that accumulate data in real time. Outcomes research uses the databases that include results and data on the use of services and characteristics of the patients to examine relations. The databases may also be used to perform epidemiological studies which describe limitation and recovery patterns, or the distribution of the determinants of disability.

In any case, in order to provide new knowledge through research, whether or not the data used were already gathered, or whether the data proceeded from new patients at the start of a study, it is important to remember that it is necessary to use appropriate sample sizes and analyses that are more complex than those provided by individual case data.

20.6.3 Assessment of the quality provided

The results accumulated in the databases of clinical centres can be used to develop quality measures, for example, by determining the proportion (adjusted) of patients with supraspinatus tendinopathies who demonstrate an improvement in the DASH, above the MCD (or MCID) in the period of x weeks.

These measures are indicators of the quality of assistance provided to the patient on behalf of the professionals and coordinators of the centre and can be, in turn, used for several purposes:

- To improve quality of care. The use of quality measures (or indicators) with this purpose requires a first evaluation and baseline of the results registered up until then to be established. Also, opportunities for improvement should be identified and consequent effort made, as well as further re-evaluation in order to assess the effect of these efforts. This process can be developed for the quality improvement, both in an institution or centre, as well as throughout several establishments.
- To provide information to the range of interested public: potential clients, consultants who purchase health services for their clients, healthcare legislators. The information may help them to compare and select providers, and even achieve applicable accreditation processes.

20.6.4 Evidence-based clinical practice (EBCP)

EBCP, also initially called 'evidence-based medicine', represents integration of the individual clinical competency with the best external clinical evidence available, together with the patient's own preferences and the centre facilities (space, equipment, time). Evidence-based medecine is an expression from the former movement for improvement of clinical quality, which was empowered by the revelation that many clinical decisions lacked foundation, and also by the considerable variability in the medical practice. This movement began in the 1960s, when the design of clinical trials began to be applied to the medical field.

EBCP requires searching for and identifying relevant studies in the literature in order to: respond to a clinical question that is posed; evaluate the studies critically; and assess the probability of applying the results of the study/studies selected to the clinical situation. This information needs to be valued by the clinician, who screens it and makes a decision considering his or her clinical experience, the availability of the centre and the needs of patients (comorbidities, pattern of disability). In this assessment it may be helpful to have a database of results from the centre,[23] as the results may contain information about what occurred in the centre, more specifically with patients who have a similar condition to those for whom the same decisions are to be applied.

The best external clinical evidence available refers to the relevant clinical research that examines the tests and measurements of the clinical exam, as well as the prognostic markers, effectiveness and safety of the treatments.[24] The practice of EBCP implies searching for the best external evidence in order to respond to clinical questions. This is not restricted to randomized controlled trials and meta-analyses, but rather the emphasis is in relation to the content of the clinical question. For example:

- In order to understand the exactness of a measurement, appropriate cross-sectional studies of patients clinically suspected of presenting the disorder in question are needed, not randomized controlled trials.

- For a question related to prognostic information, adequate patient follow-up studies are needed.
- When questions regarding treatment are posed, randomized controlled trials are preferable, as well as systematic reviews of several randomized controlled trials.

20.7 REFERENCES

1. American Physical Therapy Association. The guide to physical therapist practice. Alexandria, VA: APTA; 2001.
2. Ingersoll GL. Generating evidence through outcomes management. In: Melnyk BM, Fineout-Overholt E, editors. Evidence-based practice in nursing and healthcare: a guide to best practice. Philadelphia, PA: Lippincott, Williams & Wilkins; 2005. p. 299–332.
3. Visentini PJ, Khan KM, Cook JL, et al. The VISA score: an index of severity of symptoms in patients with jumper's knee (patellar tendinosis). Victorian Institute of Sport Tendon Study Group. J Sci Med Sport 1998;1(1):22–8.
4. Canadian Physiotherapy Association. Physical rehabilitation outcomes measures. A guide to enhanced clinical decision making. Hamilton, Ontario: CPA; 2002.
5. World Health Organization. International classification of functioning, disability, and health. Geneva: World Health Organization; 2001.
6. Fernández-López JA, Fernández-Fidalgo M, Geoffrey R, et al. Funcionamiento y discapacidad: la clasificación internacional del funcionamiento (CIF). Rev Esp Salud Pública 2009;83:775–83.
7. Jette AM, Keysor JJ. Disability models: implications for arthritis exercicse and physical activity interventions. Arthritis Rheum 2003;49:114–20.
8. Guccionne AA, Mielenz TJ, Devellis RF, et al. Development and testing of a self-report instrument to measure-actions: outpatient physical therapy improvement in movement assessment log. Phys Ther 2005;85:515–30.
9. Alonso J, Prieto L, Anto JM. The Spanish version of the SF-36 Health Survey (the SF-36 health questionnaire): an instrument for measuring clinical results. Med Clin (Barc) 1995;104:771–6.
10. Hudak PL, Amadio PC, Bombardier C. Development of an upper extremity outcome measure: the DASH (disabilities of the arm, shoulder and hand) [corrected]. The Upper Extremity Collaborative Group (UECG). Am J Ind Med 1996;29(6):602–8. Erratum in: Am J Ind Med 1996 Sep;30(3):372.
11. Budiman-Mak E, Conrad KJ, Roach K. The foot function index: a measure of foot pain and disability. J Clin Epidemiol 1991;4:561–70.
12. Stratford P, Gill C, Westaway M, et al. Assessing disability and change on individual patients: a report of a patient specific measure. Physiother Can 1995;47:258–63.
13. Robinson JM, Cook JL, Purdam C, et al. Victorian Institute Of Sport Tendon Study Group. The VISA-A questionnaire: a valid and reliable index of the clinical severity of Achilles tendinopathy. Br J Sports Med 2001;35:335–41.
14. Medina-Mirapeix F, Navarro-Pujalte E, Escolar-Reina P, et al. Mobility activities measurement for outpatient rehabilitation settings. Arch Phys Med Rehabil 2011;92:632–9.
15. Kaikkonen A, Kannus P, Jarvinen M. A performance test protocol and scoring scale for the evaluation of ankle injuries. Am J Sports Med 1994;22:462–9.
16. Guyatt GH, Sullivan MJ, Thompson PJ, et al. The 6-minute walk: a new measure of exercise capacity in patients with chronic heart failure. Can Med Assoc J 1985;132:919–23.
17. Duncan PW, Weiner DK, Chandler J, et al. Functional reach: a new clinical measure of balance. J Gerontol 1990;45:M192–7.
18. Mathias S, Nayak US, Isaacs B. Balance in elderly patients: the 'get up and go' test. Arch Phys Med Rehabil 1986;67:387–9.
19. Granger CV, Cotter AC, Hamilton BB, et al. Functional assessment scales: a study of persons with multiple sclerosis. Arch Phys Med Rehabil 1990;71:870–5.
20. Jette A, Haley S. Contemporany measurement techniques for rehabilitation outcomes assessment. J Rehabil Med 2005;37:339–45.
21. Jette A, Tao BS, Norweg A, et al. Interpreting rehabilitation outcomes measurements. J Rehabil Med 2007;39:585–90.
22. Beaton D, Katz J, Fossel A, et al. Measuring the whole or the parts? Validity, reliability and responsiveness of the Disabilities of the Arm, Shoulder and Hand outcomes measures in different regions of the upper extremity. J Hand Ther 2001;14:128–42.
23. Sackett D, Haynes B. Evidence-based-medicine: how to practice and teach EBM. 2nd ed. New York: Churchill-Livingstone; 2000.
24. Sackett D, Rosenberg W, Gray W, et al. Evidence based medicine: what it is and what it isn't. BMJ 1996;312:71–4.

20.8 APPENDIX

Appendix 1: VISA-P score

1.   For how many minutes can you sit pain free?

0 mins ☐☐☐☐☐☐☐☐☐☐☐ 100 mins   Points ☐

    0   1   2   3   4   5   6   7   8   9   10

2.   Do you have pain walking downstairs with a normal gait cycle?

strong
severe ☐☐☐☐☐☐☐☐☐☐☐ no pain   Points ☐
pain

    0   1   2   3   4   5   6   7   8   9   10

3.   Do you have pain at the knee with full active non-weightbearing knee extension?

strong
severe ☐☐☐☐☐☐☐☐☐☐☐ no pain   Points ☐
pain

    0   1   2   3   4   5   6   7   8   9   10

4. Do you have pain when doing a full weight bearing lunge?

strong
severe ☐☐☐☐☐☐☐☐☐☐☐ no pain   Points ☐
pain

    0   1   2   3   4   5   6   7   8   9   10

5. Do you have problems squatting?

Unable ☐☐☐☐☐☐☐☐☐☐☐ no problems   Points ☐

    0   1   2   3   4   5   6   7   8   9   10

6. Do you have pain during or immediately after doing 10 single leg hops?

strong severe ☐☐☐☐☐☐☐☐☐☐☐ no pain   Points ☐
pain/unable

    0   1   2   3   4   5   6   7   8   9   10

7. Are you currently undertaking sport or other physical activity?

0   ☐   Not at all

4   ☐   Modified training ± modified competition

7   ☐   Full training ± competition but not at same level as when symptoms began

10   ☐   Competing at the same or higher level as when symptoms began

8. Please complete **EITHER A, B or C** in this question.

• If you have **no pain** while undertaking sport please complete **Q8a only**.

• If you have **pain while undertaking sport but it does not stop you** from completing the activity, please complete **Q8b only**.

• If you have **pain that stops you from completing sporting activities,** please complete **Q8c only**.

8a. If you have **no pain** while undertaking sport, for how long can you train/practise?

NIL	1–5 mins	6–10 mins	7–15 mins	>15 mins	
❑	❑	❑	❑	❑	Points ❑
0	7	14	21	30	

OR

8b. If you have some pain while undertaking sport, but it does not stop you from completing your training/practice for how long can you train/practise?

NIL	1–5 mins	6–10 mins	7–15 mins	>15 mins	
❑	❑	❑	❑	❑	
0	4	10	14	20	Points ❑

OR

8c. If you have **pain which stops you** from completing your training/practice for how long can you train/practise?

NIL	1–5 mins	6–10 mins	7–15 mins	>15 mins	
❑	❑	❑	❑	❑	
0	2	5	7	10	Points ❑

TOTAL VISA SCORE ❑

Adapted from: Visentini PJ, Khan KM, Cook JL et al. The VISA score: an index of severity of symptoms in patients with jumper's knee (patellar tendinosis). Victorian Institute of Sport Tendon Study Group. J Sci Med Sport 1998;1(1):22–28.

Appendix 2: Disabilities of the Arm, Shoulder and Hand (DASH)

Please rate your ability to do the following activities in the last week by circling the number below the appropriate response.

	NO DIFFICULTY	MILD DIFFICULTY	MODERATE DIFFICULTY	SEVERE DIFFICULTY	UNABLE
1. Open a tight or new jar.	1	2	3	4	5
2. Write.	1	2	3	4	5
3. Turn a key.	1	2	3	4	5
4. Prepare a meal.	1	2	3	4	5
5. Push open a heavy door.	1	2	3	4	5
6. Place an object on a shelf above your head.	1	2	3	4	5
7. Do heavy household chores (e.g., wash walls, wash floors.)	1	2	3	4	5
8. Garden or do yard work.	1	2	3	4	5
9. Make a bed.	1	2	3	4	5
10. Carry a shopping bag or briefcase.	1	2	3	4	5
11. Carry a heavy object (over 10 lbs)	1	2	3	4	5
12. Change a lightbulb overhead.	1	2	3	4	5
13. Wash or blow dry your hair.	1	2	3	4	5
14. Wash your back.	1	2	3	4	5
15. Put on a pullover sweater.	1	2	3	4	5
16. Use a knife to cut food.	1	2	3	4	5
17. Recreational activities which require little effort (e.g., cardplaying, knitting, etc.).	1	2	3	4	5
18. Recreational activities in which you take some force or impact through your arm, shoulder or hand (e.g., golf, hammering, tennis, etc.).	1	2	3	4	5
19. Recreational activities in which you move your arm freely (e.g., playing frisbee, badminton, etc.).	1	2	3	4	5
20. Manage transportation needs (getting from one place to another).	1	2	3	4	5
21. Sexual activities.	1	2	3	4	5

	NOT AT ALL	SLIGHTLY	MODERATELY	QUITE A BIT	EXTREMELY
22. During the past week, *to what extent* has your arm, shoulder or hand problem interfered with your normal social activities with family, friends, neighbours or groups? *(circle number)*	1	2	3	4	5

	NOT LIMITED AT ALL	SLIGHTLY LIMITED	MODERATELY LIMITED	VERY LIMITED	UNABLE
23. During the past week, were you limited in your work or other regular daily activities as a result of your arm, shoulder or hand problem? *(circle number)*	1	2	3	4	5

Please rate the severity of the following symptoms in the last week. *(circle number)*

	NONE	MILD	MODERATE	SEVERE	EXTREME
24. Arm, shoulder or hand pain.	1	2	3	4	5
25. Arm, shoulder or hand pain when you performed any specific activity.	1	2	3	4	5
26. Tingling (pins and needles) in your arm, shoulder or hand.	1	2	3	4	5
27. Weakness in your arm, shoulder or hand.	1	2	3	4	5
28. Stiffness in your arm, shoulder or hand.	1	2	3	4	5

	NO DIFFICULTY	MILD DIFFICULTY	MODERATE DIFFICULTY	SEVERE DIFFICULTY	SO MUCH DIFFICULTY THAT I CAN'T SLEEP
29. During the past week, how much difficulty have you had sleeping because of the pain in your arm, shoulder or hand? *(circle number)*	1	2	3	4	5

	STRONGLY DISAGREE	DISAGREE	NEITHER AGREE NOR DISAGREE	AGREE	STRONGLY AGREE
30. I feel less capable, less confident or less useful because of my arm, shoulder or hand problem. *(circle number)*	1	2	3	4	5

DASH DISABILITY/SYMPTOM SCORE = $[\frac{(\text{sum of } n \text{ responses}) - 1}{n}] \times 25$, where n is equal to the number of completed responses.

A DASH score may <u>not</u> be calculated if there are greater than three missing items.

Adapted from: Hudak PL, Amadio PC, Bombardier C. Development of an upper extremity outcome measure: the DASH (Disabilities of the Arm, Shoulder and Hand) [corrected]. The Upper Extremity Collaborative Group (UECG). Am J Ind Med 1996;29(6):602–608. Erratum in: Am J Ind Med 1996;30(3):372.

Appendix 3: Foot Functional Index

Section 1: To be completed by patient   Name:_____ Age:____ Date:_____

Occupation:_____   Number of days of foot pain:_____(this episode)

Section 2: To be completed by patient

This questionnaire has been designed to give your therapist information as to how your foot pain has affected your ability to manage in every day life. For the following questions, we would like you to score each question on a scale from 0 (no pain) to 10 (worst pain imaginable) that best describes your foot **over the past WEEK**. Please read each question and place a number from 0–10 in the corresponding box.

No Pain 0   1   2   3   4   5   6   7   8   9   10   **Worst Pain Imaginable**

	1.	In the morning upon taking your first step?	
	2.	When walking?	
	3.	When standing?	
	4.	How is your pain at the end of the day?	
	5.	How severe is your pain at its worst?	

Answer all of the following questions related to your pain and activities **over the past WEEK**, how much difficulty did you have?   **Disability Scale**

No Difficulty 0   1   2   3   4   5   6   7   8   9   10 **So Difficult unable to do**

	6.	When walking in the house?	
	7.	When walking outside?	
	8.	When walking four blocks?	
	9.	When climbing stairs?	
	10.	When descending stairs?	
	11.	When standing tip toe?	
	12.	When getting up from a chair?	
	13.	When climbing curbs?	
	14.	When running or fast walking?	

Answer all the following questions related to your pain and activities **over the past WEEK.** How much of the time did you: **Disability Scale:**

None of the time 0   1   2   3   4   5   6   7   8   9   10 **All of the time**

	15.	Use an assistive device (cane, walker, crutches, etc) indoors?	
	16.	Use an assistive device (cane, walker, crutches, etc) outdoors?	
	17.	Limit physical activities?	

Section 3: To be completed   by physical therapist/provider SCORE:_____/170 x 100 = _____%   (SEM 5, MDC 7)

SCORE: Initial_____   Subsequent_____   Subsequent_____   Discharge_____

Number of treatment sessions :_____

Diagnosis/ICD-9 Code :_____

Adapted from: Budiman-Mak E, Conrad KJ, Roach K. The foot function index: A measure of foot pain and disability. J Clin Epidemiol 1991; 4(6): 561–570.

CHAPTER 21

MEDICAL IMAGE PROCESSING, ANALYSIS AND VISUALIZATION WITH MUSCULOSKELETAL ULTRASOUND

José Ríos Díaz • Jacinto J. Martínez Payá • Ana de Groot Ferrando • Mª Elena del Baño Aledo

A man who sets it upon himself to learn must work with as much passion as I did myself in order to find that place, and the limits of his learning are determined by his own nature.

CARLOS CASTANEDA

KEYWORDS

image analysis; echo texture; grey-level scale; histogram; look-up tables; pixel; digital image processing; image resolution; image segmentation.

21.1 ULTRASOUND IMAGE PROCESSING AND ANALYSIS

The recent developments in biomedical imaging, together with the contributions of computer and electronic engineering and other branches such as medical physics, mathematics or chemistry, have promoted the revolutionary growth of diagnostic imaging.[1]

As a result, rapid advances in technology engineering have enabled production of multidimensional high-resolution images of complex organs. Structural and functional information can be obtained for computer-assisted diagnostics and the evaluation of both treatments and interventions.[2,3]

The medical image is classified broadly within radiological sciences, mainly because most have an application in radiological diagnostics. In the clinical setting, the biomedical image of a specific organ or body part is obtained for the purpose of clinical examination which aids in the diagnosis of illness or pathology.[1,3–5]

However, medical imaging tests can also be performed with the purpose of obtaining images and information on anatomical and functional structures for research purposes, both for healthy individuals as well as those with pathology.[6] These types of studies are essential in order to deepen our understanding of the physiological processes occurring within the body which, in turn, may help with the detection of pathology, the use of preventive measures and the generation of new knowledge as a basis for further development.[7]

From a scientific point of view, the biomedical imaging field is both multidisciplinary and interdisciplinary, and has a substantial presence in the fields of physics, biology, engineering and health science.[8]

The development of a specific imaging system begins with a physiological understanding of the biological environment and its relation to the information under study obtained from an image.[1]

Once this relation is determined, research is undertaken to seek the appropriate method for obtaining the sought-after information using a specific procedure for energy transformation, commonly known as imaging physics.[9] Likewise, when an imaging method is established, the appropriate tool is designed and integrated, with an energy source, detectors and data acquisition and into an imaging system, in order to gather specific information regarding patients, all in the context of pathological research.

KEY POINTS

Image processing and analysis, when applied to ultrasound, converts ultrasound into an excellent tool for research in biomedical science.

In the context of ultrasound imaging, the last decades have seen a great development and evolution of the related equipment, offering images of high resolution and precision.[10,11] However, the performance of image analysis and other types of procedures on ultrasound is not as frequent and has not been developed as much as other techniques. This may be due to the inherent characteristics of the technique and the dependence on the sonographer and his or her skills. What clearly is a virtue and advantage from a clinical point of view, such as the dynamism and versatility of the imaging, turns into a serious inconvenience that cannot be overlooked when ultrasound is intended to be used in a more scientific context.[12]

In our research group ECOFISTEM (@ecofistem), ultrasound has been used as a tool for research in the field of physiotherapy for over 10 years. Progressively different techniques and analysis methods have also been introduced which go beyond the simple morphometric measurements created by the equipment.[13–19]

In this chapter, we will outline the basic concepts that must be acknowledged when performing image analysis in general, as well as the specific details inherent to working with images obtained by ultrasound.

21.2 THE ULTRASONOGRAPHIC IMAGE

If a good ultrasonographic image is available which is well collected with the appropriate methodology, precision and efficiency, and if this is adequately stored, it opens a world of possibilities that will enable the professional to gather information that goes beyond clinical and anatomical reasoning, converting these techniques into excellent tools for the development of research in phyisiotherapy.[20]

KEY POINTS

In order to capture an image with a method and of good quality, it's essential to be able to work with it afterwards.

21.2.1 Image capture

In the first place, when working with biomedical images, it is important to know the physical mechanism whereby a type of energy is transformed into the final image that one is going to work with. For example, in the case of radiological images (simple radiography, tomography), an electromagnetic wave (with a wavelength within the spectrum of X-rays) passes through the tissues to reach a photographic plate or a sensitive plate which is connected to a monitor which, in turn, will receive the beam, which may become

TABLE 21.1 Acoustic impedance of the different tissues

Tissue	Attenuation coefficient (dB/cm to 1 MHz)	Speed of sound propagation (m/s)
Bone	20.0	3.360
Muscle	2.5	1.580
Blood	0.20	1.570
Kidney	1.0	1.560
Liver	0.94	1.550
Brain	0.85	1.540
Fat	0.63	1.450
Water	0.002	1.480
Air	12.0	348

more or less dimmed according to the tissues passed through it. In this way, the denser tissues are represented by whiter tonalities, and those which are less dense, such as air, by tones closer to black.

By contrast, with ultrasonography, the situation is radically different: the energy which is transmitted to the tissues is of a sonic type, with frequencies much higher than the audible threshold, i.e. not of an electromagnetic[21,22] type. The sonic beam passes through tissues which, due to their histological differences, will attenuate the mechanical wave to a higher or lesser degree. It is this higher or lower resistance which physicists have named acoustic impedance (table 21.1). These differences in acoustic impedance and, therefore, in the speed with which the echoes return to the transducer, will be transformed into an image which also has multiple tones of grey. In this case, the grey tones have a completely different significance to those found using X-rays (or magnetic fields, in the case of magnetic resonance). The capacity for attenuating the sonic wave is higher in those tissues which propagate it at a higher speed. The bone has a high capacity for attenuation and, therefore, if the sound wave 'hits' a bony structure, it will not let us 'see' the structures located posteriorly and an 'acoustic shadow' will appear. Something similar happens when it hits a cavity full of air. However, if the cavity is full of static liquid, the wave will be strengthened and we will easily be able to visualize the structures that lie beneath.

In chapter 5 we have provided an indepth explanation on how to interpret a lighter level of grey (hyperechoicity) or a darker shade of grey (hypoechoicity or anechoicity) using ultrasound. Simply put, one could say that lighter shades of grey that are closer to white appear in areas rich in connective tissue and darker shades of grey are seen in areas with a higher water content.

21.2.2 Electro-acoustic-electrical transduction

The transducer is an essential element in ultrasound equipment. It essentially works in a similar way to the transducer of therapeutic ultrasound machines. The transducer contains a crystal structure through which an electric current passes, which makes it vibrate and generate a sound wave. Depending on the structure of the crystal and the characteristics of the electric current, this will vibrate with one or another frequency. This phenomenon is called piezoelectricity, and was described by Pierre and Jacques Curie (1881) on quartz, after they noted that, when mechanical forces where used, the quartz polarized and, as a result, electrical charges were generated.[21,23]

KEY POINTS

Ultrasonographic images are the result of processing the echoes received by the transducer, representing the grey-scale levels that show the differences of acoustic impedance in tissues.

The transducer on an ultrasound machine uses this mechanism in a bidirectional mechanism in order to generate the ultrasound beam and to register the echoes proceeding from the tissues and transform them, once again, into an electric signal which will ultimately translate as a digital image shown on a monitor.

21.2.3 The digital image

The digital image is a bidimensional representation that uses a numerical matrix which, in ultrasound, corresponds to the echoes formed which are, more or less, attenuated from the initial sonic beam after passing through different tissues. It is important to consider that the digital image is a discrete representation of information (non-continuous or analogic), which is formed by hundreds of elements called pixels (from picture element). Consequently, a pixel represents the lowest basic element of a digital image, which is given a numerical value and is the basic information unit within that image, for that level of resolution and quantification.[24-26]

KEY POINTS

The pixel is the basic unit of digital images and it is associated with a determined level of brightness.

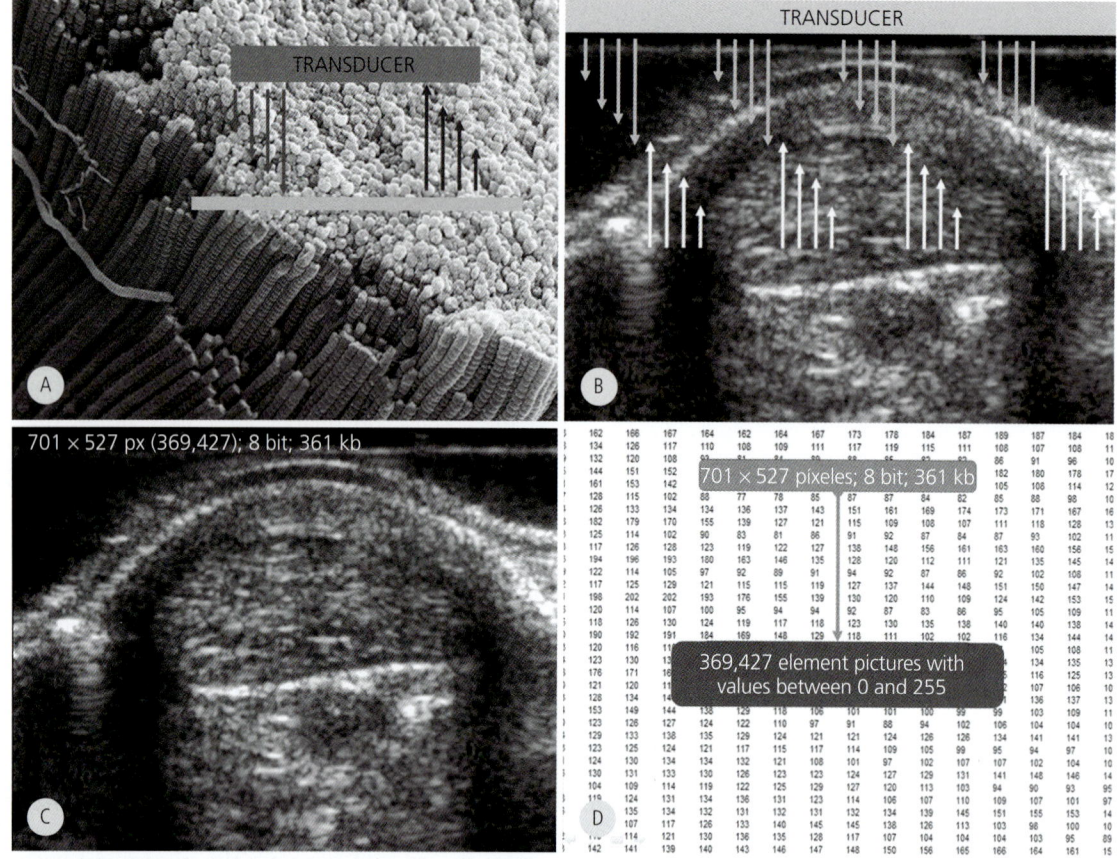

FIGURE 21.1 ■ Acquisition and construction of a digital ultrasound image. (A) The initial sonic beam passes through the tissues with different attenuation coefficients and acoustic impedance, causing a more or less marked delay in the resulting echoes (B). (C) corresponds to a transverse image of the Achilles tendon approximately 2 cm from its insertion point. The digital image is composed of a matrix of almost 370,000 pixels, each and every one of them with a grey level or tone of between 0 (black) and 255 (white). (D) Grey values from a small portion of the image represented in (C). Captured with LOGIQ-e equipment by General Electric® with transducer 12L-RS (7–13 MHz). (Colour version of figure is available online).

Each one of these elements is represented by a brightness intensity (or grey-level intensities), which allows us to interpret the structures being explored, together with the corresponding clinical and anatomical knowledge (figure 21.1). Within the field of ultrasound exploration, it is usually said that the first thing that we must ask ourselves is where and how the transducer was positioned, as a basis upon which later to reason anatomically and provide clinical conclusions.

The advantage of working with digital images is that the information provided from each one of the elements is the same. It is stored numerically and with the numbers we can perform mathematical operations, which allow us to manipulate, measure, analyse and/or modify these data matrixes. This ensemble of procedures falls within the field of image processing and analysis.

21.3 IMAGE PROCESSING

Image processing refers to the manipulation and analysis of information contained in the pixels; for example, improving, correcting, changing or analysing the image.[27,28] A simple example of these procedures can be illustrated with the analogy of a corrective lens for a vision problem: the lens performs optical processing because it acts over an optical image. As stated previously, a digital image is a matrix formed by distinct elements. When processing is performed on those elements, this is called digital image processing.

KEY POINTS

Image processing is known as the manipulation and analysis of the information contained in the digital images.

Digital processing operations can be grouped into five major categories. An indepth description would go beyond the scope of this chapter, but may be summarized as follows[27] (video 21.1).

21.3.1 Image enhancement techniques

These are used to improve some aspect relating to the quality of the image. Enhancement techniques are frequently performed in an interactive manner, so that the operator checks how to improve the quality by modifying the contrast or brightness, decreasing the noise or highlighting the borders.[29] In this type of technique, the image enhancement is subjective and depends on the judgement and experience of the operator, as there are no quantitative measures of image quality. Typically, the rate between contrast and artefacts can be measured through the receiver operating characteristic (ROC) curves generated to observe whether the changes seen in the image correspond to an improvement in the diagnosis.

Image enhancement can also be performed in the pre-processing phase, as part of an automatic analysis procedure. In this case, it is common to simplify the image considerably, producing a result which may be of little use to the human observer, but which may be useful and necessary for future analysis.

21.3.2 Image restoration

Image restoration is necessary when the method of acquiring the image produces geometric distortion or blurry images.[7,24] Geometric distortion refers to when centred objects appear non-centred, compressed or bulging outwards. It is common in magnetic resonance images to find distorted borders not discerned by the human eye, but important when seeking to combine them with computerized tomography images.

In the case of ultrasound if, during image acquisition, a low-quality image or any type of distortion is detected, it can be easily resolved simply by repeating the exploration.

21.3.3 Image analysis

The final result of image analysis operations is not usually an image, but rather numerical measurements obtained from the image data.[28–30] Some examples of analysis procedures include obtaining lengths, areas, perimeters, object classification or image segmentation.

This is one of the main applications of ultrasound. From these images it is possible to trace outlines, lines or regions of interest which will enable the measurement of lengths, perimeters and areas and echogenic parameters, as will be seen further on.

21.3.4 Image compression

Image files are generally large depending on the number of bytes they occupy. The size is not only important for the number of hard disk resources required, but also because of the time needed to transfer files from one device to another and the amount of RAM memory needed to work with ease. Numerous algorithms are available to compress images, and these can be simplified into lossy and lossless compression algorithms. The lossless algorithms are the only ones to be used in the context of biomedical image processing.[31] If lossy compressors are used, the loss of information which has been eliminated would be unrecoverable (figure 21.2).

In general terms, the image is stored in bitmap (BMP) or tagged image file format (TIFF) format, which allows for storage without loss. joint photograph experts group (JPG) or graphics interchange format (GIF) formats are avoided. If possible, save images in digital imaging and communication in medicine (DICOM) format, which stores both the data related to the patient and those of the image in the same file, even while storing a sequence (frames) of images.

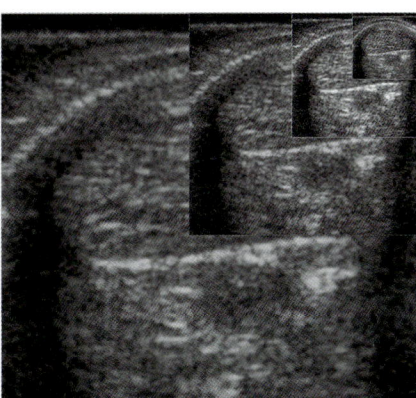

64 × 64 px
RGB; 16 kb

128 × 128 px
RGB; 64 kb

256 × 256 px
RGB; 256 kb

512 × 512 px
RGB; 1 Mb

FIGURE 21.2 ■ Representation of the same image with different sizes. Display of a transverse ultrasound image of the Achilles tendon, each sequence representing a fourth part of the preceding one. Note that by reducing the size of the matrix, the number of bits needed to store the image is also reduced. In order to work with digital images they must be stored with the highest size allowed by the original device, although this entails using a large amount of space on the hard disk. A false colour is applied to improve the contrast. Captured with LOGIQ-e equipment by General Electric® with transducer 12L-RS (7–13 MHz). Processed using *ImageJ* 1.46 with pseudocolour palettes. (Colour version of figure is available online).

21.3.5 Image synthesis

This is an area that may be less useful (and more appropriate for specialists), because it groups together the activities relating to image registration from different sources (for example, from a resonance and positron emission tomography), multidimensional visualization and three-dimensional reconstruction.[31]

When working with digital images there are several concepts that must be clear, and which are frequently confused, with regard to size, scale and resolution; this is especially important when trying to extract quantitative information.

KEY POINTS

It is necessary to differentiate between the terms of size, scale and resolution: these are concepts that are all interrelated but with varying meanings.

21.3.6 Size

The size refers to the dimensions of the image matrix (figure 21.2). The digital image has been described as a numerical matrix in which each pixel is represented by a numerical value. For image analysis software, each pixel is perfectly defined in a Cartesian system by specific coordinates defined by the row and column where it is located.[2–6]

It is simple to calculate the size of an image: normally all that is needed is to move the mouse over the image and the computer system will supply information about the dimensions of the matrix. Frequently, size is expressed by the number of pixels in rows and columns when it is less than 512×512 px. For larger sizes the result is given directly in total pixels (normally these will be seen in 'megas', megapixels or Mpx; for example, 10^6 pixels).

Regarding the size of the image, it is important to maintain the image proportions (aspect ratio) in order to avoid apparent image distortion. This is an effect that the reader will have probably experimented with at some point: when manipulating a digital image and increasing the height without modifying the width (or vice versa), the image becomes stretched out.

21.3.7 Scale

Scale refers to the relative size of the elements present in the image in relation to their normal size. There is no way of knowing the real size of the elements without a reference in the image.

This is the reason why in microscopy images there is a precept that there always be a metric reference bar.[25,27] In the case of ultrasound images, one must consider that, by changing the equipment parameters, such as the exploration depth, the scale will be modified. Many machines have a gradient on one of the sides of the images which allows for calibration of the image analysis software[31,32] when one wishes to make metric measurements (figure 21.3). However, it is advisable that, whenever an image sequence is to be used for a study in which morphometric variables are used, the same image acquisition parameters should be respected by all.[33]

KEY POINTS

A scale of reference is necessary when performing metric measurements on an image.

21.3.8 Resolution

Resolution is the size of the smallest structure that can be independently represented in the image. Resolution is a measure of the capacity to represent the original image faithfully. The resolution depends on the characteristics of the image acquisition system (commonly called resolution) and of the number of pixels and brightness used for the digitalization.[7,24,28]

In practice, there are other factors that affect resolution, but the most important ones are contrast and noise. Different situations may arise, such as having low-contrast images, which cause detail to be lost, or excessive contrast, which generally causes image elements to become superimposed. Noise refers to elements that appear in the image but that do not belong to the scene that is being represented. In the case of ultrasound, images are obtained with electromagnetic noise if the acquisition is taken close to other electronic equipment, such as plugs or outlets.[31,34]

The digitalization process consists of the transformation of the continual information contained in a real image, of an almost infinite number of light nuances and continuous graphic details, to discrete information which represents an image divided into a limited number of pixels, each one with a discrete level of brightness within a finite range of light intensity.

Thus, digitalization is made up of two different processes:
1. spatial digitalization, in which the continuous space is translated to a series of finite elements in the shape of a matrix of brightness points, pixels

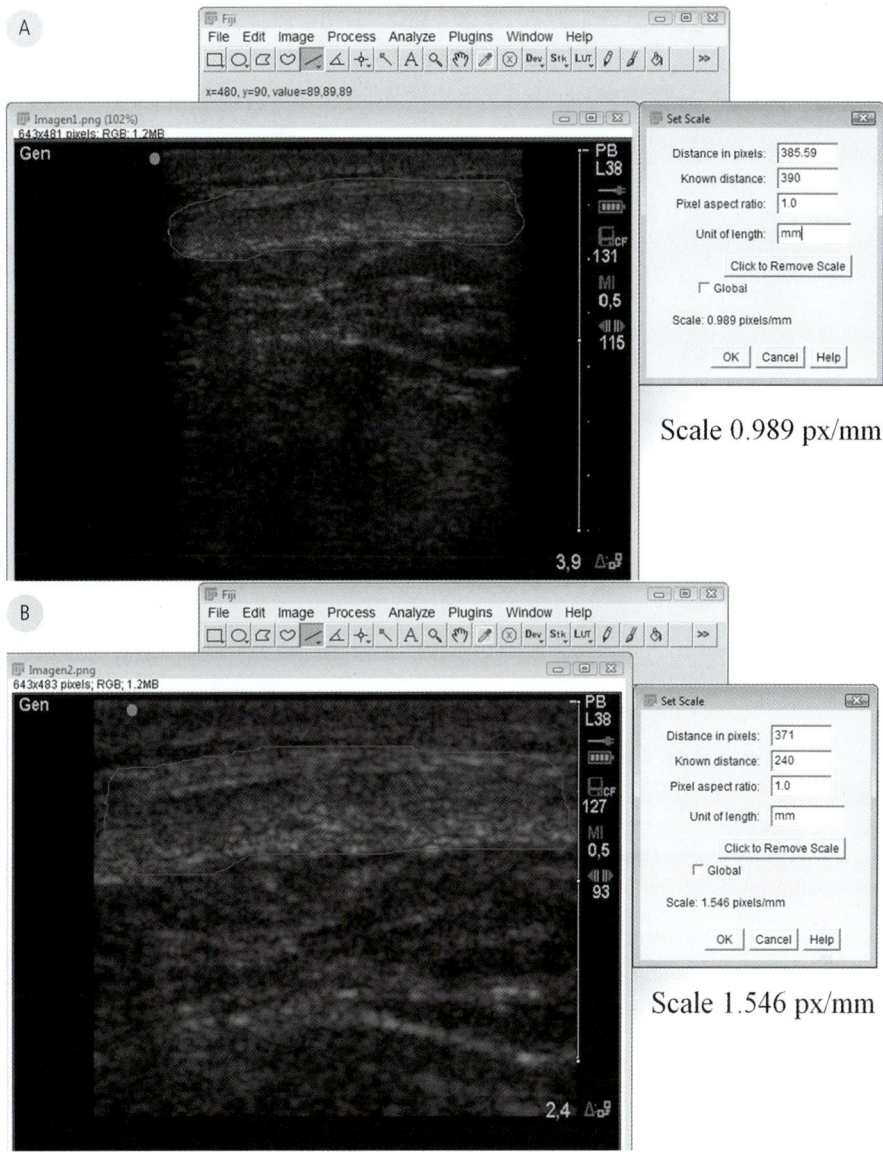

Scale 0.989 px/mm

Scale 1.546 px/mm

FIGURE 21.3 ■ Scaling of the ultrasound image. Transverse ultrasound image of the patellar tendon at 5 mm from its insertion on the patella. Note that the machine itself displays the information regarding the depth of the work and offers a scale which is highlighted in yellow. The tendon outline is highlighted in purple. (A) The depth of work at 3.9 cm provides a scale of 0.989 px/mm. (B) The depth of work at 2.4 cm provides a scale of 1.546 px/ mm. Captured with Sonosite Titan with L38 transducer. Image processing and calibration using *ImageJ* 1.46. (Colour version of figure is available online).

2. digitalization of the grey scale, the term by which the brightness represented by each pixel is known and the reflection of one or other energy, depending on what the image is representing (e.g. light, X-rays, magnetic fields, temperature, echoes).

KEY POINTS

The image resolution and the quality of detail will depend on the quality of the ultrasound machine.

These two features are related to two key questions: Can two small objects be discerned within the image? Can objects with a similar tone or colour be distinguished?

Spatial resolution is simply defined as the number of pixels by length unit. It is usually presented as pixels per inch or pixels per centimetre (figure 21.3). A standard does not exist and spatial resolution is limited by the characteristics of the image capture system used.[3,24,25]

There is an optimum value above which the human eye cannot perceive the square pixel in

651 × 445 px (23 × 16 cm) 17.7 kb   40 × 22 px (0.75 × 1 cm) 0.7 kb

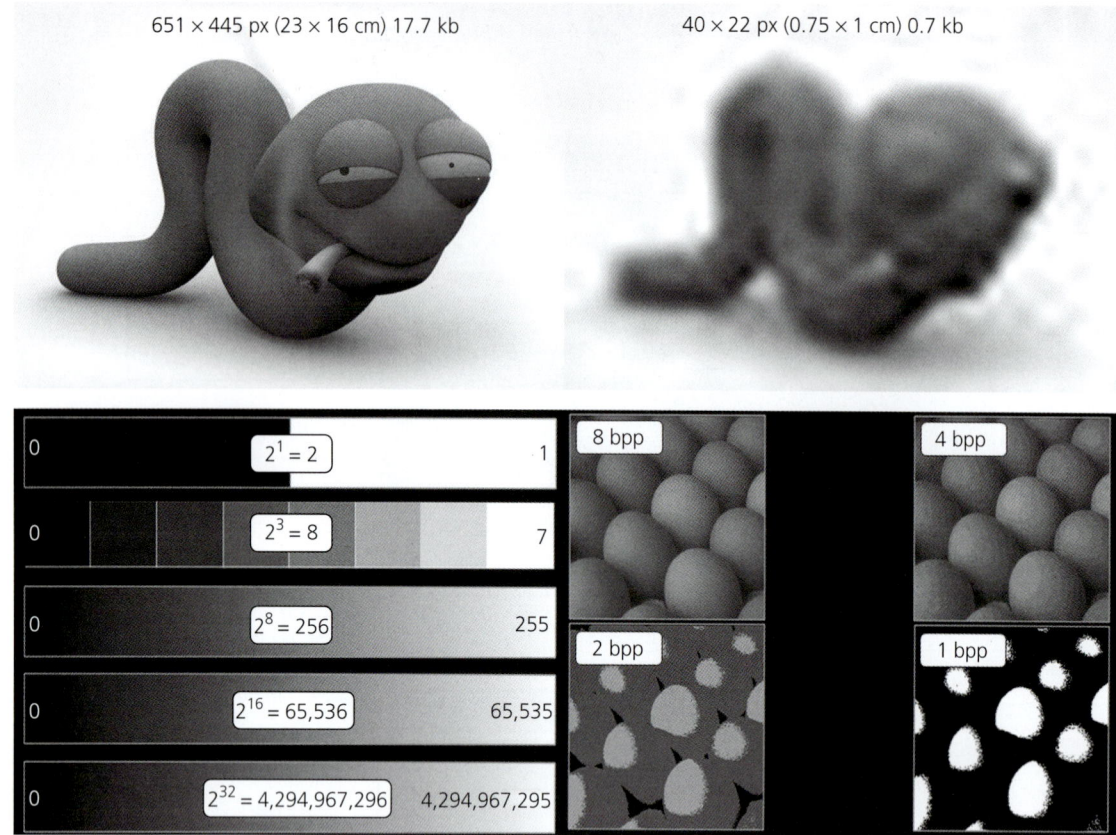

FIGURE 21.4 ■ Effects of spatial resolution and resolution of the grey level. In the sequence above, note the loss of detail when spatial resolution is reduced below what the human eye perceives to be in continuity. In the sequences below, the number of possible grey levels that a pixel can adopt are shown according to the bits of the image (bottom left) and the effect of reducing the quantification of the grey scale (bottom right).
In the image taken at 8 bits (256 possible levels of grey), the contours are easily perceived and the objects are observed with sharpness.In the image taken at 8 bits (256 possible grey levels), the contours are well defined and the objects are clear. At 4 bits (16 levels of grey), a false contour can be found on the figures. At 2 bits (four levels of grey) the loss in detail is evident and at 1 bit (binary images) the loss in detail is complete, although at times this is precisely the intention. (Colour version of figure is available online).

the image. This limit is found at around 75 px/cm (approximately 190 pixels per inch). Inferior resolutions produce distortion due to evidence of the pixel, as the element of the image is increasingly less visible as the size of the pixel increases (figure 21.4).

With low resolutions a blurring of borders occurs. For image analysis, the higher the resolution the better, albeit with the inconvenience that it comes with a higher memory storage space and RAM memory in order to manage the information.

The resolution of the grey scale is determined by the number of different values that can be adopted by the pixels that form the matrix and this, in turn, is defined by the device that gathers the intensity of the signal (the transducer on the ultrasound machine, or the CCD plate of a digital camera, for example).

It is very common to assign a value of 256 possible grey values, with each value differentiated by a different scale of grey. Typically, the zero value corresponds to absolute black and the 225 value to absolute white.[2,6,27–29] In this case this is called an 8-bit image (because $2^8 = 256$). With the development of more powerful computer equipment it is now possible to work with images of 32 or 64 bits (figure 21.4).

21.4 THE BASIS OF IMAGE PROCESSING IN GREY SCALE

21.4.1 Pseudo-colour tables

In biomedical imaging, it is common practice to apply pseudo-colour palettes (LUT: look-up tables) to an image while maintaining the

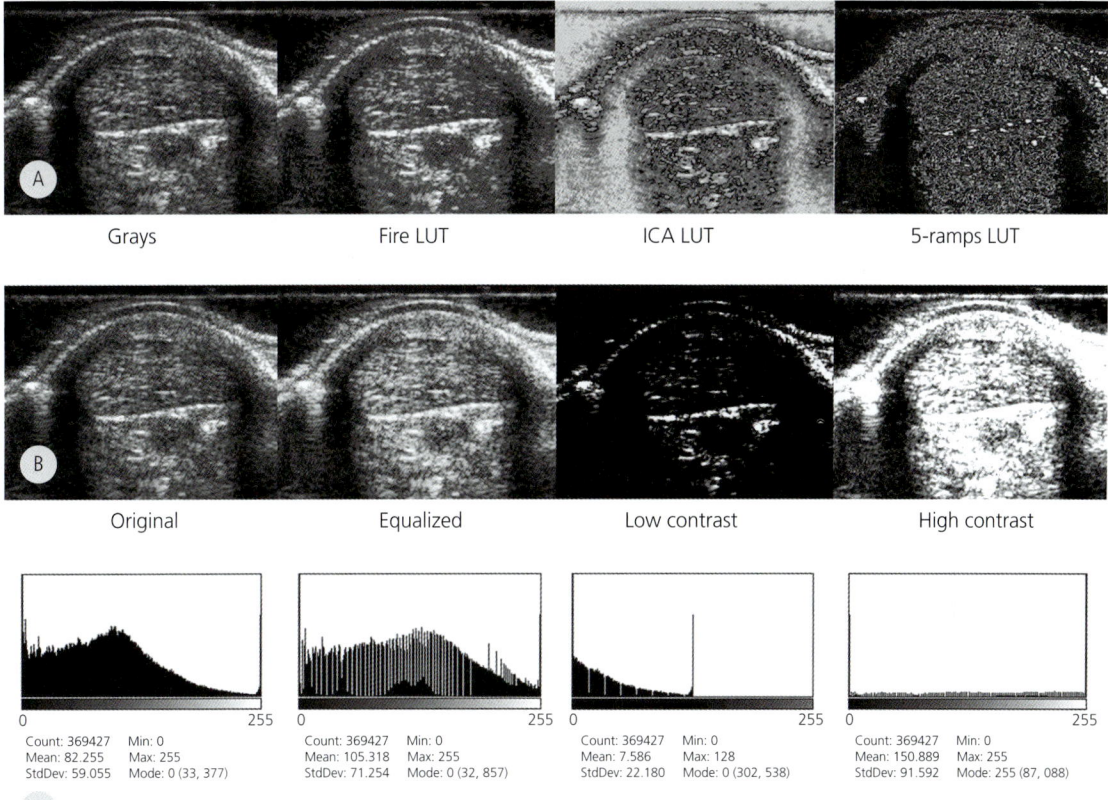

FIGURE 21.5 ■ Pseudo-colour, contrast and histogram of the grey scale. (A) Application of false colour palettes: in each of these the grey levels are substituted by different colours. The result can be more or less pleasing and sometimes this is only used for aesthetic purposes. (B) Here, the original is shown without processing, after an equalization of 10%, with low and high contrast, where the loss of information is evident. (C) Note in the histograms how, in the equalized image, the frequency of the different grey levels is levelled. The low-contrast image displays an asymmetric histogram towards black and the high-contrast image shows saturation, meaning no concrete level stands out. Captured using a LOGIQ-e device by General Electric® with transducer 12L-RS (7–13 MHz). Processing and analysis using *ImageJ* 1.46. (Colour version of figure is available online).

original 8-bit scale. Instead of assigning a grey gradient to every pixel value, a colour is assigned.[29,30,33] Some colour scales are continuous, such as the thermal colour scale, which, like the grey scale, presents a gradual range of hues. In other scales, the colour assigned to each grey value changes abruptly. The LUT can help to add impact to an image, but it must be used with caution to avoid confusing the observer (figure 21.5A) (video 21.2).

21.4.2 Image contrast

In an image it is possible to recognize an individual structure because it is differentiated from the background due to its brightness.[22,26] This grade of visibility, which represents the difference between clear and dark regions in the image, is called image contrast. If an image has low contrast it means that it is difficult to distinguish between different structures. The contrast can be affected by the image acquisition methods, as well as by the amount of elements present and the interaction between them (figure 21.5B).

21.4.3 Image histogram

A histogram is a graphic representation of a frequency distribution. In the context of an image in grey scale, the histogram is a way of representing the frequency distribution of the grey scale present in the image (figure 21.5C). Therefore, it shows how many pixels are present within a determined grey value. The information can be graphically displayed or listed as a numerical table.[26–30] In the graphic representation, the horizontal axis is used to indicate the values of the grey scale, which can be shown individually or by intervals, and the vertical axis represents the

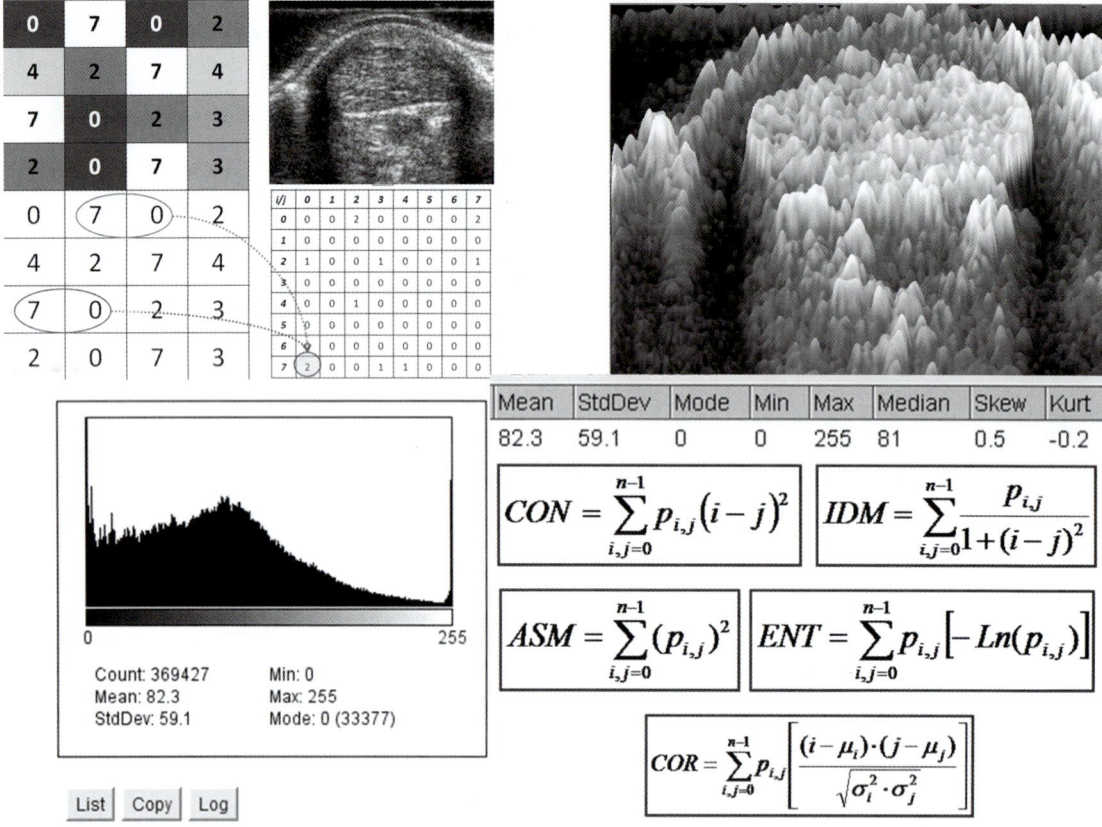

$$CON = \sum_{i,j=0}^{n-1} p_{i,j}(i-j)^2 \qquad IDM = \sum_{i,j=0}^{n-1} \frac{p_{i,j}}{1+(i-j)^2}$$

$$ASM = \sum_{i,j=0}^{n-1} (p_{i,j})^2 \qquad ENT = \sum_{i,j=0}^{n-1} p_{i,j}\left[-Ln(p_{i,j})\right]$$

$$COR = \sum_{i,j=0}^{n-1} p_{i,j}\left[\frac{(i-\mu_i)\cdot(j-\mu_j)}{\sqrt{\sigma_i^2\cdot\sigma_j^2}}\right]$$

FIGURE 21.6 ■ Echotexture analysis. Textural analysis using concurrence matrixes of the grey level is built by evaluating the grey levels of one pixel and that of its neighbours, so that information can be gathered regarding roughness, homogeneity and order, while the information obtained from the histogram is built from the individual information from each pixel. CON, contrast; IDM, inverse different moment (homogeneity); ASM, angular second moment (energy); ENT, entropy; COR, textural correlation. Captured using a LOGIQ-e device by General Electric® with transducer 12L-RS (7–13 MHz). Processing and analysis using *ImageJ* 1.46. (Colour version of figure is available online).

number of pixels for each level. Once a histogram for the underlying data has been obtained, it can be used to improve the image. The histogram can be global if it is calculated for the image as a whole, but it can also be obtained locally for a region of interest (ROI) (video 21.2).

KEY POINTS

The histogram of an image shows us the frequency distribution of the different grey levels represented in the pixels. They can be manipulated to improve or modify the image with an objective in mind.

The image contrast characteristics can be adjusted by modifying the grey values, so as to create a particular effect on the histogram.[31,32] The goal of histogram equalization is, for example, to spread out the grey intensity values

over the whole range of values, so that there are approximately the same number of pixels within each level (figure 21.5C).

21.4.4 Pixel statistics

Within this wide range of techniques we can find those that help quantify or perform operations with the numerical levels of the image's pixels.[24,28] Many of the variables thus obtained have the same meaning as in classical statistics, because they are being obtained from a matrix of numerical data (the grey levels of every single pixel that forms the image). Therefore, one can discuss middle levels, standard deviations, asymmetry coefficients and kurtosis, maximums and minimums[31,32] (video 21.2).

In the context of musculoskeletal ultrasound imaging, not many studies have explored this potential. Our group has proposed the use of the

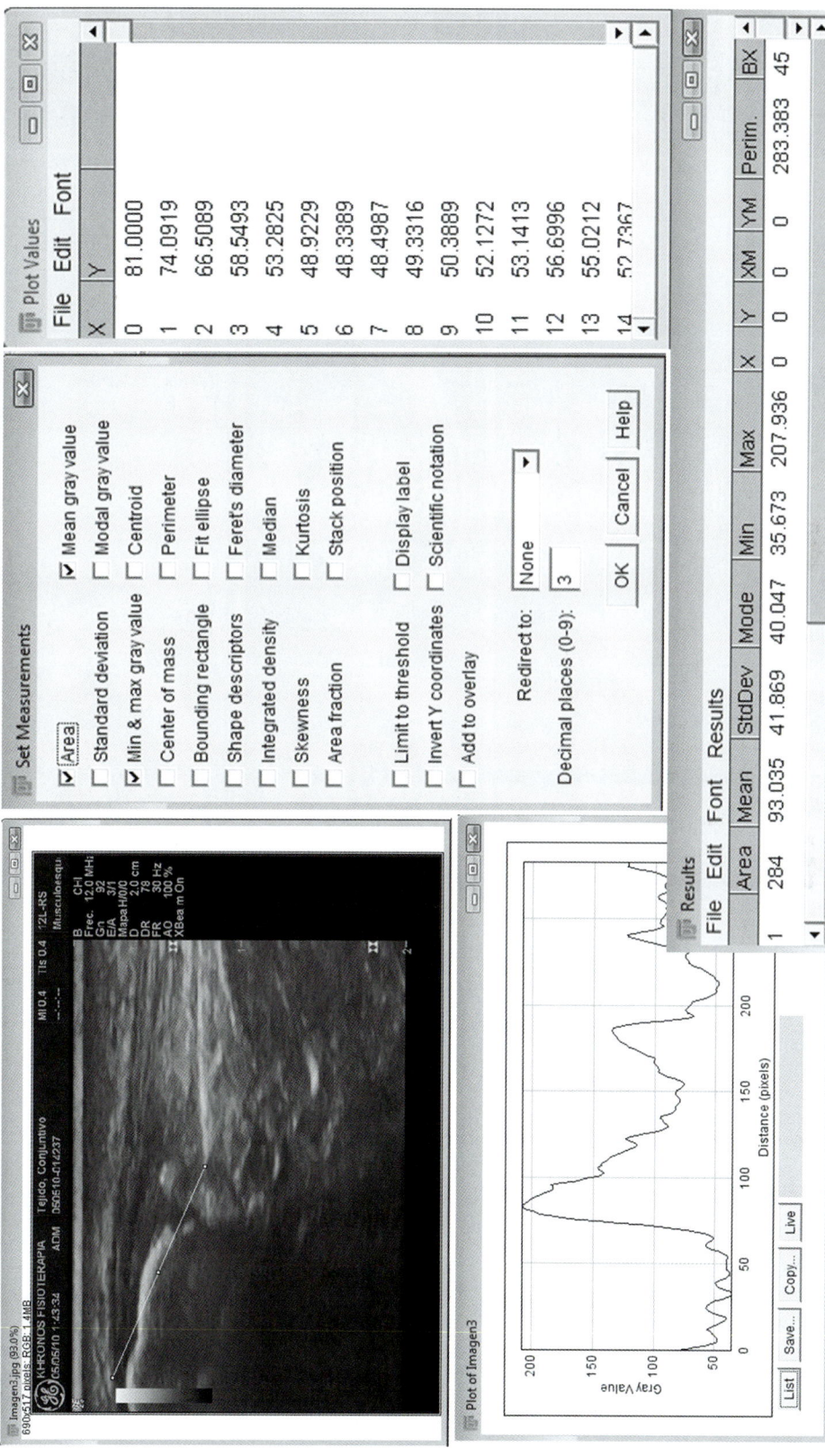

FIGURE 21.7 ■ Analysis of echogenicity. This image shows a longitudinal view of the patellar tendon at the insertion in the patella. A loss of echogenicity of the tendon can be seen, together with avulsion of the tip of the patella. Echogenicity of the region can be quantified using image analysis. The profile diagram shows changes in echogenicity and the structures crossed by the line. Values for each pixel are also obtained as well as the statistical values of the matrix. Captured using a LOGIQ-e device by General Electric® with transducer 12L-RS (7–13 MHz). Processing and analysis using *ImageJ* 1.46. (Colour version of figure is available online).

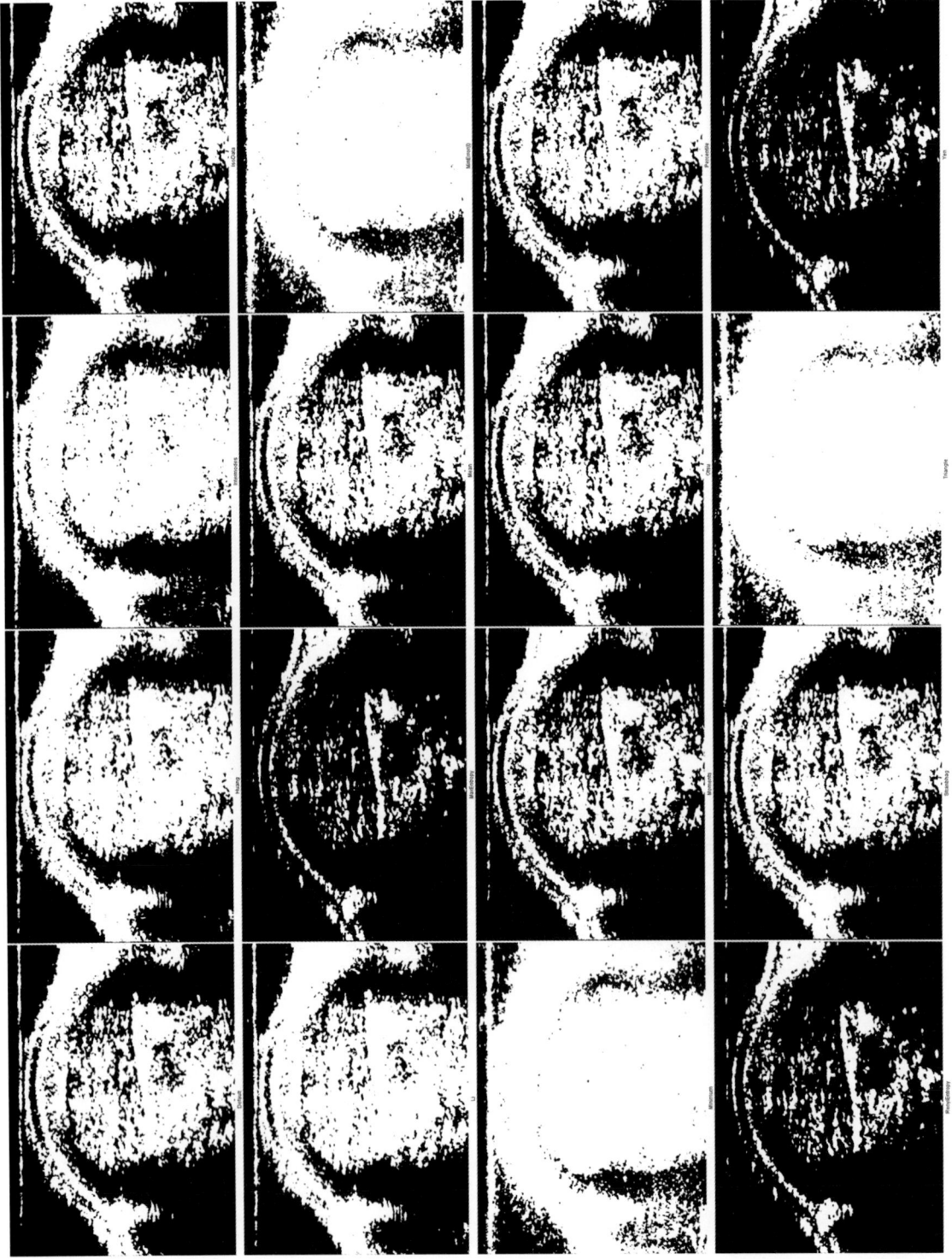

FIGURE 21.8 ■ Thresholding of the ultrasound image. The same image has been segmented using 12 different algorithms which show very different results. Captured using a LOGIQ-e device by General Electric® with transducer 12L-RS (7–13 MHz). Processing and analysis using *ImageJ* 1.46.

term quantitative analysis of echogenicity[34–37] for this type of work, which hereafter has been expanded[40] with the inclusion of textural analysis techniques using concurrence matrixes of the grey level[38,39] and the introduction of the concept of quantitative echotexture.[40–42] By means of these texture analyses, the potential of the statistics calculated on the individual pixels is improved because variables such as entropy, energy, homogeneity or textural contrast are obtained from the relationships between neighbouring pixels (figure 21.6). A recent study successfully managed to classify a battery of transverse images of the Achilles tendon according to the age of the individuals, with rates close to 100%, which would indicate that these algorithms are able to capture information of extraordinary value.[43–46]

KEY POINTS

Analyses of echotexture and quantification of echogeneicity with advanced image-processing techniques are promising advances within the research of musculoskeletal ultrasound.

If a line is drawn over a region of interest, a profile graph is obtained with the grey levels that the line passes through and this can be used to calculate the cited statistics.[32,33] On other occasions, the focus is on selecting or outlining a determined region of interest from which we can then perform these calculations (figure 21.7).

21.4.5 Image segmentation

Image segmentation consists of partitioning the image into regions or segments that become meaningful when associated with a particular application.[47,48] For example, it may be interesting to separate an injury from the rest of the image in order to carry out related measurements. This is one of the most complex tasks as there is no perfect algorithm for this and thus the result will be more or less successful depending on the characteristics of the image (figure 21.8) (video 21.3).

In order to perform these tasks, there are three segmentation methods available: manual, automatic and semiautomatic.[28] In manual segmentation, the operator decides which region is selected and which ones are excluded, and this can happen at the same time as image acquisition occurs. In contrast, in automatic and semiautomatic methods, a large amount of data needs to be previously collected (images) in order to test the method and perform the necessary adjustments. It is common for manual methods to be used in pilot studies.

However, the manual methods have serious inconveniences: they take up a lot of time, they are subject to human error and they are subjective, meaning that they have poor intraobserver reproducibility.

In semiautomatic methods, the observer begins the segmentation and afterwards only performs minor corrections.

The segmentation of ultrasound images is even more problematic (if possible), due to the characteristics inherent to the technique: there is a lack of defined borders and contours between structures, such as that which occurs in tomography or radiography.

The attempts so far regarding automatic segmentation in musculoskeletal ecography have produced moderate results[49,50] and are not completely satisfactory, therefore the analysis greatly depends on the skill and practice of the image operator (figure 21.9).

KEY POINTS

The application and creation of automatic algorithms for the detection and segmentation of ultrasound images are complicated endeavours.

21.4.6 To begin working: ImageJ

There is a great variety of commercial 'software' for image processing and analysis and undoubtedly many of these programs have very good performance. Most of these are integrated into biomedical equipment.[25,48,51]

Nevertheless, here we present free software which, beneath its simple surface, hides almost infinite potential and considerable advantages: ImageJ is an image-processing and analysis program in the public domain, written in Java and inspired by NIH Image (National Institutes of Health, USA) for Macintosh, which is now also available for Windows, Mac OS X and Linux[52] (video 21.2).

ImageJ was developed by Wayne Rasband, a special volunteer of the National Institute of Mental Health, Bethesda, Maryland, USA.[32,33]

This program can display, edit, analyse and process images, as well as enable users to save and print images of 8, 16 and 32 bits. ImageJ reads a multitude of image formats, such as TIFF, GIF, JPEG, BMP and DICOM, among others, and dynamic image sequences (stacks) are supported; these are a series of images that share the same window.

Areas and pixel statistics can be calculated in regions defined by the user, and measurements of distance and angles are also enabled.

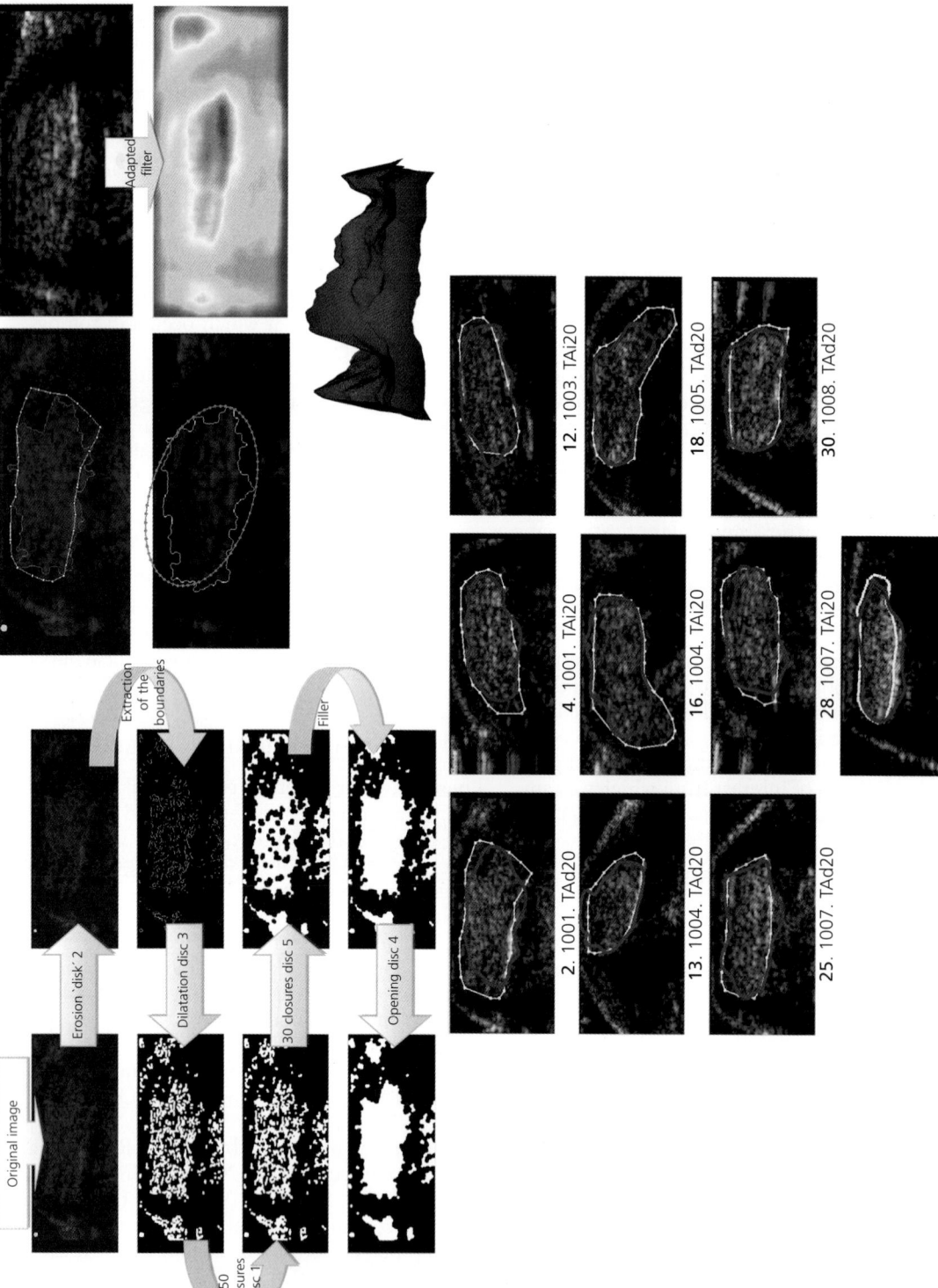

FIGURE 21.9 ■ Automatic segmentation of the contour of the Achilles tendon on ultrasound is complicated. A series of previous operations are needed and subsequently the algorithms (geodesic contours and snakes) adjust the boundary. The yellow colour indicates the traces made by an expert and trained operator; the automatic contour is shown in blue. Captured using a LOGIQ-e device by General Electric® with transducer 12L-RS (7–13 MHz). Processing and analysis using *MathLab*. (Colour version of figure is available online).

Additionally, this program supports image calibration so as to obtain the results of the measurements in real dimensions, such as millimetres or centimetres. Histograms and profile graphs can be created as well as the performance of manipulation procedures such as contrast, highlighting, softening, border detection and filters, with the possibility of performing these operations with various images at once, only dependent on the amount of memory space available.

One of the great advantages of this program is that it was designed with an architecture that provides extensibility through applications (plugins) in Java programming language, meaning that new applications can be written and programmed with the editor and compiler available. Thanks to the completely open source code, users can develop multiple applications in order to resolve specific problems and these are available to the whole community.

The software can be downloaded from http://rsbweb.nih.gov/ij/, where different applications and user tutorials can be found. A very active wiki (http://imagejdocu.tudor.lu/) community exists, where it is possible to interact with users from all around the world.

21.5 FIVE TOP TIPS FOR ULTRASOUND IMAGE ANALYSIS AND PROCESSING

To conclude this introductory chapter on ultrasound digital image processing, here are five basic recommendations for someone wishing to become familiar with these techniques.

1. Image acquisition requires special care: ultrasound has the distinct advantage of allowing for as much repetition as necessary.
2. Image storage must be performed without losing information. If necessary, image compression can be performed afterwards, but the original must be saved in its non-manipulated format.
3. The enhancing contrast or subjective manual filtering of the image is a useful tool for personal clinical evaluation; however it is important to separate this practice from the context of the quantitative analysis of results, in which a clear protocol for all the images must exist.
4. The operator must always justify the use of any image manipulation parameter, as well as ensure that the parameters can be applied to all the images.

5. Reliability and reproducibility studies are recommended, and these should include each and every one of the technicians, the acquisition method, the image operator and the analysis methods. Only in this way is it possible to avoid the typical and misleading sentence 'the study is not valid because ultrasound is very variable and technician-dependent'.

21.6 REFERENCES

1. Dhawan AP, Huang HK, Kim DS. Principles and advanced methods in medical imaging and image analysis. New York: World Scientific Publishing; 2008.
2. Dougherty G. Digital image processing for medical applications. Cambridge: Cambridge University Press; 2009.
3. Bankman IN. Handbook of medical imaging. Processing and analysis. San Diego: Academic Press; 2000.
4. Web A. Introduction to biomedical imaging. New Jersey: John Wiley; 2003.
5. Bharath AA. Introductory medical imaging. London: Morgan & Claypool Publishers; 2009.
6. Rangayyan RM. Biomedical image analysis. Boca Raton: CRC Press; 2005.
7. Suri JS, Wilson DL, Laxminarayan S. Handbook of biomedical image analysis, vol. 3. New York: Kluwer Academic; 2005.
8. Bronzino JD. The biomedical engineering handbook. 3rd ed. Boca Raton: Taylor & Francis; 2006.
9. Bushberg JT, Seibert JA, Leidholtdt EM, et al. The essential physics of medical imaging. 2nd ed. Philadelphia: Lippincott Williams & Wilkins; 2002.
10. Middleton WD, Kurtz AB, Hertzberg BS. Ecografía. Madrid: Marbán Libros; 2005.
11. Martínez-Payá JJ, editor. Anatomía ecográfica del hombro. Madrid: Médica Panamericana; 2008.
12. Acebes-Cachafeiro JC. Ecografía del aparato locomotor. Rehabilitacion (Madr) 2005;39:277–87.
13. Del Baño Aledo ME, Martínez Payá JJ, Ríos-Díaz J, et al. Aplicación en fisioterapia de la valoración cuantitativa de las características morfoecogénicas del tendón de Aquiles. Fisioterapia 2008;30:61–8.
14. Martínez-Payá JJ, Ríos-Díaz J, Palomino-Cortés MA, et al. Procesos degenerativos asintomáticos del tendón largo del bíceps braquial. Rev Fisioter (Guadalupe) 2005;4:16–30.
15. Martínez Payá JJ, Martínez Pérez LM, Ríos-Díaz J, et al. Morfología y morfometría de la corredera bicipital mediante ecografía. Rev Esp Antrop Fis 2006;26:1–10.
16. MartínezPayá JJ, Ríos-Díaz J, Martínez F, et al. Dependency of the long head of the brachial biceps and its relation to the bicipital groove. Morphological and morphometric ultrasonography study. J Bone Joint Surg Br 2006;88:327.
17. Ríos-Díaz J, Martínez-Payá JJ, de Groot-Ferrando A, et al. Nuevo método de análisis textural mediante matrices de concurrencia del nivel de gris sobre imagen ecográfica del tendón de Aquiles: diferencias entre deportistas y sedentarios. Cuest Fisioter 2009;38:68–79.
18. Ríos-Díaz J, Martínez-Payá JJ, de Groot-Ferrando A, et al. Utility of grey level co-occurrence matrices for the ultrasonographic quantitative study of the textural patterns of patellar ligament. In: Berhardt LV, editor. Advances in biology and medicine. Patellar kinematics, injuries and clinical implications. New York: Nova Science Publishers; 2012.

19. Sans N, Brasseur JL, Louatau O, et al. Ecografía tendinosa: de la imagen a la patología. Radiologia 2006;49: 165–75.

20. Valera Garrido F, Minaya Muñoz F, Sánchez Ibañez JM. Efectividad de la electrolisis percutánea intratisular (EPI®) en las tendinopatías crónicas del tendón rotuliano. Trauma Fund MAPFRE 2010;21:227–36.

21. Bruce EN. Biomedical signal processing and signal modeling. New Jersey: John Wiley; 2001.

22. Hendee WR, Ritenour ER. Medical imaging physics. 4th ed. New Jersey: John Wiley; 2002.

23. Bueno A, del Cura JL. Ecografía musculoesquelética esencial. Madrid: Editorial Médica Panamericana; 2011.

24. Russ JC. The image processing handbook. 3rd ed. Boca Raton: CRC Press; 1999.

25. Pertusa Grau JF. Técnicas de análisis de imagen. Valencia: Universitat de València; 2003.

26. Pratt WK. Digital image processing. 4th ed. New Jersey: Wiley-Interscience; 2007.

27. Glasbey CA, Horgan GW. Image analysis for the biological sciences. New Jersey: John Wiley; 1995.

28. Berry E. A practical approach to medical image processing. Boca Raton: CRC Press Taylor & Francis; 2008.

29. Bourne R. Fundamentals of digital imaging in medicine. London: Springer Verlag; 2010.

30. Suetens P. Fundamentals of medical imaging. 2nd ed. New York: Cambridge University Press; 2009.

31. Jan J. Medical image processing, reconstruction and restoration. Boca Raton: Taylor & Francis; 2006.

32. Ferreira T, Rasband W. The ImageJ 1.44 user guide. v 1.44 ed. Bethesda (Maryland): National Institute of Health; 2011.

33. Ferreira T, Rasband W The ImageJ User Guide – Version 1.44, February 2011 [actualizado Feb 2011; consultado 1 Sep 2012]. Available online at: http://imagej.nih.gov/ij/docs/user-guide.pdf.

34. Martínez Payá JJ, Ríos-Díaz J, Palomino Cortés MA, et al. Los píxeles tienen la respuesta: Análisis cuantitativo de la ecogenicidad del sistema músculo esquelético. Un nuevo sistema de prevención. In: Esparza Ros F, Fernández Jaén T, Martínez Romero JL, editors. Prevención de las lesiones deportivas. Murcia: Quaderna Editorial; 2006. p. 159–68.

35. Bovik A. The essential guide of image processing. San Diego: Academic Press; 2009.

36. Martínez Payá JJ, Ríos-Díaz J, Palomino Cortés MA, et al. Control morfométrico-ecográfico del tendón largo del bíceps braquial y de sus dependencias como sistema de prevención. In: Esparza Ros F, Fernández Jaén T, editors. Prevención de las lesiones deportivas. Murcia: Quaderna Editorial; 2006. p. 195–202.

37. Martínez-Payá JJ, Ríos-Díaz J, de Groot-Ferrando A, et al. Performance of extensor apparatus of the knee in relation to the patellar mineral density and the ultrasonographic morphology of the patellar ligament. In: Berhardt LV, editor. Advances in biology and medicine. patellar kinematics, injuries and clinical implications. New York: Nova Science Publishers; 2012.

38. Haralick RM, Shanmugam K, Dinstein I. Textural features for image classification. IEEE Trans Syst Man Cybern 1973;3:610–21.

39. Hall-Beyer M The GLCM texture tutorial. Version 2.01 February 2007 [actualizado 28 Ago 2008; consultado 1 Sep 2012]. Available online at: http://www.fp.ucalgary.ca/mhallbey/tutorial.htm.

40. Ríos-Díaz J, Martínez-Payá JJ, del Baño-Aledo ME. El análisis textural mediante matrices las matrices de concurrencia (GLCM) sobre imagen ecográfica del tendón rotuliano es de utilidad para la detección de cambios histológicos tras un entrenamiento con plataforma de vibración. Cultcienc deporte 2009;4:91–102.

41. Ríos-Díaz J, Martínez-Payá JJ, del Baño-Aledo ME, et al. Fiabilidad y reproducibilidad intra e inter observador de un método semi-automático de análisis ecográfico del tendón de Aquiles. Cuestfisioter 2010;39:190–8.

42. Ríos-Díaz J, de Groot-Ferrando A, Martínez-Payá JJ, et al. Reliability and reproducibility of a morpho-textural image analysis method over a patellar ligament ultrasonography. Reumatol Clin 2010;6:278–84.

43. Ríos-Díaz J, Martínez-Payá JJ, del Baño-Aledo ME, et al. Análisis discriminante del patrón textural ecográfico con matrices de concurrencia como nueva herramienta para el estudio del tendón. Fisioterapia. 2011;33: 157–65.

44. Theodoridis S. Koutroumbas K. Pattern recognition. 3rd ed. San Diego: Academic Press; 2006.

45. Verma B, Blumenstein M. Pattern recognition technologies and applications. New York: Information Science Reference; 2008.

46. Jähne B. Digital image processing. 5th ed. Berlin: Springer-Verlag; 2002.

47. Ye SQ. Bioinformatics: a practical approach. Boca Raton: Chapman & Hall/CRC; 2008.

48. Solomon C, Breckon T. Fundamentals of digital image processing. A practical approach with examples in MatLab. Chichester: John Wiley; 2011.

49. Bastida Jumilla MC, Morales Sánchez J, Verdú Monedero R, et al. Automatización de medidas morfológicas y ecogénicas de estructuras del aparato locomotor humano mediante procesado de imágenes ecográficas. In: Simposium Nacional de la Unión Científica Internacional de Radio (23°: 2008: Madrid). URSI 2008: XXIII Simposium Nacional de la Unión Científica Internacional de Radio, celebrado del 22 al 24 de septiembre de 2008 en Madrid. Madrid: Garcia Villalba LJ; 2008. p. 4. Available online at: http://repositorio.bib.upct.es:8080/dspace/bitstream/10317/1366/1/amm.pdf.

50. Morales Sánchez J, Verdú Monedero R, Larrey Ruiz J, et al. Morphological and echogenic measurements of structures of locomotor system by means of echographic image processing. In: Las TIC y la gestión del conocimiento en el desarrollo de la Salud: proceedings of the VII Congreso Internacional de Informática en Salud. La Habana, Cuba [consultado 1 Sep 2012]; 2009. Available online at: http://informatica2009.sld.cu/Members/jmorales/medidas-morfologicas-y-ecogenicas de-estructuras-del-aparato-locomotor-mediante-procesado-de-imagenesecograficas.

51. Bal H, Hujol J. Java for bioinformatics and biomedical applications. New York: Springer; 2007.

52. Abràmoff MD, Magalhaes PJ, Ram SJ. Image processing with ImageJ. Biophotonics International 2004;11: 36–42.

CHAPTER 22

RESOLUTION OF CLINICAL CASES

CHAPTER 4

The ultrasound findings did not correspond with the patient's clinical symptoms. An assessment of other structures suspected to be possible causes of the symptoms was performed (rotator interval, long head of biceps and the myofascial trigger point [MTrP] in the infraspinatus). Palpation of the taut band on the infraspinatus reproduced the pattern of pain. The physiotherapy diagnosis was myofascial dysfunction in the infraspinatus muscle with the presence of active trigger points. The intervention consisted of an invasive approach, performing percutaneous needle electrolysis (PNE) of the MTrP on the taut band (figure 22.1). Seven days after the physiotherapy session, the patient returned for a check-up and was found to be asymptomatic. Four weeks posttreatment the patient was called in again and a complete resolution of symptoms was confirmed.

CHAPTER 8

This clinical case report highlights the importance of a thorough anamnesis and a correct diagnosis of the myofascial pain syndrome or, in other words, of the sum of relevant MTrPs that the patient is complaining of. An incomplete anamnesis and diagnosis render the detection of the presence of a decisive MTrP on the first visit unlikely. One must assume that, apart from having had her jaw opening forced during a dentist appointment, the patient's cervical spine was also placed in a forced position for a length of time, thus also activating the MTrP of the trapezius that was responsible for the aggravation and perpetuation of the masseter MTrP. In this clinical case, the importance of the MTrPs as activators and perpetuators of other MTrPs is also stressed, in that they are able to create chains which one has to know in order to understand the clinical symptoms.

CHAPTER 9

- Muscles to be treated: the adductor pollicis, pronator teres, flexor digitorum superficialis/profundus.
- The treatment order would be as follows: first pronator teres or flexor digitorum superficialis/profundus (interchangeably, any of the two could be treated in the first place), followed by, in the second place, the adductor pollicis.

The rationale behind this choice, as explained in chapter 9, is that the patterns of both referred pain and spasm or referred inhibition have a peripheral-type dominance in most muscles. Therefore, treatment from proximal to distal could potentially facilitate a greater relaxation of the distal muscles when we move on to treat these. However, in the case of the adductor pollicis, this is the only muscle that is recommended to be treated in the first place, as occasionally its treatment generates a large opening not only of the thumb but of all the hand, together with relaxation of the entire upper limb.

CHAPTER 13

Intervention

EPI® was applied in an isolated fashion in each weekly session, together with a home programme of eccentric exercise. EPI® was performed with ultrasound guidance over the clinically relevant area of the insertion zone of the supraspinatus and over the area of fluid collection and hypervascularization. This was compatible with the diagnosis of tenosynovitis of the long head of biceps at the bicipital groove. An intensity of 2–4 mA was used for 3–10 seconds in different approaches, with the purpose of evaporating the fluid collection in real time and stimulating the repair of the tendinous insertion zone. These procedures were performed using electrotherapy

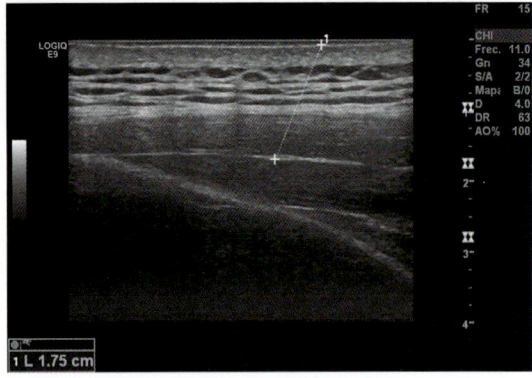

FIGURE 22.1 ■ Identification of the infraspinatus muscle for treatment with EPI®.

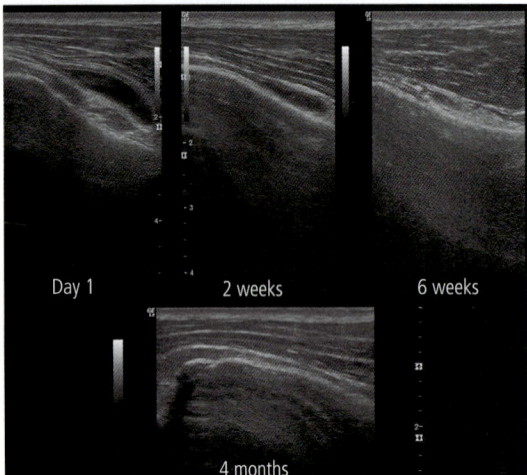

FIGURE 22.2 ■ Ultrasound image: longitudinal section with evolution of the liquid collection of the long head of biceps tendon in the short and mid term.

equipment (Cesmar Electromedicina SL, Barcelona, Spain), which produces continuous galvanic current through the cathode (modified electrosurgical scalpel with the needle) while the patient holds the anode (hand-held electrode).

Results

After three EPI® sessions, the patient was discharged. A significant clinical improvement in function was noted: orthopaedic tests were negative and the total disappearance of fluid collection in the area was observed. The follow-up 6 weeks postdischarge did not reveal any relapses (figure 22.2).

EPI® has been demonstrated to reach the affected tissue and provoke a local inflammatory process, allowing for the phagocytosis and repair of the degenerated tissue, with functional changes in the short term, hence the fact that it

can be used as an effective therapy to resolve this clinical situation.

In tendons that have a sheath, such as the long head of biceps or the tibialis posterior tendons, tenosynovitis processes are frequently difficult to resolve. In these cases, the effect of the evaporation in real time (which EPI® can provoke) constitutes an attractive treatment option, especially when considering the chronic nature of these processes and the effectiveness and safety of the technique.

CHAPTER 14

Intervention

Four days after the injury the first session of EPI® was applied. This was repeated 7 days later (in total, two EPI® sessions were administered and other therapies were not associated). EPI® was performed with ultrasound guidance over the clinically relevant area in the area of poor scarring in order to stimulate correct tissue proliferation, and over the area of haematic collection and oedema. This coincided with the area that was re-torn with an intensity of 2–4 mA for 3–10 seconds using different approaches, with the object of evaporating the haematoma in real time and stimulating the repair of the muscle area.

In between EPI® treatment sessions, the patient was recommended to perform gentle eccentric exercises of the affected area. In this sense, the treatment protocol was not modified with regard to the first damage that occurred in the region.

Results

After two EPI® sessions, the patient presented a highly significant clinical improvement of function and an improvement of the structure of the tissue assessed under ultrasound. Magnetic resonance imaging (MRI) was repeated 1 week later, and 2 weeks after performing the first MRI. Forty-eight hours after the application of the first EPI® session, the result of the MRI was as follows:

> the study was performed according to the usual protocol. Notable improvement of the injury described in the medial soleus, with only two small images remaining of residual appearance measuring approximately 15 mm with a considerable reduction of the peripheral oedema. Interfascial collections are not found. Conclusion: significant improvement of the recurrent soleus rupture.

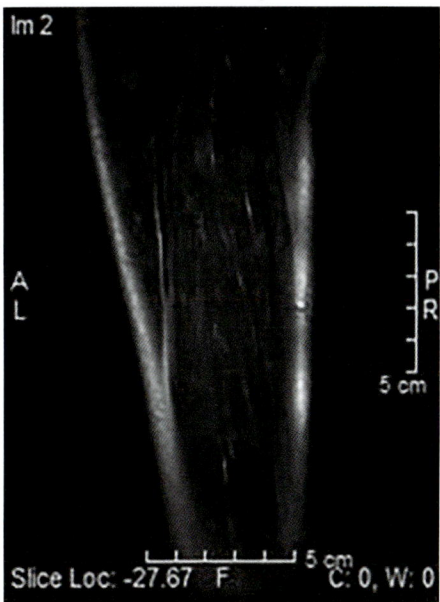

FIGURE 22.3 ■ Magnetic resonance image: posterior leg region where regeneration of the soleus appears in the internal middle one-third portion.

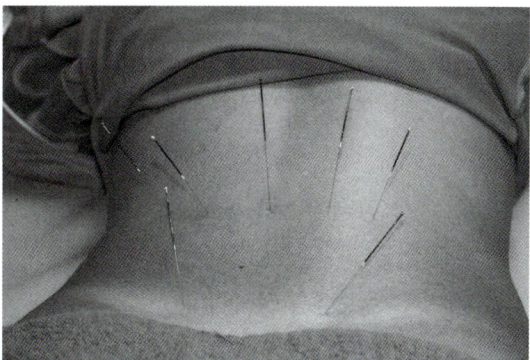

FIGURE 22.4 ■ Acupuncture application over the lumbar region.

Forty-eight hours after the second EPI® application, the result of the MRI indicated: 'improvement in the described lesion is observed compared to previous studies at the level of the medial and the middle third of the soleus. The remaining muscle is normal' (figure 22.3).

From the point of view of function, the manual strength tests failed to reproduce the pain after the application of the first EPI® session.

The follow-up in the following 6 weeks after discharge revealed zero recurrence.

The initial phase of all repair processes within a muscle lesion is characterized by inflammation and the formation of a haematoma. Classically, physiotherapy techniques have attempted to control (not inhibit) the initial inflammatory process and stimulate the correct tissue proliferation. The risk was associated with an irregular organization of the collagen tissue due to the persistence of the overlying haematoma. In these circumstances, EPI® is able to act upon the oedema and the haematic collection in the early phase, thus minimizing the risks and acting on the affected tissue in real time.

CHAPTER 15

In view of the results, initial treatment with acupuncture was decided upon, using the technique of tendinomuscular meridians for irradiated pain in the points (figure 15.34):

- UB-67: *ying* and tonification of the affected meridian (in this case the urinary bladder)
- UB-64V: *yuan* of the bladder
- KD-4: *luo* of the kidney.

Painful points of the irradiated area that corresponded with acupuncture points of the affected meridian (GB-34, UB-57, UB-56) and painful points under palpation of the lumbar area (*a'shi*) were treated with the dispersion technique, even though these did not correspond with classical acupuncture points.

The patient received two weekly sessions of acupuncture, with a marked improvement in the irradiated pain in the third session. Therefore treatment continued with a focus on the low-back pain and sacroiliac pain.

A tonification treatment of KD Yang was applied, with the aim of energetically strengthening the kidney (figure 22.4) as this could have been the cause of the asthenia and lumbar sensations, while, at the same time, local symptomatic treatment of the low-back pain was applied on the following points:

- GV-4 (life gate): KD Yang tonifying treatment
- UB-23 (*back-shu* point of the kidney): stimulates the *yang* of the kidney
- UB-52: reinforces the previous point.

Two transfixed needles were also applied in both sacroiliac joints in a caudal direction, stimulating the points found on the sacral foramina at the same time.

Treatment was reinforced between sessions with the application of two therapy needles applied semipermanently in both sacroiliac joints.

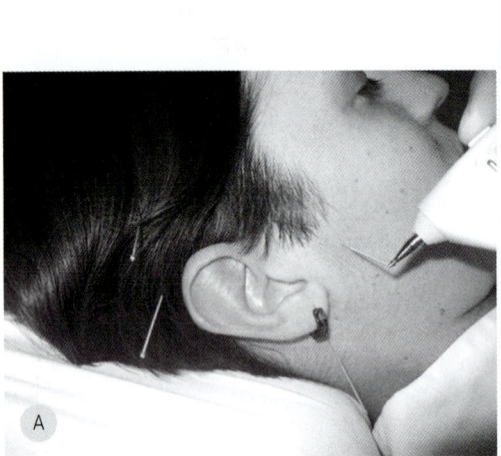

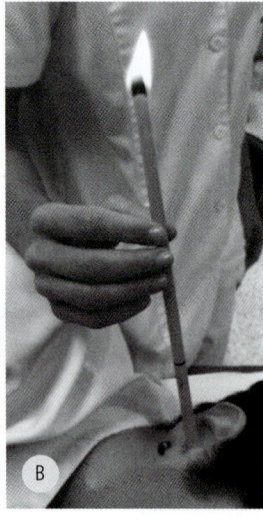

FIGURE 22.5 ■ (A) Electrical stimulation and (B) moxibustion. (Colour version of figure is available online).

CHAPTER 16

After assessing the patient, electroacupuncture treatment was applied on the following points:

- the tendinomuscular meridian or *San Jiao* is one of the meridians responsible for the symptoms in the ear and corresponds with a territory of distal arm irradiation: SJ1, SJ3, SJ4, PC6
- local *ashi* points: along the right upper limb, with electrodispersion parameters
- local points: GB2, SJ21, SI19, located anterior to the tragus at the ear
- monopolar stimulation (retroauricular points) in the *San Jiao* meridian (one retroauricular distance) and in the gall bladder meridian (two retroauricular distances). The most active points are chosen and stimulated selectively (figure 22.5A)
- bilateral KD-3 and KD-7 (with tonification parameters), aimed at tonifying the kidney *yin* (according to traditional Chinese medicine, the kidney is believed to open into the ear).

In the following physiotherapy sessions, the anterior treatment was combined with manual acupuncture in the following points:

- bilateral LI-4 (due to its direct action upon the head and the face)
- GB-20 (special action over the cervical spine and suboccipital insertions).

Auriculotherapy (*shenmen* points, kidney, adrenal sympathetic) in the lateral ear on the same side.

Hollow ginger moxa inside the ear (figure 22.5B).

CHAPTER 17

The patient came to us seeking pain relief at least until the decision of whether or not to be operated on was made. He was tired of taking oral medication for such a long time.

The patient was informed of the treatment, and the fact that it would not impede him with regard to surgery (that is, if the neurophysiologist's reports recommended surgery) and that we were only going to treat the symptoms so that he could live the most normal life possible.

After examining the patient, the following protocol was established:

- week 1: mesotherapy following the Ordiz points (figures 15.6 and 15.7) Traumeel® + Spascupreel®
- week 2: Traumeel® + Zeel® + Discus®
- week 3: Traumeel® + Zeel® + Discus®.

Twenty-four hours after the first session, the patient confirmed an improvement in his symptoms, although this was difficult to assess as he had exercised quite vigorously that week, although he did report a decrease in the oral intake of non-steroidal anti-inflammatory drugs (NSAIDs) thanks to a decrease in perceived pain.

After the following two sessions the patient noticed a marked decrease in pain. Although he wasn't able to give up the oral NSAIDs completely, he was able to decrease the intake to only occasionally. The pain reduced enough to allow for a return to training, although not for longer than 20 minutes.

CHAPTER 18

This patient presented with the classical picture of subacromial bursitis following excessive overuse. She underwent one injection and two follow-up sessions of physiotherapy when she was discharged with advice to come back immediately if the pain recurred. She has been symptom-free for over 3 years now.

The advantage of deposition of a medium-acting corticosteroid via injection is that it rapidly addresses the issue of inflammation of the synovial lining of the bursa. This is extremely cost-effective as it saves many sessions of physiotherapy and results in reduced morbidity.

However, it does not address the cause of the condition, and the literature confirms this; the evidence is that corticosteroid injections do work, but only for a short while. If the cause is not explained and coping mechanisms are not given to the patient once the anti-inflammatory effect has occurred, symptoms can recur.

Corticosteroid injections therefore do not supplant the physiotherapist; they are merely a rapid and simple way of eliminating painful symptoms so that proper retraining can take place. This allows for greater professional satisfaction for the clinician, extensive cost savings for health services and faster relief for the patient.

Physiotherapists in the UK have been receiving training in musculoskeletal injections since 1995, when I presented the first course in Birmingham, England.

My hope is that one day all musculoskeletal physiotherapists will include this additional skill in their armoury of treatment options.

CHAPTER 19

The key message from this typical midportion Achilles tendon case is that high-volume image-guided injections permitted a reduction in symptom response to impact loading that was critical in allowing this patient to return to running gradually.

GLOSSARY

Aberrant hyperinnervations: a phenomenon that can appear in cases of regeneration following paralysis, in which an erroneous direction of the growing nerve fibres occurs (i.e. involving the fibres of a mistaken muscle, or a tactile receptor placed in an inappropriate location).

Activity limitation: the difficulties that a person may have in performing activities.

Acute injury: the initial immediate phase post-injury, where autologous repair mechanisms take place to control the inflammatory process and pain.

Adverse event: any harmful effect, however small, when it is not intended and non-therapeutic.

Algorithm: procedure of processing or working instructions that, thanks to their great precision, can be executed independently via a mechanical or electronic device.

Aliasing: produces softer curves adjusting the outline between the background and the region of pixels that is flattened. Generally, the intensity of the pixel or the opacity is adjusted in order to achieve a gentler transition with the background.

Allopathy: therapy that uses remedies that produce effects in a healthy state that are different from the effects produced by the disease to be treated.

Anaphylaxis: the reactions mediated by subtypes of the IgE and IgG antibodies. Prior sensitization to the allergen must exist, which produces specific immunoglobulins for the antigen; the later exposure to the allergen generates an anaphylactic reaction. Many cases of anaphylaxis occur, however, with no previous history of exposure to any allergens.

Anatomical terminology: the anatomical terminology (AT) is the international rule on human anatomical terminology published in 1998. In April 2011, the anatomical terminology was published online (http://www.unifr.ch/ifaa/) by the Federative International Programme for Anatomical Terminology (FIPAT).

Anisotropy: artifact that triggers changes in the echogenicity of tissues depending on the ultrasound beam angle. Normally, this is due to the lack of perpendicularity in the exploration. This shows up as a loss of echogenicity and may lead to an error in interpretation as it could be confused with a pathological image. Although this phenomenon may appear in muscles, ligaments and nerves, it appears most frequently in the tendon, due to the spiral shape that the collagen fibres of the long muscle tendons acquire in the insertion areas. Its presence can be confused with a case of tendinosis.

Antisepsis: method consisting of fighting or preventing infectious conditions by destroying the microbes that cause it.

Arcuate line: the arcuate line of the abdomen is a horizontal line that marks the inferior limit of the posterior layer of the sheath of the rectus abdominis muscle.

Artefact: unexpected images that appear in the normal ultrasound that do not correspond with normal structures and which may lead to confusion.

Asepsis: the ensemble of scientific procedures designed to protect the body from infectious germs. Applied mainly to sterilization of surgical material.

Aspect ratio: the relation between the vertical and horizontal dimensions of an image.

Axial resolution: the possibility of the ultrasound device visualizing two different structures located one above the other (y-axis) and in a direction that is parallel to the ultrasound beam. When the frequency is increased, the axial resolution increases but the depth of penetration of the ultrasound beam decreases. At low frequencies, the ultrasound beam penetrates more, while axial resolution decreases.

Basic research: the scientific research that is performed without an immediate practical purpose, with the aim of increasing the knowledge of the fundamental principles of nature or reality itself. The relationship between basic and applied science (which is the opposite concept) is crucial for the interrelation known as research and development or research, development and innovation (R + D or R + D + i).

Biological accident: an exposure that can lead to an infection by the human immunodeficiency virus (HIV), the hepatitis B virus (HBV) or the hepatitis C virus (HCV) via a percutaneous wound (needle or cut with a sharp object) or via contact with a mucous membrane or broken skin with blood, tissue or any other body fluid that is potentially infected.

Burst: stimulation using pulses or bursts.

Byte: packet of binary data formed by 8 bits. A byte can represent values of 0–255 and, therefore, may represent 256 symbols, numbers or colours.

Calibration: the comparison between an instrument with the standard. The standard is considered as a reference and the most accurate measure.

Carotid sheath: fascial conduit at the neck that contains the common carotid artery followed by the internal carotid, the internal jugular vein and the vagus nerve.

Clinical reasoning: the process of reflecting and making decisions regarding the patient's treatment and assessment, performed by the professional within a clinical context, based on relevant available knowledge (information, procedures, concepts) and clinical skills. This process is based on three main elements: one's own knowledge, the associated thought processes (cognition) and reflection (thinking) upon the thought process itself (metacognition).

Colour: one of the most difficult terms to define, digitally code and reproduce. The main reason is because colour is a perceptive phenomenon and cannot be described in a totally objective manner.

Colour channel: where information is stored for each of the primary components of the colour in a colour model. For example, the red, green, blue (RGB) colour model has three separate channels for red, green and blue.

Comet tail: an artifact that appears when the ultrasound beam hits a narrow and highly echogenic interphase which causes a series of linear echoes behind it. This is very characteristic in the presence of highly echogenic foreign bodies, as well as small air bubbles found within a solid medium. This artifact is very useful for revealing osteosynthesis material.

Competencies: the professional responses that individuals provide according to the requirements of their work duties. These involve a basis of knowledge, abilities (knowing what to do), attitudes and behaviour (knowing how to behave) that are all interrelated.

Compression: a data codification process performed so that the amount of information is reduced in order to obtain smaller files. Compression techniques can be classified into techniques with loss (not to be recommended in image analysis) and without loss.

Contrast: the difference in luminance between the regions of interest of an image.

Cronbach's alpha: a reliability coefficient that provides an estimate of internal consistency among items.

Cun/tsun: a term that describes a measurement unit or relative distance, equivalent to 1 inch.

Cutaneous trigger point: painful site found on the skin tissue which evokes referred pain in response to the application of pressure or another mechanical stimulus. According to studies by Sinclair (1949), referred pain produced from cutaneous trigger points is of a throbbing type with moderately severe intensity. Some of the areas in which the referred pain is produced are found within the same metameric distribution as the original site; however others do not present any segmentary relation to it. In these areas a modulation of the sensation is found (sensitivity to the referred pressure or to the referred dysaesthesia).

Cytokines: proteins that regulate the function of the cells that produce them or other cell types. These are the agents responsible for intercellular communication, that induce activation of specific membrane receptors and functions such as proliferation and cellular differentiation, chemotaxis, growth and modulation of the immunoglobulin secretion. These are mainly produced by lymphocytes and activated macrophages, although they may also be produced by polymorphonuclear lymphocytes, endothelial and epithelial cells and adipocytes of connective tissue. Depending on which cell produces them, these are called lymphokines (lymphocytes), monokines (monocytes, precursors of macrophages), adipokines (adipose cells or adipocytes) or interleukins (haematopoietic cells). Their main action is regulation of inflammation mechanisms. There are both proinflammatory and anti-inflammatory cytokines.

DASH (Disabilities of the Arm, Shoulder and Hand): this is a specific measurement tool for assessing the quality of life related to disorders of the upper limb. This self-administered questionnaire assesses the upper limb as a functional unit and enables quantification and comparison of the repercussion of the various processes that affect different regions of the limb. It was developed following an initiative by the American Academy of Orthopaedic Surgeons and has been translated into different languages with various transcultural adaptations.

Deep fascia: a layer of dense fibrous connective tissue that generates compartments, forms intermuscular septa and surrounds the muscles, bones, nerves and blood vessels.

Dermis: internal layer of the two main skin layers. The dermis is formed of connective tissue, blood vessels, sebaceous and sweat glands, nerves, hair follicles and other structures. It is made of a thin outer layer called the papillary dermis and an inner thick layer called the reticular dermis. Its upper border is the epidermis while the lower border is known as the hypodermis. This is the application site used in mesotherapy.

Dermometer: a device similar to that used for measuring skin conductivity or resistance, used to explore the skin surface seeking points with great conductance (of low skin resistance). Apparently, these are commonly found above myofascial trigger points. Some dermometers are enabled for electrotherapy, commonly continuous currents (8–10 Hz).

Drug vector: a type of drug used in mesotherapy, not for its pharmacological properties, but rather due to the fact that it helps other drugs to become diffused into the body thanks to its influence upon the ionic properties of the cell membrane. This is the case with lidocaine and procaine.

Echogenicity: the capacity for reflexion and acoustic impedance of the tissues when these are crossed by an ultrasound beam. The greater the echogenicity of the tissue (greater capacity of reflexion and acoustic impedance), the whiter and hyperechoic it will appear. In contrast, with less echogenicity (less capacity for reflexion and acoustic impedance), the tissue appears more black and hypoechoic. Based on the greater or lesser echogenicity of the tissues, the following types of images are distinguished: (1) anechoic or anechogenic image, black image; (2) hypoechoic or hypoechogenic image, with a tendency towards black; (3) hyperechoic or hyperechogenic image, very white image; (4) isoechoic or isoechogenic image, the same echogenicity between two tissues; (5) homogeneous image, and (6) heterogeneous image.

Effectiveness: related to the possibility of an individual or collective benefitting from a health intervention according to the normal conditions of clinical practice.

Efficacy: the impact or effect of an action performed for the purpose of influencing the level of health or well-being of the population in the best possible conditions or experimental conditions (optimal conditions). This responds to the question: what is the expected capacity of a health intervention (under ideal conditions of use and application) to improve the health level of an individual or group?

Efficiency: achieving a concrete result based on a minimal amount of resources or obtaining the maximum benefit from a limited amount of resources. Efficiency considers the expenses or costs in relation to the efficacy or effectiveness achieved.

Electrolysis: the process that separates the elements of a compound using electricity. This entails the capture of electrodes via cations in the cathode (a reduction process) and the liberation of electrons by the anions in the anode (oxidation). This process, applied to sodium chloride and the water that is found in the tissues of our body, makes them break down into their basic chemical elements, which rapidly regroup to form completely new substances.

Electromagnetic spectrum: the model for describing and classifying the complete range of electromagnetic radiation, ranging from maximum frequency and thus greater energy (gamma rays) to, at the other extreme, minimal frequency and therefore less energy (radio waves).

Electrospray: a parameter used in high-frequency electroacupuncture for the sedation of acute or subacute pain (*yang*-type pain).

Epifascial: the subcutaneous structure embedded in the superficial fascia.

Epitenon: the peripheral cover of some tendons. It is a sheath of lax connective tissue that covers the tendon in all its length. It contains blood vessels, lymph vessels and nervous fibres that cross it in order to reach the tendon.

Fascia: the sheath of connective tissue located below the skin that surrounds the organs, muscle groups, muscles, blood vessels and nerves, and covers the spaces that would otherwise be empty (the thoracic, abdominal, pelvic cavities), linking some structures with others, enabling them to slide slowly between themselves. There are different types of fascia, classified according to the tissue that they are made from, the anatomical localization and their functions.

Fascia lata: a sheath of deep fascia that covers the thigh.

Fibroadipose septum: intermuscular connective tissue that is hyperechoic under ultrasound and becomes extramuscular at the origin of the tendon. Its relation with the muscle fibres is that of a true myotendinous junction, and therefore this is one of the weak points of muscles. Common injuries involving the septum appear on the rectus femoris and hamstring muscles.

Fibrotic scar: poor elastic repair. An increase in collagen is usually produced inside and between the cells and tissues. This reduces tissue movement and may cause injuries due to elongation and pain.

Fischer technique for segmental spinal sensitization treatment: the diagnosis of the presence of segmental spinal sensitization by exploring the existence of hyperalgesia and/or allodynia in the dermatome, the myotome and the sclerotome of the different metameric segments of a selected patient. Once the segmental levels affected by segmental spinal sensitization have been diagnosed, a therapeutic protocol is applied, consisting of infiltration of local anaesthetic in the interspinous and supraspinous ligaments of the sensitized segmental levels, followed by infiltration in the other trigger points (myofascial or not myofascial) of peripheral structures, corresponding with the myotomes and sclerotomes of the segments affected by segmental spinal sensitization. Although Fischer recommends the use of infiltration, both he (Fischer 2001, 2007, personal communications) and other followers (Imamura 2007; Shah 2007, 2010, personal communications) admit that positive results can also be obtained using dry needling.

Frequency: the frequency of an ultrasound wave consists of the number of cycles or changes in pressure occurring in 1 second. The frequency is quantified in cycles per second or hertz. It is determined by a source that emits noise and by the medium via which it is travelling.

Galvanism: a form of electrotherapy that involves a sustained and interrupted flow of electrons from the negative to the positive pole (unchanging polarity) and which produces a chemical response below the electrodes.

Gauge: an indicator of the width of a needle. This is expressed as a number followed by a 'G'. A greater number before the 'G' indicates less width.

Goal: the expected result after the process of care provided to a patient. The goals indicate a change in the body structures or functions, the limited activities or the restrictions in participation, and are measurable in a concrete time frame.

Grey scale: the manner of codifying the colour of an image that only has black, white and shades of gray. The most common way of visualizing this is using 8 bits per pixel, which provides 256 levels of intensity.

Growth factors: the ensemble of molecules with a protein nature and the ability to act upon the cell cycle during processes of cellular repair and regeneration.

Histogram: in the field of digital image processing, a histogram is a graph that represents the statistical frequency of the grey scale or the colour values of an image, as well as the range of contrast and brightness. In a colour image a histogram can be created using information regarding all the possible colours or three histograms, one for each of the individual colour channels.

Homeopathy: a healing system for illnesses based on the application of minimal doses of the same substances that, in greater quantities, would produce in a healthy person the same or similar symptoms to those that one wishes to treat.

IEEE: a non-profit organization that gathers a worldwide professional association for the advancement of technology in areas that range from aerospatial systems, computation and telecommunications to biomedical engineering. The IEEE was originally the acronym of the Institute of Electrical and Electronics Engineers. Currently, the areas of interest have expanded to cover a wide array of fields, and therefore it is simply known as IEEE.

Iliotibial tract: fibrous longitudinal reinforcement on the lateral surface of the fascia lata.

Image: the graphic representation of an object. The digital image is the representation of that object via a matrix of pixels.

Impairment: a problem affecting the functions (of the body systems) or the body structures (of organs or limbs).

Insertional trigger point: hyperalgic site found on the myotendinous junction and/or in the bony insertion of the taut band. It is painful under palpation and may cause spontaneous pain, with an area of referred pain that is less distant and widespread than the central myofascial trigger points. This is a type of enthesopathy caused by a central trigger point, which is explained by the degenerative changes and ensuing liberation of nociceptive and sensitizing substances that can cause maintained tension of the taut band at its insertion points.

Interface: the limit that exists between two media with different sonic resistance that are pierced by a beam.

International Classification of Functioning, Disability and Health (ICF): a classification developed by the World Health Organization, with the objective of providing a common, trustworthy, standardized language that is transculturally applicable and that enables the description of human functioning and disability. It is formed of two main parts: the first regarding functioning and disability, with two components: (1) body functions and structures; and (2) activities and participation, and the second regarding the so-called contextual factors, with two components: (1) environmental factors; and (2) personal factors.

Interrater reliability: the consistency among scores given by different examiners who are assessing the same object or response. This is determined by comparing the scores assigned to a group at a specific point in time.

Intraclass correlation coefficient: a family of correlation coefficients that enable the measurement of reliability between two or more repeated measures.

Intrarater reliability: the consistency with which an examiner assigns scores to an object or response on two or more occasions.

Intratissue: directed to the affected tissue within the body via a local application.

Intratissue Percutaneous Electrolysis (EPI®): invasive physiotherapy technique consisting of the application of a continuous current via a puncture needle that acts as a negative electrode (cathode) and which, via sonographic control, will provoke an electrochemical reaction in the degenerated region of the tendon.

Isoechoic: also known as isoechogenic. In ultrasound, due to the characteristics of the tissues, structures are observed with similar echogenicities. If we add to this the morphological similarities of the same, a thorough knowledge of the explored area is compulsory. In this manner, the following are considered to be isoechoic: (1) the tendons, the ligaments and the nerves; and (2) the arteries and veins.

Jump sign: general painful response shown by patients consisting of an avoidance of the painful stimulus causing the patient to wince or vocalize. In this context, this refers to the response upon the pressure of the myofascial trigger point.

Lateral resolution: the ability of the ultrasound device to distinguish between two objects found one beside the other at the same depth in a perpendicular direction from the ultrasound beam (x-axis). When the frequency is increased, lateral resolution increases, but the penetration depth of the ultrasound beam decreases.

Lipolytic effect: an effect characterized by destruction of the adipose cell and its posterior elimination.

Local twitch response: involuntary, brief, transient and isolated contraction of the fibres that form the taut band in response to an appropriate stimulus, especially if this is applied over the myofascial trigger point. This can be provoked manually and via the rapid insertion of a needle.

Matrix metalloproteinases (MMP): a family of at least 20 extracellular enzymes with proteolytic activity. Among their functions, they are responsible for the degradation of collagen together with the inactivation of the alpha-1 antitrypsin and the activation of tumour necrosis factor-α. One of the best known is collagenase.

Measurement: assigning numbers to an object, event or person in order to quantify or qualify it according to measurement rules.

Mesotherapy: the treatment of diseases using various intradermal injections with small doses of different medicines that are practised on the affected region.

Mirror image: artifact that is produced when an interphase is found in front of another curved and hyperechogenic image, so that the same image can be observed at the other side of the said surface.

Monopolar electromyography needle: needle-shaped electrode that is inserted into the skeletal muscle in order to register its bioelectric activity. It is a solid needle with an insulated coating that completely covers it, except for the tip. It registers the difference in potential between the electrode tip and an electrode placed in the skin.

Moxibustion: a technique of traditional Chinese medicine that uses the pressed root of the mugwort plant, which is shaped like a cigar and is known as moxa.

Muscle injury: painful anomaly that is produced at the muscle level. Muscle injuries are generally self-limited and can be classified into: (1) direct injuries (contusions and lacerations); and (2) indirect injuries (lesions due to elongation, delayed-onset muscle soreness [DOMS] and compartmental syndrome).

Muscle regeneration: regeneration is the reactivation of development processes in order to restore missing tissue. As a result of this repair process, the muscle tissue develops properties that render it indistinguishable from the original tissue.

Musculoskeletal ultrasound: a simple, non-invasive imaging procedure that uses the echoes produced by an ultrasound emission directed over a body or object as a source of data, in order to form an image of the organs or internal masses with different purposes. The ultrasound image in physiotherapy is a tool that enables the performance of a dynamic, fast, efficient and innocuous study in real time together with comparative examinations that can be used as an extension of the physiotherapy assessment and diagnosis in order to assess the musculoskeletal tissue objectively, register the evolution of the lesion and validate the different physiotherapy therapeutic techniques, thus improving the possibilities of professional success.

Myofascial pain syndrome (MPS): a specific non-inflammatory condition characterized by a regional pain that commonly presents in specific areas of the body. A highlighted characteristic of MPS is the presence of one or several myofascial trigger points – discrete, hyperirritable nodules found within a taut band of skeletal muscle.

Needle: a filament made of metal or another hard material, of a relatively small size, generally straight, sharp at one end and with the other ending in an eye or loop for threading a needle. The parts of the needle are the tail, handle, junction area, shaft and tip.

NSAIDs: the acronym for non-steroidal anti-inflammatory drugs, which are chemical substances with an anti-inflammatory, analgesic and antipyretic effect. These reduce the inflammatory symptoms and provide pain and fever relief, respectively. The term 'non-steroidal' refers to the fact that the clinical effects are similar to those of corticoids, although without the side effects. As analgesics, they are characterized by not belonging to the class of narcotics and they act by blocking the synthesis of prostaglandins. The most widespread examples of this type of drugs are aspirin, ibuprofen and naxoprene.

Patellar ligament: prolongation of the ligament of the quadriceps tendon from the inferior pole of the patella to the tibial tuberosity.

Percutaneous: substance, drug or procedure that is effected, occurring or performed through the skin. Regarding the technique of Intratissue Percutaneous Electrolysis (EPI®),

this refers to the application performed through the skin using a needle.

Periosteal trigger point: hyperalgic site found on the periosteum which evokes referred pain in response to the application of pressure or another mechanical stimulus. Under experimental circumstances, evoked pain from periosteal trigger points is usually severe and with consistent locations, although the extension of the pain depends on the intensity of the stimulus. In a similar manner to the myofascial trigger points, the periosteal trigger points produce hypersensitivity in the muscles and bony prominences of the referred area, as well as frequent autonomic reactions (e.g. sweating, paleness, nausea).

Physiotherapy care process: the ensemble of interventions or procedures performed or prescribed by the physiotherapist in order to care for patients and cure their health problems. A care process must be centred on the patient and provide effective responses for the patient's needs, values and preferences.

Pixel: a single point or picture element of an image. A rectangular image may be composed of thousands of pixels, each representing the colour of the image in a given situation. The value of a pixel is generally comprised of various channels, with colours made up of components of red, green and blue, and sometimes their alpha (transparency), or made up of a single component if the image is in grey scale. Furthermore, similarly to the fact that the bit is the smallest information unit that a computer can process, a pixel is the smallest element that the hardware and software of the screen and printer can manipulate when creating graphics.

Platelet-rich plasma: concentrated suspension of centrifuged blood that contains great amounts of thrombocytes; these in turn can liberate great amounts of growth factors.

Puncture: the introduction of a sharp tool, such as a needle, into tissue, organ or cavity.

Qi: the Chinese term that describes the energy generated by the metabolic processes.

Referred pain: pain perceived in an area different to the area causing the pain, and that does not follow an innervation pattern.

Region of interest (ROI): any portion of an image that is selected for processing or measurement procedures or in order to perform any action upon it.

Reliability: the reliability of a measure refers to the consistency of results when measuring the same characteristic or process under consistent conditions. This must not be confused with the term accuracy, which provides information regarding how close a measured value is to the reality, and which depends on the measurement tool. Along these lines, the term precision is used to refer to the reproducibility of measures.

Residues manager: the person or entity, public or private, that performs any of the operations involved in the handling of waste, whether or not they are the producers of the same.

Resolution: image resolution indicates the amount of detail that can be appreciated in an image. A greater resolution equals an image with greater detail or visual quality.

Reverberation: a phenomenon that occurs when the ultrasound beam that returns to the transducer is partially reflected and bounces back towards the interior of the body, where it makes contact again with the original interphase, thus causing it to return once more to the transducer. The device interprets that this portion of the beam has travelled a double distance in relation to the initial echo. In the screen a second line will appear at a double depth in relation to the real interphase.

ROC analysis: acronym for receiver operating characteristic (ROC) and commonly known as ROC curves. According to the theory of signal detection, it is a graphic representation of sensitivity, as opposed to specificity for a binary classification system, according to the variation in discrimination threshold, which can also be interpreted as the result of the percentage of true positives compared to the percentage of false positives. In this manner, a tool for selecting the optimal models is available. This is usually used in diagnostic decision making.

Saphenous hiatus: an oval-shaped opening in the superomedial part of the fascia lata of the thigh, 3–4 cm inferolateral to the pubic tubercle. It is crossed by the greater saphenous vein, the superficial epigastric artery, the external pudendal artery and the femoral branch of the genitofemoral nerve.

Scar tissue trigger point: hyperalgesic site found on a scar, which commonly evokes referred pain in response to the application of pressure or another mechanical stimulus. According to Simons et al. (1999), the scar tissue trigger points found on the skin and the mucous membranes produce sensations of stinging, itchiness or electric tingling.

Segmental spinal sensitization: state of hyperactivity of the dorsal horn caused by the bombardment of nociceptive impulses proceeding from damaged or sensitized tissue.

Sonoelastography: an imaging technique that uses Doppler ultrasound in order to estimate the peak displacement of the tissue under a harmonic externally induced vibration. The common understanding is that the healthy and pathological tissues respond differently to this excitation. Sonoelastography assesses the elasticity of the tissues and translates their stiffness to a colour scale that ranges from blue (greater resistance) to red (less resistance). Currently this is being applied to muscles and tendons.

Sonographic transducer: this is one of the key elements of ultrasound and is based on the piezoelectric effect. Transducers have a double function: in the first place, they transform the electrical energy that they receive into sound energy (generated by ultrasound, via quartz crystals), and afterwards, they recapture the reflected ultrasound beams from the different tissues, transforming them into electrical energy that, once processed, provides an ultrasound image. Four main models of transducers can be found: (1) linear (locomotor system); (2) convex (abdominal); (3) endocavity (endoanal or endovaginal); and (4) sectorial (cardiac) transducers.

Superficial fascia: a layer of lax connective and mainly adipose connective tissue (although in specific areas, such as the eyelids and others, there is a lack of adipose tissue), found beneath the skin and superficial to the deep fascia. Besides its subcutaneous presence, it is also found internally, covering viscera and glands, vasculonervous bundles and, in general, in locations where it covers spaces that are otherwise unoccupied.

Taut band: ensemble of contiguous skeletal muscle fibres that presents increased tension compared to that of the surrounding muscle.

Tendinitis: clinical picture characterized by the presence of inflammation in the tendon.

Tendinopathy: term used as a synonym of tendinosis in reference to a chronic tendon problem.

Tendinosis: clinical picture characterized by angiofibroblastic hyperplasia: functional changes in the tendons, collagen degradation, hypervascularization and proliferation of ground substance.

Test–retest reliability: the consistency of a measure to be repeated from one time to another.

Thread needling: perforating techniques that have an entrance and exit point.

Thresholding: an image-processing method that creates a bitonal or binary image where two levels are assigned to pixels that are above or below the specified threshold value, which causes some pixels to turn black and others white. This can be performed manually, semi-automatically or automatically, for which a large number of methods or algorithms have been developed.

Titin: structural protein of muscle fibre with a high molecular weight, it is endosarcomeric and not involved in muscle contraction. This protein connects the myosin to the Z line of the sarcomere.

Tonification point: point via which the energetic channel of a meridian can be increased.

Transverse fascia: the transverse fascia (or fascia transversalis) is a thin connective layer that is found in the inner surface of the transversus abdominis and the extraperitoneal fascia. It is part of the general fascial layer that lines the abdominal walls, and is directly continuous with the fascia of the quadratus lumborum, iliacus, psoas major and pelvis. In the groin region, the transverse fascia is thicker and denser, but it becomes finer as it ascends towards the diaphragm, where it is continuous with the fascia that covers the inferior surface of this muscle.

Triple burner: a term found in traditional Chinese medicine that describes the three types of metabolism: (1) respiratory; (2) digestive; and (3) excretory.

Tumour necrosis factor-α (TNF-α): this factor belongs to a group of cytokines that stimulate the acute phase of the inflammatory reaction. This is a glucopeptidic hormone formed by 185 amino acids, deriving from a propeptide formed by 212 amino acids. Some cells synthesize shorter isoforms of the molecule.

Ultrasound: high-frequency sound waves (above the audible level) and with a low wavelength (depending on the medium they have to cross).

'Wand' effect: according to the 'wand' effect, described by Daniel Dennett, when an object is touched via a stick held by the hand, a series of complex kinaesthetic and tactile mechanisms are triggered which allow one to feel through the wand, experiencing the (false) sensation that there are nerve terminals in its tip.

Waste: any substance or object which the owner disposes of or which the person has the intention or obligation of disposing of.

Waste owner: the producer of the waste or the physical person or legal entity that has them in their power and that does not have a licence as waste handler.

Waste producer: any physical or legal entity whose activity, excluding refuse derived from household waste, produces waste. In different centres, clinics and hospitals, the title of waste producer is given to those professionals who are responsible for the activities that generate these and, in particular, the physiotherapist responsible for the corresponding physiotherapy service.

Xue: Chinese term referring to the blood in the body.

Zhang-fu: theory of the organs and viscera according to traditional Chinese medicine. Related to the cycles of the five elements and the correspondences between the elements in nature with the internal organs of the human being.

INDEX

Page numbers followed by "*f*" indicate figures, "*t*" indicate tables, and "*b*" indicate boxes.